MENOPAUSE PRACTICE

A Clinician's Guide
6th Edition

MENOPAUSE PRACTICE

A Clinician's Guide
6th Edition

Editor-in-Chief
Carolyn J. Crandall, MD, MS, NCMP

Associate Editors

Gloria A. Bachman, MD; Stephanie S. Faubion, MD, MBA, FACP, NCMP, IF; Wendy Klein, MD, FACP;

James H. Liu, MD, NCMP; JoAnn E. Manson, MD, DrPH, NCMP; Joanne Mortimer, MD, FACP;

JoAnn V. Pinkerton, MD, NCMP; Nanette F. Santoro, MD; Jan L. Shifren, MD, NCMP; Rebecca C. Thurston, PhD

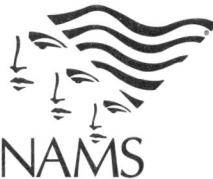

NAMS
THE NORTH AMERICAN
MENOPAUSE SOCIETY

The North American Menopause Society
Pepper Pike, Ohio

The North American Menopause Society
30100 Chagrin Blvd, Suite 210
Pepper Pike, OH 44124, USA
Tel: 440-442-7550
E-mail: info@menopause.org
Web: www.menopause.org

The information presented in this clinician's guide
is provided as a compilation of the existing state of
knowledge on the subject matter. It is not meant to
substitute for the provider's experience and judgment
brought to each clinical situation.

The field of menopause management is constantly
changing. As with all reference resources, this guide
reflects the best understanding of the science of menopause
management at the time of publication, but it should be
used with the clear understanding that continuing research
and clinical experience may result in new knowledge.

NAMS uses *AMA Manual of Style,* 10th edition, for its language and style formats
Cover and text design and layout by Clarence D Meriweather
ISBN 978-0-578-53228-8
Printed in the United States of America

Contributors

NAMS greatly appreciates the efforts of all contributors to the content of *Menopause Practice: A Clinician's Guide.*

Rebecca H Allen, MD, MPH
Warren Alpert Medical School
 of Brown University
Women and Infants Hospital
Providence, Rhode Island

Idoroenyi Amanam, MD
City of Hope National Medical Center
Duarte, California

Dina N Anderson, MD
Mount Sinai Hospital
New York

David F Archer, MD, NCMP
Eastern Virginia Medical School
Norfolk, Virginia

Gloria A Bachmann, MD
Rutgers Robert Wood Johnson
 Medical School
New Brunswick, New Jersey

Marcella Calfon Press, MD, PhD
Ronald Reagan UCLA Medical Center
Los Angeles, California

Janet S Carpenter, PhD, RN, FAAN
Indiana University-Purdue University
Indianapolis School of Nursing
Indianapolis, Indiana

Carolyn J Crandall, MD, MS, NCMP
David Geffen School of Medicine
 at University of California
Los Angeles, California

Mihaela Cristea, MD
City of Hope National Medical Center
Duarte, California

Carrie Cwiak, MD, MPH
Emory University School of Medicine
Atlanta, Georgia

Samar R El Khoudary, PhD, MPH, BPharm, FAHA
University of Pittsburgh
Pittsburgh, Pennsylvania

Evyatar Evron, MD
David Geffen School of Medicine at UCLA
Santa Monica, California

Marwan Fakih, MD
City of Hope National Medical Center
Duarte, California

Stephanie S Faubion, MD, MBA, FACP, NCMP, IF
Mayo Clinic
Rochester, Minnesota

Heather E Fields, MD
Mayo Clinic Arizona
Scottsdale, Arizona

Carolyn Goh, MD
UCLA Medical Center
Santa Monica, California

Steven R Goldstein, MD, FACOG, CCD, NCMP
New York University School of Medicine
New York

Jun Gong, MD
Cedars-Sinai Medical Center
Los Angeles, California

Clarisa R Gracia, MD, MSCE
University of Pennsylvania
Philadelphia, Pennsylvania

Minda A Green, PhD
Drexel University College of Medicine
Philadelphia, Pennsylvania

Tamara B Horwich, MD, MS
Ahmanson-UCLA Cardiomyopathy Center
Los Angeles, California

Lina Huang, MD, FRCSC
McGill University
Montreal, Quebec, Canada

Michelle Jacobson, MD, FRCSC
Latrobe Hospital
Latrobe, Pennsylvania

Jae Jung, MD, PhD
Norton Cancer Institute
Louisville, Kentucky

Risa Kagan, MD, FACOG, CCD, NCMP
University of California San Francisco
Sutter East Bay Physicians
 Medical Foundation
Berkeley, California

Scott Kahan, MD, MPH
Johns Hopkins Bloomberg School
 of Public Health
Washington, DC

Andrew M Kaunitz, MD, NCMP
University of Florida College of Medicine-
 Jacksonville
Jacksonville, Florida

Susan Kellogg Spadt, PhD, CRNP, IF, FCST, CSC
Drexel University College of Medicine
Rosemont, Pennsylvania

Anita M Kelsey, MD, FACC, FASE
St Francis Hospital and Medical Center
Hartford, Connecticut

Sheryl A Kingsberg, PhD
Case Western Reserve University
 School of Medicine
Cleveland, Ohio

Wendy Klein, MD, MACP
Virginia Commonwealth University
 School of Medicine
Richmond, Virginia

Juliana (Jewel) M Kling, MD, MPH
Mayo Clinic Arizona
Scottsdale, Arizona

Howard M Kravitz, DO, MPH
Rush Medical College
Chicago, Illinois

Elizabeth Kusturiss, MSN, CRNP, IF
Center for Pelvic Medicine
Rosemont, Pennsylvania

James H Liu, MD, NCMP
University Hospitals Case Medical Center
MacDonald Women's Hospital
Case Western Reserve University
    School of Medicine
Cleveland, Ohio

Pauline M Maki, PhD
University of Illinois at Chicago
Chicago, Illinois

JoAnn E Manson, MD, DrPH, NCMP
Brigham and Women's Hospital
Harvard Medical School
Boston, Massachusetts

Michael R McClung, MD
Founding Director, Oregon
    Osteoporosis Center
Portland, Oregon

Denise M Millstine, MD
Mayo Clinic Arizona
Scottsdale, Arizona

Gita D Mishra, PhD
School of Public Health,
    University of Queensland
Queensland, Australia

Joanne Mortimer, MD, FACP
City of Hope Comprehensive
    Cancer Center
Duarte, California

Jeri W Nieves, PhD
Columbia University
New York

Ana E Núñez, MD
Drexel University College of Medicine
Philadelphia, Pennsylvania

Bruce Patsner, MD, JD
Inova Fairfax Women's Hospital
Falls Church, Virginia
Virginia Commonwealth University
    School of Medicine
Richmond, Virginia
George Washington University
    School of Medicine
Washington, DC

Jelena M Pavlović, MD, PhD
Albert Einstein College of Medicine
Montefiore Headache Center
New York

Anne Peters, MD
Keck School of Medicine
    of the University of Southern California
Los Angeles, CA

JoAnn V Pinkerton, MD, NCMP
University of Virginia Health System
Charlottesville, Virginia

Michael Policar, MD, MPH
University of California
San Francisco, California

Jennifer G Robinson, MD, MPH
University of Iowa
Iowa City, Iowa

Tami Rowen, MD
University of California
San Francisco, California

Nanette F Santoro, MD
University of Colorado School of Medicine
Aurora, Colorado

Jenifer Sassarini, MBChB, PhD, MRCOG
University of Glasgow School of Medicine
Scotland, United Kingdom

Sheila Sahni, MD
Garden State Heart Center
Clark, New Jersey

Ellen W Seely, MD
Harvard Medical School
Brigham and Women's Hospital
Boston, Massachusetts

Jan L Shifren, MD, NCMP
Harvard Medical School
Massachusetts General Hospital
Boston, Massachusetts

Chrisandra L Shufelt, MD, MS, FACP, NCMP
Cedars-Sinai Medical Center
Los Angeles, California

Claudio N Soares, MD, PhD, FRCPC, MBA
Queen's University School of Medicine
Kingston, Ontario, Canada

Anna Sokalska, MD, PhD
University of Pennsylvania
Philadelphia, Pennsylvania

Daphne Stewart, MD, MS
City of Hope Comprehensive
    Cancer Center
Duarte, California

Cynthia A Stuenkel, MD, NCMP
University of California, San Diego
La Jolla, California

Emily D Szmuilowicz, MD, MS
Feinberg School of Medicine
Northwestern University
Chicago, Illinois

Rebecca C Thurston, PhD
University of Pittsburgh
Pittsburgh, Pennsylvania

L Elaine Waetjen, MD
University of California Davis
    Medical Center
Sacramento, California

Karol E Watson, MD, PhD
David Geffen School of Medicine at UCLA
Los Angeles, California

Fiona M Watt, B Med Sci, MBBS, PhD
King's College
London, United Kingdom

Wendy Wolfman, MD, FRCSC
Mount Sinai Hospital
Toronto, Ontario, Canada

Acknowledgments

NAMS extends great appreciation for the review and approval of the members of the 2018-2019 NAMS Board of Trustees.

NAMS is grateful to Amag Pharmaceuticals, Inc, for the unrestricted grant funding that supported in part the development costs for this *Clincian's Guide*. This company exercised no control over its content.

Continuing Medical Education Information and Disclosures

This essential guide to menopause management for all healthcare providers who treat or counsel women at midlife and beyond is certified as an enduring continuing medical education (CME) activity.

Release date: September 25, 2019
Expiration date: September 25, 2022

The North American Menopause Society (NAMS) is accredited by the Accreditation Council for Continuing Medical Education (ACCME) to provide continuing medical education for physicians.

NAMS designates this enduring activity for a maximum of 26.0 *AMA PRA Category 1 Credits*™. Physicians should claim only the credit commensurate with the extent of their participation in the activity.

Other healthcare providers who participate in this enduring activity will receive a certificate of participation. For nurses and other learners who need to report contact hours of pharmacotherapeutics education, NAMS has determined that this enduring activity includes a maximum of 19.0 hours of pharmacotherapeutics education.

Learning Objectives

At the conclusion of this enduring activity, participants should be able to
- Initiate discussion with patients on menopause and healthy aging, including its effect on quality of life and sexuality
- Perform appropriate clinical assessments to diagnose conditions of menopause and aging, assess health risks, and identify any contraindications to medications
- Discuss a full range of management options with patients on the basis of their health risks, goals, and preferences
- Collaborate with other healthcare professionals to offer effective, individualized therapy for menopause symptoms and conditions
- Counsel and encourage patients to achieve a healthy lifestyle

Commercial Support

This CME activity is supported in part by unrestricted grant funding from Amag Pharmaceuticals, Inc.

Claiming CME Credit

To claim CME credit, please read and study the entire *Clinician's Guide* and complete and submit the evaluation online to NAMS by the expiration date of September 25, 2022. Certificates will be issued to those who complete the online evaluation. The evaluation with instructions on submission begins on page 339.

Disclosure Statement and Disclosures

To help ensure that its CME activities are free of commercial bias, NAMS has a process in which everyone in a position to control the content of a CME activity, whether involved in its development, management, presentation, or evaluation, are required to disclose all "relevant financial relationships" with any "commercial interest." Any actual or potential conflicts of interest that exist as a result of such financial relationships are resolved before the CME activity begins. Depending on the nature of the conflict, resolutions may include, but are not limited to, communicating obligations and restrictions to the participant, altering his/her role within the activity, reviewing his/her content for possible revision, and monitoring his/her participation. Resolving conflicts of interest may also include identifying an alternative faculty member, assigning a different topic, or having an effective peer review of the content of the activity so that any promotional content can be eliminated. The Society's Disclosure Form requests all those in a position to control the content of a CME to indicate their understanding of and willingness to comply with each of these statements:

- The content and/or presentation of the information (slides, abstracts, handouts) with which I am involved will promote quality or improvements in healthcare and will not promote a specific proprietary business interest of a commercial interest. Content for this activity, including any presentation of therapeutic options, will be well-balanced, evidence-based, and free of inappropriate commercial influence.

- Educational materials with which I am involved, such as slides, posters, abstracts, and handouts, will not contain any commercial logos, advertising, or product-group messages.

- I have not and will not accept any honoraria, additional payments, or reimbursements for this CME activity beyond that that has been agreed to directly with NAMS.

- I understand that NAMS may need to review my presentation and/or content before the activity, and I will provide educational content in advance as requested.

- I have obtained the right or permission, where necessary, to use all digital images and photos presented in my instructional material, both electronic and printed, as defined by US Copyright law.

- I agree that the materials in my presentation are in compliance with the Health Insurance Portability and Accountability Act (HIPAA) and any other applicable laws governing the use and disclosure of patient information.

- If I am presenting at a live event, I understand that a monitor from NAMS may be attending the event to ensure that my presentation is educational and not promotional in nature.

- If I am providing recommendations involving clinical medicine, they will be based on evidence that is accepted within the profession of medicine as adequate justification for their indications

and contraindications in the care of patients. All scientific research referred to, reported, or used in this activity in support of justification of a patient care recommendation will conform to the generally accepted standards of experimental design, data collection, and analysis.

- If I am discussing specific healthcare products or services, I will use generic names to the extent possible. If I need to use trade names, I will use trade names from several companies when available and not only trade names from any single company.

- If I have been trained or used by a commercial interest or its agent as a speaker (eg, speakers' bureau) for any commercial interest, the promotional aspects of that presentation will not be included in any way within this activity.

- If I am presenting research funded by a commercial interest, the information presented will be based on generally accepted scientific principles and methods and will not promote the commercial interest of the funding company.

For the contributors

Dr. Anderson reports Speaker/Trainer: Allergan. Dr. Archer reports Board of Directors: *InnovaGyn*; Consultant: *AbbVie, Agile Therapeutics, Evestra, Exeltis, InnovaGyn, Radius Health, TherapeuticsMD*; Research Support: *AbbVie, Bayer Healthcare, Endoceutics, Glemnark, Radius Health, Shionogi, TherapeuticsMD*; Stock/Ownership: *Agile Therapeutics, InnovaGyn*. Dr. Cristea reports Speaker: *Astra Zeneca*, Dr. Cwiak reports Advisory Board: *Medicines 360*; Research Funding: *Contramed, Medicines 360; Royalties: Springer*. Dr. Faubion reports Consultant/Advisory Board: *Amag, Mithra*. Dr. Goldstein reports Consultant: *Cook Ob/Gyn, Cooper Surgical; Equipment Loan: GE Ultrasound*. Dr. Huang reports Advisory Board/Speaker: *Pfizer, Sandoz*. Dr. Jung reports Speaker: *Amgen*; Principal Investigator, *Merck, Regeneron*. Dr. Kagan reports Advisory Board: *Amag, Lupin, P&G, Radius;* Consultant: *Amag, Amgen, Cooper Surgical, Heron Therapeutics, Therapeutics MD*; Speaker: *Amag, Astellas, Cooper Surgical, Therapeutics MD*; Research Fees paid to ABSMC Research Institute: *Endoceutics*. Dr. Kahan reports Consultant: *Novo Nordisk, Takeda, Eisai, Orexigen*. Dr. Kaunitz reports Advisor/Consultant: *Amag, Mithra, Pfizer*; Research Grants paid to the University of Florida: *Allergan, Endoceutics, Medicines360, Myovant*; Royalties: UpToDate. Dr. Kellogg Spadt reports Consultant: *Materna,*

Contents

Tables and Figures

5. Other Common Symptoms in Midlife Women

6. Diseases Common in Midlife Women

10. Vitamins, Minerals, and Other Dietary Supplements

11. Prescription Therapies

Menopause

Menopause Demographics, Staging, and Terminology

Every woman who survives the middle-age stage of life will experience menopause, usually when aged between 40 and 58 years. Worldwide, populations are projected to age over the coming decades, with the number of women aged 50 years and older expected to grow significantly. In 1990, 471 million women worldwide were aged at least 50 years. In 2015, this number increased by 82.6% worldwide (861 million in 2015), which corresponds to a 2.4% increase per year on average.[1]

By the year 2020, the number of US women who will be aged at least 50 years is estimated to be 64 million.[2] This number is expected to increase to close to 90 million by 2060. The overall life expectancy for US females is 81.2 years, which has been unchanged since 2012.[3] The probability of survival from age 50 to 80 years in US women was estimated to be 67.2% in 2013; US women who survive to age 50 are expected to live an average of 33.3 more years.[4] With increasing life expectancy, many women will spend up to 40% of their lives in postmenopause, with more than 60% surviving at least until the age of 80 years.

Similarly, more Canadian women will experience menopause over the coming decades. In 2016, about 39% of Canadian women were aged at least 50 years. This number is projected to increase to 43% in 2038; assuming medium growth rate.[5,6] With the remarkable increase in life expectancy at birth of 23.0 years for Canadian women (from 60.6 y in 1920-1922 to 83.6 y in 2009-2011), many Canadian women also will spend up to 40% of their lives postmenopause.[7]

Staging

Menopause marks an important stage in a woman's life, characterized by changes in bleeding patterns, hormone levels, body composition, and psychosocial well-being. A standard reproductive staging system and universally accepted menopause terminology are critical to advancing clinicians' and researchers' understanding of this inevitable event.

In 2001, the Stages of Reproductive Aging Workshop (STRAW) established basic terminology and a staging system to characterize the last 10 to 15 years of a woman's reproductive aging.[8] STRAW was refined in 2011 to include data-driven adjustments to the original staging system (STRAW+10).[9]

STRAW+10 is now considered to be the gold standard for characterizing reproductive aging, from the reproductive years through menopause. It divides the reproductive-aging continuum into seven stages—five before and two after the final menstrual period (Figure 1).[9]

Terminology

Climacteric. The term *climacteric* has been defined as the period of endocrinologic, somatic, and transitory psychologic changes that occur at the time of menopause. The term is sometimes used interchangeably with *perimenopause.*

Early menopause and late menopause. *Early menopause* and *late menopause* are vague terms that can be used to describe menopause that occurs earlier or later within the normal range of ages at the final menstrual period (FMP). Menopause is usually considered early when the FMP occurs before age 45 and late when it occurs after age 54.

Early postmenopause and late postmenopause. STRAW +10 classified postmenopausal women as in *early postmenopause* if they are within 8 years of their FMP; otherwise, they are classified as in *late postmenopause.* Unlike early postmenopausal women, late postmenopausal women experience more limited or no further changes in reproductive endocrine function but greater effects of the somatic aging process.

Induced menopause. *Induced menopause* is defined as the cessation of menses that comes after either surgical removal of both ovaries (bilateral oophorectomy, with or without hysterectomy) or iatrogenic ablation of ovarian function (by chemotherapy, pelvic radiation, or other forms of ovarian toxicity). Bilateral oophorectomy is the most common cause of induced menopause.

Menopause transition. According to STRAW+10, the *menopause transition* is defined as the time before the FMP when the menstrual cycle becomes variable or other menopause-related symptoms begin. Based on the degree of variability of the menstrual cycle, women could be classified as being in the early (7 or more days persistent difference in cycle lengths from previous normal cycle) or late (60 or more days of amenorrhea, observed at least one time) transition stages.

Natural menopause. *Natural menopause* is defined as the permanent cessation of menses because of loss of ovarian follicular activity. Occurrence of natural menopause can only be determined retrospectively after 12 consecutive months of amenorrhea after the FMP. For some women, menstrual-bleeding criteria cannot be used to define menopause, and the diagnosis can be supported with criteria including history of bilateral oophorectomy, symptoms, or measurement of endocrine markers.

Perimenopause. The term *perimenopause* literally means "around menopause." It begins with the onset of intermenstrual cycle irregularities (±7 d) or other menopause-related symptoms and extends beyond the FMP to

Figure 1. The Stages of Reproductive Aging Workshop + 10 Staging System

Stage	−5	−4	−3b	−3a	−2	−1	+1a	+1b	+1c	+2
Terminology	REPRODUCTIVE				MENOPAUSE TRANSITION		POSTMENOPAUSE			
	Early	Peak	Late		Early	Late	Early			Late
					Perimenopause					
Duration	variable				variable	1-3	2 (1+1)		3-6	Remaining lifespan
PRINCIPAL CRITERIA										
Menstrual cycle	Variable to regular	Regular	Regular	Subtle changes in flow/ length	Variable length Persistent ≥7-day difference in length of consecutive cycles	Interval of amenorrhea of ≥60 days				
SUPPORTIVE CRITERIA										
Endocrine FSH AMH Inhibin B			Low Low	Variableª Low Low	↑ Variableª Low Low	↑ >25IU/Lᵇ Low Low	↑ Variableª Low Low	Stabilizes Very low Very low		
Antral follicle count			Low	Low	Low	Low	Very low	Very low		
DESCRIPTIVE CHARACTERISTICS										
Symptoms						Vasomotor symptoms Likely	Vasomotor symptoms Most likely			Increasing symptoms of urogenital atrophy

↑ indicates elevated.
a. Blood draw on cycle days 2-5.
b. Approximate expected level based on assays using current international pituitary standard.
Abbreviations: AMH, antimüllerian hormone; FMP, final menstrual period; FSH, follicle-stimulating hormone.
Adapted from Harlow SD, et al.[9] © North American Menopause Society.

Menarche

FMP (0)

include the 12 months after menopause, thus lasting 1 year longer than the menopause transition. Perimenopause is a clinically useful term because it encompasses the highly symptomatic years.

Postmenopause. The term *postmenopause* refers to the stage of life after menopause.

Premature menopause/Premature ovarian failure/ Primary ovarian insufficiency. These terms all refer to menopause that occurs before age 40. Because premature cessation of ovarian function may not always be permanent and because of the negative implication of the term "failure," *primary ovarian insufficiency* (POI) has emerged as the preferred terminology.[10] Several studies, including the Study of Women's Health Across the Nation (SWAN), indicate that the percentage of US women experiencing POI is approximately 1%. Applying this 1% estimate to the projected number of US women who will be aged 15 to 44 years in 2020 (approximately 65 million), approximately 650,000 US women will experience POI. This number will increase to almost 730,000 women by 2060.[2] It has been recommended by The North American Menopause Society and the American Congress of Obstetricians and Gynecologists that the term premature ovarian failure no longer be used.

Premenopause. The term *premenopause* refers to the stage of life that precedes menopause.

As women traverse the menopause, several physical and psychological alterations happen. Women and their healthcare providers may be challenged to distinguish menopause-related changes from those attributable to normal aging. A number of endocrine systems manifest age-related changes that may or may not have their onset during the menopause transition. Furthermore, concurrent medical disorders such as obesity, diabetes mellitus (DM), dyslipidemia, thyroid disease, and hypertension often develop during midlife and may influence reproductive aging.

Stages of Reproductive Aging

Aging is a natural, time-related, genetically determined and environmentally modified process of deterioration of the physiological functions.

Women are born with a finite number of oocytes that decline over a woman's lifetime. The ovaries of a female fetus contain 6 to 7 million oocytes at approximately 20 weeks' gestation, 1 to 2 million at birth, and 300,000 to 500,000 at the onset of puberty. About 400 to 500 oocytes will be ovulated, but most oocytes are lost through apoptosis.[11] Loss of oocytes from ovulation and atresia characterize reproductive aging.

Although menopause is ultimately defined by ovarian follicular exhaustion, several observations suggest that abnormal estradiol-positive feedback mechanisms and an attenuated luteinizing hormone (LH) surge contribute to reproductive aging, independent of ovarian failure.[12,13] The wide range of age at which menopause occurs (40-58 y) indicates that chronologic age is not a useful predictor of reproductive senescence. Despite improvements in overall longevity, reproductive senescence occurs earlier than failure of other organ systems.[12]

To provide nomenclature and encourage consistency in research and reporting, a standardized definition of reproductive aging based on menstrual-cycle bleeding criteria and follicle-stimulating hormone (FSH) levels was initially proposed by STRAW in 2001 and was subsequently validated.[8,14-16] In 2011, the multidisciplinary, multinational, STRAW+10 workshop reevaluated the criteria for the staging system and incorporated new data related to FSH, antral follicle count (AFC), antimüllerian hormone (AMH), and inhibin B, as well as evidence regarding postmenopause changes in FSH and estradiol levels.[9] Data from several cohort studies on midlife women (SWAN, the Tremin Research Program on Women's Health, the Melbourne Women's Midlife Health Project, the Seattle Midlife Women's Health Study, the Michigan Bone Health and Metabolic Study, the Biodemographic Models of Reproductive Aging, and the Penn Ovarian Aging Study) were analyzed and adopted by consensus. Menstrual-cycle criteria remain the most important staging criteria.

STRAW+10 staging is applicable to women regardless of demographics, age, body mass index (BMI), and lifestyle characteristics. Special considerations apply to some clinical situations. The course of reproductive aging in women with POI compared with that of healthy women appears to be more variable, including potential episodes of resumption of menstrual cycles.[17]

Menstrual-cycle criteria cannot be applied to women who do not have regular menstrual cycles. Menstrual-bleeding criteria also cannot be used in staging women after hysterectomy or endometrial ablation; therefore, reproductive aging can be assessed using endocrine markers. However, endocrine evaluation is not recommended for at least 3 months after surgery, given the fact that FSH levels may be transiently elevated after pelvic surgery.[18]

The STRAW+10 writing group acknowledged particular challenges in evaluating reproductive aging in women with chronic illnesses and those undergoing chemotherapy.[9]

The STRAW+10 staging system has seven stages, each with specific clinical criteria, endocrine parameters, and characteristic markers of reproductive aging. Five stages precede and two come after the final menstrual period. Stages −5 to −3 comprise the reproductive interval; −2 to −1, the menopause transition; and +1 to +2, postmenopause (Figure 1).[9] It must be emphasized that not all healthy women follow this pattern. Most women progress from one stage to the next; however, there are women who can move back and forth between stages or skip a stage.

Reproductive stages (STRAW+10 stages −5, −4, −3b, and −3a)

The reproductive phase includes three stages: early (stage −5), peak (stage −4), and late (stages −3b and −3a).[9] Menarche is considered as entry into stage −5. It usually takes several years to assume regular menstrual cycles, which should then occur every 21 to 35 days for a number of years and is a landmark of stages −4 and −3b.

The late reproductive stage (STRAW+10 stage −3) marks the time when fecundability begins to decline and a woman may begin to notice changes in her menstrual cycles.[9] Critical endocrine changes relevant to fertility occur before changes in the menstrual cycle are noted. The late reproductive stage has been divided into two phases: −3b and −3a.

In −3b, the earlier phase, menstrual cycles and early follicular-phase FSH remain normal. However, AMH and AFC are low. Most studies suggest that inhibin B is also low.[19-21]

The late reproductive stage (stage −3a) is characterized by subtle menstrual-cycle changes in flow and length, with increasing frequency of shorter cycles, variable FSH levels, and other markers of ovarian aging being low.

Endocrine and ultrasound evaluation

Cycle day 3 FSH is the most commonly used test of ovarian reserve.[22] The increase in FSH contributes to the advancement of follicles leaving the resting phase. The estradiol level in the early follicular phase is either normal or elevated. Aromatase expression increases with age in regularly cycling women and compensates for the known age-related decrease in granulosa cell number in the dominant follicle.[23] FSH should therefore be interpreted in conjunction with an estradiol level. Elevated estradiol can suppress FSH, giving "falsely" normal FSH levels.

Antimüllerian hormone is produced by the granulosa cells of preantral and small antral follicles, many of which are unmeasured by ultrasound. Its most important clinical application is based on its ability to represent the number of preantral and antral follicles[24] and predict the response to ovarian hyperstimulation[25] or assess iatrogenic damage (radiation, chemotherapy, uterine artery embolization, and ovarian surgery) to ovarian follicle reserve.[26] Antimüllerian hormone levels capture quantitative but not qualitative data on ovarian reserve. Age-dependent decline in oocyte quality may be related to various factors: deterioration of the integrity and function of the meiotic spindle; impairment of the selection process, allowing poor-quality oocytes to develop to the dominant follicle; cumulative damage to the oocyte with age; and decreased quality of granulosa cells.[27-29]

Data on the relationship between AMH and natural fertility at different stages of reproductive life are limited. One large study demonstrated that AMH levels were not associated with fertility (time to pregnancy) in couples without a diagnosis of infertility attempting conception.[30] Thus, ovarian reserve testing is not recommended as a screening tool to predict infertility in the general population.

Information about AMH levels across the female reproductive lifespan comes primarily from aggregate data from several studies.[31-33] One model shows that the peak AMH concentration is observed at 24.5 years, with a strong correlation between AMH and the number of follicles from the time of the peak levels until menopause.[32] However, from birth to the time of peak AMH, lower levels may not correlate with follicle numbers. Thus, caution is recommended in interpreting AMH levels in girls and in women aged younger than 25 years.[34]

There is high interindividual variability in AMH secondary to the significant differences in the number of small follicles. Most studies demonstrate relatively stable AMH throughout the menstrual cycle; however, some studies suggest that intracycle variability may be somewhat greater in younger women with high levels compared with older women with lower levels.[35]

Antimüllerian hormone levels also may be influenced by exogenous hormone use. This should be taken into consideration when interpreting values in the clinical setting. As demonstrated in several studies, AMH levels can be 29.8% to 50% lower in hormone contraception users and can increase after discontinuation.[36-40] Similarly, lower AMH levels also have been observed during pregnancy, especially in the second and third trimesters.[41]

Available data are conflicting in terms of the relationship between AMH, BMI, and smoking.[42] Some ethnic variations have been observed, with white women having higher AMH levels than black and Hispanic women.

Antral follicle count, as defined by the number of ultrasound-detectable follicles 2 mm to 10 mm, and AMH are both useful markers of ovarian response to controlled ovarian stimulation.[43] Antral follicles are sensitive to FSH. They correlate with the number of primordial follicles and are considered to represent the available pool of follicles.

Despite the strong correlation between AFC and AMH, they provide complementary information and should not be interpreted interchangeably. Antral follicle count demonstrates the number of viable follicles, which are potentially losing ability to produce AMH but will respond to the gonadotropins and the cohort of nonviable atretic follicles, whereas AMH provides information on very small, partially unmeasured by ultrasound, and nonatretic follicles.[43,44]

Menopause transition (STRAW+10 stages –2 and –1)

The menopause transition is characterized by menstrual cycle irregularity, reflecting an increase in variability of hormone secretion and inconsistent ovulation.[45] The transition culminates with menopause, the complete cessation of menses. There is no specific endocrine marker of the early or late transition.[46]

Early menopause transition (stage –2)

Consistent with the original STRAW classification and the ReSTAGE Collaboration,[8,15,16] the formal onset of the early menopause transition as defined in STRAW+10 is marked by a persistent difference of 7 days or more in the length of consecutive cycles.[9] Persistence is defined as recurrence within 10 cycles of the first variable-length cycle. Cycles in the early menopause transition are also characterized by elevated but variable early follicular-phase FSH levels and low AMH levels and AFC.

Late menopause transition (stage –1)

According to STRAW+10 and consistent with the original STRAW and ReSTAGE criteria for the late menopaus transition is 60 or more consecutive days of amenorrhea.[9] One such episode is sufficient to stage women aged 45 years and older. For women aged 40 to 44 years, recurrence of an episode of amenorrhea of 60 days or longer within a year improves prediction of entry into the late menopause transition. Menstrual cycles are characterized by

increased variability in cycle length, extreme fluctuations in hormone levels, and increased prevalence of anovulation. FSH levels fluctuate between postmenopause and those consistent with the reproductive stages. A serum FSH level of 25 IU/L or higher in a random blood draw has been incorporated into the STRAW+10 classification criteria as an independent marker for the late menopause transition. This stage is estimated to last, on average, 1 to 3 years.

Clinical implications

An explanation for elevated serum estradiol levels during some cycles in the menopause transition reflects a physiologic phenomenon termed *luteal out-of-phase* (LOOP) event (Figure 2).[22,47] In a LOOP cycle, which occurs in about one in four cycles in women studied during the early menopause transition (and approximately one-third of women in the late menopause transition), elevated FSH levels are adequate to recruit a second follicle during the luteal phase of an ongoing cycle.[22] Recruitment of a second follicle results in a follicular phase-like rise in estradiol secretion superimposed on the mid- to late-luteal phase of the ongoing ovulatory cycle. FSH levels drop to midreproductive levels during the menstrual and follicular phases of the subsequent cycle, and estradiol levels peak during the subsequent menstrual phase. Concurrent with persistent estradiol elevations are marked falls in luteal progesterone. About half the time, an LH surge and ovulation occur within the first 5 days of the cycle. As a result, the final length of the second cycle is unusually short (<21 d). If ovulation does not occur, estradiol levels drop until the onset of a new follicular phase, and the resulting cycle is then longer than average (>36 d).

Overproduction of estradiol by an enlarged cohort of recruited follicles or a LOOP cycle may result in mastalgia, migraine, menorrhagia, growth of uterine fibroids, or endometrial hyperplasia. Conversion of androgen to estrogen through aromatization increases with age and body weight, another mechanism resulting in elevated estradiol levels during the menopause transition.[48] Women with a longer menopause transition might experience increased exposure to unopposed estrogen and an increased risk for reproductive cancers.[49]

Despite the reduction in fertility with reproductive aging, women should be aware that pregnancy can occur until menopause, at least based on the hormone dynamics of the menstrual cycles that have been observed. In one study of the menopause transition, 25% of all cycles longer than 60 days were ovulatory.[50] The average day of ovulation occurred on day 27 of the cycle. In other studies, approximately 40% to 60% of cycles were anovulatory,[45] but several oocytes may be released during other cycles, perhaps accounting for the increased incidence of twins born to midlife women. Evaluation of menstrual-cycle dynamics in women approaching menopause in SWAN indicated that an ovulatory pattern is present in most cycles up to the time of the FMP.[51]

As women progress through the menopause transition, the number of anovulatory cycles increases.[52] As anticipated, progesterone levels are low during anovulatory cycles. Measures of overall progesterone secretion show a linear decline from STRAW+10 stages −3 to −1 and +1.[50,52] In other studies, progesterone levels are reduced late in the menopause transition or not reduced at all in ovulatory cycles.[45,53]

Estradiol levels also vary: in anovulatory cycles that ended in bleeding, estradiol levels are comparable with those of women who had ovulated. In cycles without bleeding, estradiol levels are low, approximately one-third the level characteristic for ovulatory cycles. Women who are obese are more likely to have anovulatory cycles characterized by high estradiol levels.[52,54] Women who are obese also are more likely to have lower premenopause yet higher postmenopause estradiol levels compared with women of normal weight.[55,56]

Women of different ethnic groups demonstrate similar patterns of hormone changes with the menopause transition, but the concentration of hormones differs.[57] Chinese and Japanese women have lower estradiol levels than white, black, and Hispanic women. FSH concentrations are higher in black women than in women of other ethnicities. The ethnic differences are independent of menopause status.

The longitudinal Melbourne Women's Midlife Health Project that followed women through the menopause transition demonstrated that testosterone levels did not change over time.[58] Other studies evaluating testosterone concentrations during the menopause transition present conflicting data.

Figure 2. A Luteal Out-of-Phase (Loop) Event

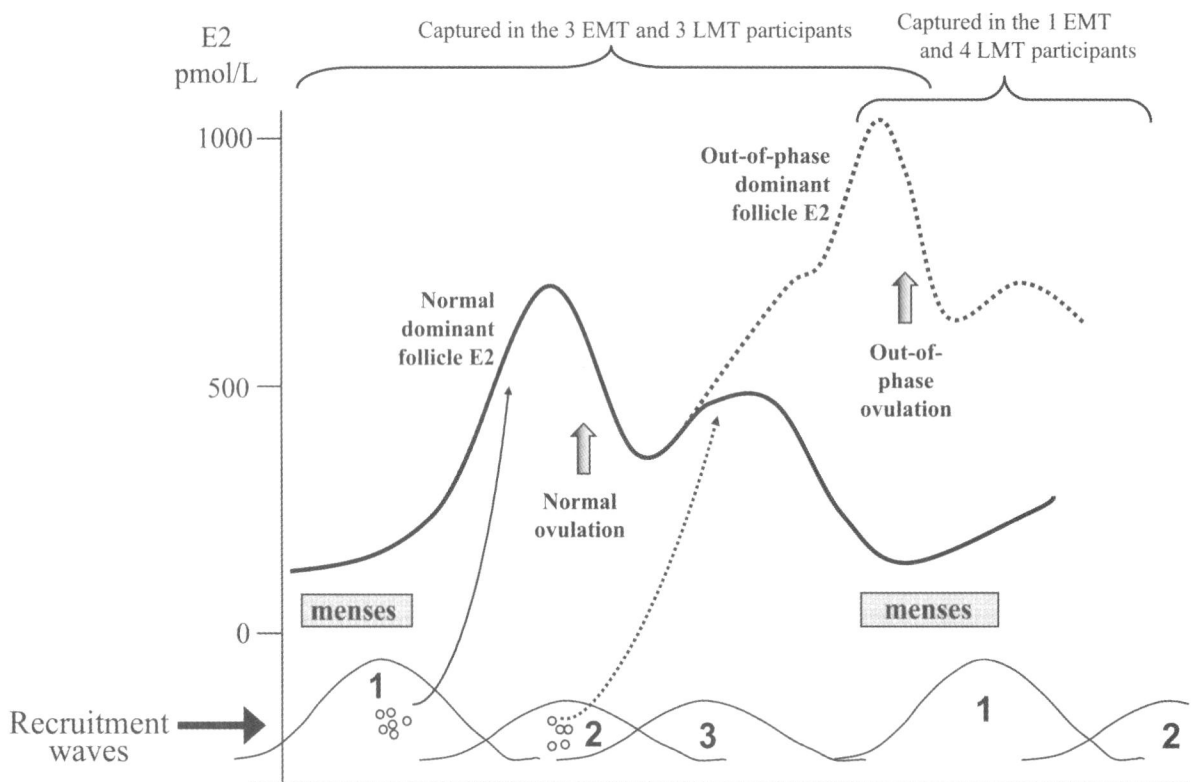

Abbreviations: E2, estradiol; EMT, early menopause transition; LMT, late menopause transition.
From Hale GE, et al.[22] © North American Menopause Society.

In one small study, the midcycle rise of free testosterone and androstenedione, characteristic of younger (19-37 y), regularly cycling women, was found to be consistently and significantly absent in older (43-47 y), regularly cycling women.[59] Total testosterone levels and sex hormone-binding globulin (SHBG) did not differ significantly in any cycle stage between older and younger women. Data from the Rancho Bernardo Study suggest that reduction in testosterone levels at menopause may be transient and followed by normalization in older women.[60] In a large cross-sectional Australian study, serum androgen levels were shown to decline with age from the early reproductive years without changing at the menopause transition.[61] As in the Rancho Bernardo study, testosterone levels increased slightly during the seventh decade of life.

In the Melbourne Women's Midlife Health Project, the menopause transition was associated with a drop in the levels of SHBG.[58] During the 4 years before menopause to 2 years after menopause, SHBG levels decreased by approximately 40%. The greatest change occurred 2 years before menopause and was concurrent with a dramatic decline in serum estradiol. Reduced SHBG levels alter the free androgen index, calculated as the ratio of testosterone to SHBG. The index rises by nearly 80% during the menopause transition, with the maximal change occurring 2 years before the FMP.

Postmenopause
(STRAW+10 stages +1a, +1b, +1c, and +2)

The hallmark for initiation of postmenopause is the FMP. There is no single specific endocrine marker of postmenopause.[46]

Early postmenopause
(stages +1a, +1b, and +1c)

During the first 2 years of early postmenopause, FSH continues to rise and estradiol continues to decrease.[9] STRAW stage +1a is defined as the 12 months after the FMP, which is also defined as the end of perimenopause. Stage +1b encompasses the second postmenopause year and ends at the time point at which FSH and estradiol levels begin to stabilize. Vasomotor symptoms (VMS) are most likely to occur during stages +1a and +1b, which in general last 2 years. During the 3- to 6-year period defined as stage +1c, high FSH levels and low estradiol levels stabilize.

Late postmenopause (stage +2)

Stage +2 begins 5 to 8 years after the FMP and continues for the remaining lifespan.[9] Further changes in reproductive endocrine function are limited, and somatic aging

predominates. This phase is marked by increasing genitourinary symptoms; however, some studies demonstrated decreases in FSH level in more elderly women.

Endocrine findings during postmenopause include elevated FSH and LH, with FSH levels consistently greater than 20 mIU/mL starting approximately 4 years after menopause. Postmenopause estradiol levels range from 10 pg/mL to 25 pg/mL, and estrone levels average 30 pg/mL but may be higher in women who are obese because aromatization increases in proportion to adipose tissue volume.[62]

Transient elevations of estradiol in postmenopausal women may reflect activity in a residual follicle, but such activity does not usually result in ovulation. At least one such case, however, has been formally reported,[63] and many clinicians can attest to at least one woman who has described a "normal" menstrual cycle accompanied by premenstrual molimina and normal pattern of menstrual bleeding after menopause. These episodes, nevertheless, constitute unscheduled postmenopausal bleeding and as such must be formally evaluated.

The postmenopausal ovary continues to produce androstenedione and testosterone. Higher levels of androgens in some postmenopausal women might reflect ovarian stromal hyperplasia and luteinization.[64]

In the Rancho Bernardo Study, women aged 50 to 89 years with intact ovaries had total testosterone levels that increased with age, reaching premenopause levels by age 70, with relatively stable levels thereafter.[60] In a report from the Cardiovascular Health Study, total testosterone levels declined with age until age 80, whereas free testosterone levels did not vary by age.[65] White ethnicity, lower BMI, oral estrogen, and corticosteroid use were each associated with lower testosterone levels in women aged older than 65 years.

Surgical menopause results in lower testosterone levels. In the Rancho Bernardo study, women who had undergone bilateral oophorectomy with hysterectomy had testosterone levels that did not vary with age and were 40% to 50% lower than levels in women with an intact uterus and ovaries.[60]

Physiology of the Menopause Transition

The hypothalamic-pituitary-ovarian (HPO) axis undergoes a series of changes as a woman traverses menopause. The primary driver of change is ovarian follicular depletion, which begins even before birth and results in a progressive, exponential loss of follicles over a woman's lifetime.[11,66] Follicle dysfunction precedes the near-complete exhaustion that occurs at menopause, and several patterns of change have been described along with an overall progression.

The normal menstrual cycle in midreproductive life

An idealized menstrual cycle is 28 days long, with a follicular phase that lasts for 14 days and a luteal phase that also lasts for 14 days (Figure 3). Early follicular-phase FSH levels rise slightly, which i nitiates a wave of folliculogenesis. As a dominant follicle is selected, estradiol rises exponentially until the midcycle peak (day 13). This peak in estradiol initiates an LH, and to a lesser extent, FSH surge on day 14. The LH surge completes the process of ovulation and corpus luteum formation, and progesterone production rises dramatically over the course of the luteal phase, peaking at about days 20 to 22 and declining thereafter in the absence of a pregnancy. All of these cardinal hormone events are affected by the changes of the menopause transition.

The early transition (STRAW+10 stage −2)

The early transition may be best conceptualized as a state of "compensated failure" of the HPO axis. The decrease in follicle numbers and size of the follicle cohort results in a reduction in circulating inhibin B and AMH, both of which are granulosa cell products and both of which help to restrain follicle growth.[67] In early reproductive life, higher levels of AMH and inhibin B help protect the entire follicle pool in the ovary and limit the number of follicles in the "growing pool" each month, preventing a woman from ovulating all of her ovarian follicles over just a few menstrual cycles.[68] With aging, the loss of inhibin B releases FSH from inhibitory restraint, allowing growth of the remaining, diminished follicle pool.[67] The loss of AMH also releases the primordial ovarian follicles from growth inhibition, a mechanism that has been shown in the mouse[68] and implied in humans.[69] Although these two changes in hormone secretion make more follicles available for ovulation and maintain regular cyclicity, they do so at the cost of accelerated follicle atresia.[66]

The early menopause transition is characterized by an increase in cycle irregularity by 7 or more days or an occasional "skipped" menstrual period without amenorrhea of 60 days or more in duration.[9] In this part of the transition, women do not have consistently low estradiol levels, although some of the classic symptoms of menopause begin to increase in prevalence. FSH and follicular-phase

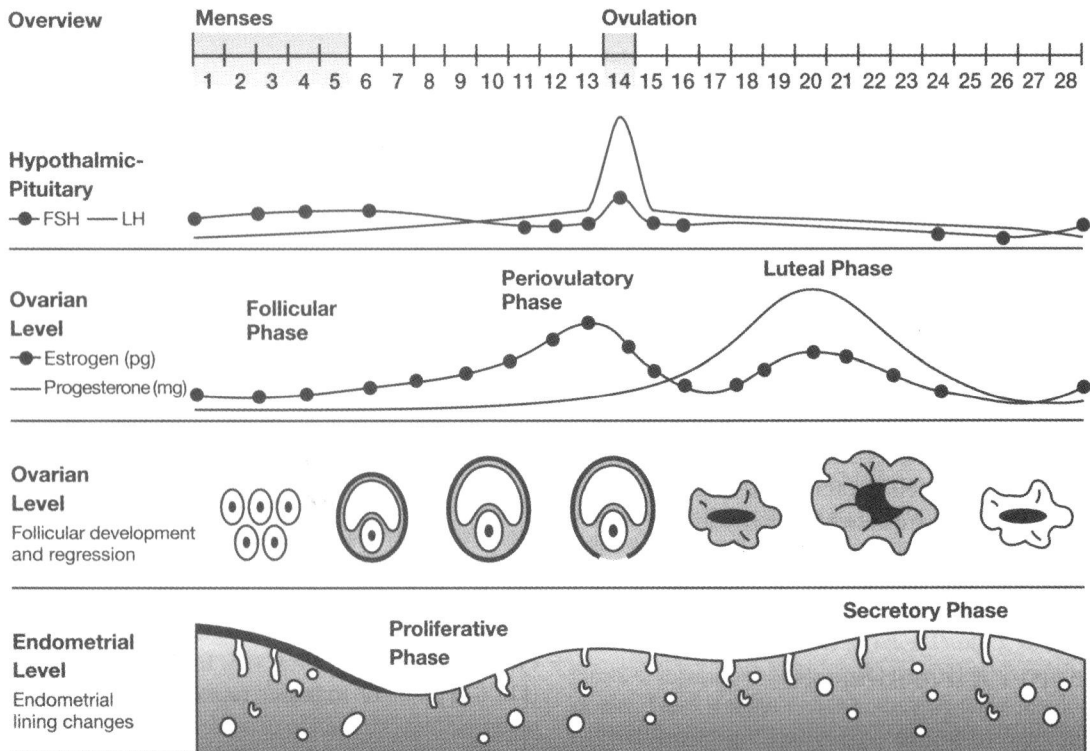

Figure 3. The Menstrual Cycle

estradiol are intermittently elevated, and sometimes luteal phase estradiol can be elevated compared with normally cycling midreproductive-aged women.[70] Menstrual-cycle length shortens because the follicular phase of the cycle becomes compressed.[71] The process of follicle growth is accelerated,[72] but follicles reach a smaller peak diameter than they do in midreproductive-aged women.[73] Folliculogenesis even appears to occur in the luteal phase preceding the subsequent cycle.[22,74] The net result of these changes is that women spend more time in the luteal phase of the cycle, which can lead to more premenstrual symptoms and more frequent menstrual periods.

Additional phenomena include ovulatory failures. These can happen via two mechanisms. In one case, there can be follicle growth, estradiol secretion, and an LH surge but no corpus luteum formation.[73] In the other, an LH surge fails to occur despite apparently normal estrogen production.[75] The latter situation, failure to mount an LH surge in the face of adequate estrogen exposure, indicates that there is hypothalamic-pituitary dysfunction that accompanies the menopause transition. The HPO axis may become less sensitive to estrogen as a woman ages, and this may contribute to the cycle irregularity of the menopause transition.

The late transition (STRAW+10 stage –1)

By the late transition, follicular depletion drops below a critical threshold, and the compensatory mechanisms that kept menstrual cyclicity relatively regular during the early transition can no longer keep pace. The follicle cohort becomes critically low, and folliculogenesis is intermittent. The late transition is marked by amenorrhea of longer than 60 days, and estrogen deficiency symptoms become much more prevalent as women go for longer lengths of time without sufficient estradiol production. When follicular growth does occur, failure of robust ovulation is more likely, and progesterone production over the luteal phase decreases.[52] Eventually, follicle numbers become so low that folliculogenesis cannot occur, and estradiol and progesterone production essentially ceases. For the first year after the final menses, estrogen production appears to occur at variable levels, but no progesterone production is observed, and women remain amenorrheic.[76]

Laboratory testing to determine a woman's menopause stage is fraught with potential pitfalls. FSH levels are notoriously variable both from cycle to cycle and day to day across a menstrual cycle. Although a very high FSH level can help predict that a woman is likely to be menopausal, a normal or low FSH is not informative.[67] Attention has turned to the use of AMH as a potentially superior marker of time to menopause.[77] Some investigators have reported that the change in AMH over time also may be helpful in predicting menopause[78]; however, this marker has not yet been demonstrated to correlate with the STRAW stages of reproductive aging and requires validation in further clinical studies before it can be recommended for clinical use.

It is important to remember that these mechanisms apply only to women who have had relatively regular menstrual cycles throughout their reproductive lives. Women with amenorrhea syndromes have been studied only minimally. Polycystic ovary syndrome (PCOS), for example, is present in 5% to 20% of women, depending on the exact definition used.[79,80] There is evidence that the progression to menopause for these women, although it involves the same physiologic fundamentals, is later in life and can be preceded by an appearance of regular menstrual cycling—for the first time in their lives.[81] These late reproductive-aged cycles can be fertile and may represent a brief period of time in which a woman with PCOS "escapes" from the chronic suppression of follicle growth brought about by elevated AMH levels.

The life course of women with functional hypothalamic amenorrhea, which is present in 3% to 5% of the population, is virtually unstudied. However, with reproductive aging, despite reduced central neural gonadotropin-releasing hormone drive, FSH may still rise, and follicle growth could theoretically occur. The clinical point is that amenorrhea syndromes should not be assumed to be fixed and irreversible, because the reproductive background changes with time.

Adrenal Physiology and Menopause

The adrenal gland is composed of two functionally and embryologically distinct parts known as the adrenal cortex and the adrenal medulla.[82] The adrenal cortex produces three main types of hormones: glucocorticoids (cortisol and corticosterone), produced in the zona fasciculata; mineralocorticoids (predominantly aldosterone), produced in the zona glomerulosa; and sex steroids (primarily androgens), produced in the zona reticularis. The adrenal medulla produces and secretes catecholamines (epinephrine, norepinephrine, and to a lesser extent, dopamine) in response to stimulation by sympathetic neurons. Dehydroepiandrosterone (DHEA), dehydroepiandrosterone sulfate (DHEAS), and androstenedione, often referred to as adrenal androgens, are precursor hormones produced in the adrenal gland that are enzymatically converted to active androgens or estrogens in the peripheral tissues.

Aldosterone secretion from the zona glomerulosa is regulated by three main factors: 1) angiotensin II (as part of the renin-angiotensin-aldosterone system in which renin secreted in response to decreased renal arterial blood pressure from the renal juxtaglomerular cells converts angiotensinogen to angiotensin I, which in turn is converted by angiotensin-converting enzyme into angiotensin II); 2) potassium concentration (direct effect); and 3) adrenocorticotropic hormone secreted by the anterior pituitary (to a lesser degree).[82]

Glucocorticoid secretion from the zona fasciculata is regulated primarily by adrenocorticotropic hormone secreted from the anterior pituitary, which in turn is stimulated by corticotropin-releasing hormone and arginine vasopressin as part of the hypothalamic-pituitary-adrenal (HPA) axis.

Corticotropin-releasing hormone secretion and resulting adrenal glucocorticoid secretion are influenced by circadian rhythms as well as by stressors. Cortisol exerts negative inhibitory feedback on the secretion of both corticotropin-releasing hormone and adrenocorticotropic hormone. Adrenal androgen secretion is regulated by adrenocorticotropic hormone.[83]

Most of serum cortisol circulates bound to cortisol binding globulin. Oral estrogen increases cortisol-binding globulin and, as a result, total cortisol concentration, as does the marked increase in estrogen that occurs during pregnancy.[84] Tamoxifen increases serum cortisol concentration by a similar mechanism.[85] In contrast, transdermal estrogen, which does not increase cortisol-binding globulin, has minimal effect on serum cortisol concentration.[84] Salivary cortisol concentration, which reflects the free rather than total serum cortisol concentration, is not influenced by estrogen use.

Effect of aging on adrenal function

Numerous studies have demonstrated that circulating levels of DHEAS decrease with age in both men and women,[58,61,86] beginning in the early to mid-twenties.[61,86] In women participating in SWAN, cross-sectional analyses confirmed the well-established age-related fall in circulating DHEAS levels, although longitudinal analyses of women undergoing the menopause transition demonstrated a transient increase in circulating DHEAS levels in the late menopause transition (Figure 4).[87,88] The transient increase in DHEAS over the menopause transition also occurs in women who have undergone bilateral salpingo-oophorectomy (BSO), supporting an adrenal origin of this phenomenon.[89] Whether this transient increase in DHEAS bears physiologic significance is unknown. Studies evaluating changes in cortisol concentration over the menopause transition have been conflicting. Although an analysis of

the SWAN cohort showing a transient increase in DHEAS over the menopause transition did not show an accompanying change in cortisol concentration,[88] a transient rise in urinary cortisol was observed in the late menopause transition in the Seattle Midlife Women's Health Study.[90]

Studies examining the relationships between VMS and HPA axis activation have been conflicting. Although VMS have been positively associated with urinary cortisol,[91] and night sweat "bother" has been associated with higher plasma cortisol levels,[92] cortisol levels were not associated with VMS severity in perimenopausal and early postmenopausal women participating in the Seattle Midlife Women's Health Study.[93,94]

Relationships between LH/HPA axis and adrenal steroids

It has long been known that the adrenal cortex has receptors for LH.[95] Despite this knowledge, the role of LH and its receptor in modulating adrenal gland function has remained unclear. Several interactions between LH and adrenal steroid production in pathologic states have been demonstrated. There are several case reports of adrenal tumors that grew or first appeared during pregnancy and were demonstrated to be stimulated by human chorionic gonadotropin, which has homology with LH and binds to the same receptor. In some of the cases, the excess in adrenal steroids resolved at the end of pregnancy[96] and recurred in subsequent pregnancies.[97] A case report of a woman with bilateral adrenal hyperplasia showed that LH stimulated cortisol production and that suppression of LH with leuprolide also suppressed cortisol production.[98]

Whether LH and adrenal steroids are related in non-pathologic conditions has also been investigated. A study of postmenopausal women demonstrated that higher serum LH levels were correlated with higher urinary cortisol levels and lower urinary aldosterone levels.[99] A positive relationship between LH levels up to 41 IU/L, but not higher, and serum cortisol was also demonstrated in a group of 112 postmenopausal woman.[100] In addition, LH levels were reported to correlate with levels of DHEAS. These studies suggest that LH may play a role in modulating levels of adrenal steroids in perimenopausal and postmenopausal women. Details of this regulation require further investigation.

Exogenous DHEA therapy

Although it is well established that circulating levels of adrenal androgens decline with age, supplementation with exogenous DHEA is not recommended in the general population because of the lack of evidence for efficacy coupled with the absence of data assuring long-term safety.[101] Dehydroepiandrosterone sulfate levels are also lower in women with both primary and secondary adrenal insufficiency, because the adrenal glands represent the predominant source of DHEA and DHEAS production. Studies evaluating the efficacy of exogenous DHEA treatment in women with adrenal insufficiency, however, have produced conflicting results.[102] Furthermore, the potential risks of treatment, including androgenic adverse effects, lack of strict regulation of quality and content of DHEA supplements, and the unknown long-term safety profile of treatment, need to be considered.

One small randomized, controlled trial (RCT) of women with adrenal insufficiency found that women randomized to DHEA treatment experienced improvements in well-being and sexuality,[103] but other studies have reported conflicting results.

A systematic review and meta-analysis of RCTs examining DHEA treatment effects in women with adrenal insufficiency concluded that DHEA treatment led to small improvements in quality of life and depression but no significant benefits in terms of anxiety and sexual well-being.[102] The authors therefore concluded that the available evidence does not support routine use of DHEA in women with adrenal insufficiency.

Similarly, a systematic review and meta-analysis of DHEA use in postmenopausal women with normal adrenal function found no evidence of improvement in sexual symptoms, serum lipids, serum glucose, weight, or bone mineral density (BMD).[104] Routine DHEA use in postmenopausal women is not recommended.[105] Local vaginal therapy with DHEA has been proven to improve vaginal pain and dyspareunia.

Adrenal fatigue

The term *adrenal fatigue* has been promulgated by popular media to describe a purported scenario in which chronic exposure to long-term physical, emotional, or

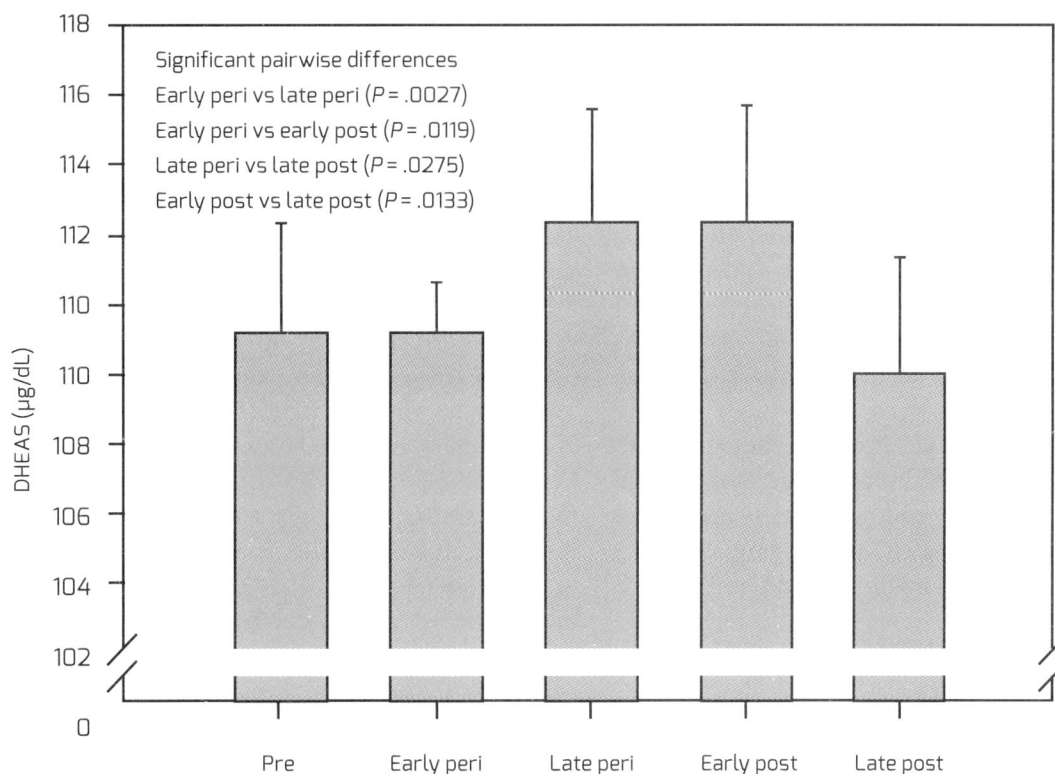

Figure 4. Adjusted Mean DHEAS by Menopause Status in SWAN

Significant pairwise differences
Early peri vs late peri ($P = .0027$)
Early peri vs early post ($P = .0119$)
Late peri vs late post ($P = .0275$)
Early post vs late post ($P = .0133$)

DHEAS (μg/dL)

Pre | Early peri | Late peri | Early post | Late post

Cross-sectional analyses confirmed the well-established age-related fall in circulating DHEAS levels. Longitudinal analyses of women undergoing the menopause transition demonstrated a transient increase in circulating DHEAS levels in the late menopause transition.
Abbreviations: DHEAS, dehydroepiandrosterone sulfate; SWAN, Study of Women's Health Across the Nation.
Adapted from Crawford S, et al.[87] Used with permission. Copyright © 2009 by The Endocrine Society.

psychological stress leads to downregulation of the HPA axis and resulting fatigue of the adrenal glands.[106,107] There is no diagnostic test for adrenal fatigue, although some practitioners employ salivary cortisol day curves using unsubstantiated reference ranges that can engender abnormal results in healthy people. Symptoms of adrenal fatigue, including fatigue, difficulty sleeping, and mood disturbances, are nonspecific and common to many medical conditions as well as to everyday life.

Despite the permeation of this purported condition throughout the media and in health books, evidence of its existence is lacking to date. This unproven diagnosis must be distinguished from true adrenal insufficiency, a well-characterized medical condition resulting from hypofunction of the adrenal glands or pituitary gland that is diagnosed by low serum cortisol levels at baseline or in response to adrenocorticotropic hormone stimulation, for which glucocorticoid replacement therapy is essential. Known potential risks of glucocorticoid therapy include osteoporosis, hyperglycemia, myopathy, and psychiatric symptoms; in the absence of a proven medical condition that warrants glucocorticoid therapy, the risks of therapy are not justified. Furthermore, it is well-known that long-term exogenous glucocorticoid therapy can cause adrenal insufficiency via suppression of the HPA axis. Ironically, this in turn prevents the adrenal glands from adequately responding to physical stress and can be life-threatening if unrecognized or undertreated. Another "cost" of diagnosis is distraction from the recognition and appropriate treatment of another underlying and potentially treatable condition, such as depression, obstructive sleep apnea, or another medical problem.

A 2016 systematic review concluded that most studies describing adrenal fatigue lacked quantitative assessment of adrenal function by accepted methodology and produced conflicting results.[107] Based on the lack of substantive evidence, the authors concluded that adrenal fatigue does not exist. The Endocrine Society has agreed with the conclusion that there is "no substantiation that 'adrenal fatigue' is an actual medical condition."[106]

Primary Ovarian Insufficiency and Early Menopause

Primary ovarian insufficiency (POI) is a distinct clinical entity with multiple etiologies, characterized by hypergonadotrophic hypogonadism in women aged younger than 40 years (previously known as *premature ovarian failure*). The term POI is preferred to the term *premature ovarian failure* because the condition is neither always complete ovarian failure nor always permanent.[108]

Primary ovarian insufficiency is thought to affect approximately 1% of US women by age 40, which is approximately two standard deviations below the median age at menopause.[109,110] Early menopause occurs in approximately 3% of the population aged between 40 and 45 years.[109] Primary ovarian insufficiency also is present in approximately 1 in 1,000 women aged younger than 30 years and 1 in 10,000 women aged younger than 20 years.[111]

Despite episodes of amenorrhea and elevated FSH levels, ovulation in women with POI may occur intermittently and unpredictably for several years. It is estimated that 25% of women with POI will experience at least one spontaneous return of ovarian function.[112] In women with POI who have a normal karyotype, one-half may still have ovarian follicles capable of functioning intermittently. A pregnancy rate of 5% to 10% has been reported in one systematic review.[113] Other data suggest that spontaneous pregnancy rates are closer to 3% to 5%.[112,114] In a large proportion of women diagnosed with spontaneous POI, the etiology behind the syndrome remains undiagnosed, and the term idiopathic POI is appropriate.[110]

Early menopause

Early menopause is defined as menopause occurring between the ages of 40 and 45 years. It occurs naturally in 3% to 5% of the population, but more commonly early menopause is surgical.[109,115] Although no specific diagnostic workup is necessary for women with early menopause, these women are also at increased risk for the long-term effects of early estrogen deficiency compared with women who experience menopause at the average age. Multiple medical societies, including The North American Menopause Society, the International Menopause Society, the American College of Obstetricians and Gynecologists, the American Society for Reproductive Medicine, the British Medical Society, and the Society of Obstetricians and Gynaecologists of Canada, as well as the Endocrine Society, support the philosophy of the use of hormone therapy (HT) for women with POI and early menopause until the average age of menopause.[116-118]

Etiologies of POI and early menopause

Primary ovarian insufficiency has multiple etiologies, including genetic (X-chromosome related and autosomal), autoimmune, toxic, infectious, metabolic, and iatrogenic causes (Table 1).[108,109,113,119-126] About a third of cases appear to be familial, with at least one affected female relative.[127]

Genetic

Genetic factors can affect gonadal development, DNA replication or meiosis and repair, hormone signaling, immune function, and metabolism.[114] Women with primary amenorrhea will have a higher incidence of karyotypic abnormalities (21%) compared with women who present with secondary amenorrhea (11%).[110,128,129] If a Y chromosome is found, gonadectomy is recommended because of the elevated risk of gonadoblastoma.[130]

Turner syndrome. Turner syndrome, the most common identifiable genetic disorder for POI, refers to the complete or partial loss of one X chromosome. It has been postulated to occur because of the reduction of X-linked genes that escape X inactivation or the lack of the matching X gene pair at meiosis.[131] Other X chromosome abnormalities associated with POI include triple X, mosaics, deletions, isochromosomes, microdeletions, translocations, and point mutations. Rare single nucleotide variations in both X and autosomes have been discovered by new genetic tools and analysis of candidate genes in mice models of infertility.

Turner syndrome occurs in 1 in 2,500 to 3,000 births, although 99% of Turner syndrome fetuses are associated with miscarriage.[132] Phenotypic expression includes—among others—POI, short stature, lymphedema (commonly webbed neck), cardiac (coarctation of the aorta, bicuspid aortic valve) and renal anomalies, endocrine dysfunction, wide-spaced nipples and shield chest, cubitus valgus, short fourth metacarpal, and auditory or ophthalmologic problems.[132,133] Women with complete monosomy X develop a normal complement of primordial follicles but undergo accelerated follicular atresia, usually resulting in prepubertal primary ovarian insufficiency. Women with Turner mosaicism, often because of point mutations, may have spontaneous menarche or may present at varying ages with POI.[134]

In women with clinical suspicion, primary amenorrhea, or hypergonadotropic POI, a karyotype should be offered. On diagnosis, a multidisciplinary approach is recommended.[135] In the case of delayed puberty, girls with Turner syndrome should be treated with estrogen replacement, beginning at age 12. The recommended treatment includes transdermal estradiol at gradually increasing doses over 2 years to a target dose of 100 µg of estradiol. On menarche, progestogen replacement is added.

Table 1. Known Causes of POI and Early Menopause

Genetic disorders

- X chromosome disorders (monosomy, trisomy, or translocations, deletions), reduced gene dosage, nonspecific impairment of meiosis, and accelerated atresia
- Specific genetic disorders on the long arm of the X chromosome (POF1, POF2, and FMR1 genes)
- Autosomal genes such as FOXL2 that codes for the forkhead transcription factor that plays a major role in development of the ovary
- Mutations involving enzymes important for reproduction
  - Galactosemia
  - 17α-hydroxylase deficiency (CYP17A1)
  - Aromatase deficiency
- Mutations involving reproductive hormones, their receptors, and actions
  - FSH receptor mutations
  - Mutations involving postreceptor steps in FSH actions
  - LH-receptor mutations

Associated autoimmune disorders

- Autoimmune polyendocrine syndromes
  - Hypothyroidism
  - Adrenal insufficiency
  - Hypoparathyroidism
  - Type 1 DM
- Dry eye syndrome
- Myasthenia gravis
- Rheumatoid arthritis
- Systemic lupus erythematosus
- Congenital thymic aplasia

Miscellaneous disorders

- Metabolic syndromes
- Infections (mumps, HIV)
- Idiopathic

Iatrogenic causes

- Pelvic radiation
- Chemotherapy (alkylating agents)
- Surgical menopause
  - Oophorectomy
  - Ovarian cystectomy
  - Consequence of hysterectomy or uterine artery embolization

Abbreviations: DM, diabetes mellitus; FMR1, fragile X mental retardation 1; FOXL2, forkhead box L2; FSH, follicle-stimulating hormone; HIV, human immunodeficiency virus; POF1, premature ovarian failure 1; POF2, premature ovarian failure 2; POI, primary ovarian insufficiency.

Nelson LM[108]; Luborsky JL, et al[109]; van Kasteren YM, et al[113]; Aittomäki K, et al[119]; Latronico AC, et al[120]; Vegetti W, et al[121]; Harris SE, et al[122]; Progetto Menopausa Italia Study Group[123]; Rebar RW[124]; Vearncombe KJ[125]; Vujovic S.[126]

The benefits of estrogen replacement include development of secondary sex characteristics and maximal bone density accrual.[133,136,137] There is no role for delaying estrogen therapy (ET) to maximize height with growth hormone treatment; this approach has a deleterious effect on building maximal bone density.[133,138] For young women with primary ovarian insufficiency, adequate calcium and vitamin D are recommended.[110] Girls with Turner syndrome should continue to be monitored through adulthood for cardiovascular disease (CVD), fracture risk, impaired glucose tolerance, celiac disease, hypothyroidism, hepatic dysfunction, and dyslipidemia. Women with Turner syndrome have a higher incidence of not only type 2 DM and congenital heart problems but also coronary artery disease, cerebrovascular disease, and mortality because of cardiometabolic complications.[139] It is recommended to continue estrogen-progestogen therapy until an appropriate age for menopause.[133,137] Women should be evaluated and counseled about their own personal risks if contemplating pregnancy via egg donation.

Fragile X syndrome. Fragile X syndrome is an X-linked inherited cause of POI in premutation carriers because of a mutation of the fragile X mental retardation 1 (FMR1) gene.[140] The premutation is carried by 1 in 200 women.[141] The syndrome accounts for about 11.5% of familial POI but only 3% of sporadic POI and therefore has become one of the most common known genetic causes.[131] Normally, there are 5 to 45 copies of the CGG trinuclear repeat in the 5' area region of chromosome X. When there are more than 200 repeats, the full syndrome of fragile X syndrome with mental disability and autism, more commonly in men, occurs.[142] When there are 55 to 200 repeats, or a "premutation allele," there is an approximately 20% chance of developing POI.[143] There is also a 16% risk of developing ataxia as the woman ages.[142] It is recommended that women with POI be screened for the fragile X premutation because of the implications for their offspring and families.[108]

Autosomal defects

Autosomal defects caused by mutations in various genes have been found to be associated with POI. These are rare causes of POI. The presence of other phenotypic abnormalities in association with POI should prompt referral to a genetic counselor for consideration of additional genetic panels for investigation.

Autoimmune

Autoimmune oophoritis is a rare cause of POI, occurring in 4% of women with spontaneous POI and adrenal antibodies.[108] It also may occur in type 1 and type 2 polyglandular autoimmune failures. The development of autoimmune POI usually precedes adrenal failure, which can be life-threatening. Therefore, it is recommended that the presence of steroidal antibodies prompt referral for careful follow-up by an endocrinologist.

Toxic, infectious, and metabolic

Mumps has been the classic but rare example of an infectious disease associated with oophoritis and potentially POI. When a postpubertal girl develops mumps-related parotitis, oophoritis should be suspected when lower abdominal tenderness or ovarian pain occurs.[144] HIV infections have been associated with a higher incidence of early menopause, either because of the infection or the use of antiretroviral medications.[145] Polycyclic aromatic hydrocarbons released into the environment by fossil fuel combustion or through tobacco smoke also have been identified as potential contributors to POI development.[146] From the evaluation of a nationwide population study, the incidence of POI was found to be higher in women with PCOS.[147] The apparent paradox of women with an excess of follicles experiencing an earlier-than-normal menopause is unexplained in this study; however, the incidence of hysterectomy may have been higher in women with PCOS.

Iatrogenic

Early menopause can be medically or surgically induced. Iatrogenic menopause occurs as a result of bilateral oophorectomies or oophorocystectomies or with gonadotoxic chemotherapy or radiation.

Surgical menopause. Women with surgical menopause experience an abrupt nonreversible drop in hormones (estrogen, progesterone, and androgens). One in eight US women will have their ovaries removed for benign reasons before natural menopause.[148] Many oophorectomies occur at the time of hysterectomy and are done in women with normal ovaries. In women at high risk of breast and ovarian cancer, such as carriers of *BRCA1* and *BRCA2* gene mutations, early elective oophorectomy does offer a significant reduction in all-cause mortality by age 70.[149] Elective bilateral oophorectomies done at the time of benign hysterectomy in premenopausal women aged younger than 45 years has been shown to lead to numerous negative long-term outcomes, such as increased risk of all-cause mortality (hazard ratio [HR], 1.41), coronary heart disease (HR, 1.26), and CVD (HR, 1.84) and worse bone health, menopause symptoms, and mood symptoms.[148] There was also a higher incidence of Parkinson disease and cognitive impairment.[150] In cases for which elective oophorectomy is being considered, the benefits and risks must be carefully reviewed and discussed with the woman. If elective bilateral oophorectomy is performed, ET may be considered until the average age of menopause to mitigate the negative health outcomes of early surgical menopause.

Chemotherapy and radiation-induced menopause. Eighty percent of childhood patients with cancer now survive, and it is estimated that 1 in 168 US women between the ages of 20 and 39 years will develop cancer yearly.[151] Types of chemotherapy used in women with cancer have variable gonadotoxic effects, depending on the type, previous ovarian reserve, dosage, and the age of administration.[152] Women who undergo allogeneic stem cell transplant for various hematologic disease and malignancy are at particularly high risk for POI after induction with whole-body radiation and chemotherapy.[153]

Diagnosis of POI and early menopause

The standard diagnostic criterion for menopause (12 mo with no menses) as applied to women aged 40 years and older does not apply to younger women. Unfortunately, there is no characteristic menstrual history preceding either POI or early menopause. Some women have typical menopause symptoms, at least intermittently, whereas others do not. Another group of women who present for advice are women who have decreased ovarian reserve found during infertility evaluations.

The European Society of Human Reproduction and Embryology guidelines for POI recommend these diagnostic criteria: 1) the presence of menstrual disturbance such as oligomenorrhea or amenorrhea for at least 4 months, and 2) an elevated FSH level more than 25 IU/L on two occasions at least 4 weeks apart.[110]

Severe menopause symptoms often occur in women who experience induced menopause by oophorectomy, chemotherapy, or radiotherapy. Symptoms include hot flashes, mood changes, depression, insomnia, and a lack of energy. Some may experience joint pain or symptoms of genitourinary syndrome of menopause (vaginal dryness, burning, painful intercourse). The timeframe of onset of symptoms to progression of early menopause is unpredictable. Because early estrogen deficiency has a negative effect on bone density and possibly on cognitive function and sexual function, repeated testing and a timely diagnosis is warranted.[150,154-156] A careful history and physical examination are needed to rule out other

causes of menstrual dysfunction, particularly secondary amenorrhea (Table 2).[108]

Initial laboratory evaluation after a negative pregnancy test includes serum prolactin, FSH, estradiol, and thyroid-stimulating hormone and is warranted for any woman aged younger than 40 years who misses three or more consecutive menstrual cycles.[157] Additional laboratory tests should be performed to exclude a variety of other causes (Table 3).

Transvaginal ultrasound imaging is useful to provide information regarding the ovarian volume and AFC.[108] A karyotype and fragile X premutation testing is recommended after the diagnosis of POI is made. The implications of chromosome abnormality or fragile X premutation should be discussed before the test is performed. Karyotype testing is helpful in diagnosing familial syndromes that include POI and identifying a Turner mosaic or translocation condition. Patients with positive adrenal antibodies should follow-up with an endocrinologist.

Table 2. Differential Diagnosis of Secondary Amenorrhea

Low FSH conditions

- Pregnancy
- Hypothalamic amenorrhea
  - Secondary to constitutional disorder
    - Uncontrolled DM
    - Celiac disease
  - Extremes of lifestyle
    - Exercise
    - Caloric restriction
    - Perceived stress
  - Lesions of the hypothalamus/pituitary
  - GnRH agonist/antagonist therapy
- Hyperprolactinemia
- Hypothyroidism and hyperthyroidism
- PCOS

Elevated FSH condition

- POI

Abbreviations: DM, diabetes mellitus; FSH, follicle-stimulating hormone; GnRH, gonadotropin-releasing hormone; POI, primary ovarian insufficiency; PCOS, polycystic ovary syndrome.
Nelson LM.[108]

Whether HT is administered, baseline BMD testing is recommended and should be repeated every 5 years.[108,110] In younger patients, attention should be given to the Z-score for their age and ethnic group rather than the T-score. Bisphosphonates (FDA pregnancy risk category C) should be avoided in young women, because many are hoping for conception. Animal studies with bisphosphonates suggest teratogenicity, with consequences on fetal growth and skeletal development. In humans, preconception and first trimester use of bisphosphonates have been associated with adverse pregnancy outcomes.[158]

First-degree relatives of women with POI should consider the increased risk of earlier menopause or fertility preservation measures when deciding when to have a family.[110]

Management of POI and early menopause

Primary ovarian insufficiency is a devastating diagnosis for a young woman. Many women see multiple clinicians before the diagnosis is made, and many are unhappy with how the diagnosis was conveyed. Specialized multidisciplinary clinics have been initiated to provide compassionate expert care for these women, with the goal of providing diagnosis, emotional support, general information, and encouragement about fertility options as well as to tailor individual prescriptions for optimal outcomes. Women diagnosed with POI should be counseled appropriately regarding the diagnosis, its etiologies, and the subsequent effects not only on fertility but also on long-term sequelae including longevity, quality of life, mood, cognition, bone health, cardiovascular health, and sexuality.

Hormone therapy

Physiologic estrogen and progestogen therapy mitigate the long-term effects of estrogen depravation on various organ systems and is considered standard of care for women with POI. Many women are reluctant to initiate HT because of the propagation of the dangers of HT after the publication of the results of the Women's Health Initiative in 2002.[159] However, HT for these young women is true "replacement therapy" and should be compared with the use of other steroid replacement therapies in other endocrine organs. These women will require long-term therapy that should be reevaluated yearly and possibly altered as the woman's medical and social needs change.

Hormone therapy for secondary amenorrhea and oligomenorrhea

Because women with secondary amenorrhea and oligomenorrhea are younger than typical menopausal women, many experts recommend treating with the equivalent

---

Table 3. Clinical Evaluation in Women With Suspected POI

- Complete history and physical examination
- Family history of early menopause
- LH, FSH, estradiol, and prolactin levels
- If FSH initially elevated, repeat FSH and estradiol levels on at least 2 occasions, usually 1 month apart
- Karyotype (consider molecular cytogenetic studies of the X chromosome)
- FMR1 gene premutation testing
- Adrenal antibodies (evaluate adrenal reserve with ACTH testing if positive)
- TSH and thyroid peroxidase antibodies
- Fasting blood glucose
- Serum calcium and phosphorus concentrations
- Pelvic ultrasound

Not indicated

- Progesterone withdrawal test
- Ovarian antibodies
- Ovarian biopsy

Abbreviations: ACTH, adrenocorticotropic hormone; FMR1, fragile X mental retardation 1; FSH, follicle-stimulating hormone; LH, luteinizing hormone; POI, primary ovarian insufficiency; TSH, thyroid-stimulating hormone.

---

of the 100 µg transdermal estradiol patch, or 1.25 mg conjugated equine estrogens, or 2 mg of estradiol orally to approximate the average estrogen level produced in a reproductive-stage menstrual cycle (100 pm/L or 387 pml/L). If the uterus is present, a cyclical progestogen should be added for 12 days of the month.[160] Note that at these higher doses of estrogen, additional progestin is needed to prevent hyperplasia.

If the woman does not want to risk becoming pregnant in the situation of intermittent menses, hormone contraception can be used to provide hormone replacement.[161-163] Emerging evidence, however, suggests that physiologic HT is superior to hormone contraceptives.[163] Another option for women with heavier menses or intolerance to progestins is an intrauterine progestin system combined with transdermal estrogen.[164] An advantage of HT is that it is prescribed in a regimen of continuous ET, whereas in women taking the oral contraceptive pill, there can be a week-long hormone-free interval in therapy, amounting to 3 months of estrogen deficiency per year and possibly resulting in monthly symptoms of estrogen withdrawal during the hormone-free week.

Alternatives include the use of continuous or extended-cycle oral contraceptive pills. Therapies should be reviewed annually.[110]

For women experiencing an early menopause, especially if aged younger than 45 years, the benefits of using HT until the average age of natural menopause are believed to outweigh the risks. There is no evidence that HT increases the risk of breast cancer in this age group. In one population-based cohort of 1,003 women with POI, there was a decreased incidence of breast cancer (odds ratio, 0.59).[165]

Ramifications of POI and early menopause

Life expectancy
Many of the studies about the ramifications of early menopause on life expectancy are accrued from observational studies and large epidemiologic international databases of women with very long-term follow-ups. The Mayo Clinic Cohort Study of Oophorectomy and Aging[166] and the Nurses' Health Study (up to 28 y),[167] as well as a 2016 large meta-analysis that included 23 studies,[148] have confirmed earlier mortality, primarily because of CVD, in women who are rendered menopausal by surgery before the age of 45. This excess mortality from CVD is most pronounced for women who undergo oophorectomy and do not have subsequent ET.

Women experiencing early menopause or POI may experience significant psychological consequences.[168] For some women, particularly those who are younger, the diagnosis can precipitate a range of emotions, including grief, sadness, and diminished self-esteem. In an older study of early menopausal women caused by BSO, anxiety and depression were significantly greater after BSO and reduced with estrogen use.[169] Spontaneous POI may be associated with an increased lifetime risk for major depression, as well as poorer psychosocial adjustment.[170-171] Several studies show an increased risk of depression and anxiety in women with earlier menopause caused by BSO.[172-173] One study did not show improvement with ET.[172] Therefore, it is important to offer psychological support for concerns about early loss of fertility, self-image, and sexual function and be sensitive to mood changes in these women. Adequate HT to reduce menopause symptoms and possibly improve mood is suggested.

Fertility
Whenever possible, counseling regarding childbearing options should be provided before any chemotherapy, radiation, or surgery that may induce menopause. Clinicians should consider referral to a fertility specialist in all situations in which early loss of fertility is possible. Options for preserving fertility include ovarian hyperstimulation with oocyte retrieval followed by oocyte or embryo cryopreservation, ovarian tissue cryopreservation, ovarian suppression with hormones, ovarian transposition, and conservative gynecologic surgery (eg, trachelectomy for cervical cancer). However, diminished ovarian reserve correlates with poor pregnancy rates with all these options, and not all options are available for all women.

Because of the possibility of spontaneous and unexpected pregnancy, women with POI should be counseled early in their course of treatment regarding their desire to conceive. If pregnancy is not desired, oral contraceptives, barrier methods, or an intrauterine device are suggested to prevent the unlikely occurrence of an unintentional pregnancy. Oral contraceptives provide additional benefits, including relief of VMS and vaginal dryness and maintenance of BMD. A discussion of contraception is especially important for women who carry the FMR1 gene, who carry a higher risk for a child with mental retardation.

REFERENCES

1. United Nations. Population Division. Department of Economic and Social Affairs. *World Population Prospects: The 2017 Revision*. File POP/15-3: Annual female population by five-year age group, region, subregion and country, 1950-2100 (thousands). Estimates, 1950-2015. June 2017. https://esa.un.org/unpd/wpp/Download/Standard/Population/. Accessed March 1, 2019.

2. US Census Bureau, Population Division. *2014 National Population Projections Tables*. Table 9. Projections of the population by sex and age for the United States: 2015 to 2060 (NP2014-T9). Revised May 9, 2017. www.census.gov/data/tables/2014/demo/popproj/2014-summary-tables.html. Accessed March 1, 2019.

3. Arias E, Heron M, Xu J; Division of Vital Statistics. *United States Life Tables, 2013*. National Vital Statistics Reports. Vol 66, No 3. Hyattsville, MD: National Center for Health Statistics. April 11, 2017. www.cdc.gov/nchs/data/nvsr/nvsr66/nvsr66_03.pdf. Accessed March 1, 2019.

4. Kochanek KD, Murphy SL, BS, Xu J, Tejada-Vera B; Division of Vital Statistics. *Deaths: Final Data for 2014*. National Vital Statistics Reports. Vol 65, No 4. Hyattsville, MD: National Center for Health Statistics. June 30, 2016. Updated April 3, 2017. www.cdc.gov/nchs/data/nvsr/nvsr65/nvsr65_04.pdf. Accessed March 1, 2019.

5. Statistics Canada. *Projected Population by Projection Scenario, Age, and Sex as of July 1, Canada, Provinces, and Territories, Annual (Persons)*. CANSIM database. Table 052-0005. Last modified September 17, 2014. http://www5.statcan.gc.ca/cansim/a26?lang=eng&id=520005. Accessed March 1, 2019.

6. Statistics Canada. *Population by Sex and Age Group*. CANSIM database. Table 051-0001. Last modified September 27, 2017. http://www.statcan.gc.ca/tables-tableaux/sum-som/l01/cst01/demo10a-eng.htm. Accessed March 1, 2019.

7. Statistics Canada. *Life Expectancy 1920-1922 to 2009-2011*. Canadian Megatrends website. Last modified March 3, 2017. http://www.statcan.gc.ca/pub/11-630-x/11-630-x2016002-eng.htm. Accessed March 1, 2019.

8. Soules MR, Sherman S, Parrott E, et al. Executive summary: Stages of Reproductive Aging Workshop (STRAW) Park City, Utah, July, 2001. *Menopause*. 2001;8(6):402-407.

9.   Harlow SD, Gass M, Hall JE, et al; STRAW 10 Collaborative Group. Executive summary of the Stages of Reproductive Aging Workshop + 10: addressing the unfinished agenda of staging reproductive aging. *Menopause*. 2012;19(4):387-395.

10.   Torrealday S, Pal L. Premature menopause. *Endocrinol Metab Clin North Am*. 2015;44(3):543-557.

11.   Baker TG. A quantitative and cytological study of germ cells in human ovaries. *Proc R Soc Lond B Biol Sci*. 1963;158:417-433.

12.   Neal-Perry G, Nejat E, Dicken C. The neuroendocrine physiology of female reproductive aging: an update. *Maturitas*. 2010;67(1):34-38.

13.   Veldhuis JD. Changes in pituitary function with ageing and implications for patient care. *Nat Rev Endocrinol*. 2013;9(4):205-215.

14.   Harlow SD, Cain K, Crawford S, et al. Evaluation of four proposed bleeding criteria for the onset of late menopausal transition. *J Clin Endocrinol Metab*. 2006;91(9):3432-3438.

15.   Harlow SD, Crawford S, Dennerstein L, Burger HG, Mitchell ES, Sowers MF; ReSTAGE Collaboration. Recommendations from a multi-study evaluation of proposed criteria for staging reproductive aging. *Climacteric*. 2007;10(2):112-119.

16.   Harlow SD, Mitchell ES, Crawford S, Nan B, Little R, Taffe J; ReSTAGE Collaboration. The ReSTAGE Collaboration: defining optimal bleeding criteria for onset of early menopausal transition. *Fertil Steril*. 2008;89(1):129-140.

17.   Bidet M, Bachelot A, Bissauge E, et al. Resumption of ovarian function and pregnancies in 358 patients with premature ovarian failure. *J Clin Endocrinol Metab*. 2011;96(12):3864-3872.

18.   Qu X, Cheng Z, Yang W, Xu L, Dai H, Hu L. Controlled clinical trial assessing the effect of laparoscopic uterine arterial occlusion on ovarian reserve. *J Minim Invasive Gynecol*. 2010;17(1):47-52.

19.   Santoro N, Adel T, Skurnick JH. Decreased inhibin tone and increased activin A secretion characterize reproductive aging in women. *Fertil Steril*. 1999;71(4):658-662.

20.   Reame NE, Wyman TL, Phillips DJ, de Kretser DM, Padmanabhan V. Net increase in stimulatory input resulting from a decrease in inhibin B and an increase in activin A may contribute in part to the rise in follicular phase follicle-stimulating hormone of aging cycling women. *J Clin Endocrinol Metab*. 1998;83(9):3302-3307.

21.   Klein NA, Illingworth PJ, Groome NP, McNeilly AS, Battaglia DE, Soules MR. Decreased inhibin B secretion is associated with the monotropic FSH rise in older, ovulatory women: a study of serum and follicular fluid levels of dimeric inhibin A and B in spontaneous menstrual cycles. *J Clin Endocrinol Metab*. 1996;81(7):2742-2745.

22.   Hale GE, Hughes CL, Burger HG, Robertson DM, Fraser IS. Atypical estradiol secretion and ovulation patterns caused by luteal out-of-phase (LOOP) events underlying irregular ovulatory menstrual cycles in the menopausal transition. *Menopause*. 2009;16(1):50-59.

23.   Shaw ND, Srouji SS, Welt CK, et al. Compensatory increase in ovarian aromatase in older regularly cycling women. *J Clin Endocrinol Metab*. 2015;100(9):3539-3547.

24.   Hansen KR, Hodnett GM, Knowlton N, Craig LB. Correlation of ovarian reserve tests with histologically determined primordial follicle number. *Fertil Steril*. 2011;95(1):170-175.

25.   Broer SL, van Disseldorp J, Broeze KA, et al; IMPORT Study Group. Added value of ovarian reserve testing on patient characteristics in the prediction of ovarian response and ongoing pregnancy: an individual patient data approach. *Hum Reprod Update*. 2013;19(1):26-36.

26.   Gracia CR, Sammel MD, Freeman E, et al. Impact of cancer therapies on ovarian reserve. *Fertil Steril*. 2012;97(1):134-140.e131.

27.   Gougeon A, Chainy GB. Morphometric studies of small follicles in ovaries of women at different ages. *J Reprod Fertil*. 1987;81(2):433-442.

28.   Volarcik K, Sheean L, Goldfarb K, Woods L, Abdul-Karim FW, Hunt P. The meiotic competence of in-vitro matured human oocytes is influenced by donor age: evidence that folliculogenesis is compromised in the reproductively aged ovary. *Hum Reprod*. 1998;13(1):154-160.

29.   Warburton D. Biological aging and the etiology of aneuploidy. *Cytogenet Genome Res*. 2005;111(3-4):266-272.

30.   Steiner AZ, Pritchard D, Stanczyk FZ, et al. Association between biomarkers of ovarian reserve and infertility among older women of reproductive age. *JAMA*. 2017;318(14):1367-1376.

31.   Wallace WH, Kelsey TW. Human ovarian reserve from conception to the menopause. *PLoS One*. 2010;5(1):e8772.

32.   Kelsey TW, Wright P, Nelson SM, Anderson RA, Wallace WH. A validated model of serum anti-müllerian hormone from conception to menopause. *PLoS One*. 2011;6(7):e22024.

33.   Kelsey TW, Anderson RA, Wright P, Nelson SM, Wallace WH. Data-driven assessment of the human ovarian reserve. *Mol Hum Reprod*. 2012;18(2):79-87.

34.   Fleming R, Kelsey TW, Anderson RA, Wallace WH, Nelson SM, et al. Interpreting human follicular recruitment and antimullerian hormone concentrations throughout life. *Fertil Steril*. 2012;98(5):1097-1102.

35.   Sowers M, McConnell D, Gast K, et al. Anti-Müllerian hormone and inhibin B variability during normal menstrual cycles. *Fertil Steril*. 2010;94(4):1482-1486.

36.   van den Berg MH, van Dulmen-den Broeder E, Overbeek A, et al. Comparison of ovarian function markers in users of hormonal contraceptives during the hormone-free interval and subsequent natural early follicular phases. *Hum Reprod*. 2010;25(6):1520-1527.

37.   Bentzen JG, Forman JL, Pinborg A, et al. Ovarian reserve parameters: a comparison between users and non-users of hormonal contraception. *Reprod Biomed Online*. 2012;25(6):612-619.

38.   Dólleman M, Verschuren WM, Eijkemans MJ, et al. Reproductive and lifestyle determinants of anti-Mullerian hormone in a large population-based study. *J Clin Endocrinol Metab*. 2013;98(5):2106-2115.

39.   Kallio S, Puurunen J, RuokonenA, Vaskivuo T, Piltonen T, Tapanainen JS. Antimüllerian hormone levels decrease in women using combined contraception independently of administration route. *Fertil Steril*. 2013;99(5):1305-1310.

40.   Birch Petersen K, Hvidman HW, Forman JL, et al. Ovarian reserve assessment in users of oral contraception seeking fertility advice on their reproductive lifespan. *Hum Reprod*. 2015;30(10):2364-2375.

41.   Köninger A, Kauth A, Schmidt B, et al. Anti-Mullerian-hormone levels during pregnancy and postpartum. *Reprod Biol Endocrinol*. 2012;11:60.

42.   Seifer DB, Golub ET, Lambert-Messerlian G, et al. Variations in serum müllerian inhibiting substance between white, black, and Hispanic women. *Fertil Steril*. 2009;92(5):1674-1678.

43.   Genro VK, Grynberg M, Scheffer JB, Roux I, Frydman R, Fanchin R. Serum anti-Müllerian hormone levels are negatively related to follicular output rate (FORT) in normo-cycling women undergoing controlled ovarian hyperstimulation. *Hum Reprod*. 2011;26(3):671-677.

44.   Mutlu MF, Erdem M, Erdem A, et al. Antral follicle count determines poor ovarian response better than anti-Müllerian hormone but age is the only predictor for live birth in in vitro fertilization cycles. *J Assist Reprod Genet*. 2013;30(5):657-665.

45.   Hale GE, Zhao X, Hughes CL, Burger HG, Robertson DM, Fraser IS. Endocrine features of menstrual cycles in middle and late reproductive age and the menopausal transition classified according to the Staging of Reproductive Aging Workshop (STRAW) staging system. *J Clin Endocrinol Metab*. 2007;92(8):3060-3067.

46.   Burger HG, Hale GE, Dennerstein L, Robertson DM. Cycle and hormone changes during perimenopause: the key role of ovarian function. *Menopause*. 2008;15(4 pt 1):603-612.

47.   Hale GE, Robertson DM, Burger HG. The perimenopausal woman: endocrinology and management. *J Steroid Biochem Mol Biol*. 2014;142:121-131.

48.   Welt CK, Jimenez Y, sluss PM, Smith PC, Hall JE. Control of estradiol secretion in reproductive ageing. *Hum Reprod*. 2006;21(8):2189-2193.

49.   O'Connor KA, Ferrell RJ, Brindle E, et al. Total and unopposed estrogen exposure across stages of the transition to menopause. *Cancer Epidemiol Biomarkers Prev*. 2009;18(3):828-836.

50.   O'Connor KA,Ferrell R, Brindle E, et al. Progesterone and ovulation across stages of the transition to menopause. *Menopause*. 2009;16(6):1178-1187.

51.   Santoro N, Crawford SL, El Khoudary SR, et al. Menstrual cycle hormone changes in women traversing the menopause: Study of Women's Health Across the Nation. *J Clin Endocrinol Metab*. 2017;102(7):2218-2229.

52. Santoro N, Crawford SL, Lasley EL, et al. Factors related to declining luteal function in women during the menopausal transition. *J Clin Endocrinol Metab.* 2008;93(5):1711-1721.

53. Hale GE, Burger HG. Hormonal changes and biomarkers in late reproductive age, menopausal transition and menopause. *Best Pract Res Clin Obstet Gynaecol.* 2009;23(1):7-23.

54. Santoro N, Lasley B, McConnell D, et al. Body size and ethnicity are associated with menstrual cycle alterations in women in the early menopausal transition: The Study of Women's Health across the Nation (SWAN) Daily Hormone Study. *J Clin Endocrinol Metab.* 2004;89(6):2622-2631.

55. Freeman EW, Sammel MD, Lin H, Gracia CR. Obesity and reproductive hormone levels in the transition to menopause. *Menopause.* 2010;17(4):718-726.

56. Randolph JF Jr, Zheng H, Sowers MR, et al. Change in follicle-stimulating hormone and estradiol across the menopausal transition: effect of age at the final menstrual period. *J Clin Endocrinol Metab.* 2011;96(3):746-754.

57. Randolph JF Jr, Sowers M, Bondarenko IV, Harlow SD, Luborsky JL, Little RJ. Change in estradiol and follicle-stimulating hormone across the early menopausal transition: effects of ethnicity and age. *J Clin Endocrinol Metab.* 2004;89(4):1555-1561.

58. Burger HG, Dudley EC, Cui J, Dennerstein L, Hopper JL. A prospective longitudinal study of serum testosterone, dehydroepiandrosterone sulfate, and sex hormone-binding globulin levels through the menopause transition. *J Clin Endocrinol Metab.* 2000;85(8):2832-2838.

59. Mushayandebvu T, Castracane VD, Gimpel T, Adel T, Santoro N. Evidence for diminished midcycle ovarian androgen production in older reproductive aged women. *Fertil Steril.* 1996;65(4):721-723.

60. Laughlin GA, Barrett-Connor E, Kritz-Silverstein D, von Mühlen D. Hysterectomy, oophorectomy, and endogenous sex hormone levels in older women: the Rancho Bernardo Study. *J Clin Endocrinol Metab.* 2000;85(2):645-651.

61. Davison SL, Bell R, Donath S, Montalto JG, Davis SR. Androgen levels in adult females: changes with age, menopause, and oophorectomy. *J Clin Endocrinol Metab.* 2005;90(7):3847-3853.

62. Lobo RA. Menopause and aging. In: Strauss JF III, Barbieri RL. *Yen & Jaffe's Reproductive Endocrinology: Physiology, Pathophysiology, and Clinical Management.* 7th ed. Philadelphia, PA: Elsevier Saunders; 2014:308-339.

63. Seungdamrong A, Weiss G. Ovulation in a postmenopausal woman. *Fertil Steril.* 2007;88(5):1438 e1431-1432.

64. Rinaudo P, Strauss JF 3rd. Endocrine function of the postmenopausal ovary. *Endocrinol Metab Clin North Am.* 2004;33(4):661-674.

65. Cappola AR, Ratcliffe SJ, Bhasin S, et al. Determinants of serum total and free testosterone levels in women over the age of 65 years. *J Clin Endocrinol Metab.* 2007;92(2):509-516.

66. Hansen KR, Knowlton NS, Thyer AC, Charleston JS, Soules MR, Klein NA. A new model of reproductive aging: the decline in ovarian non-growing follicle number from birth to menopause. *Hum Reprod.* 2008;23(3):699-708.

67. Burger HG, Dudley EC, Robertson DM, Dennerstein L. Hormonal changes in the menopause transition. *Recent Prog Horm Res.* 2002;57:257-275.

68. Durlinger AL, Gruijters MJ, Kramer P, et al. Anti-müllerian hormone inhibits initiation of primordial follicle growth in the mouse ovary. *Endocrinology.* 2002;143(3):1076-1084.

69. Mumford SL, Legro RS, Diamond MP, et al. Baseline AMH level associated with ovulation following ovulation induction in women with polycystic ovary syndrome. *J Clin Endocrinol Metab.* 2016;101(9):3288-3296.

70. Santoro N, Brown JR, Adel T, Skurnick JH. Characterization of reproductive hormonal dynamics in the perimenopause. *J Clin Endocrinol Metab.* 1996;81(4):1495-1501.

71. Lenton EA, Landgren BM, Sexton L, Harper R. Normal variation in the length of the follicular phase of the menstrual cycle: effect of chronological age. *Br J Obstet Gynaecol.* 1984;91(7):681-684.

72. Klein NA, Battaglia DE, Fujimoto VY, Davis GS, Bremner WJ, Soules MR. Reproductive aging: accelerated ovarian follicular development associated with a monotropic follicle-stimulating hormone rise in normal older women. *J Clin Endocrinol Metab.* 1996;81(3):1038-1045.

73. Santoro N, Isaac B, Neal-Perry G, et al. Impaired folliculogenesis and ovulation in older reproductive aged women. *J Clin Endocrinol Metab.* 2003;88(11):5502-5509.

74. Vanden Brink H, Robertson DM, Lim H, et al. Associations between antral ovarian follicle dynamics and hormone production throughout the menstrual cycle as women age. *J Clin Endocrinol Metab.* 2015;100(12):4553-4562.

75. Weiss G, Skurnick JH, Goldsmith LT, Santoro NF, Park SJ. Menopause and hypothalamic-pituitary sensitivity to estrogen. *JAMA.* 2004;292(24):2991-2996. Erratum in: *JAMA.* 2005;293(2):163. *JAMA.* 2007;298(3):288.

76. Metcalf MG, Skidmore DS, Lowry GF, Mackenzie JA. Incidence of ovulation in the years after the menarche. *J Endocrinol.* 1983;97(2):213-219.

77. Finkelstein JS, Lee H, Burnett-Bowie S-A, et al. Utility of anti-mullerian hormone (AMH) for predicting the time to the final menstrual period: the Study of Women's Health Across the Nation (SWAN) [abstract]. Endocrine Society's 98th Annual Meeting and Expo; April 1-4, 2016; Boston, MA. Abstract OR21-6.

78. Freeman, EW, Sammel MD, Lin H, Boorman DW, Gracia CR. Contribution of the rate of change of antimüllerian hormone in estimating time to menopause for late reproductive-age women. *Fertil Steril.* 2012;98(5):1254-1259.e1-2.

79. Azziz R, Woods KS, Reyna R, Key TJ, Knochenhauer ES, Yildiz BO. The prevalence and features of the polycystic ovary syndrome in an unselected population. *J Clin Endocrinol Metab.* 2004;89(6):2745-2749.

80. Sirmans SM, Pate KA. Epidemiology, diagnosis, and management of polycystic ovary syndrome. *Clin Epidemiol.* 2013;6:1-13.

81. Brown ZA, Louwers YV, Fong SL, et al. The phenotype of polycystic ovary syndrome ameliorates with aging. *Fertil Steril.* 2011;96(5):1259-1265.

82. Stewart PM, Newell-Price J. The adrenal cortex. In: Melmed S, Polonsky KS, Larsen PR, Kronenberg HM, eds. *Williams Textbook of Endocrinology.* 13th ed: Philadelphia, PA: Elsevier; 2016:490-555.

83. Molina PE. Adrenal gland. Chap 6. In: *Endocrine Physiology.* 4th ed. New York, NY: McGraw-Hill;2013. https://accessmedicine.mhmedical.com/content.aspx?bookid=507&sectionid=42540506. Accessed March 19, 2019.

84. Qureshi AC, Bahri A, Breen LA, et al. The influence of the route of oestrogen administration on serum levels of cortisol-binding globulin and total cortisol. *Clin Endocrinol (Oxf).* 2007;66(5):632-635.

85. Rossi E, Morabito A, Di Rella F, et al. Endocrine effects of adjuvant letrozole compared with tamoxifen in hormone-responsive postmenopausal patients with early breast cancer: the HOBOE trial. *J Clin Oncol.* 2009;27(19):3192-3197.

86. Orentreich N, Brind JL, Rizer RL, Vogelman JH. Age changes and sex differences in serum dehydroepiandrosterone sulfate concentrations throughout adulthood. *J Clin Endocrinol Metab.* 1984;59(3):551-555.

87. Crawford S, Santoro N, Laughlin GA, et al. Circulating dehydroepiandrosterone sulfate concentrations during the menopausal transition. *J Clin Endocrinol Metab.* 2009;94(8):2945-2951.

88. McConnell DS, Stanczyk FZ, Sowers MR, Randolph JF Jr, Lasley BL. Menopausal transition stage-specific changes in circulating adrenal androgens. *Menopause.* 2012;19(6):658-663.

89. Lasley BL, Crawford SL, Laughlin GA, et al. Circulating dehydroepiandrosterone sulfate levels in women who underwent bilateral salpingo-oophorectomy during the menopausal transition. *Menopause.* 2011;18(5):494-498.

90. Woods NF, Carr MC, Tao EY, Taylor HJ, Mitchell ES. Increased urinary cortisol levels during the menopausal transition. *Menopause.* 2006;13(2):212-221.

91. Cagnacci A, Cannoletta M, Caretto S, Zanin R, Xholli A, Volpe A. Increased cortisol level: a possible link between climacteric symptoms and cardiovascular risk factors. *Menopause.* 2011;18(3):273-278.

92. Gordon JL, Rubinow DR, Thurston RC, Paulson J, Schmidt PJ, Girdler SS. Cardiovascular, hemodynamic, neuroendocrine, and inflammatory markers in women with and without vasomotor symptoms. *Menopause.* 2016;23(11):1189-1198.

93. Woods NF, Cray L, Mitchell ES, Herting JR. Endocrine biomarkers and symptom clusters during the menopausal transition and early postmenopause: observations from the Seattle Midlife Women's Health Study. *Menopause.* 2014;21(6):646-652.

94. Woods NF, Mitchell ES, Smith-Dijulio K. Cortisol levels during the menopausal transition and early postmenopause: observations from the Seattle Midlife Women's Health Study. *Menopause.* 2009;16(4):708-718.

95. Pabon JE, Li X, Lei ZM, Sanfilippo JS, Yussman MA, Rao CV. Novel presence of luteinizing hormone/chorionic gonadotropin receptors in human adrenal glands. *J Clin Endocrinol Metab.* 1996;81(6):2397-2400.

96. Close CF, Mann MC, Watts JF, Taylor KG. ACTH-independent Cushing's syndrome in pregnancy with spontaneous resolution after delivery: control of the hypercortisolism with metyrapone. *Clin Endocrinol (Oxf).* 1993;39(3):375-379.

97. Kasperlik-Zaluska AA, Szczupacka I, Leszczynska-Bystrzanowska J, Drus-Przybyszewska G. Pregnancy-dependent Cushing's syndrome in three pregnancies. *BJOG.* 2000;107(6):810-812.

98. Lacroix A, Hamet P, Boutin JM. Leuprolide acetate therapy in luteinizing hormone-dependent Cushing's syndrome. *N Engl J Med.* 1999;341(21):1577-1581.

99. Saxena AR, Seely EW. Luteinizing hormone correlates with adrenal function in postmenopausal women. *Menopause.* 2012;19(11):1280-1283.

100. Alevizaki M, Saltiki K, Mantzou E, Anastasiou E, Huhtaniemi I. The adrenal gland may be a target of LH action in postmenopausal women. *Eur J Endocrinol.* 2006;154(6):875-881.

101. Wierman ME, Arlt W, Basson R, et al. Androgen therapy in women: a reappraisal: an Endocrine Society clinical practice guideline. *J Clin Endocrinol Metab.* 2014;99(10):3489-3510.

102. Alkatib AA, Cosma M, Elamin MB, et al. A systematic review and meta-analysis of randomized placebo-controlled trials of DHEA treatment effects on quality of life in women with adrenal insufficiency. *J Clin Endocrinol Metab.* 2009;94(10):3676-3681.

103. Arlt W, Callies F, van Vlijmen JC, et al. Dehydroepiandrosterone replacement in women with adrenal insufficiency. *N Engl J Med.* 1999;341(14):1013-1020.

104. Elraiyah T, Sonbol MB, Wang Z, et al. Clinical review: The benefits and harms of systemic dehydroepiandrosterone (DHEA) in postmenopausal women with normal adrenal function: a systematic review and meta-analysis. *J Clin Endocrinol Metab.* 2014;99(10):3536-3542.

105. Davis SR, Panjari M, Stanczyk FZ. Clinical review: DHEA replacement for postmenopausal women. *J Clin Endocrinol Metab.* 2011;96(6):1642-1653.

106. Seaborg E. The myth of adrenal fatigue. *Endocrine News.* September 2017. https://endocrinenews.endocrine.org/myth-adrenal-fatigue. Accessed March 19, 2019.

107. Cadegiani FA, Kater CE. Adrenal fatigue does not exist: a systematic review. *BMC Endocr Disord.* 2016;16(1):48.

108. Nelson LM. Clinical practice. Primary ovarian insufficiency. *N Engl J Med.* 2009;360(6):606-614.

109. Luborsky JL, Meyer P, Sowers MF, Gold EB, Santoro N. Premature menopause in a multi-ethnic population study of the menopause transition. *Hum Reprod.* 2003;18(1):199-206.

110. European Society for Human Reproduction and Embryology (ESHRE) Guideline Group on POI, Webber L, Davies M, et al. ESHRE guideline: management of women with premature ovarian insufficiency. *Hum Reprod.* 2016;31(5):926-937.

111. Falorni A, Brozzetti A, Aglietti MS, et al. Progressive decline of residual follicle pool after clinical diagnosis of autoimmune ovarian insufficiency. *Clin Endocrinol (Oxf).* 2012;77(3):453-458.

112. Bachelot A, Nicolas C, Bidet M, et al. Long-term outcome of ovarian function in women with intermittent premature ovarian insufficiency. *Clin Endocrinol (Oxf).* 2017;86(2):223-228.

113. van Kasteren YM, Schoemaker J. Premature ovarian failure: a systematic review on therapeutic interventions to restore ovarian function and achieve pregnancy. *Hum Reprod Update.* 1999;5(5):483-492.

114. Tucker EJ, Grover SR, Bachelot A, Touraine P, Sinclair AH. Premature ovarian insufficiency: new perspectives on genetic cause and phenotypic spectrum. *Endocrine Rev.* 2016;37(6):609-635.

115. Faubion SS, Kuhle CL, Shuster LT, Rocca WA. Long-term health consequences of premature or early menopause and considerations for management. *Climacteric.* 2015;18(4):483-491.

116. Practice Committee of American Society for Reproductive Medicine. Current evaluation of amenorrhea. *Fertil Steril.* 2008;90 (5 suppl):S219-S225.

117. Committee on Gynecologic Practice. Committee Opinion No. 698: hormone therapy in primary ovarian insufficiency. *Obstet Gynecol.* 2017;129(5):e134-e141.

118. The NAMS 2017 Hormone Therapy Position Statement Advisory Panel. The 2017 hormone therapy position statement of The North American Menopause Society. *Menopause.* 2017;24(7):728-753.

119. Aittomäki K, Lucena JL, Pakarinen P, et al. Mutation in the follicle-stimulating hormone receptor gene causes hereditary hypergonadotropic ovarian failure. *Cell.* 1995;82(6):959-968.

120. Latronico AC, Chai Y, Arnhold IJ, Liu X, Mendonca BB, Segaloff DL. A homozygous microdeletion in helix 7 of the luteinizing hormone receptor associated with familial testicular and ovarian resistance is due to both decreased cell surface expression and impaired effector activation by the cell surface receptor. *Mol Endocrinol.* 1998;12(3):442-450.

121. Vegetti W, Marozzi A, Manfredini E, et al. Premature ovarian failure. *Mol Cell Endocrinol.* 2000;161(1-2):53-57.

122. Harris SE, Chand AL, Winship IM, Gersak K, Aittomäki K, Shelling AN. Identification of novel mutations in FOXL2 associated with premature ovarian failure. *Mol Hum Reprod.* 2002;8(8):729-733.

123. Progetto Menopausa Italia Study Group. Premature ovarian failure: frequency and risk factors among women attending a network of menopause clinics in Italy. *BJOG.* 2003;110(1):59-63.

124. Rebar RW. Premature ovarian failure. *Obstet Gynecol.* 2009;113(6): 1355-1363.

125. Vearncombe KJ, Pachana NA. Is cognitive functioning detrimentally affected after early, induced menopause? *Menopause.* 2009;16(1):188-198.

126. Vujovic S. Aetiology of premature ovarian failure. *Menopause Int.* 2009;15(2):72-75.

127. Janse F, Knauff EA, Niermeijer MF, et al; Dutch Premature Ovarian Failure Consortium. Similar phenotype characteristics comparing familial and sporadic premature ovarian failure. *Menopause.* 2010;17(4):758-765.

128. Jiao X, Qin C, Li J, et al. Cytogenetic analysis of 531 Chinese women with premature ovarian failure. *Hum Reprod.* 2012;27(7):2201-2207.

129. Kalantari H, Madani T, Zari Moradi S, et al. Cytogenetic analysis of 179 Iranian women with premature ovarian failure. *Gynecol Endocrinol.* 2013;29(6):588-591.

130. Liu AX, Shi HY, Cai ZJ, et al. Increased risk of gonadal malignancy and prophylactic gonadectomy: a study of 102 phenotypic female patients with Y chromosome or Y-derived sequences. *Hum Reprod.* 2014;29(7):1413-1419.

131. Rossetti R, Ferrari I, Bonomi M, Persani L. Genetics of primary ovarian insufficiency. *Clin Genet.* 2017;91(2):183-198.

132. Morgan T. Turner syndrome: diagnosis and management. *Am Fam Physician.* 2007;76(3):405-410.

133. Bondy CA; Turner Syndrome Study Group. Care of girls and women with Turner syndrome: a guideline of the Turner Syndrome Study Group. *J Clin Endocrinol Metab.* 2007;92(1):10-25.

134. Castronovo C, Rossetti R, Rusconi D, et al. Gene dosage as a relevant mechanism contributing to the determination of ovarian function in Turner syndrome. *Hum Reprod.* 2014;29(2):368-379.

135. Trolle C, Hjerrild B, Cleemann I, Mortensen KH, Grayholt CH. Sex hormone replacement in Turners syndrome. *Endocrine.* 2012:41(2):200-219.

136. Pinsker JE. Clinical review: Turner syndrome: updating the paradigm of clinical care. *J Clin Endocrinol Metab.* 2012;97(6):E994-E1003.

137. Gravholt CH, Andersen NH, Conway GS, et al; International Turner Syndrome Consensus Group. Clinical practice guidelines for the care of girls and women with Turner syndrome: proceedings from the 2016 Cincinnati International Turner Syndrome Meeting. *Eur J Endocrinol.* 2017;177(3):G1-G70.

138. Bakalov VK, Bondy CA. Fracture risk and bone mineral density in Turner syndrome. *Rev Endocr Metab Disord.* 2008;9(2):145-151.

139. Castelo-Branco C. Management of Turner syndrome in adult life and beyond. *Maturitas.* 2014;79(4):471-475.

140. Rousseau F, Rouillard P, Morel ML, Khandjian EW, Morgan K. Prevalence of carriers of premutation-size alleles of the FMR1 gene—and implications for the population genetics of the fragile X syndrome. *Am J Hum Genet*. 1995;57(5):1006-1018.

141. Tassone F, Long KP, Tong TH, et al. FMR1 CGG allele size and prevalence ascertained through newborn screening in the United States. *Genome Med*. 2012;4(12):100.

142. Hagerman R, Hagerman P. Advances in clinical and molecular understanding of the FMR1 premutation and fragile X-associated tremor/ataxia syndrome. *Lancet Neurol*. 2013;12(8):786-796.

143. Cronister A, Schreiner R, Wittenberger M, Amiri K, Harris K, Hagerman RJ. Heterozygous fragile X female: historical, physical, cognitive, and cytogenetic features. *Am J Med Genet*. 1991;38(2-3):269-274.

144. Morrison JC, Givens JR, Wiser WL, Fish SA. Mumps oophoritis: a cause of premature menopause. *Fertil Steril*. 1975;26(7):655-659.

145. Tariq S, Anderson J, Burns F, Delpech V, Gilson R, Sabin C. The menopause transition in women living with HIV: current evidence and future avenues of research. *J Virus Erad*. 2016;2(2):114-116.

146. Matikainen T, Perez GI, Jurisicova A, et al. Aromatic hydrocarbon receptor-driven Bax gene expression is required for premature ovarian failure caused by biohazardous environmental chemicals. *Nat Genet*. 2001;28(4):355-360.

147. Pan ML, Chen LR, Tsao HM, Chen KH. Polycystic ovarian syndrome and the risk of subsequent primary ovarian insufficiency: a nationwide population-based study. *Menopause*. 2017;24(7):803-809.

148. Evans EC, Matteson KA, Orejuela FJ, et al; Society of Gynecologic Surgeons Systematic Review Group. Salpingo-oophorectomy at the time of benign hysterectomy: a systematic review. *Obstet Gynecol*. 2016;128(3):476-485.

149. Finch AP, Lubinski J, Møller P, et al. Impact of oophorectomy on cancer incidence and mortality in women with a *BRCA1* or *BRCA2* mutation. *J Clin Oncol*. 2014;32(15):1547-1553.

150. Rocca WA, Bower JH, Maraganore DM, et al. Increased risk of cognitive impairment or dementia in women who underwent oophorectomy before menopause. *Neurology*. 2007;69(11):1074-1083.

151. Noone AM, Howlader N, Krapcho M, et al, eds. *SEER Cancer Statistics Review, 1975-2015*. Bethesda, MD: National Cancer Institute; 2017. Updated September 10, 2018. https://seer.cancer.gov/csr/1975_2015/. Accessed March 19, 2019.

152. Garrido-Oyarzun MF, Castelo-Branco M. Controversies over the use of GnRH agonists for reduction of chemotherapy-induced gonadotoxicity. *Climacteric*. 2016,19(G):522 525. Accessed March 19, 2019.

153. Guida M, Castaldi MA, Rosamilio R, Giudice V, Orio F, Selleri C. Reproductive issues in patients undergoing hematopoietic stem cell transplantation: an update. *J Ovarian Res*. 2016;9(1):72.

154. Gallagher JC. Effect of early menopause on bone mineral density and fractures. *Menopause*. 2007;14(3 pt 2):567-571.

155. Kalantaridou SN, Vanderhoof VH, Calis KA, Corrigan EC, Troendle JF, Nelson LM. Sexual function in young women with spontaneous 46,XX primary ovarian insufficiency. *Fertil Steril*. 2008;90(5):1805-1811.

156. van der Stege JG, Groen H, van Zadelhoff SJ, et al. Decreased androgen concentrations and diminished general and sexual well-being in women with premature ovarian failure. *Menopause*. 2008;15(1):23-31.

157. Rebar RW, Connolly HV. Clinical features of young women with hypergonadotropic amenorrhea. *Fertil Steril*. 1990;53(5):804-810.

158. McNicholl DM, Heaney LG. The safety of bisphosphonate use in pre-menopausal women on corticosteroids. *Curr Drug Saf*. 2010;5(2):182-187.

159. Rossouw JE, Anderson GL, Prentice RL, et al; Writing Group for the Women's Health Initiative. Risks and benefits of estrogen plus progestin in healthy postmenopausal women: principal results from the Women's Health Initiative randomized controlled trial. *JAMA*. 2002;288(3):321-333.

160. Sullivan SD, Sarrel PM, Nelson LM. Hormone replacement therapy in young women with primary ovarian insufficiency and early menopause. *Fertil Steril*. 2016;106(7):1588-1599.

161. Langrish JP, Mills NL, Bath LE, et al. Cardiovascular effects of physiological and standard sex steroid replacement regimens in premature ovarian failure. *Hypertension*. 2009;53(5):805-811.

162. Crofton PM, Evans N, Bath LE, et al. Physiological versus standard sex steroid replacement in young women with premature ovarian failure: effects on bone mass acquisition and turnover. *Clin Endocrinol (Oxf)*. 2010;73(6):707-714.

163. O'Donnell RL, Warner P, Lee RJ, et al. Physiological sex steroid replacement in premature ovarian failure: randomized crossover trial of effect on uterine volume, endometrial thickness and blood flow, compared with a standard regimen. *Hum Reprod*. 2012;27(4):1130-1138.

164. Wildemeersch D. Safety and comfort of long-term continuous combined transdermal estrogen and intrauterine levonorgestrel administration for postmenopausal hormone substitution—a review. *Gynecol Endocrinol*. 2016;32(8):598-601.

165. Wu X, Cai H, Kallianpur A, et al. Impact of premature ovarian failure on mortality and morbidity among Chinese women. *PLoS One*, 2014;9(3):e89597.

166. Rocca WA, Grossardt BR, de Andrade M, Malkasian GD, Melton LJ 3rd. Survival patterns after oophorectomy in premenopausal women: a population-based cohort study. *Lancet Oncol*. 2006;7(10):821-828.

167. Parker WH, Fesjabuch D, Broder MS, et al. Long-term mortality associated with oophorectomy compared with ovarian conservation in the Nurses' Health Study. *Obstet Gynecol*. 2013;121(4):709-716.

168. Liao KL, Wood N, Conway GS. Premature menopause and psychological well-being. *J Psychosom Obstet Gynaecol*. 2000;21(3):167-174.

169. Nathorst-Böös J, von Schoultz B, Carlstrom K. Elective ovarian removal and estrogen replacement therapy—effects on sexual life, psychological well-being and androgen status. *J Psychosom Obstet Gynaecol*. 1993;14(4):283-293.

170. Schmidt PJ, Luff JA, Haq NA, et al. Depression in women with spontaneous 46, XX primary ovarian insufficiency. *J Clin Endocrinol Metab*. 2011;96(2):E278-E287.

171. Mann E, Singer D, Pitkin J, Panay N, Hunter MS. Psychosocial adjustment in women with premature menopause: a cross-sectional survey. *Climacteric*. 2012;15(5):481-489.

172. Rocca WA, Grossardt BR, Geda YE, et al. Long-term risk of depressive and anxiety symptoms after early bilateral oophorectomy. *Menopause*. 2008;15(6):1050-1059.

173. Rocca WA, Gazzuola-Rocca L, Smith CY, et al. Accelerated accumulation of multimorbidity after bilateral oophorectomy: a population-based cohort study. *Mayo Clinic Proc*. 2016;91(11):1577-1589.

Midlife and Aging-Related Body Changes

Vulvovaginal Changes

To understand the changes to the vulva and vagina during menopause, it is important to review the relevant anatomy and histology, because these features of the vagina and vulva are what make them uniquely sensitive to the physiologic changes of menopause. Although vulvovaginal changes during menopause universally occur, not all women become symptomatic or require clinical intervention.

The vagina, which is of müllerian origin,[1-3] is composed of an adventitial layer of connective tissue, then smooth muscle; the inner lumen is made up of a lamina propria underlying the nonkeratinized stratified squamous epithelium. The epithelial layer is hormone sensitive and made up of a basal layer of cells, a parabasal and glycogen-containing layer, and a superficial layer. Although the vulva is nonkeratinized, the labia minora do contain sweat and sebaceous glands, unlike the vagina. Bartholin glands are tubuloalveolar glands, and their excretory ducts are lined by transitional-type epithelium.

The role of hormones and the vulva and vagina

Historically, the hormone focus regarding vulvar and vaginal health has been on the degree of estrogenic stimulation. It is well established that there are receptors for estrogen throughout the vagina, vulva, urethra, and even in the trigone of the bladder.[4-7] The roles of estrogen are numerous, including maintaining blood flow to the vulvovaginal tissue, the collagen within the epithelium, and the hyaluronic acid and mucopolysaccharides within the moistened epithelial surfaces. Estrogen also plays a role in supporting the microbiome and protecting the tissue from pathogens.[5,6,8]

One of the unique features of the vagina is its acidity (average pH, 4.5), which is maintained by the presence of lactobacilli that convert glucose into lactic acid.[9] It should be noted that although a predominance of lactobacillus usually indicates a lower vaginal pH and low Nugent score, not all types of lactobacillus are equally effective at lowering vaginal pH. As well, the Nugent score becomes higher in vaginal microbiomes communities that are made up of more anaerobes. The glycogen in the epithelial layer is important for maintaining vaginal health by providing the substrate for the lactobacilli to produce lactic acid. This feature is thought to be specific to the human vagina because most other mammals have much higher vaginal pH values.

Although estrogen is important in maintaining vulvovaginal health, there are emerging data that androgens also have a role. All three layers of the vagina have been shown to have androgen receptors (ARs); in addition, androgens have been shown in animal studies to stimulate nerve fibers as well as mucification of the epithelium.[5]

The role of the microbiome in the vulva and vagina

Bacteria, especially *Lactobacillus*, have long been known to play a role in maintaining vaginal health. Although there are numerous types of bacteria, lactobacilli appear to play a key role in that they form *community state types* within the vagina. Community state types are characterized by the proportion of different lactobacilli as well as by other less common organisms.[10]

Although lactobacilli are key, one well-described community state type shows fewer lactobacilli and a predominance of other, anaerobic organisms, including *Mobiluncus* and *Atopobium vaginae*.[10] There have been community state types described that have focused on different *Gardnerella* subtypes as well.[11] These community state types appear to be reflective of vaginal health.

Within vaginal secretions are lymphocytes, neutrophils, macrophages, and Langerhans cells, all of which are known to play a role in preventing infection in the human body.[12] Studies have shown that there is a change in the presence of these inflammatory cells during the menstrual cycle and that the lymphocytic population is highly sensitive to vaginal pH.

What are the vulvovaginal changes that occur during menopause?

Menopause is a physiologic transition in women that leads to a drop in ovarian steroid hormone production because of oocyte depletion. Women also can undergo medical or surgical menopause, which leads to a much more abrupt change in hormone levels. With menopause as well as with aging, there is a decrease in levels of estrogen and dehydroepiandrosterone.

Given the role of estrogen and dehydroepiandrosterone on the maintenance of vaginal epithelial tissue, there is a thinning of the most superficial layer in women with menopause and aging.[13] This thinning is exacerbated by a subsequent loss in elasticity, and one of the usual manifestations noted on pelvic exam is the loss or absence of rugae. These hormone changes may lead to an overall narrowing of the vaginal canal and poor distention. For some women, pain with any form of vaginal penetration occurs because of these changes. The *genitourinary syndrome of menopause* refers to the genital and urinary symptoms that women may experience with the gonadal hormone decline that accompanies menopause. (See also "Genitourinary Syndrome of Menopause" in Chapter 4.)

There also are changes that occur to the epithelial layers of the vulva. Although the vulva doesn't have the same muscular and connective tissue layers or elasticity compared with the vagina, the epithelial layers are rich in hormone receptors (HRs), thus the thinning of vulvar tissue can lead to clinical effects on not only the external genitalia but also on the urethra and bladder, given the similar anatomic histology and sensitivity to hormones.[14]

The decrease in the glycogen content of the hormonally deprived epithelium causes a decrease in the substrate used to support the vaginal lactobacilli. This in turn leads to a decreased amount of lactic acid and thus an increase in the vaginal pH routinely seen in menopause.[15] The higher pH predisposes the vagina to an increase in lymphocytes and plasma cells that may translate into unwanted vaginal discharge.[8] There also is a decrease in physiologic vaginal secretions. The underlying mechanism may be decreased gene expression of the extracellular vaginal matrix in postmenopausal women.[7]

The urinary tract, especially the urethra and bladder, also have HRs. As the vagina narrows, the urethra moves closer to the introitus. Vaginal atrophy is associated with higher rates of urinary tract infections, frequency, urgency, and dysuria because of these changes.[16] Some data have shown that local vaginal estrogen but not systemic estrogen appears to improve urinary stress incontinence.[17] (See also "Urinary Incontinence" and "Other Urinary Tract Symptoms" in Chapter 4.) Additionally, there is evidence that shows a role for HRs in the muscles of the pelvic floor, which may explain increased pelvic organ prolapse in menopause. (See also "Pelvic Pain" in Chapter 5.) Some data suggest that local estrogen treatment may be effective in preventing prolapse.[18]

The changes to the vulvovaginal tissue that occur during menopause are part of a complex interplay among steroid hormones, cellular properties, and the microbiome.[8] The more that is understood about the important and unique properties of the vagina and how it changes during menopause, the more some of the common medical conditions that are a result of changes in vulvovaginal health during menopause can be managed for women who are symptomatic.

Body Weight

Obesity in the United States disproportionately affects women. The 2013-2014 US age-adjusted prevalence of obesity (body mass index [BMI] $\geq$30 kg/m^2) was 40.4% in women compared with 35% in men. There has been continued increasing prevalence in women, but not men, over the decade between 2005 and 2014.[19] Prevalence of severe obesity (BMI $\geq$40 kg/m^2) is nearly double in women (9.9%) compared with men (5.5%) and continues to increase. Prevalence of abdominal (or central) obesity, which is more consistently associated with obesity-related comorbidities than is BMI, has increased even more significantly and much more strongly affects women. Abdominal obesity prevalence in women from 2011 to 2012 was 64.7% compared with 43.5% in men, increasing from 55.4% in women and 37.1% in men from 1999 to 2000.[20]

Weight gain and menopause

Many women gain weight during the menopause transition.[21] It is not yet entirely clear what is responsible for this weight gain. In most cases, it is unlikely that menopause itself or the use of hormone therapy (HT) is directly responsible.[22,23] Weight gain during the menopause transition seems to be related mostly to aging and lifestyle. Lean body mass decreases with age, which is compounded by increasingly sedentary lifestyles as most women age. Less energy expenditure via decreased intentional and spontaneous physical activity tends to increase fat mass and weight gain in older women.[24] Menopause symptoms may affect weight indirectly, such as with disturbed sleep patterns secondary to vasomotor symptoms (VMS) and mood changes, which can interfere with healthy lifestyle habits and weight-management behaviors.[25]

Body composition and fat distribution change significantly during menopause. Women are significantly more likely to experience increased abdominal and visceral fat during the menopause transition. Postmenopausal women may be less likely to lose visceral fat during intentional weight reduction compared with premenopausal women.[26,27] Several studies have shown that menopause is associated with increased fat in the abdominal region as well as decreased lean body mass, independent of age.[28]

The change in distribution of fat from subcutaneous stores to visceral abdominal fat may have detrimental metabolic effects. Increased trunk-mass-to-leg-fat-mass ratio has been associated with increases in blood pressure, fasting glucose, and abnormal lipoprotein profiles.[29] Women who have obesity with increased visceral adipose tissue stores compared with subcutaneous abdominal adipose tissue are more likely to have obesity-related cardiometabolic conditions, including type 2 diabetes mellitus (DM), metabolic syndrome, hepatic steatosis, and aortic plaque.[30]

The effects of HT on weight are conflicting.[31,32] In the Postmenopausal Estrogen/Progestin Interventions trial (N=847 aged 45-64 y), women using estrogen with or without progestogen weighed, on average, 2.2 lb (1 kg) less than placebo recipients at the end of the 3-year trial.[33] No difference in weight was noted between the groups using estrogen therapy (ET) or estrogen-progestogen therapy (EPT). In the Women's Health Initiative (WHI) trial of 10,739 postmenopausal women aged 50 to 79 years randomized to conjugated equine estrogens (CEE) 0.625 mg daily or placebo, BMI had increased 0.5 kg/m^2 in both groups by the 6-year follow-up.[34] Waist circumference increased 1.4 cm in the CEE group and 1.9 cm in the placebo group, not statistically significant.

Risks of overweight

Regardless of sex, higher levels of body weight and body fat are associated with increased risk for numerous adverse health consequences such as cardiovascular disease (CVD), type 2 DM, hypertension, several cancers, osteoarthritis, and premature mortality.[35,36] Postmenopausal women

who have obesity have a higher rate of breast cancer than postmenopausal women of normal weight.[37,38]

Elevated BMI and adiposity are also associated with more frequent or severe VMS.[39-41] Weight gain over midlife may increase the likelihood of reporting VMS. However, this association appears to reverse as women transition through the menopause, with indication that higher BMI or adiposity is associated with fewer VMS when women are postmenopausal.[42-44]

This reversal of the relation between adiposity and VMS, depending on menopause stage, parallels those for the relation between BMI and estradiol: premenopausal and perimenopausal women who are obese have lower estradiol levels than women who are not obese, but postmenopausal women who are obese have the highest estradiol levels compared with women who are not obese.[45,46]

There is a lack of well-designed randomized trials to test the effect of weight loss or dietary changes on VMS, but there is some indication that weight loss in women who have excess weight and/or a reduced-fat diet with increased intake of fruit, vegetables, and whole grains may improve the occurrence of VMS,[47,48] particularly for women earlier in the menopause transition. However, fully powered trials designed to test weight loss for VMS reduction are needed to conclusively address the effect of weight loss on VMS.

Underweight can also be a health concern. In addition to psychosocial concerns, such as eating disorders and body image dysmorphia, in some cases overdieting or excessive weight loss in premenopausal women leads to temporary cessation of menstrual cycles and consequently an increased risk for osteoporosis later in life.[49]

Optimization of body weight

Managing weight in perimenopausal and postmenopausal women is essential. The advice to eat a healthy diet, increase physical activity, and minimize weight gain is appropriate for almost all women at or above a healthy weight. For women with excess weight, weight loss is generally indicated. Moderate weight loss often leads to significant health improvements. As little as a 3% sustained body weight loss improves glycemic control and triglycerides and decreases risk for type 2 DM.[50] Weight loss of 5% to 10% further reduces hyperglycemia and triglycerides; improves blood pressure, low-density and high-density lipoprotein cholesterol ranges, and liver function and fatty liver disease; reduces functional limitations and chronic pain; and decreases the need for hypertension, type 2 DM, and lipid medications in many women.[50-52]

25

The Diabetes Prevention Program demonstrated that moderate lifestyle intervention that led to 7% weight loss over 6 months, with about half this weight loss being maintained more than 4 years, led to a 58% decreased progression to type 2 DM.[53] For every kilogram of weight loss, there was a 16% reduced risk of developing type 2 DM.[54] Moreover, a reduced risk for type 2 DM was maintained for more than a decade, despite much of the weight being regained over time.[55]

The US Preventive Services Task Force recommends that clinicians offer comprehensive lifestyle interventions to all women with obesity.[56,57] Joint guidelines issued by the American College of Cardiology, the American Heart Association, and the Obesity Society recommend programs led by trained interventionists that provide at least 14 sessions over 6 months.[52] The American Diabetes Association recommends at least 16 sessions over 6 months for women with excess weight and type 2 DM.[58] Additional participation in a comprehensive weight-loss maintenance program or ongoing counseling is recommended in order to minimize weight regain.[52]

Behavior therapy for weight management

Several counseling strategies are valuable for guiding women to manage weight. Motivational interviewing can improve behavior counseling in women who are ambivalent about behavior change and has been shown to improve weight-loss outcomes.[59-61] This technique is a collaborative, client-centered process that focuses on assisting and guiding women to build motivation and supports personalized problem-solving to achieve behavior change and weight loss. The "5 As" framework for behavior change (Table 1),[62] initially developed for smoking-cessation counseling, has been adapted for behavior therapy for obesity, in which healthcare professionals provide brief counseling and arrange additional care as needed. Components of behavior therapy for obesity and weight loss include goal setting, self-monitoring, addressing barriers, problem-solving, positive reinforcement, and ongoing support.

The primary target for behavior change is to create an energy deficit by addressing caloric intake and energy expenditure.[52] A caloric reduction of 500 to 750 calories per day is estimated to lead to weight loss of 1 to 1.5 lb per week in the short term, with the rate of weight loss decreasing asymptotically over time.[63] This typically translates to a rule-of-thumb caloric intake goal of 1,200 to 1,500 calories per day for most women.

Clinically meaningful weight loss can occur across a broad range of macronutrient compositions.[52] For example, in a study that examined four diets that varied in fat

Table 1. The "5 As" Framework for Behavior Change

- **Assess.** Measurement of BMI, identification of comorbid conditions known to interfere with weight loss (depression, sleep disorders, chronic pain, stress, binge eating), and discussion about readiness for change.

- **Advise.** Counseling about the benefits of weight loss and behavior changes.

- **Agree.** Establish weight-loss goals that are specific, measurable, attainable, relevant, and time based. Establishing attainable weight-loss goals is important because women often expect to lose far more weight than is reasonable. Self-monitoring of weight, nutrition, and/ or physical activity is a key part of maintaining positive behavior changes.

- **Assist.** A problem-solving process in which barriers to achieving weight loss are identified and resolved. Identifying the underlying causes of, and contributors to, weight problems in individual women can help them achieve weight loss.

- **Arrange.** On the basis of an assessment of a woman's progress, women may be referred to more intensive or specialized treatment. Referral options include dietitians, hospital-based programs, behavior-medicine providers, and evidenced-based commercial weight loss programs.

Abbreviation: BMI, body mass index.
Fitzpatrick SL, et al.[62]

content (20-40%), protein (15-25%), and carbohydrates (35-65%), there was similar weight loss and no difference in hunger or satiety ratings among the interventions over 2 years.[64] Thus, a key factor of diet choice is patient preference. However, there is a wide interindividual variation in weight loss between groups, and there is mounting evidence that certain physiologic factors affect responsiveness to different dietary patterns. For example, women with insulin resistance tend to respond better to either lower carbohydrate or lower glycemic-index dietary patterns compared with women with normal insulin sensitivity.[65-67] Additionally, some studies suggest that slightly elevated protein intake results in greater reduction in weight, fat mass, and triglyceride levels.[68] A higher-protein diet also was shown to improve weight loss as well as total body fat reduction compared with a high-fiber diet in women who were overweight and obese.[69]

Regular exercise is particularly valuable to help minimize weight gain in midlife women. Aerobic and resistance exercises are both beneficial, and resistance-type exercise, such as strength training exercises, may be particularly helpful to improve lean body mass and body fat.[70] In a randomized study of 107 postmenopausal women, resistance exercise plus calorie restriction resulted in greater losses in fat-mass parameters than did calorie restriction alone.[71] To address energy expenditure, aerobic physical activity on par with at least 30 minutes of brisk walking on most days of the week (≥150 min/wk) is recommended to help achieve an energy deficit.[52] Higher levels of activity (200-300 min/wk) are recommended over the long term in order to prevent weight regain. Strength and resistance training stimulate muscle production and may improve osteopenia.[72] Finding exercises that fit individual limitations, abilities, and preferences and/or supervision by an experienced fitness instructor with a prescribed exercise program can help improve adherence.

Commercial weight-loss programs that have evidence to support their efficacy and safety are an option to provide a comprehensive lifestyle program. However, the amount of weight loss women can expect to achieve with these programs is likely less than they expect.[73] A meta-analysis of 13 randomized, controlled trials (RCTs) of commercial weight-loss programs found that among the most popular programs, weight loss at 1 year ranged from 2.6% for Weight Watchers to 4.9% for Jenny Craig compared with controls. Few commercial programs had long-term data available.

Very-low-calorie diets (variably defined as 800 to <1,000 kcal/d) are viable options in some women but should be provided only within the context of a high-intensity lifestyle intervention and close medical monitoring.[52] Women should be supervised by trained practitioners in a medical-care setting, because rapid weight loss has the potential for medical complications such as gallstones and electrolyte disturbances. Total meal replacement with a very-low-calorie diet over 3 months has the potential to achieve 10% to 15% weight loss,[74] but it may result in substantial weight regain, especially in the absence of a maintenance program.[52,58]

Of particular significance to the population of perimenopausal and postmenopausal women are strategies to prevent CVD, which is the leading cause of death for North American women. General diet and lifestyle recommendations from the American Heart Association (Table 2),[75] if rigorously applied with other lifestyle recommendations, will significantly decrease the risk for CVD and noncardiac disease as well.[75-77]

Obesity and sleep

Inadequate or disordered sleep is associated with obesity and weight gain. Poor sleep leads to a range of appetitive,

---

Table 2. General Diet and Lifestyle Recommendations From the American Heart Association

- Maintain a healthy body weight.
- Consume a diet rich in vegetables and fruits. Whole fruit is preferred over fruit juice because it contains more fiber and is digested slower.
- Choose whole-grain, high-fiber foods.
- Consume fish, especially oily fish, at least twice a week.
- Limit intake of saturated and *trans* fat.
- Minimize intake of sugar-sweetened beverages. Evidence suggests that calories consumed as liquids have less satiety than those from solid foods.
- Choose and prepare foods with less salt. Reduced sodium intake can prevent hypertension, act as an adjunct to antihypertensive medication, and facilitate hypertension control.
- Consume alcohol in moderation. Alcohol can be addictive, and high intake has been associated with serious health and social consequences. The American Cancer Society recommends that women limit alcohol intake to no more than one drink per day.
- Minimize eating foods prepared outside the home if you are not provided an ingredients list. Many restaurants today note ingredients and calories. Foods prepared outside the home or take-out foods generally tend to come in large portions, have high-energy density, and are often also high in saturated fat, *trans* fat, cholesterol, added sugars, and sodium and low in fiber and micronutrients.

American Heart Association Nutrition Committee, et al.[75]

---

immune, stress, and inflammatory mediators that may contribute to weight gain.[78] Sleep deprivation is associated with increased cortisol, lower thyrotropin, lower leptin, reduced glucose tolerance and insulin sensitivity, and decreased energy expenditure.[79-81] A 2006 study reported an association between reduced sleep and increased weight gain in more than 68,000 women followed in the Nurses' Health Study (median follow-up, 12 y). Investigators found that women who slept 5 hours or fewer gained 2.5 lb (1.14 kg) more than those sleeping 7 hours. Women sleeping 6 hours gained 1.6 lb (0.71 kg) more than those sleeping 7 hours.[82] Of note, VMS may cause poor or fragmented sleep, which may then affect risk for weight gain. (See also "Sleep Disturbance" in Chapter 5.)

Pharmacologic interventions

Pharmacotherapy is indicated as an adjunct to behavior counseling in women with a BMI of 30 kg/m^2 or higher

CHAPTER 2

and those with a BMI of 27 kg/m² or higher with at least one obesity-related comorbidity (eg, type 2 DM, hypertension, hyperlipidemia).[51] Similar to treatments for other behavior-related health conditions such as pharmacotherapy for hypertension or type 2 DM, the benefits of medication are most often lost if the treatment is discontinued. Thus, women who respond to treatment, which is often defined as at least a 5% weight loss after 3 months of treatment, should continue the medication, with goals of continuous weight loss and maintenance of lost weight. In those who respond to treatment, average weight loss with long-term medications range from 5% to 15%, depending on the medication and population studied. All obesity medications are contraindicated in pregnancy.

Phentermine and diethylpropion are sympathomimetic drugs that work as appetite suppressants. Because of the abuse potential associated with these medications, they are approved only for short-term use.

Orlistat is a pancreatic lipase inhibitor that decreases the absorption of ingested fat. In one trial, orlistat plus behavior counseling led to an approximately 10% body weight loss over 1 year, with most of this weight kept off for more than 4 years.[83] In 3,305 participants randomized to orlistat or placebo, far more participants in the orlistat group completed the trial (52%) compared with the placebo group (34%), and weight loss in the orlistat group at year 1 (10.6 kg) and year 4 (5.8 kg) significantly exceeded placebo (6.2 kg and 3.0 kg, respectively). Far more participants who took orlistat lost at least 5% of their body weight at both 1 year (72.8% vs 45.1%) and 4 years (52.8% vs 37.3%) of treatment. Risk of progression to type 2 DM was reduced by 45% in participants with baseline impaired glucose tolerance and 37% overall in the orlistat group compared with the placebo group. The most common adverse events (AEs) are gastrointestinal (GI) related, including diarrhea and flatulence, when consuming large amounts of fat while taking the medication.[84] Because orlistat binds to fat-soluble vitamins, women are at risk for deficiencies; thus, they should be advised on a nutritionally balanced, reduced-fat, reduced-calorie diet, and they should take a multivitamin that contains fat-soluble vitamins separately from the medication.

Lorcaserin is a selective serotonin 2c receptor agonist that stimulates the serotonin 2c receptors in the appetite center of the brain. Treatment with lorcaserin leads to an approximately nearly 7% body weight loss, on average, in women completing 1 year of treatment, with far more women achieving clinically meaningful weight loss compared with placebo (66.4% vs 32.1% lost ≥5% body weight; 36.2% vs 13.6% lost ≥10% body weight).[85]

Several intermediate cardiovascular risk factors, including blood pressure, heart rate, lipids, and glycemic control, improve with the weight loss. Patients with type 2 DM had 0.9% glycated hemoglobin improvement, which is more than expected from moderate weight loss alone and on par with many type 2 DM medications.[86]

Lorcaserin is classified as a schedule IV substance. Dosing is either 10 mg twice daily or 20 mg extended release (ER) once daily.[87] The most common AEs are headache, dizziness, fatigue, nausea, dry mouth, and constipation. Caution is necessary if women are being treated with serotonergic or antidopaminergic medications, which can rarely precipitate serotonin syndrome or neuroleptic malignant syndrome. Other warnings include caution in women with valvular heart disease, congestive heart failure, or psychiatric disorders and those at risk for priapism.

Phentermine-topiramate ER takes advantage of the additive weight-loss effects of these two agents. Phentermine, a sympathomimetic amine, decreases appetite and leads to short-term weight loss. Topiramate, which has multiple mechanisms of action, is approved for migraine and seizure prevention. On average, topiramate leads to relatively little weight loss by itself. Together, however, these medications lead to impressive weight loss at low doses. In the SEQUEL trial, a 2-year evaluation of phentermine-topiramate ER versus placebo, participants treated with the medication lost approximately 10% of body weight, on average, compared with less than 2% weight loss in the placebo group.[88] Participants treated with the medication also had improved cardiometabolic markers, including reduced blood pressure and lipids, and progression to type 2 DM was reduced by 76% compared with placebo in participants treated with the top dose of the medication. The most common AEs are paresthesia, dizziness, dysgeusia, insomnia, constipation, and dry mouth.

Phentermine-topiramate ER is classified as a schedule IV substance. Because topiramate is a known teratogen (which can cause cleft lip or palate), pregnancy should be ruled out before starting the medication, and women of childbearing age should use contraception and have monthly pregnancy testing during use.[89]

Naltrexone-bupropion sustained-release (SR) leads to much greater weight loss than either agent alone. Bupropion, a dopamine and norepinephrine reuptake inhibitor, has been approved by FDA for depression and smoking cessation. Naltrexone, an opioid-receptor antagonist, has long been used for the treatment of addictions. In clinical trials, weight loss in participants who completed

1 year of treatment with naltrexone-bupropion SR was approximately 8.2% of baseline body weight compared with 1.4% with placebo, and when combined with intensive lifestyle intervention, naltrexone-bupropion SR use led to a 12% weight loss compared with 7% weight loss in the counseling plus placebo group.[90,91] Measures of food cravings also were improved across the clinical trials, which may be related to the effects of naltrexone and/or bupropion in the mesocorticolimbic dopamine system and other brain areas related to reward-driven behaviors.[92] The most common AEs are nausea, constipation, diarrhea, headache, and vomiting. Contraindications include uncontrolled hypertension, seizure disorders, chronic opioid pain medication use, and monoamine oxidase inhibitor use.[93]

Liraglutide 3.0 mg, a glucagon-like peptide 1 receptor agonist previously FDA approved at 1.8 mg for diabetes treatment, also is approved for chronic weight management. Unlike other medications, liraglutide requires injectable administration through a small needle delivered subcutaneously to the abdomen, arm, or thigh. In one trial, treatment with liraglutide 3.0 mg led to approximately 9% weight loss compared with 3% with placebo in participants completing 1 year of treatment.[94] Nearly two-thirds of participants treated with liraglutide 3.0 mg lost at least 5% of initial body weight compared with less than one-third in the placebo group. In participants with prediabetes at baseline, 71% treated with liraglutide no longer had prediabetes at the end of year 1 compared with 39% in the placebo group.[95] At 3 years out, there was nearly an 80% decreased progression to type 2 DM compared with placebo. The most common AEs include nausea and GI complaints.[96] Hypoglycemia also may occur, particularly in women on antidiabetic medications, and may be severe in women concomitantly treated with sulfonylureas or insulin. This medication should not be used in women with a history of medullary thyroid carcinoma, multiple endocrine neoplasia type 2, or acute pancreatitis. (See also "Metabolic Syndrome, Prediabetes, and Diabetes" in Chapter 8.)

Bariatric surgery

Several bariatric surgical procedures are used for the treatment of severe obesity. Bariatric surgery is indicated for women with a BMI of 40 kg/m^2 or higher or for women with a BMI of 35 kg/m^2 or higher with at least one obesity-related comorbidity who have failed conservative treatment.[52] The most common bariatric surgeries are vertical sleeve gastrectomy and Roux-en-Y gastric bypass. Laparoscopic gastric banding is no longer commonly used because of poor long-term outcomes. Long-term data on bariatric surgery are impressive, with average 2-year weight losses of 25% and 32% of body weight for vertical sleeve gastrectomy and Roux-en-Y gastric bypass, respectively.[97] Additionally, most women show improvement or resolution in numerous comorbid conditions, including type 2 DM, hypertension, obstructive sleep apnea, and hyperlipidemia, and several studies have shown long-term mortality improvements.[97,98] Perioperative complications with bariatric surgeries in experienced surgical teams have declined and are similar to those seen with other common abdominal surgeries.[99]

Skin Changes

For both women and men, their genetic makeup (intrinsic aging) combined with environmental and lifestyle choices (extrinsic aging) influence the clinical changes in the largest organ in one's body, the skin.

Ultraviolet (UV) exposure, smoking, pollution, poor diet, sleep deprivation, and anything else that increases free-radical production are examples of extrinsic aging. For women, the precipitous decline in beta-estradiol released from the ovaries is the single most important endogenous factor influencing cutaneous changes during menopause. Decreases in progesterone play a lesser role. A drop in pituitary growth hormone that promotes cellular division and regeneration by direct binding to growth HRs or indirectly via hepatic insulin-like growth factor 1 production also have a minor influence on skin degeneration during this critical time.[100]

All these factors contribute to adverse skin changes, with the face being the most obvious area of the body for which menopausal women often seek medical advice. Facial aging, overall, is caused by changes in various tissue layers, including the skin (epidermis and dermis), subcutaneous fat, muscle, and bone.[101] Fluctuations in one tissue layer affects the others, making visible aging a dynamic and complex process.

Estrogen influence on cellular metabolism and clinical effect

Collagen provides the infrastructure for elastin, hyaluronic acid, and other glycosaminoglycans that primarily make up the extracellular dermal matrix. There are estrogen receptors (ERs) on cellular components in the dermis.[102] As menopause approaches and estrogen levels fall, there is a resultant significant decrease in fibroblast activity, and less collagen is produced (Table 3).[103] Additionally, there is increased breakdown of existing collagen via collagen metabolism enzymes (matrix metalloproteinases and collagenase). The end result is decreased production and increased degradation.

Dermal thinning from collagen loss reduces the skin's ability to retain elasticity (from elastin) and moisture (from glycosaminoglycans and hyaluronic acid). Glycosaminoglycan production decreases with menopause, and existing elastin fibers become thick and clumpy with a decreased capacity to stretch. The net effect is formation of lines and wrinkles and skin laxity.

A second important effect of glycosaminoglycans and hyaluronic acid in the dermal extracellular matrix are their humectant qualities. This is an affinity to bind with water. Its abundance in youth keeps the skin looking moist and hydrated.

With aging, the culmination of these factors causes a significant increase in transepidermal water loss. Lack of estrogen also causes a decrease in sebum production. The combination of these two effects leads to skin-barrier disruption and dryness of the skin.

Estrogens also influence the dermal vascular system. The drop in estradiol reduces blood flow and decreases angiogenesis. This decrease in oxygenation to the capillaries of the stratum spinosum and basal-cell layer of the epidermis contributes to epidermal thinning and a decreased cell turnover rate via effects on the keratinocyte.

Additionally, loss of estrogen decreases cellular growth factors and repair enzymes, causing increased skin fragility, easy bruising, and impaired wound healing.

Finally, the maintenance of melanocytes (cells that manufacture the pigment melanin) is under the control of estrogens. Estrogen exerts a regulatory effect on the production of melanin when young skin is exposed to UV light. As menopause ensues, this regulation dwindles, and melanocyte activity increases on UV light-exposed skin, causing blotchiness and dyschromia.[104]

Changes in cutaneous support structures (fat and bone)

A youthful appearance greatly depends on having the correct amount of facial fat in the right anatomical compartments. The "triangle of youth" inverts with age as significant shifts occur in deeper structures during menopause. In youth, the two points of the triangle base lie across the upper face with full cheekbones, and the pointy apex is by the chin. As we age, the fullness shifts toward the bottom of the face, and the cheekbone area becomes hollow. Hence, the pointy apex inverts to the top of the face between the eyebrows, and the "heavier" base sits by the sagging lower face because of the changes. Redistribution, accumulation, and atrophy of fat lead to facial volume loss.[105] The forehead and cheek area lose fat with age, whereas the mouth and jaw regions gain fat. Additionally, the areas of fat tend to become further apart. Instead of a smooth, almost contiguous layer, the fat pads pull away from each other and tend to appear as separate structures.[106] These fat-pad modifications lead to contour deformities and centrofacial hollowing.

There also is a significant loss of facial bone with age. Skeletal aging of the face can be caused by the changes in

Table 3. Estrogen Drop Effects on Skin During Menopause	
Cause	**Effect**
Decreased fibroblast activity/collagen loss	Lines and wrinkles, volume loss
Disrupted elastin	Skin less elastic "stretched out rubber band"
Decreased GAG production	Skin less hydrated and plump "grape to raisin"
Disruption of melanocyte regulation	Blotchiness and dyschromia on sun-exposed areas
Decreased blood flow and cellular oxygenation effects on keratinocyte	Epidermal thinning ("thin skin"), easy bruising, increased visibility of veins and bony landmarks
Disruption of cellular growth factors and repair enzymes	Increased skin fragility and impaired wound healing
Accelerated lipoatrophy	Facial hollowing
Fat pad modification	Contour deformities
Bone resorption	Eyelid sagging/hooding, jowling, folds, and shadow creation

Abbreviation: GAG, glycosaminoglycan.
Wilkinson HN, et al.[103]

the relative dynamics of bone expansion and resorption. Bone resorption leads to biometric volume loss.[106] Without the structural support of bone, there are noticeable changes in the layers of overlying soft tissue and skin.

Estrogen depletion influences bone resorption. Contraction of periorbital bone leads to eyelid hooding and increased visibility of infraorbital fat pads as they lose their bony malar support. Similarly, centromaxillary resorption leads to the development of deepened nasolabial folds, and shortening of the bony mandible leads to the appearance of jowls because the loss of structural support causes the redundant skin to hang over itself, creating a fold. Last, perioral bone loss causes the upper lip to elongate and get flatter. With less support from the underlying ostium, the skin droops, and the distance between the nasal tip and the upper lip increases.

Universal recommendations, practical advice, cosmetic interventions

Proper ultraviolet light protection or avoidance

The single best way to maintain healthy skin is to block harmful UV rays. Ultraviolet B (UVB) rays (290-320 nm) cause sunburn. Sunburn is an example of oxidative stress on the skin, leading to free-radical production and cellular apoptosis (cell death), primarily on the keratinocyte. Longer ultraviolet A (UVA) rays (320-400 nm) are the primary contributors to aged-looking skin, melanocyte effects, and the cellular damage that serves as a precursor to cell signaling, causing carcinogenesis. Long-term UV light exposure causes cumulative negative effects on the appearance of one's skin. Lines, wrinkles, rough texture, and brown spots are all a result of cumulative UV damage. In susceptible women, it is also the leading cause of nonmelanoma skin cancer, primarily basal-cell and squamous-cell carcinoma. Both benign (seborrheic keratosis, angiomas, solar lentigo) and malignant (basal-cell carcinoma, squamous-cell carcinoma, malignant melanoma) effects develop more frequently in the typical age bracket of someone in menopause.

A common complaint at an office visit will be the development of new "growths" on the face and body, especially the upper body. A tan, warty papule could clinically resemble a benign seborrheic keratosis, but on a sundamaged area also could (rarely) be a verrucous squamous-cell carcinoma. Similarly, a smooth, pink papule on the face or nose is usually a benign angiofibroma/flat wart but also can rarely be a basal-cell carcinoma, especially if there is a telangiectasia within the papule or it appears pearly. Solar lentigos can occasionally be asymmetric and multicolored, heightening a suspicion for a superficial spreading melanoma or a lentigo maligna melanoma. If there are any clinical questions differentiating benign from malignant growths, a referral to a dermatologist or a small shave biopsy is warranted.

Use of sunscreen

Ultraviolet exposure and proper sunscreen use should be discussed at every well-woman visit. For prevention of skin cancer, as well as hindering skin aging and photodamage, every woman should consider applying a physical-based sunblock every day throughout the year. Ultraviolet A rays stay constant throughout the seasons and can penetrate window glass. Chemical-based sun blocks are effective UVB blockers but are fairly ineffective blocking UVA. Unfortunately, American standards of sun protection factor (SPF) only measure UVB. Once an SPF of 30 is attained, 95% of UVB is blocked. This is the reason a woman who uses an SPF 80 may still get a suntan. The US chemical-based sun blocks (which absorb UV rays) do not filter UVA rays effectively, regardless of SPF number. Zinc or titanium oxide are the most effective physical-based sun blocks (which scatter or reflect UV rays) available in the United States. Many companies have micronized the particles and have added a subtle tint so that a 16% concentration goes on more like a makeup primer than a thick paste.

Reapplying every 2 to 3 hours during outdoor activities also is essential. Other advancements in solar protection include more fashionable broad-brimmed hats and UV protection factor clothing. Sun avoidance during the peak hours of 11 AM to 3 PM also is advisable.

Diet and smoking

Not only is counseling regarding a healthy diet and healthy lifestyle good for overall health, but the benefits may extend to a healthier skin as well. The benefits of a healthy diet in type 2 DM management and improved cardiovascular effects have been recognized for decades. Similarly, avoidance of smoking is beneficial, especially for pulmonary health. Benefits may extend to skin health because smoking is a vasoconstrictor.

Emollients and other topical agents

Any moisturizer that minimizes transepidermal water loss appears to make the skin appear more hydrated. Most cream-based moisturizers (ones that do not easily pour out of a bottle) contain ingredients that mimic the youthful epidermis (ie, ceramides, glycerin, shea butter). Adding a humectant molecule to the topical agent (ie, hyaluronic acid) will attract water and make the skin more hydrated.

A frequently used intervention to reverse cutaneous changes in the skin of women as they age is the application of topical retinoids. Data suggest that topical retinoids have an effect on most components of the skin, including the keratinocyte, the melanocyte, and the pilosebaceous unit.[107] Retinoids may cause increases in angiogenesis and decreases in the matrixmetalloproteinases, which are responsible for the degradation of collagen.

The AE of employing topical retinoids on the face is tolerability. Effective, stable, topical retinoids (usually prescription-strength tazarotene, adapelene, or tretinoin) cause facial irritation or excessive dryness, especially during the first 3 months of use, but usually resolve after this time period.

Steps to increasing tolerability include starting three-times-per-week application, slowly increasing over time to more frequent application, culminating in once-daily usage. Another strategy is to start with weaker concentrations or applying a facial moisturizer first to decrease absorption until the skin adapts to retinoid usage. Alternatively, one can start with a weaker, less-stable, over-the-counter retinol and, over time, switch the cosmeceutical to a pharmaceutical strength.

The second most studied topical agent is the family of alpha- and beta-hydroxy topical acid preparations. They primarily work on the epidermal layers, causing a smoothing effect on texture via keratinocyte effects. They appear to be less effective than retinoids but typically have better tolerability.

Targeted in-office therapies

A tailored, individualistic approach is best for addressing women's concerns during menopause, because each woman will notice different things, especially on her face during this time. Many choose to address one primary concern (ie, brown spots), whereas others want to discuss multiple interventions often relating to the changes in the different tissue layers (ie, rough skin, fine lines, and sagging). Most of these procedures are considered elective and are usually done in offices that are set up to do these types of interventions. If you do not do this work, it is best to identify and work with centers from which you have good outcomes data.

Epidermal and superficial dermal repair

Peeling agents are widely used to improve skin texture and normalize pigmentary alterations and dyschromias from hormone surges. Superficial agents, namely glycolic, salicylic, and lactic acids, are applied in the office in various concentrations and lengthening times to cause a

light desquamation and are frequently used as an adjunct to at-home topical regimens. Limitations are burning, stinging, prolonged erythema, and uneven penetration, especially if using a topical retinoid at home. Widely used agents such as the Vi peel combine various stronger ingredients (trichloroacetic acid, phenol, retinoic acid) in a proprietary blend that provides a slower, steady penetration and deeper, prolonged desquamation without pigmentary changes. Combination peeling agents containing resorcinol, lactic, and salicylic acid (Jessner's or modified Jessner's solution) are used to penetrate deeper than hydroxy acids alone. Trichloracetic acid also is used in-office in concentrations from 10% to 30% for full-face, medium-depth peeling. Trichloracetic acid 20% to 30% also can be applied with a cotton swab to remove unwanted brown spots without the downtime of full-face peeling. Common limitations are prolonged healing and postprocedure pigmentary alteration.

Developed in the early 2000s, fractional lasers create thousands of microscopic thermal columns of damage per square centimeter, without overlap.[108] This then turns on a fibroblastic response to stimulate collagen formation via a wound-healing process. Deeper fractionated lasers work via the same theory but penetrate deeper into the dermis and create more zones of damage.

Vascular-specific (potassium-titanyl-phosphate or pulsed dye) lasers are additional therapeutic options for women who simply want to target nonglobal concerns such as facial telangectasias.[109] Intense pulsed-light treatments are nonlaser-based technologies that can specifically target hemoglobin (vascular) or melanin (pigment) chromophores with varying wavelength hand pieces for specific concerns

Filling agents and toxins

Aesthetic technology was revolutionized in the 1990s with the introduction of botulinum toxin purified protein extract injections to smooth lines created from hyperdynamic muscles by temporarily blocking acetylcholine release at the neuromuscular junction. Around the same time, an onslaught of injectable filling agents became available to eradicate static lines on the face. Available toxin extracts used in the United States have a 3- to 4-month duration of action. A topical formulation as well as a longer-acting injectable form are in the pipeline and may be commercially available within the next few years.

Most dermal filling agents today are comprised of hyaluronic acid gels of nonanimal origin. They temporarily (6-18 mo duration) fill a line, wrinkle, or fold or are used for lip augmentation. Most of the gel particles used for these indications have rheologic properties of medium to high cohesively and low to medium gel hardness[110] and provide natural-looking results that may last from 6 to 18 months.

Over repetitive use, most women feel that the results from these toxins and fillers tend to last longer and longer. For example, after using toxins three times a year for 2 to 3 years, some women may follow-up twice the next year. For toxin therapy, this is likely because of women's "retraining" how they use their various facial muscles with certain expressions when muscular capacity is diminished in one area. This is commonly noted in the frontalis region of the forehead. Even after the toxin effect has worn off, the rhytids in that area do not come back to the same degree as before.

For filling agents, repetitive tissue trauma from the needle insertion used to deliver the filling agent will cause fibroblasts to create collagen via a wound-healing response, thereby making the line less visible even after the agent has been metabolized away.

The various interventions will have different periods of effectiveness. The most temporary interventions are the hyaluronic acid fillers, which typically are effective from 6 to 18 months.[111] Synthetic fillers may not need to be repeated as frequently because they are usually not systemically absorbed.

Deep dermal and subcutaneous repair

Radiofrequency delivers energy to heat dermal tissue while bypassing the skin's surface. This energy causes a wound contraction and tissue remodeling in the deep dermal layer. Over 6 to 9 months' time, improvements can be seen in fine lines and wrinkles in various parts of the face.

Focused ultrasound delivers thermal energy to exact depths of the dermis or subcutaneous tissue to cause a contraction and stimulate collagen production while bypassing superficial structures. Unlike the quick results of toxins and gel fillers, these in-office treatments work via fibroblast stimulation, a physiologic cellular response that typically takes 6 to 9 months to show full clinical effects. Treatments range from full-face therapy to targeted areas such as eyelid hooding or neck sagging. Responses also are more variable and depend on a woman's wound-healing cellular pathways.

Support structure repair
Collagen stimulators

Collagen stimulators such as poly L lactic acid diminish facial wrinkles by restoring the underlying structure of the skin. The particles are deposited either into the subcutaneous fat layer or the supraperiosteal plane, depending on the region of the face. This causes a foreign body-type reaction that turns on fibroblasts to make new collagen in the corresponding deep tissue plane, thereby volumizing that area. Typically, three treatments are performed 2 to 3 months apart; clinical results have been shown in FDA trials to last 25 months.[112] Improvements are seen in folds, contour, and shadowing as the deeper planes are thickened.

Modified hyaluronic acids

In 2010, hyaluronic acid gel agents modified for injection into deeper planes were introduced.[113] These particles were customized for lift and duration up to 2 years. A mixture of low- and high-molecular-weight hyaluronic acid particles were formulated to be an efficiently and tightly cross-linked gel. These gels are commonly used for volume loss in the midface and can restore the craniofacial skeletal plane to a more youthful frame by increasing tissue mass in the supraperiostial plane.

In the past, a deeper volumizing agent made of calcium hydroxylapetite was commonly used for injection into this deeper plane. Most practitioners who care for women wanting intervention use either one of these molecules in practice today. An added benefit of the entire family of hyaluronic gel agents is that they can be reversed or dissolved away with the administration of injected hyaluronidase. This is useful if the product is injected incorrectly or inadvertently injected into an artery, a medical emergency that can lead to ischemia, tissue necrosis, and even blindness if it flows retrograde into the ophthalmic artery. Therefore, having a trained clinician who does this regularly should be encouraged for your patients considering this intervention. However, women should be made aware of the costs, because these interventions are considered elective or cosmetic. Most women will have to pay for these skin-care interventions out of pocket.

Future considerations

Each passing year is met with rapid advancements in science and technology. Because in-office therapies, especially cosmetic ones, are tailored to each individual woman, a corresponding evolution is occurring in the area of precision medicine. Optimal therapies will be based on the context of a woman's genetic component or other molecular or cellular analyses. Identifying woman-specific defects and then replenishing (via stem-cell therapy or targeted intravenous infusion) are examples of potential future medical advances that can be extrapolated from general health concerns into cutaneous maintenance and antiaging algorithms.

Hair Changes

Some women experience thinning of hair on the scalp and/or unwanted growth of hair on the face (hirsutism) in midlife and associate these hair changes with menopause. The hair loss phenomenon has been called *androgenetic alopecia*, although multiple factors beyond genetic predisposition and local androgen metabolism, including growth factors (especially cytokines), other hormones,[114] and stress may be involved. To complicate matters, chronic illness, medications, and supplements often contribute to hair loss.

Generally, it has been postulated that the increase in the ratio of androgen to estrogen during the menopause transition may influence the hair changes observed, and some women respond well to antiandrogen treatments; however, that response is inconsistent, pointing to a more complex pathophysiology that has yet to be elucidated. Furthermore, the cause of the variability in end-organ sensitivity of the pilosebaceous unit to circulating androgens (ie, frontal vs occipital scalp; scalp vs facial hair) remains unclear.[115]

Ultimately, hair growth aberrations can have significant psychological consequences that affect body image, self-esteem, quality of life,[116] and emotional well-being, possibly leading to anxiety and depression.[117] These adverse consequences may not correlate with the clinical severity of the hair loss.[116] This underscores the importance of proactive discussion, and when requested by the woman, effective medical management and appropriate and timely referral for specialty care.

Causes of hair loss

The onset of hair loss during and after the menopause transition may be caused by a variety of conditions. *Female pattern hair loss* (FPHL) and *telogen effluvium* (TE) are the most common causes. In FPHL, the altered estrogen-to-androgen ratio may play a role in pathogenesis, leading to gradual hair thinning. A sudden onset of hair shedding characterizes TE, a disruption of the hair cycle that occurs several months after a major life stressor or because of chronic illness or prescribed medications known to promote hair loss such as anticoagulants and beta-blockers. The two often coexist, and a striking progression of FPHL or unmasking of FPHL may occur after an acute TE episode.

In FPHL, the hair thins mainly on the crown of the scalp. It usually starts with a widening through the center hair part. The frontal hairline remains intact, and the hair loss rarely progresses to total or near total baldness as it might in male pattern hair loss (MPHL). Male pattern hair loss can also occur in women, although not common, involving vertex balding and bitemporal recession. Another form of hair loss, *frontal fibrosing alopecia* (FFA), occurs predominantly in postmenopausal women. Other causes of hair loss, including thyroid disease, various cicatricial (scarring) alopecias, trichotillomania, alopecia neoplastica, tinea capitis, and alopecia areata are less common but should be considered in the differential diagnosis when evaluating patients for hair loss.

Frontal fibrosing alopecia deserves special attention because it has become more common in the years since it was first described in 1994.[118] It is an inflammatory cicatricial permanent alopecia, characterized by frontotemporal recession,[119] follicular hyperkeratosis, perifollicular erythema,[120] and diffuse bilateral eyebrow, eyelash, and/or body hair loss. Postmenopausal women are most commonly affected, although men and younger women may be affected as well. Current data are insufficient to establish any racial or ethnic differences in disease prevalence. The pathogenesis is poorly understood; however, it is postulated to be an autoreactive immune response against an unknown antigen, with endogenous or exogenous agents proposed as potential triggers.[121] There has been mixed data regarding sunscreen as a potential trigger.[122,123] Titanium nanoparticles have been identified in the hair shafts of patients with FFA; however, it is unclear whether these are causative or incidental.[124] The effectiveness of treatment with finasteride (although not FDA approved for women) in some patient groups suggests that androgens also might be partially involved in disease pathogenesis.[125]

Pathophysiology

The pathophysiology of FPHL is not completely understood, and there is evidence to suggest that genetic, hormone, and environment factors are involved.[126]

In a normal adult scalp, approximately 80% to 90% of hair is in the anagen (growth) phase, 1% to 2% in the catagen (transitional) phase, and 10% to 20% is in the telogen (resting) phase. The premature termination of the anagen phase is a landmark event in the development of FPHL.[127] The delay between the end of the telogen phase and the beginning of a new anagen phase also is observed in disease pathogenesis; however, the mechanisms through which hormone factors may lead to these changes within the follicles have yet to be fully understood.

Although estrogen receptors (ERs) and androgen receptors (ARs) have been found on hair follicles, the exact mechanism of action of estrogen on hair follicles is unknown. It is believed to protect against hair loss, with the ER pathway involved in telogen-anagen follicle cycling. This is illustrated by women's increased hair density during pregnancy from prolongation of anagen and the postpartum TE (gravidarum) that accompanies the decline in maternal estrogen levels. The protective effect of estrogen has been further suggested by a study investigating aromatase levels in follicles of women with FPHL.[128] The enzyme levels on the frontal scalp region were found to be half as high as those of the occipital region, and six times greater than the levels found on the frontal follicles of men.

Nevertheless, although other studies have demonstrated equivocal evidence regarding estrogen as a potential stimulator or inhibitor of hair growth,[129] therapy with estrogen has failed to consistently promote hair growth in postmenopausal women, thus further questioning the precise role it plays in FPHL.

Androgens, importantly dihydrotestosterone, which is converted from testosterone by 5α-reductase at the hair follicle level, act via the AR. Androgens have differential effects on hair follicles, depending on their body site, and cause progressive miniaturization and shortening of the anagen phase of susceptible hair follicles on the scalp.[130] The androgen effect is well documented in genetically susceptible males and is known to cause hair loss, although its role in FPHL is less clear.

During postmenopause, testosterone levels decrease but not as significantly as estrogen levels, therefore leading to a hypoestrogenemic and a relative hyperandrogenic state that may lead to patterned hair loss (PHL) in susceptible persons.[131] In a study of a group of premenopausal women with FPHL, the ratio of estrogen to androgen was found to be significantly lower than in the control group and was suggested as the hair loss trigger.[132]

Microinflammation of the hair follicles, or mild lymphohistiocytic inflammatory infiltrates located in the peri-infundibular region, is often seen with hair miniaturization on scalp biopsies. External factors such as UV radiation, environmental pollutants, and inhabitants of the skin microbiota and follicle may be implicated in the induction of this microinflammatory process.[133] The significance of this inflammatory process in the development of FPHL, as well as its relationship to the miniaturization process and the hormone elements implicated in disease pathogenesis, is uncertain.

Although FPHL appears to run in families, especially in cases of early onset,[134] very little is known regarding the genetic basis and inheritance pattern of the condition. The high prevalence of FPHL and the fact that it manifests with varying degrees of intensity and different ages of onset suggest a polygenic pattern with incomplete penetrance.[135] The strongest evidence of genetic involvement in the development of PHL comes from studies involving the AR gene in men, where the *AR/EDA2R* region is most strongly implicated. Because the AR gene is found on the X chromosome but similar balding phenotypes are often observed in fathers and sons, the current hypothesis points to polygenic inheritance rather than the commonly held theory of direct maternal transmission.[126] Although there is less overall genetic evidence in FPHL, the AR gene has been implicated in both FPHL[135] and in hirsutism.[136,137]

Several environment risk factors have been investigated. A study conducted on identical twins points to several environment factors possibly associated with FPHL, including longer sleep duration, higher levels of stress, smoking, DM, and hypertension.[138] Low ferritin levels and low vitamin D levels also have been associated with FPHL, but there are no studies showing that supplementation is consistently helpful in treatment.

In the menopause transition, FPHL is the most likely diagnosis for hair thinning and alopecia. History, examination, and when indicated, laboratory investigations should confirm the diagnosis and exclude other disorders. It is important to note that analogous to their male counterparts, women with early onset PHL appear to have a higher prevalence of hypertension and hyperaldosteronemia than do age-matched controls.[139] Although specific studies in menopausal women are lacking, blood pressure screening in all women presenting with PHL may be worthwhile for earlier diagnosis and treatment of unsuspected hypertension.

Clinical history and examination

A complete medical history and review of systems should be performed. Detailed female history is important, including menstrual history, number of pregnancies and/or miscarriages, age at menopause, menopause symptoms, HT use, and associated symptoms of androgen excess such as acne, seborrhea, and hirsutism. Family history should be obtained, focusing on PHL, autoimmune conditions, thyroid disorders, and malignancies. Further potential hair loss triggers, including medication history, severe illness, surgery, or weight loss, should be sought, as well as dietary and hair care history.

Clinical examination should confirm the distinctive pattern of loss over the crown, with the widening of the central part and retention of the frontal hairline seen in FPHL, and exclude other types of hair loss, including a cicatricial alopecia such as FFA with loss of visible follicular openings. Women can also show a male-type pattern of alopecia with vertex balding and bitemporal recession.

Other signs of hyperandrogenism should be screened for, including acne, seborrhea, obesity, clitoromegaly, increased muscle mass, deepened voice, and hirsutism. Hair pull test results may be positive early in FPHL but are usually negative in women experiencing hair loss for an extended period of time.[140] A positive hair pull test may indicate another diagnosis such as TE, which can be acute (<6 mo) or chronic (>6 m). Lateral eyebrow hair loss is typical of hypothyroidism, but patchy or diffuse eyebrow loss along with body hair loss can be seen in FFA and alopecia areata.

Laboratory investigations

In women presenting with significant hair loss or alopecia, pathologic causes should be excluded at least on the basis of a thorough history, physical examination, and review of systems. Baseline studies can include a complete blood count, a comprehensive metabolic panel, thyroid function tests (thyroid-stimulating hormone, thyroxine levels), and iron, ferritin, and zinc levels to screen for systemic disease, thyroid disease, and nutritional deficiency. In women with FPHL and other signs of androgen excess, an androgen screen is important to exclude an androgen-secreting tumor or other endocrinopathy. A total and free testosterone level and levels of sex hormone-binding globulin and DHEA can identify high androgen levels. Levels of testosterone and DHEA greater than 140 ng/dL to 200 ng/dL (4.85-6.9 nmol/L) and 700 μg/dL (19 μmol/L), respectively, are suggestive of an ovarian or adrenal tumor.[141,142] Further investigation, such as autoimmune screening and referral to an endocrinologist, may be required but should be done on the basis of relevant signs or symptoms.

A scalp biopsy, if indicated, can confirm the diagnosis of FPHL, with miniaturization of terminal hair follicles into vellus hairs, leading to a diagnostic ratio of terminal to vellus hairs of less than 4:1.[143] Biopsies for hair loss are best processed both horizontally and vertically and interpreted by a dermatopathologist with experience in hair loss disorders. A scalp biopsy also can be helpful to evaluate for inflammation and to rule out other causes of hair loss such as FFA, which is characterized by perifollicular scarring and lymphocytic inflammation.

The diagnostic yield for finding a laboratory abnormality in most patients with FPHL is low; generally, women with a sudden advanced presentation of FPHL or with clinical signs and symptoms of virilization or endocrinopathy show an abnormality.

Treatment

The goal of all treatment options for FPHL is to prevent progression of the hair loss rather than to promote hair regrowth. The same is true for FFA. Nutritional deficiencies should be corrected, and multivitamin supplements can be given to support hair regrowth, although there is no strong evidence that vitamins or supplements improve FPHL. Hypervitaminosis A can be detrimental to hair growth, but adequate vitamin A is important for normal hair cycling.[144-146] There is little to no evidence to support the use of biotin in hair growth, and high doses can influence laboratory tests, so biotin supplementation is not routinely recommended.

Minoxidil

Topical minoxidil remains the only FDA-approved treatment for FPHL. It is commonly used in combination with oral antiandrogens. Topical minoxidil is beneficial for hair regrowth as a nonspecific hair-growth promoter.[140,147] Although it has been used for more than 30 years, there is limited understanding about its mechanism of action; it prolongs the anagen phase of the hair cycle and increases follicle size. One study has suggested that minoxidil promotes stem-cell differentiation via adenosine triphosphate synthase.[148] For FPHL, a 2% solution and a 5% foam are approved by FDA. The men's formulation comes in 5% solution and foam and can be used in women as well; they are often more readily available.

Facial hypertrichosis, contact dermatitis, and irritation are possible AEs.[149] Although once-daily use of the 5% foam was not found to be significantly more effective than twice-daily use of the 2% solution, the foam was generally considered more cosmetically acceptable. Contact dermatitis and irritation are more likely with both the 2% and 5% solution. Facial hypertrichosis is more common with all 5% preparations than with 2%. All AEs completely resolve with discontinuation. Many patients experience the "dread shed," an initial shedding that lasts about 1 to 2 months; ultimately, this is allowing for new growth. Stabilization of hair loss or improvement of hair growth takes at least 4 to 6 months.

tumor DHEA > 700

Testosterone > 140-200

Hair growth-promoting agents with variable evidence to support their use include low-level laser therapy and platelet-rich plasma therapy. Hair transplantation is an option for some women who retain thicker hair in the occipital scalp, although many women with FPHL have thinning diffusely throughout the scalp. Where appropriate, specific hairstyling, topical camouflage fibers/makeup, or hairpieces can be recommended.[140]

Hormone treatments

Because of the likely hormone component of FPHL, two types of hormone treatments have been studied for hair loss: antiandrogens and ET. However, their use has not been evaluated in RCTs and is based only on small studies. Hormone agents for the treatment of FPHL are used off-label.

Antiandrogens. Antiandrogens compete with circulating androgens for the high-affinity AR.[140,150]

Spironolactone competitively blocks the AR and suppresses ovarian androgen synthesis.[150] Although it has been used in doses of 50 mg to 200 mg daily as an antiandrogen for FPHL, it is not FDA approved.[140,150,151] Hyperkalemia is a risk; baseline and continued monitoring of serum potassium is recommended.[152] Other AEs include fatigue, postural hypotension, and liver abnormalities.[140,150,152] Spironolactone was found to be tumorigenic and teratogenic in animal studies,[152] but several large studies have shown no association between spironolactone and estrogen-dependent tumors in postmenopausal women.[153-155]

Finasteride, a type II 5α-reductase inhibitor, prevents conversion of testosterone to the more potent DHEA.[156] Finasteride is government approved and effective for treatment of MPHL, but it is not approved for any indication in women.

Estrogen therapy. In some women, cessation of ET, as well as hormone contraception, can precipitate hair shedding and unmask FPHL. Estrogen therapy, if appropriate to continue prescribing, sometimes supports hair growth as it supports other skin structures.[157] However, it is not consistently effective for hair loss problems.[158]

Adjunctive therapies

Bimatoprost is a prostaglandin analog/prodrug used to control the progression of glaucoma and in the management of ocular hypertension. In December 2008, the indication to lengthen eyelashes was approved by FDA.[159] It has not been found to be effective for FPHL in the concentration approved for eyelash growth (0.03%).

Over-the-counter *ketoconazole shampoo* 2% has been used as an antiandrogen and has been suggested to reduce shedding and promote hair growth in MPHL through androgen-dependent pathways.[160] A study of antidandruff shampoos containing 1% zinc pyrithione also was suggestive of potential hair growth.[161] Hair count results showed a sustained improvement in hair growth with daily use. These shampoos are known to be anti-inflammatory and may improve the microinflammation seen in FPHL. Alternatively, coexisting seborrheic dermatitis may exacerbate hair loss, and its proper treatment also may improve hair growth. Scalp health is important to maintain in any treatment regimen for hair loss.

Another treatment option includes the low-energy laser-light products that are available for treatment of alopecia.[162] They are designed as a hairbrush/comb, band, or helmet that shines red light directly on the scalp. One such handheld, noninvasive device was cleared by FDA for safety for men in 2007 and for women with FPHL in 2011. There is one multicenter trial showing a minor but statistically significant benefit.[163]

Camouflaging topical sprays, powders, or keratin fibers may be alternatives to achieve sufficient density for FPHL.[164] Many brands are available over the counter. Hairpieces or extensions can also be helpful but may cause traction alopecia or breakage of hair.

Cell-mediated treatments for androgenetic alopecia

There are two main experimental approaches to cell-mediated treatments for androgenetic alopecia: the direct injection of cultured cells or the use of cell-secreted factors as a hair growth-promoting product. Preclinical studies have shown that cells from the hair follicle mesenchyme cells can be cultured and used to induce new hair follicle formation.[165] The injected cells also can increase the size of the resident hair follicles. Alternatively, cells are cultured, and the culture supernatant is processed to produce a compound rich in hair growth-promoting factors for use in treatment. These cell-mediated treatment approaches may be available in a few years. Also, platelet-rich plasma isolated from whole blood associated with multiple growth factors is currently gaining popularity in the marketplace.[166] There may be benefit; however, there are no standardized protocols and very few RCTs.

Hirsutism

Coarse facial hairs in women typically arise in areas of the body where the hair follicles are the most androgen-sensitive, including the chin, upper lip, and cheeks.[167] Hirsutism affects between 5% and 15% of women. Except for rare cases of virilizing tumors or adrenal hyperplasia caused by enzymatic defects, hirsutism is caused mainly by ovarian androgen overproduction (polycystic ovary syndrome [PCOS]) or by peripheral hypersensitivity to normal levels of circulating androgen (idiopathic hirsutism). The role of androgens in women with hirsutism is further evidenced by the reduction in hair density that can be attained with antiandrogen treatments, including hormone contraceptives with low androgenicity.

Most women with hirsutism have an exaggerated response to androgens as a result of enhanced local 5α-reductase activity. Other clinical disorders that have been observed with acute or transient androgen excess include FPHL, seborrhea (oily face and scalp, frequently with associated seborrheic dermatitis), and acne. If chronic androgen excess exists, PCOS is the most common cause (70-80% of cases); androgen-secreting tumors, androgenic drug intake, and endocrinopathies are less frequent causes.[167] Polycystic ovary syndrome is associated with insulin resistance, which must be screened for in suspected cases.

Facial hair in menopause

Another hair-growth phenomenon of concern to many women is the appearance of fine hairs ("peach fuzz") on the face, most commonly on the upper lip and chin but sometimes generalized in appearance. Rapidly growing, large "rogue hairs" can sometimes be found on the chin. The growth of unwanted hair is common, and sometimes occurs long before menopause. Unfortunately, treatment of FPHL with topical or oral minoxidil may increase facial hair.

Management of hirsutism

The first step in management should focus on any underlying cause, the woman's goals and expectations, and the degree of patient distress. The diagnostic evaluation should focus on confirming the condition and the presence of excess levels of androgen. Other associated abnormalities and conditions, including ovulatory dysfunction, adrenal hyperplasia, DM, and thyroid hormone abnormalities, need to be ruled out.

Treatment modalities encompass a combination of therapies, including hormone drugs, peripheral androgen blockage, and mechanical depilation. For most women, the initiation of pharmacologic therapy followed by direct hair removal is recommended. In postmenopausal women without an underlying tumor, antiandrogens such as spironolactone and 5α-reductase inhibitors (eg, finasteride) may be tried.[168,169] Direct hair removal methods include plucking, waxing, or shaving. Shaving is less traumatic than the other methods, but it may lead to folliculitis and ingrown hairs. Bleaching is also useful, particularly for mild conditions. Chemical depilatory agents may irritate the skin, especially facial skin. Electrolysis can usually destroy terminal hairs after 6 months of treatment. Electrolysis can be complicated by folliculitis and postinflammatory dyspigmentation.

Laser treatment is effective for large areas but can only be used on darkly pigmented hair.[170] Dyspigmentation, hypertrophic scars, and thermal burns (blistering, ulceration) can occur as AEs of laser treatment.[171] Other uncommon AEs may include premature graying of hair and tunneling of hair under the skin.[172] Also, paradoxical hypertrichosis is a rare AE seen in patients treated with intense pulsed-light devices, diode lasers, and alexandrite lasers.[173]

Estrogen therapy may delay the progression of hirsutism, but it will not change coarse terminal hairs into softer and less noticeable vellus hairs.

REFERENCES

1. Cohen Sacher B. The normal vulva, vulvar examination, and evaluation tools. *Clin Obstet Gynecol.* 2015;58(3):442-452.

2. Kurita T. Developmental origin of vaginal epithelium. *Differentiation.* 2010;80(2-3):99-105.

3. Cai Y. Revisiting old vaginal topics: conversion of the Müllerian vagina and origin of the "sinus" vagina. *Int J Dev Biol.* 2009;53(7):925-934.

4. Kelley C. Estrogen and its effect on vaginal atrophy in post-menopausal women. *Urol Nurs.* 2007;27(1):40-45.

5. Labrie F, Martel C, Pelletier G. Is vulvovaginal atrophy due to a lack of both estrogens and androgens? *Menopause.* 2017;24(4):452-461.

6. Lev-Sagie A. Vulvar and vaginal atrophy: physiology, clinical presentation, and treatment considerations. *Clin Obstet Gynecol.* 2015;58(3):476-491.

7. Shynlova O, Bortolini MA, Alarab M. Genes responsible for vaginal extracellular matrix metabolism are modulated by women's reproductive cycle and menopause. *Int Braz J Urol.* 2013;39(2):257-267.

8. Muhleisen AL, Herbst-Kralovetz MM. Menopause and the vaginal microbiome. *Maturitas.* 2016;91:42-50.

9. Mirmonsef P, Hotton AL, Gilbert D, et al. Free glycogen in vaginal fluids is associated with Lactobacillus colonization and low vaginal pH. *PLoS One.* 2014;9(7):e102467.

10. Ravel J, Gajer P, Abdo Z, et al. Vaginal microbiome of reproductive-age women. *Proc Natl Acad Sci U S A.* 2011;108(suppl 1):4680-4687.

11. Albert AY, Chaban B, Wagner EC, et; Vogue Research Group. R. A study of the vaginal microbiome in healthy Canadian women utilizing cpn60-based molecular profiling reveals distinct gardnerella subgroup community state types. *PLoS One.* 2015;10(8):e0135620.

12. Patton DL, Thwin SS, Meier A, Hooton TM, Stapleton AE, Eschenbach DA. Epithelial cell layer thickness and immune cell populations in the normal human vagina at different stages of the menstrual cycle. *Am J Obstet Gynecol.* 2000;183(4):967-973.

13. Weber MA, Diedrich CM, Ince C, Roovers JP. Focal depth measurements of the vaginal wall: a new method to noninvasively quantify vaginal wall thickness in the diagnosis and treatment of vaginal atrophy. *Menopause.* 2016;23(8):833-838.

14. Mac Bride MB, Rhodes DJ, Shuster LT. Vulvovaginal atrophy. *Mayo Clin Proc*. 2010;85(1):87-94.

15. Miller EA, Beasley DE, Dunn RR, Archie EA. Lactobacilli dominance and vaginal pH: why is the human vaginal microbiome unique? *Front Microbiol*. 2016;7:1936.

16. Constantine GD, Bruyniks N, Princic N, et al. Incidence of genitourinary conditions in women with a diagnosis of vulvar/vaginal atrophy. *Curr Med Res Opin*. 2014;30(1):143-148.

17. Cody JD, Jacobs ML, Richardson K, Moehrer B, Hextall A. Oestrogen therapy for urinary incontinence in post-menopausal women. *Cochrane Database Syst Rev*. 2012;10:CD001405.

18. Ismail SI. Bain C, Hagen S. Oestrogens for treatment or prevention of pelvic organ prolapse in postmenopausal women. *Cochrane Database Syst Rev*. 2010;(9):CD007063.

19. Flegal KM, Kruszon-Moran D, Carroll MD, Fryar CD, Ogden CL. Trends in obesity among adults in the United States 2005-2014. *JAMA*. 2016;315(21):2284-2291.

20. Ford ES, Maynard LM, Li C. Trends in mean waist circumference and abdominal obesity among US adults, 1999-2012. *JAMA*. 2014;312(11):1151-1153.

21. Kapoor E, Collazo-Clavell ML, Faubion SS. Weight gain in women at midlife: a concise review of the pathophysiology and strategies for management. *Mayo Clin Proc*. 2017;92(10):1552-1558.

22. Milewicz A, Tworowska U, Demissie M. Menopausal obesity—myth or fact? *Climacteric*. 2001;4(4):273-283.

23. Crawford SL, Casey VA, Avis NE, McKinlay SM. A longitudinal study of weight and the menopause transition: results from the Massachusetts Women's Health Study. *Menopause*. 2000;7(2):96-104.

24. Douchi T, Yamamoto S, Yoshimitsu N, Andoh T, Matsuo T, Nagata Y. Relative contribution of aging and menopause to changes in lean and fat mass in segmental regions. *Maturitas*. 2002;42(4):301-306.

25. Broomberger JT, Matthews KA, Schott LL, et al. Depressive symptoms during the menopausal transition: the Study of Women's Health Across the Nation (SWAN). *J Affect Disord*. 2007;103(1-3)267-272.

26. Lovejoy JC, Champagne CM, de Jonge L, Xie H, Smith SR. Increased visceral fat and decreased energy expenditure during the menopausal transition. *Int J Obes (Lond)*. 2008;32(6):949-958.

27. Park HS, Lee KU. Postmenopausal women lose less visceral adipose tissue during a weight reduction program. *Menopause*. 2003;10(3):222-227.

28. Franklin RM, Ploutz-Snyder L, Kanaley JA. Longitudinal changes in abdominal fat distribution with menopause. *Metabolism*. 2009;58(3):311-315.

29. Park JK, Lim YH, Kim KS, et al. Body fat distribution after menopause and cardiovascular disease risk factors: Korean National Health and Nutrition Examination Survey 2010. *J Womens Health (Larchmt)*. 2013;22(7):587-594.

30. Neeland IJ, Ayers CR, Rohatqi AK, et al. Associations of visceral and abdominal subcutaneous adipose tissue with markers of cardiac and metabolic risk in obese adults. *Obesity (Silver Spring)*. 2013;21(9):E439-E447.

31. Thorneycroft IH, Lindsay R, Pickar JH. Body composition during treatment with conjugated estrogens with and without medroxyprogesterone acetate: analysis of the Women's Health, Osteoporosis, Progestin, Estrogen (HOPE) trial. *Am J Obstet Gynecol*. 2007;197(2):137.e1-e7.

32. Utian WH, Gass ML, Pickar JH. Body mass index does not influence response to treatment, nor does body weight change with lower doses of conjugated estrogens and medroxyprogesterone acetate in early postmenopausal women. *Menopause*. 2004;11(3):306-314.

33. Barrett-Connor E, Slone S, Greendale G, et al. The Postmenopausal Estrogen/Progestin Interventions Study: primary outcomes in adherent women. *Maturitas*. 1997;27(3):261-274.

34. Bonds DE, Lasser N, Qi L, et al. The effect of conjugated equine oestrogen on diabetes incidence: the Women's Health Initiative randomised trial. *Diabetologia*. 2006;49(3):459-468.

35. Folsom AR, Kushi LH, Anderson KE, et al. Associations of general and abdominal obesity with multiple health outcomes in older women: the Iowa Women's Health Study. *Arch Intern Med*. 2000;160(14):2117-2128.

36. Calle EE, Rodriguez C, Walker-Thurmond K, Thun MJ. Overweight, obesity, and mortality from cancer in a prospectively studied cohort of US adults. *N Engl J Med*. 2003;348(17):1625-1638.

37. Eliassen AH, Colditz GA, Rosner B, Willett WC, Hankinson SE. Adult weight change and risk of postmenopausal breast cancer. *JAMA*. 2006;296(2):193-201.

38. Velie E, Kulldorff M, Schairer C, Block G, Albanes D, Schatzkin A. Dietary fat, fat subtypes, and breast cancer in postmenopausal women: a prospective cohort study. *J Natl Cancer Inst*. 2000;92(10):833-839.

39. Thurston RC, Sowers MR, Sternfeld B, et al. Gains in body fat and vasomotor symptom reporting over the menopausal transition: the study of Women's Health Across the Nation. *Am J Epidemiol*. 2009:170(6):766-774.

40. Thurston RC, Sowers MR, Chang Y, et al. Adiposity and reporting of vasomotor symptoms among midlife women: the Study of Women's Health Across the Nation. *Am J Epidemiol*. 2008;167(1):78-85.

41. Gold EB, Block G, Crawford S, et al. Lifestyle and demographic factors in relation to vasomotor symptoms: baseline results from the Study of Women's Health Across the Nation. *Am J Epidemiol*. 2004;159(12):1189-1199.

42. Gold EB, Crawford SL, Shelton JF, et al. Longitudinal analysis of changes in weight and waist circumference in relation to incident vasomotor symptoms: the Study of Women's Health Across the Nation (SWAN). *Menopause*. 2017;24(1):9-26.

43. Thurston RC, Chang Y, Mancuso P, Matthews KA. Adipokines, adiposity, and vasomotor symptoms during the menopause transition: findings from the Study of Women's Health Across the Nation. *Fertil Steril*. 2013;100(3):793-800.

44. Thurston RC, Santoro N, Matthews KA. Adiposity and hot flashes in midlife women: a modifying role of age. *J Clin Endocrinol Metab*. 2011;96(10):E1588-E1595.

45. Freeman EW, Sammel MD, Lin H, Gracia CR. Obesity and reproductive hormone levels in the transition to menopause. *Menopause*. 2010;17(4):718-726.

46. Randolph JF Jr, Zheng H, Sowers MR, et al. Change in follicle-stimulating hormone and estradiol across the menopausal transition: effect of age at the final menstrual period. *J Clin Endocrinol Metab*. 2011;96(3):746-754.

47. Huang AJ, Subak LL, Wing R, et al; Program to Reduce Incontinence by Diet and Exercise Investigators. An intensive behavioral weight loss intervention and hot flushes in women. *Arch Intern Med*. 2010;170(13):1161-1167. Erratum in: *Arch Intern Med*. 2010;170(17):1601.

48. Kroenke CH, Caan BJ, Stefanick ML, et al. Effects of dietary intervention and weight change on vasomotor symptoms in the Women's Health Initiative. *Menopause*. 2012;19(9):980-988.

49. Marcus MD, Bromberger JT, Wei HL, Brown C, Kravitz HM. Prevalence and selected correlates of eating disorder symptoms among a multiethnic community sample of midlife women. *Ann Behav Med*. 2007;33(3):269-277.

50. Jensen MD, Ryan DH, Apovian CM, et al; American College of Cardiology/American Heart Association Task Force on Practice Guidelines; Obesity Society. 2013 AHA/ACC/TOS guideline for the management of overweight and obesity in adults: a report of the American College of Cardiology/American Heart Association Task Force on Practice Guidelines and the Obesity Society. *J Am Coll Cardiol*. 2014;63(25 pt B):2985-3023. Erratum in: *J Am Coll Cardiol*. 2014;63(25 pt B):3029-3030.

51. Apovian CM, Aronne LJ, Bessesen DH, et al; Endocrine Society. Pharmacological management of obesity: an Endocrine Society clinical practice guideline. *J Clin Endocrinol Metab*. 2015;100(2):342-362.

52. American College of Cardiology/American Heart Association Task Force on Practice Guidelines, Obesity Expert Panel, 2013. Expert panel report: guidelines (2013) for the management of overweight and obesity in adults. *Obesity (Silver Spring)*. 2014;22(suppl 2):S41-S410.

53. Knowler WC, Barrett-Connor E, Fowler SE, et al; Diabetes Prevention Program Research Group. Reduction in the incidence of type 2 diabetes with lifestyle intervention or metformin. *N Engl J Med.* 2002;346(6):393-403.

54. Hamman RE, Wing RR, Edelstein SL, et al. Effect of weight loss with lifestyle intervention on risk of diabetes. *Diabetes Care.* 2006;29(9):2102-2107.

55. Diabetes Prevention Program Research Group, Knowler WC, Fowler SE, et al. 10-year follow-up of diabetes incidence and weight loss in the Diabetes Prevention Program Outcomes Study. *Lancet.* 2009;374(9702):1677-1686. Erratum in: *Lancet.* 2009;374(9707):2054.

56. US Preventive Services Task Force. Screening for obesity in adults: recommendations and rationale. *Ann Intern Med.* 2003;139(11):930-932.

57. Moyer VA; US Preventive Services Task Force. Screening for and management of obesity in adults: US Preventive Services Task Force recommendation statement. *Ann Intern Med.* 2012;157(5):373-378.

58. American Diabetes Association. 6. Obesity management for the treatment of type 2 diabetes. *Diabetes Care.* 2016;39(suppl 1):S47-S51.

59. Armstrong MJ, Mottershead TA, Ronksley PE, Sigal RJ, Campbell TS, Hemmelgarn BR. Motivational interviewing to improve weight loss in overweight and/or obese patients: a systematic review and meta-analysis of randomized controlled trials. *Obes Rev.* 2011;12(9):709-723.

60. Pollak KI, Alexander SC, Coffman CJ, et al. Physician communication techniques and weight loss in adults: Project CHAT. *Am J Prev Med.* 2010;39(4):321-328.

61. Barnes RD, Ivezaj V. A systematic review of motivational interviewing for weight loss among adults in primary care. *Obes Rev.* 2015;16(4):304-318.

62. Fitzpatrick SL, Wischenka D, Appelhans BM, et al; Society of Behavioral Medicine. An evidence-based guide for obesity treatment in primary care. *Am J Med.* 2016;129(1):115.e1-e7.

63. Hall KD, Sacks G, Chandramohan D, et al. Quantification of the effect of energy imbalance on bodyweight. *Lancet.* 2011;378(9793):826-837.

64. Sacks FM, Bray GA, Cary VJ, et al. Comparison of weight-loss diets with different compositions of fat, protein, and carbohydrates. *N Engl J Med.* 2009;360(9):859-873.

65. Ebbeling CB, Leidig MM, Feldman HA, Lovesky MM, Ludwig DS. Effects of a low-glycemic load vs low-fat diet in obese young adults: a randomized trial. *JAMA.* 2007;297(19):2092-2102. Erratum in: *JAMA.* 2007;298(6):627.

66. Pittas AG, Das SK, Hajduk CL, et al. A low-glycemic load diet facilitates greater weight loss in overweight adults with high insulin secretion but not in overweight adults with low insulin secretion in the CALERIE trial. *Diabetes Care.* 2005;28(12):2939-2941.

67. Cornier MA, Donahoo WT, Pereira R, et al. Insulin sensitivity determines the effectiveness of dietary macronutrient composition on weight loss in obese women. *Obes Res.* 2005;13(4):703-709.

68. Wycherley TP, Moran LJ, Clifton PM, Noakes M, Brinkworth GD. Effects of energy-restricted high-protein, low-fat compared with standard-protein, low-fat diets: a meta-analysis of randomized controlled trials. *Am J Clin Nutr.* 2012;96(5):1281-1298.

69. Te Morenga LA, Levers MT, Williams SM, Brown RC, Mann J. Comparison of high protein and high fiber weight-loss diets in women with risk factors for the metabolic syndrome: a randomized trial. *Nutr J.* 2011;10:40.

70. Donnelly JE, Blair SN, Jakicic JM, Manore MM, Rankin JW, Smith BK; American College of Sports Medicine. American College of Sports Medicine position stand. Appropriate physical activity intervention strategies for weight loss and prevention of weight regain for adults. *Med Sci Sports Exerc.* 2009;41(2):459-471.

71. Brochu M, Malita MF, Messier V, et al. Resistance training does not contribute to improving the metabolic profile after a 6-month weight loss program in overweight and obese postmenopausal women. *J Clin Endocrinol Metab.* 2009;94(9):3226-3233.

72. Watson SL, Weeks BK, Weis LJ, Horan SA, Beck BR. Heavy resistance training is safe and improves bone, function, and stature in postmenopausal women with low to very low bone mass: novel early findings from the LIFTMOR trial. *Osteoporos Int.* 2015;26(12):2889-2894.

73. Gudzune KA, Doshi RS, Mehta AK, et al. Efficacy of commercial weight-loss programs: an updated systematic review. *Ann Intern Med.* 2015;162(7):501-512. Erratum in: Correction. *Ann Intern Med.* 2015.

74. Lean M, Brosnahan N, McLoone P, et al. Feasibility and indicative results from a 12-month low-energy liquid diet treatment and maintenance programme for severe obesity. *Br J Gen Pract.* 2013;63(607):e115-e124.

75. American Heart Association Nutrition Committee, Lichtenstein AH, Appel LJ, et al. Diet and lifestyle recommendations revision 2006: a scientific statement from the American Heart Association Nutrition Committee. *Circulation.* 2006;114(1):82-96. Erratum in: *Circulation.* 2006;114(1):e27; *Circulation.* 2006;114(23):e629.

76. Appel LJ, Brands MW, Daniels SR, Karanja N, Elmer PJ, Sacks FM; American Heart Association. Dietary approaches to prevent and treat hypertension: a scientific statement from the American Heart Association. *Hypertension.* 2006;47(2):296-308.

77. Kris-Etherton P, Eckel RH, Howard BV, St Jeor S, Bazzarre TL; Nutrition Committee Population Science Committee and Clinical Science Committee of the American Heart Association. AHA science advisory: Lyon Diet Heart Study. Benefits of a Mediterranean-style, National Cholesterol Education Program/American Heart Association Step I dietary pattern on cardiovascular disease. *Circulation.* 2001;103(13):1823-1825.

78. Kahan S. Obesity and sleep: an evolving relationship. *Sleep Health.* 2017;3(5):381-382.

79. Spiegel K, Leproult R, Van Cauter E. Impact of sleep debt on metabolic and endocrine function. *Lancet.* 1999;354:1435-1439.

80. Spiegel K, Knutson K, Leproult R, Tasali E, Van Cauter E. Sleep loss: a novel risk factor for insulin resistance and type 2 diabetes. *J Appl Physiol.* 2005;99(5):2008-2019.

81. Taheri S, Lin L, Austin D, Young T, Mignot E. Short sleep duration is associated with reduced leptin, elevated ghrelin, and increased body mass index. *PLoS Med.* 2004;3:e62.

82. Patel SR, Malhotra A, White DP, Gottlieb DJ, Hu FB. Association between reduced sleep and weight gain in women. *Am J Epidemiol.* 2006;164(10):947-954.

83. Torgerson JS, Hauptman J, Boldrin MN, Sjöström L. XENical in the prevention of diabetes in obese subjects (XENDOS) study: a randomized study of orlistat as an adjunct to lifestyle changes for the prevention of type 2 diabetes in obese patients. *Diabetes Care.* 2004;27(1):155-161. Erratum in: *Diabetes Care.* 2004;27(3):856.

84. Xenical [package insert]. South San Francisco, CA: Genentech USA; 2016.

85. Smith SR, Weissman NJ, Anderson CM, et al; Behavioral Modification and Lorcaserin for Overweight and Obesity Management (BLOOM) Study Group. Multicenter, placebo-controlled trial of lorcaserin for weight management. *N Engl J Med.* 2010;363(3):245-256.

86. O'Neil PM, Smith SR, Weissman NJ, et al. Randomized placebo-controlled clinical trial of lorcaserin for weight loss in type 2 diabetes mellitus: the BLOOM-DM study. *Obesity (Silver Spring).* 2012;20(7):1426-1436.

87. Belviq [package insert]. Zofingen, Switzerland: Arena Pharmaceuticals; 2017.

88. Garvey WT, Ryan DH, Look M, et al. Two-year sustained weight loss and metabolic benefits with controlled-release phentermine/topiramate in obese and overweight adults (SEQUEL): a randomized, placebo-controlled, phase 3 extension study. *Am J Clin Nutr.* 2012;95(2):297-308.

89. Qysmia [package insert]. Campbell, CA: Vivus; 2012.

90. Apovian CM, Aronne L, Rubino D, et al; COR-II Study Group. A randomized, phase 3 trial of naltrexone SR/bupropion SR on weight and obesity-related risk factors (COR-II). *Obesity (Silver Spring).* 2013;21(5):935-943.

91. Wadden TA, Foreyt JP, Foster GD, et al. Weight loss with naltrexone SR/bupropion SR combination therapy as an adjunct to behavior modification: the COR-BMOD trial. *Obesity (Silver Spring)*. 2011;19(1):110-120.

92. Billes SK, Sinnayah P, Cowley MA. Naltrexone/bupropion for obesity: an investigational combination pharmacotherapy for weight loss. *Pharmacol Res*. 2014;84:1-11.

93. Contrave [package insert]. Deerfield, IL: Takeda Pharmaceuticals; 2014.

94. Pi-Sunyer X, Astrup A, Fujioka K, et al; SCALE Obesity and Prediabetes NN8022-1839 Study Group. A randomized, controlled trial of 3.0 mg of liraglutide in weight management. *N Engl J Med*. 2015;373(1):11-22.

95. le Roux C, Astrup A, Fujioka K, et al; SCALE Obesity Prediabetes NN8022-1839 Study Group. 3 years of liraglutide versus placebo for type 2 diabetes risk reduction and weight management in individuals with prediabetes: a randomised, double-blind trial. *Lancet*. 2017;389(10077):1399-1409.

96. Victoza [package insert]. Bagsvaerd, Denmark; 2017.

97. Sjöström L, Narbro K, Sjöström CD, et al; Swedish Obese Subjects Study. Effects of bariatric surgery on mortality in Swedish obese subjects. *N Engl J Med*. 2007;357(8):741-752.

98. Buchwald H, Avidor Y, Braunwald E, et al. Bariatric surgery: a systematic review and meta-analysis. *JAMA*. 2004;292(14):1724-1737.

99. Birkmeyer NJ, Dimick JB, Share D, et al; Michigan Bariatric Surgery Collaborative. Hospital complication rates with bariatric surgery in Michigan. *JAMA*. 2010;304(4):435-442.

100. Zouboulis CC, Makrantonaki E. Hormonal therapy of intrinsic aging. *Rejuvenation Res*. 2012;15(3):302-312.

101. Coleman SR, Grover R. The anatomy of the aging face: volume loss and changes in 3-dimensional topography. *Aesthet Surg J*. 2006;26(1S):S4-S9.

102. Raine-Fenning NJ, Brincat MP, Muscal-Baron Y. Skin aging and menopause: implications for treatment. *Am J Clin Dermatol*. 2003;4(6):371-378.

103. Wilkinson HN, Hardman MJ. The role of estrogen in cutaneous ageing and repair. *Maturitas*. 2017;103:60-64.

104. Verdier-Sévrain, Bonté F, Gilchrest B. Biology of estrogens in skin: implications for skin aging. *Exp Dermatol*. 2005; 15(2):83-94.

105. Donofrio LM. Fat distribution: a morphologic study for the aging face. *Dermatol Surg*. 2000;26:1107-1112.

106. Vlegger D, Fitzgerald R. Dermatological implications on skeletal aging: a focus on supraperiosteal volumization for perioral rejuvenation. *J Drugs Dermatol*. 2008;7(3):209-220.

107. Darlenski R, Surber C, Fluhr JW. Topical retinoids in the management of photodamaged skin: from theory to evidence-based practical approach. *Br J Dermatol*. 2010;163(6):1157-1165.

108. US Food and Drug Administration. Medical lasers. www.fda.gov/Radiation-EmittingProducts/RadiationEmittingProductsandProcedures/SurgicalandTherapeutic/ucm115910.htm. Last updated May 14, 2018. Accessed April 8, 2019.

109. Bernstein EF. The pulsed-dye laser for treatment of cutaneous conditions. *G Ital Dermatol Venereol*. 2009;144(5):557-572.

110. Pierre S, Liew S, Benadin A. Basics of dermal filler rheology. *Dermatol Surg*. 2015;41(suppl 1):120-126.

111. Brandt FS, Cazzaniga A. Hyaluronic acid gel fillers in the management of facial aging. *Clin Interv Aging*. 2008;3(1):153-159.

112. Ezzat WH, Keller GS. The use poly-L-lactic acid filler in facial aesthetics. *Facial Plast Surg*. 2011;27(6):503-509.

113. Sundaram H, Voigts B, Beer K, Meland M. Comparison of the rheological properties of viscosity and elasticity in two categories of soft tissue fillers: calcium hydroxylapatite and hyaluronic acid. *Dermatol Surg*. 2010;36(suppl 3):1859-1865.

114. Deplewski D, Rosenfield RL. Role of hormones in pilosebaceous unit development. *Endocr Rev*. 2000;21(4):363-392.

115. Rosenfield RL. Hirsutism and the variable response of the pilosebaceous unit to androgen. *J Investig Dermatol Symp Proc*. 2005;10(3):205-208.

116. Reid EE, Haley AC, Borovicka JH, et al. Clinical severity does not reliably predict quality of life in women with alopecia areata, telogen effluvium, or androgenic alopecia. *J Am Acad Dermatol*. 2012;66(3):e97-e102.

117. Schmitt JV, Ribeiro CF, Souza FH, Siqueira EB, Bebber FR. Hair loss perception and symptoms of depression in female outpatients attending a general dermatology clinic. *An Bras Dermatol*. 2012;87(3):412-417.

118. Kossard S. Postmenopausal frontal fibrosing alopecia. Scarring alopecia in a pattern distribution. *Arch Dermatol*. 1994;130(6):770-774. Erratum in: *Arch Dermatol*. 1994;130(11):1407.

119. Vano-Galvan S, Saceda-Corralo D, Moreno-Arrones OM, Camacho-Martinez FM. Updated diagnostic criteria for frontal fibrosing alopecia. *J Am Acad Dermatol*. 2018;78(1):e21-e22.

120. Vano-Galvan S, Molina-Ruiz AM, Serrano-Falcon C, et al. Frontal fibrosing alopecia: a multicenter review of 355 patients. *J Am Acad Dermatol*. 2014;70(4):670-678.

121. Assouly P, Reygagne P. Lichen planopilaris: update on diagnosis and treatment. *Semin Cutan Med Surg*. 2009;28(1):3-10.

122. Seegobin SD, Tziotzios C, Stefanato CM, Bhargava K, Fenton DA, McGrath JA. Frontal fibrosing alopecia: there is no statistically significant association with leave-on facial skin care products and sunscreens. *Br J Dermatol*. 2016;165(6):1407-1408.

123. Cranwell WC, Sinclair R. Frontal fibrosing alopecia: regrowth following cessation of sunscreen on the forehead [published online ahead of print June 12, 2018]. *Autralas J Dermatol*.

124. Brunet-Possenti F, Deschamps L, Colboc H, et al. Detection of titanium nanoparticles in the hair shafts of a patient with frontal fibrosing alopecia. *J Eur Acad Dermatol Venereol*. 2018;32(12):e442-e443.

125. Tosti A, Piraccini BM, Iorizzo M, Misciali C. Frontal fibrosing alopecia in postmenopausal women. *J Am Acad Dermatol*. 2005;52(1):55-60.

126. Ramos PM, Miot HA. Female pattern hair loss: a clinical and pathophysiological review. *An Bras Dermatol*.2015;90(4):529-543.

127. Cotsarelis G, Millar SE. Towards a molecular understanding of hair loss and its treatment. *Trends Mol Med*.2001;7(7):293-301.

128. Sawaya ME, Price VH. Different levels of 5alpha-reductase type I and II, aromatase, and androgen receptor in hair follicles of women and men with androgenetic alopecia. *J Invest Dermatol*. 1997;109(3):296-300.

129. Yip L, Rufaut N, Sinclair R. Role of genetics and sex steroid hormones in male androgenetic alopecia and female pattern hair loss: an update of what we now know. *Australas J Dermatol*. 2011;52(2):81-88.

130. Kaufman KD. Androgens and alopecia. *Mol Cell Endocrinol*. 2002;198(1-2):89-95.

131. Nathan L. Menopause and postmenopause. In: DeCherney AH, Nathan L, Goodwin TM, Laufer N, Roman A, eds. *Current Diagnosis and Treatment: Obstetrics and Gynecology*. 11th ed. New York: McGraw Hill Medical; 2012:948-970.

132. Riedel-Baima B, Riedel A. Female pattern hair loss may be triggered by low oestrogen to androgen ratio. *Endocr Regul*. 2008;42(1):13-16.

133. Mahé Y F, Michelet JF, Billoni N, et al. Androgenetic alopecia and microinflammation. *Int J Dermatol*. 2000;39(8):576-584.

134. Paik JH, Yoon JB, Sim WY, Kim BS, Kim NI. The prevalence and types of androgenetic alopecia in Korean men and women. *Br J Dermatol*. 2001;145(1):95-99.

135. Redler S, Brockschmidt FF, Tazi-Ahnini R, et al. Investigation of the male pattern baldness major genetic susceptibility loci AR/EDA2R and 20p11 in female pattern hair loss. *Br J Dermatol*. 2012;166(6):1314-1318.

136. Calvo RM, Asunción M, Sancho J, San Millán JL, Escobar-Morreale HF. The role of the CAG repeat polymorphism in the androgen receptor gene and of skewed X-chromosome inactivation, in the pathogenesis of hirsutism. *J Clin Endocrinol Metab*. 2000;85(4):1735-1740.

137. Weintrob N, Eyal O, Slakman M, et al. The effect of CAG repeats length on differences in hirsutism among healthy Israeli women of different ethnicities. *PLoS One*. 2018;13(3):e0195046.

138. Gatherwright J, Liu MT, Gliniak C, Totonchi A, Guyuron B. The contribution of endogenous and exogenous factors to female alopecia: a study of identical twins. *Plast Reconstr Surg*. 2012;130(6):1219-1226.

139. Arias-Santiago S, Gutiérrez-Salmerón MT, Buendía-Eisman A, Girón-Prieto MS, Naranjo-Sintes R. Hypertension and aldosterone levels in women with early-onset androgenetic alopecia. *Br J Dermatol*. 2009;162(4):786-789.

140. Olsen EA, Messenger AG, Shapiro J, et al. Evaluation and treatment of male and female pattern hair loss. *J Am Acad Dermatol*. 2005;52(2):301-311.

141. Sarfati J, Bachelot A, Coussieu C, Meduri G, Touraine P; Study Group Hyperandrogenism in Postmenopausal Women. Impact of clinical, hormonal, radiological, and immunohistochemical studies on the diagnosis of postmenopausal hyperandrogenism. *Eur J Endocrinol*. 2011;165(5):779-788.

142. Waggoner W, Boots LR, Azziz R. Total testosterone and DHEAS levels as predictors of androgen-secreting neoplasms: a populational study. *Gynecol Endocrinol*. 1999;13(6):394-400.

143. Sperling LC, Cowper SE, Knopp EA. *An Atlas of Hair Pathology With Clinical Correlations*. 2nd ed. Boca Raton, FL: CRC; 2012.

144. Cheruvattath R, Orrego M, Gautam M, et al. Vitamin A toxicity: when one a day doesn't keep the doctor away. *Liver Transpl*. 2006;12(12):1888-1891.

145. Duncan FJ, Silva KA, Johnson CJ, et al. Endogenous retinoids in the pathogenesis of alopecia areata. *J Invest Dermatol*. 2013;133(2):334-343.

146. Holler PD, Cotsarelis G. Retinoids putting the "a" in alopecia. *J Invest Dermatol*. 2013;133(2):285-286.

147. Lucky AW, Piacquadio DJ, Ditre CM, et al. A randomized, placebo-controlled trial of 5% and 2% topical minoxidil solutions in the treatment of female pattern hair loss. *J Am Acad Dermatol*. 2004;50(4):541-553.

148. Goren A, Naccarato T, Situm M, Kovacevic M, Lotti T, McCoy J. Mechanism of action of minoxidil in the treatment of androgenetic alopecia is likely mediated by mitochondrial adenosine triphosphate synthase-induced stem cell differentiation. *J Biol Regul Homeost Agents*. 2017;31(4):1049-1053.

149. Blume-Peytavi U, Hillmann K, Dietz E, Canfield D, Garcia Bartels N. A randomized, single-blind trial of 5% minoxidil foam once daily versus 2% minoxidil solution twice daily in the treatment of androgenetic alopecia in women. *J Am Acad Dermatol*. 2011;65(6):1126-1134.

150. Sinclair R, Wewerinke M, Jolley D. Treatment of female pattern hair loss with oral antiandrogens. *Br J Dermatol*. 2005;152(3):466-473.

151. Scheinfeld N. A review of hormonal therapy for female pattern (androgenic) alopecia. *Dermatol Online J*. 2008;14(3):1.

152. Burova EP. Antiandrogens. In: Wakelin SH, Maibach HI, eds. *Handbook of Systemic Drug Treatment in Dermatology*. London: Thieme; 2002:32-40.

153. Mackenzie IS, Morant SV, Wei L, Thompson AM, MacDonald TM. Spironolactone use and risk of incident cancers: a retrospective, matched cohort study. *Br J Clin Pharmacol*. 2017;83(3):653-663.

154. Biggar RJ, Andersen EW, Wohlfahrt J, Melbye M. Spironolactone use and the risk of breast and gynecologic cancers. *Cancer Epidemiol*. 2013;37(6):870-875.

155. Mackenzie IS, Macdonald TM, Thompson A, Morant S, Wei L. Spironolactone and risk of incident breast cancer in women older than 55 years: retrospective, matched cohort study. *BMJ*. 2012;13;345:e4447.

156. Trüeb RM; Swiss Trichology Study Group. Finasteride treatment of patterned hair loss in normoandrogenic postmenopausal women. *Dermatology*. 2004;209(3):202-207.

157. Mirmirani P. Managing hair loss in midlife women. *Maturitas*. 2013;74(2):119-122.

158. Herskovitz I, Tosti A. Female pattern hair loss. *Int J Endocrinol Metab*. 2013;11(4):e9860.

159. Banaszek A. Company profits from side effects of glaucoma treatment. *CMAJ*. 2011;183(14):E1058.

160. Hugo Perez BS. Ketocazole as an adjunct to finasteride in the treatment of androgenetic alopecia in men. *Med Hypotheses*. 2004;62(1):112-115.

161. Berger RS, Fu JL, Smiles KA, et al. The effects of minoxidil, 1% pyrithione zinc and a combination of both on hair density: a randomized controlled trial. *Br J Dermatol*. 2003;149(2):354-362.

162. Leavitt M, Charles G, Heyman E, Michaels D. HairMax LaserComb laser phototherapy device in the treatment of male androgenetic alopecia: a randomized, double-blind, sham device-controlled, multicentre trial. *Clin Drug Investig*. 2009;29(5):283-292.

163. Jimenez JJ, Wikramanayake TC, Bergfeld W, et al. Efficacy and safety of a low-level laser device in the treatment of male and female pattern hair loss: a multicenter, randomized, sham device-controlled, double-blind study. *Am J Clin Dermatol*. 2014;15(2):115-127.

164. Atanaskova Mesinkovska N, Bergfeld WF. Hair: what is new in diagnosis and management? Female pattern hair loss update: diagnosis and treatment. *Dermatol Clin*. 2013;31(1):119-127.

165. McElwee KJ, Kissling S, Wenzel E, Huth A, Hoffmann R. Cultured peribulbar dermal sheath cells can induce hair follicle development and contribute to the dermal sheath and dermal papilla. *J Invest Dermatol*. 2003;121(6):1267-1275.

166. Takikawa M, Nakamura S, Nakamura S, et al. Enhanced effect of platelet-rich plasma containing a new carrier on hair growth. *Dermatol Surg*. 2011;37(12):1721-1729.

167. Azziz R. The evaluation and management of hirsutism. *Obstet Gynecol*. 2003;101(5 pt 1):995-1007.

168. Barrionuevo P, Nabhan M, Altayar O, et al. Treatment options for hirsutism: a systematic review and network meta-analysis. *J Clin Endocrinol Metab*. 2018;103(4):1258-1264.

169. Spritzer PM, Lisboa KO, Mattiello S, Lhullier F. Spironolactone as a single agent for long-term therapy of hirsute patients. *Clin Endocrinol (Oxf)*. 2000;52(5):587-594.

170. Hovenic W, DeSpain J. Laser hair reduction and removal. *Facial Plast Surg Clin North Am*. 2011;19(2):325-333.

171. Alster TS, Khoury RR. Treatment of laser complications. *Facial Plast Surg*. 2009;25(5):316-323.

172. Rasheed AI. Uncommonly reported side effects of hair removal by long pulsed-alexandrite laser. *J Cosmet Dermatol*. 2009;8(4):267-274.

173. Desai S, Mahmoud BH, Bhatia AC, Hamzavi IH. Paradoxical hypertrichosis after laser therapy: a review. *Dermatol Surg*. 2010;36(3):291-298.

3

Vasomotor Symptoms

Prevalence

Vasomotor symptoms (VMS; hot flashes and night sweats) are the most commonly reported symptoms of the menopause transition. By 2025, an estimated 21 million US women and 1.1 billion women around the world will experience menopause-related VMS.[1] Women's individual experiences of VMS vary, but hot flashes are characterized by a sudden intense sensation of heat in the upper body, particularly the face, neck, and chest. Each hot flash episode typically lasts between 1 and 5 minutes and may be accompanied by perspiration, chills, anxiety, and occasionally, heart palpitations.[2] A *night sweat* refers to a hot flash that occurs during sleep.

A number of established methods are used to assess VMS, from subjective questionnaire-based symptom scales, such as the Greene Climacteric Scale,[3] to physiological measures using skin conductance.[4,5] Subjective symptom scales are the most commonly used, but the prevalence of reported VMS is affected by variations in questions on the frequency and severity of symptoms used in each scale. The responses are also affected by the time frame covered—typically either for VMS experienced over the last 2 weeks or over the last 12 months—the longer time frame tends to result in more symptoms and may be subject to recall bias. Hot flash severity, using FDA categories, are often classified as mild (sensation of heat without sweating), moderate (sensation of heat with sweating, able to continue activity), or severe (sensation of heat with sweating, causing cessation of activity). Such methodologic differences between studies, including in the definitions of menopause status, have introduced variation into estimates of the timing, frequency, and severity of VMS experienced by women across populations.

Pattern of vasomotor symptoms over the menopause transition

The US Study of Women's Health Across the Nation (SWAN), a large cohort study of women transitioning through menopause that included a racially/ethnically diverse sample, found that 60% to 80% of women experience VMS at some point during the menopause transition, with prevalence rates varying by racial/ethnic group.[6,7] In the initial SWAN survey of 16,065 women aged 40 to 55 years, black women reported VMS most frequently (46%), followed by Hispanic (35%), white (31%), Chinese (21%), and Japanese (18%) women.[8] Japanese women were also least likely to describe their symptoms as bothersome.[9] Another study found that black women had a longer duration of VMS than white women.[10]

The various reasons involved in these differences remain unclear, including the influence of cultural variations in how women perceive and report VMS. In SWAN, however, after controlling for key covariates such as body weight and smoking, racial/ethnic differences in VMS persisted.[6,7]

The prevalence of VMS changes throughout the menopause transition.[11] A systematic international review of studies found that the percentage of women who reported hot flashes increased from around 21% in premenopause to 41% during perimenopause and remained at 42% postmenopause.[12] A similar pattern is seen in other studies, with 20% to 40% of premenopausal women reporting VMS, increasing to 60% to 80% of women in perimenopause and through to postmenopause, with variations across racial/ethnic groups.[6,13]

43

The duration of VMS is longer than previously believed. The Penn Ovarian Aging Study found that women experience moderate to severe VMS for a median of 10 years.[10] In SWAN, women reported frequent VMS for a median of 7 years and 4.5 years after the final menstrual period.[14] Most black women have these symptoms for more than a decade. In both studies, women who began having VMS early in the transition had them the longest.

Women show pronounced variations in the trajectory of symptoms. From a major Australian longitudinal study of more than 5,000 women through the menopause transition, analysis of the probability of experiencing VMS in the past year generated four distinct groups: mild (42% of women), moderate (18%), early severe (11%), and late severe (29%) (Figure).[11] The mild group saw little change in their symptoms, whereas the moderate group peaked within 4 years postmenopause. Women in the early group had the highest probability of VMS just before or at menopause, whereas the late group saw the probability of VMS continue to grow through perimenopause and then peak slowly well into postmenopause, with a clear decline in symptoms occurring more than 7 years after menopause. Other studies have reported similar findings, especially with a distinct group of women who continue to experience severe or frequent VMS many years into postmenopause.[15,16]

Risk factors
Evidence for a wide range of risk factors for VMS has emerged from multiple large-scale prospective studies. For some, the associations persist after controlling for confounding factors, but in most cases, the underlying causes or mechanisms at work still remain unclear.

Socioeconomic factors
Findings from the United Kingdom, Australia, and the United States all show that women with lower educational attainment or lower socioeconomic position report VMS more often than their counterparts with higher education or higher socioeconomic position.[6,17] SWAN also found that women with lower income or who reported difficulty in paying for basics were more likely to report VMS than other women.[6]

Obesity
Obesity was once thought to offer some measure of protection against VMS, given the peripheral conversion of androgens to estrone in adipose tissue. Studies subsequently

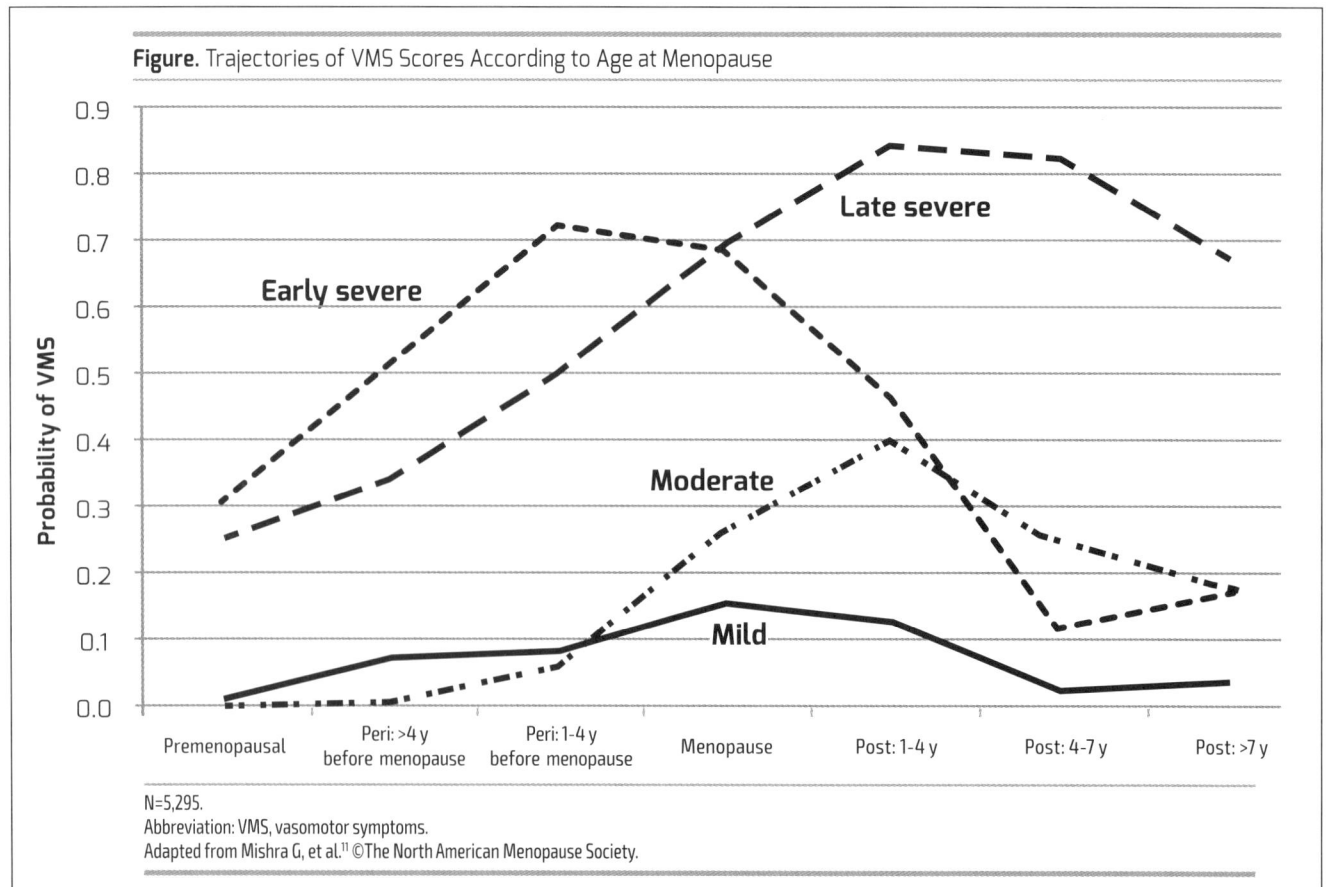

Figure. Trajectories of VMS Scores According to Age at Menopause

Early severe

Late severe

Moderate

Mild

Probability of VMS

Premenopausal | Peri: >4 y before menopause | Peri: 1-4 y before menopause | Menopause | Post: 1-4 y | Post: 4-7 y | Post: >7 y

N=5,295.
Abbreviation: VMS, vasomotor symptoms.
Adapted from Mishra G, et al.[11] ©The North American Menopause Society.

challenged that notion, with a number of studies showing women with a higher body mass index (BMI) more likely to report VMS.[7,18] Furthermore, one meta-analysis found that the women who were obese were nearly twice as likely to experience hot flashes as women with a normal BMI.[19] In a detailed study of a subsample of women from SWAN, it was found that a higher percentage of body fat and abdominal adiposity were linked to increased odds of reporting VMS.[20,21] However, data point to a likely reversal of the direction of the relation between adiposty and VMS by age or menopause stage. Higher adiposity in women who are younger or early in the menopause transiton is associated with increased VMS, whereas higher adiposity when women are older or well into their postmenopause years are associated with decreased VMS.[22-24] Notably, this reversal of the relation between adiposity and VMS over the menopause transition parallels those between adiposity and circulating estadiol.[25]

Health behaviors

Because health behaviors are modifiable and can be included in preventive health initiatives, their potential links with VMS are of considerable interest. For example, cigarette smoking is consistently shown to increase the risk of VMS.[7,26,27] Compared with never smokers, women who were former smokers were 30% more likely to experience VMS, whereas current smokers were almost twice as likely to report them.[27] A dose-response relationship also has been found between pack-years of smoking and increased risk of VMS.[28]

The evidence for associations of other health behaviors and the risk of VMS is both weaker and mixed. Some studies have found that heavy or high-risk drinking is linked with VMS.[26,29,30] In SWAN, alcohol intake and other dietary factors were not associated with VMS after accounting for confounding factors such as education, smoking, and BMI.[31] Conversely, a detailed study of dietary patterns of Australian women found that diets characterized by fruit or Mediterranean-style items were linked with lower risk of VMS, whereas high-fat and high-sugar diets were associated with increased risk.[32]

Physical activity—another key health behavior—also does not show a consistent link with VMS in SWAN and other studies, after adjusting for confounding factors.[7] Although physical activity can have positive benefits for mood and sleep, a systematic review has found that exercise was not an effective treatment for VMS.[33]

Hysterectomy

Vasomotor symptoms tend to be more frequent and severe after hysterectomy or oophorectomy. Specifically, women who have had a hysterectomy with bilateral oophorectomy (both ovaries removed) experienced more frequent and severe menopause symptoms than women who experienced natural menopause.[34] In addition, a prospective study of women in Australia shows that even for those who had a hysterectomy with ovarian conservation (before age 50 y) have a higher risk of experiencing both hot flashes and night sweats that persist for well over a decade.[35]

Vasomotor symptoms and health-related outcomes

Studies on US women have shown a clear effect of VMS on key quality-of-life outcomes, including sleep, mood (depressive symptoms), and cognitive function.[7] Findings from SWAN have associated VMS with all aspects of sleep disturbance related to poor sleep continuity and quality, including falling asleep, staying asleep, and early morning awakening.[36] Findings from InterLACE, a large international collaboration that has combined data from more than 230,000 middle-aged women across 20 cohort and cross-sectional studies,[37] also indicate that women with often/severe VMS at baseline were more likely to have subsequent depressed mood compared with those without VMS, but this association can be largely explained by the difficulty in sleeping.[38] (See also "Sleep Disturbance" in Chapter 5.)

Mounting evidence points to links between VMS and the risk of two main physical health outcomes: cardio-vascular disease (CVD) and poor bone health. Findings from a large meta-analysis show that women with VMS had an unfavorable CVD risk profile (higher systolic and diastolic blood pressures, more adverse circulating total cholesterol profiles, a more insulin-resistant profile) compared with women without VMS.[39-42] Associations with measures of subclinical CVD conditions have been observed in US women.[43,44] Further, studies have found associations for VMS with lower bone mineral density, osteoporosis, and even bone fractures.[45,46]

Etiology

Despite their ubiquity, the precise underlying physiology of VMS remains poorly understood. It is likely that VMS reflect multiple interactive physiologic processes.

Ovarian estrogen

It has long been thought that the declines in ovarian estradiol are likely important to VMS. Whereas all women experience declines in estradiol, not all women experience VMS. Studies find that the correlation between VMS and circulating estradiol levels is modest,[47] yet it is possible that the degree of change in estrogens over the menopause transition is important to VMS. For example, in a study of 204 Melbourne Women's Midlife Health Project participants, a more pronounced change in estradiol over time (steep slope of change in an S-shaped curve) was associated with more severe VMS.[48] However, estrogens alone typically do not explain VMS, and it is clear that other physiologic mechanisms are likely involved.

Thermoregulation

Thermoregulatory models of VMS postulate that they are acute heat-dissipation events occurring in the context of altered thermoregulatory functioning in symptomatic women. According to this model, the thermoneutral zone of menopausal women is narrowed, and small perturbations in body temperature, particularly over this zone, trigger an acute heat-dissipation event in the form of a hot flash.[49] Heat-dissipation responses are controlled in humans by the medial preoptic area of the hypothalamus, with effectors including cutaneous vessels for vasodilation and vasoconstriction.[50] Therefore, a dysfunction in thermoregulation in the hypothalamic control center, its messengers (adrenergic neurons controlling vasoconstriction and cholinergic neurons controlling vasodilation), or the effectors (cutaneous vessels) may underlie VMS. Early evidence for this model comes from a series of laboratory and field studies.[51]

Kisspeptin-neurokinin B-dynorphin

Vasomotor symptoms likely originate centrally, reflecting alterations in hypothalamic thermoregulatory processes.[51] It is well accepted that menopause is associated with increased hypothalamic gonadotropin-releasing hormone (GnRH) secretion, resulting in high gonadotropin (eg, follicle-stimulating hormone) concentrations. Neurokinin B, a neuropeptide found in the hypothalamic infundibular nucleus, is a key proximate regulator of GnRH secretion. Neurokinin B is part of the same functional neuron network that also secretes neuropeptide kisspeptin and the opioid dynorphin; together they are called kisspeptin-neurokinin B-dynorphin (KNDy) neurons.[52] KNDy neurons project to the median preoptic nucleus,[53] the key hypothalamic site of thermoregulatory neuronal pathways.

Postmortem studies have shown hypertrophy of these KNDy neurons in postmenopausal women, with expression of estrogen receptor-α messenger RNA but not GnRH messenger RNA.[54] There is also evidence of increased neurokinin B and kisspeptin gene expression without neuron loss.[52] Similar changes are observed in comparable brain structures with ovariectomy of young monkeys.[55] KNDy neurons express estrogen receptor-α and are responsive to estrogen.[56] In monkeys, estrogen suppressed neurokinin B and kisspeptin expression.[57] These findings suggest that increased neurokinin B gene expression in the hypothalamus in women is secondary to estrogen withdrawal.

Further evidence comes from rodent studies. Rats use their tails as their main effector of thermoregulation; therefore, measures of tail skin temperature and vasodilation have been used as animal models of VMS. Ovariectomized rats without estrogen replacement show a shift in the thermoneutral zone,[58] similar to that demonstrated in postmenopausal women.[59]

Studies have demonstrated increased tail skin temperature in rats with central administration of kisspeptin[60] and increased tail vasodilation with senktide (a neurokinin B agonist) injected directly into the median preoptic nucleus.[61] Conversely, selective KNDy neuron ablation results in reduced cutaneous vasodilation and responsiveness to estrogen.[62]

Further data come from humans. In an observational study of 17,695 postmenopausal women participating in the Women's Health Initiative, genetic variation in the tachykinin receptor 3 (TACR3) locus was associated with higher likelihood of having VMS.[63] Notably, TACR3 encodes the neurokinin 3 receptor, the preferred binding site for neurokinin B. Finally, data have demonstrated induction of VMS in healthy premenopausal women with administration of neurokinin B[64] and amelioration of VMS in healthy postmenopausal women with a neurokinin B antagonist.[65] Thus, there is accumulating evidence that KNDy neurons are involved in thermoregulation and VMS.

Serotonin

Serotonin may play a role in VMS. Selective serotonin-reuptake inhibitors (SSRIs) designed to increase the available serotonin at the serotonergic synapse have been shown in placebo-controlled trials to have some efficacy in reducing the number and severity of VMS.[66] Serotonin, involved in mood, anxiety, sleep, and sexual behavior, is thought to play a key role in thermoregulation.

Early animal studies suggested that increases in hypothalamic release of serotonin resulted in an increase in body temperature and that control of core temperature was as a result of fine balance of serotonin receptor 5-HT, epinephrine, and norepinephrine.[67,68]

A series of subsequent studies demonstrated the importance of the serotonin receptor subtypes 5-HT1A and 5-HT2A to thermoregulation.[69-71] For example, direct stimulation of the 5-HT2A receptor can induce hyperthermia in rodents,[72] and peripheral administration of 5-HT1A agonists to humans and rodents can reduce core body temperature, which can be blocked by 5-HT1A antagonists.[73] However, the precise involvement of 5-HT and its receptors in the physiology of VMS is not well understood. Several theories have been proposed,[74] but the role of serotonin in central regulatory pathways is complex, and further study regarding the role of 5-HT and its receptors in VMS is required.

Peripheral autonomic and central adrenergic nervous system

Several lines of work underscore the importance of the autonomic nervous system, which includes sympathetic and parasympathetic branches, to VMS. Early studies implicated the monoamine norepinephrine in the manipulation of central thermoregulatory function and VMS. Animal studies indicated that intrahypothalamic injection of norepinephrine can narrow the thermoregulatory zone. Some evidence in humans indicated that in symptomatic postmenopausal women, VMS could be provoked with the α2-adrenergic antagonist yohimbine and ameliorated with the α-adrenergic agonist clonidine; these agents may act to modify the thermoneutral zone.[59,75]

Other studies have emphasized the importance of sympathetic adrenergic vasoconstrictor nerves, and sympathetic vasodilator nerves control the cutaneous circulation, which plays an important role in thermoregulation and potentially VMS. Sympathetic vasoconstrictor nerves release norepinephrine, which interacts with postsynaptic α1- and α2-receptors on cutaneous arterioles. In a thermoneutral environment, there is tonic activation of the vasoconstrictor system. Large increases in skin blood flow, such as with health loss, are mediated primarily (80-90%) by activation of sympathetic vasodilator nerves in the skin.[50]

Early studies indicated increased blood flow to the forearm and hand during a hot flash[76] and a diminished vasoconstrictor response to cold in women with VMS.[77] In studies measuring skin blood flow using laser Doppler imaging with iontophoresis, women with severe VMS had increased skin blood flow compared with their matched contemporaries with no VMS.[78] Other studies further underscored the importance of alterations in sympathetic nerve activity to the skin in VMS-associated alterations in skin blood flow.[79]

Autonomic control of cardiac function has also been implicated in the etiology of VMS. Significant decreases in cardiac vagal (parasympathetic) control acutely during the VMS have been observed both in laboratory and ambulatory studies.[80,81] Changes in cardiac vagal control have also been observed with VMS during wake and sleep, even in women not aware of their VMS.[82]

Other central nervous system processes

Other central nervous system processes have been implicated in VMS. Functional neuroimaging has demonstrated a rise in brainstem activity preceding the detectable onset of a hot flash, followed by activity in the insula and prefrontal cortices.[83,84] These data suggest that pre-VMS brainstem activity may reflect the functional origins of VMS and activity in the insula and prefrontal cortices, the phenomenologic correlates of VMS. Thus, alterations in brain activity is observed acutely during the hot flash episode.

Other work has compared indices of brain health in women with various levels of VMS frequency. These studies suggest that more physiologically measured VMS have been associated with greater default mode network connectivity, particularly networks supporting the hippocampus.[85] The default mode network is a network of brain regions that are active during rest in the absence of external stimuli, hyperactivity of which is characteristic of major depressive disorder and other psychiatric conditions. Initial work links more physiologically measured VMS during sleep with greater white matter hyperintensities,[86] an indicator of brain small vessel disease linked to future stroke, cognitive decline, and dementia.[87] Therefore, there may be a link between VMS and brain health, although the mechanism remains to be elucidated.

Additional physiologic processes

Several other physiologic changes have been observed in conjunction with VMS. However, whether these processes are part of the physiology of VMS, are a correlate of VMS, or are a consequence of VMS remain to be clarified.

Hypothalamic-pituitary-adrenal axis

It has been suggested that VMS may be associated with cortisol and dysregulated function of the hypothalamic-pituitary-adrenal axis. Notably, hypothalamic-pituitary-adrenal axis dysregulation is a feature of a range of acute and chronic stress conditions. In the Seattle Midlife Women's Health Study, overnight urinary cortisol levels were found to increase during the late perimenopause and were highest in women with more severe VMS.[88] Others using small samples support an acute cortisol response to VMS in symptomatic women.[30,89] A study of midlife women demonstrated that a higher frequency of VMS with higher hair cortisol and more severe and bothersome VMS were associated with a flatter diurnal cortisol slope.[90] However, findings of a link between VMS and cortisol are mixed,[91] requiring more rigorous investigation.

Endothelial dysfunction

Endothelial injury and dysfunction is an initiating event in atherosclerosis and a significant predictor of cardiovascular events.[92] In the SWAN Heart Study, a reduced brachial artery flow-mediated dilation was found, indicating poorer endothelial function in women with VMS relative to women without VMS, controlling for CVD risk factors and endogenous estradiol.[43] Another study similarly demonstrated that severity of VMS was the most important independent predictor of endothelial dysfunction in this group of midlife women.[93] Further, altered arterial blood flow in women with VMS has been found.[94] In two other studies, one of which used physiologic measures of VMS, VMS early in the menopause transition were associated with poorer endothelial function.[95,96] Conversely, *greater* subcutaneous vessel response to endothelial dependent and independent vasodilation agents in women with VMS was found.[78] Thus, VMS, particularly when occurring early in the menopause transition, may be accompanied by altered vascular and particularly endothelial function, but further research is merited.

Inflammation and clotting

Several other studies have linked VMS to a more proinflammatory or procoagulant profile. Several studies have linked VMS to adverse alterations in the inflammatory cascade, such as IL-8 and tumor necrosis factor-a.[97,98] In SWAN, women who reported VMS were found to have a more procoagulant profile (higher Factor VIIc, tPA-ag).[99] Other studies report no significant relationship between VMS and proinflammatory cytokines.[100,101] Data on the effects of VMS on systemic inflammation and clotting warrant further study.

The precise underlying physiology of VMS has not yet been fully identified and likely involves a complex interplay between central nervous system and peripheral physiologic processes. There have been notable advances in the understanding of the likely neurobiology of VMS. As this work continues, a more complete understanding of the physiology of VMS can be leveraged to inform new, promising treatments for this common menopause symptom.

Treatment

Most women will experience VMS at some point during the menopause transition. However, historically, menopause-related VMS were trivialized, ridiculed, attributed to emotional instability and insanity, and responsible for broken family relations.[102] Some people continue to question whether VMS are real,[103] even though scientists have objectively measured them with physiological monitoring devices since the late 1970s.[104] These issues are compounded by the fact that their underlying physiology is not fully understood. (See also "Etiology" in this chapter.)

Severe symptoms may continue to be undertreated. In the early 2000s, hormone therapy (HT) use drastically declined after new data on its risks were published.[105] However, healthcare providers are now being encouraged to prescribe HT on the basis of individual patient needs.[106] In developing countries, undertreatment of severe symptoms may be a bigger issue. For example, in a 2016 population-based survey of more than 1,500 Bangladeshi women, none were taking prescription therapies for their VMS,[107] although many prescription therapies are known to be efficacious.

Confusion about menopause and proven treatments for VMS are persistent problems for healthcare providers, women, and their partners.[106,108,109] Confusion is likely exacerbated by inadequate amounts of understandable, culturally appropriate, and accurate information.[108,110] A study of healthcare providers found that 81% of 100 physicians-in-training (residents) reported having limited training in menopause medicine, and 50% reported low comfort with managing menopause symptoms.[111] Communication about nonhormone treatment is often inadequate as well,[112] and gynecologists and primary care providers say misunderstandings from confusing messages about menopause are the most difficult part of communicating with menopausal women.[113]

Prescription therapies

Hormone therapy

Hormone therapy is FDA approved as first-line therapy for relief of VMS. Hormone therapy includes estrogen therapy (ET), estrogen-progestogen therapy (EPT), and estrogen-receptor agonists and antagonists (ERAAs). In women with a uterus, EPT or conjugated equine estrogens plus bazedoxifene (an ERAA) should be used to provide endometrial protection. When FDA-approved estrogen therapy trials were subjected to meta-analysis, there were no significant differences in effectiveness between estradiol and conjugated equine estrogens for VMS.[106] However, estradiol showed more robust effects on anxiety and depressive symptoms and therefore may provide additional benefits in multisymptomatic women. (See also Chapter 9, "Prescription Therapies.")

Estrogen alone or combined with progestogen reduces VMS frequency by 75% and significantly reduces VMS severity. Progestogens alone are also effective in treating VMS, but there are no long-term safety data available. A 3-month study showed no clinically significant effects on cardiovascular health of oral micronized progesterone 300 mg per day.[114]

In another RCT, oral micronized progesterone 300 mg per day was significantly more efficacious than placebo in reducing VMS frequency and VMS severity after 4 and 8 weeks of treatment.[115] Discontinuation because of AEs affected 11% of the progesterone group and 7% of the placebo group.

The lowest, most-effective dose of HT should be used and may take 6 or more weeks to take effect. About 50% of women will experience a return of VMS when HT is discontinued. Compounded hormones are not recommended because of safety concerns, unless a woman cannot tolerate other hormone therapies.

Paroxetine

Paroxetine is an SSRI commonly used to manage depression.[116] It is the only nonhormone medication approved by FDA for reducing VMS. Paroxetine salt 7.5 mg or paroxetine 10 mg to 25 mg per day has sustained benefits in reducing VMS for up to 24 weeks,[117,118] reduces VMS-related sleep problems,[119,120] and is generally very well tolerated.

The efficacy of paroxetine for VMS has been demonstrated in several studies.[116,121] An additional trial done in 80 survivors of gynecologic cancer who had completed postcancer treatment showed that paroxetine significantly reduced VMS frequency and severity after 4 and 16 weeks of treatment and nighttime awakenings caused by VMS at 16 weeks.[120] It was well tolerated, with no serious adverse events (AEs).

Paroxetine may have use in helping women reduce VMS-associated sleep problems. In a pooled report combining two studies of postmenopausal women with moderate to severe VMS, paroxetine significantly reduced hot flash-related nighttime awakenings and increased the numbers of hours of sleep (sleep duration) by week 4 compared with placebo.[119] Benefits for nighttime awakenings were sustained through 12 or 24 weeks of treatment. (See also "Sleep Disturbance" in Chapter 5.)

Other selective serotonin-reuptake inhibitors and serotonin norepinephrine-reuptake inhibitors

There is evidence for the efficacy of other SSRIs and serotonin norepinephrine-reuptake inhibitors (SNRIs) for reducing VMS. Large randomized, controlled trials (RCTs) show that daily doses of citalopram (10-20 mg), escitalopram (10-20 mg), desvenlafaxine (100-150 mg), and venlafaxine (37.5-150 mg) reduce hot flash frequency and severity.[122-125]

Using data from 899 symptomatic women, a pooled analysis of individual-level data showed that after 8 weeks of treatment, escitalopram (10-20 mg), venlafaxine (75 mg), and low-dose 17-β estradiol (0.5 mg) were all effective and comparable in reducing hot flash frequency (1.4 VMS/d; 1.8 VMS/d; and 2.4 VMS/d, respectively).[126]

On the basis of these studies, SSRIs and SNRIs look to be effective for relief of VMS. The efficacy and toxicity of an SSRI/SNRI may vary on the basis of a woman's pharmacogenetic profile,[127] but such genomic profiling may not be widely available.

Gabapentinoids

Evidence from large RCTs shows that gabapentin (600-2,400 mg) reduces VMS.[128-131] An RCT of 79 Iranian women were randomized to receive gabapentin 300 mg per day for 4 weeks followed by fluoxetine 20 mg per day for an additional 4 weeks or fluoxetine, then gabapentin.[132] Each 4-week intervention period was followed by a 2-week washout period. Compared with fluoxetine, gabapentin demonstrated greater reductions in Greene Climacteric scale hot flash severity (55-68% vs 20-23%) and night sweat severity (56-62% vs 18-41%). Adverse events were tremors with gabapentin (n=4) and lack of appetite with fluoxetine (n=3). This study did not include asssement with a hot flash diary as reported in most other trials.

Clonidine

There is evidence that clonidine reduces VMS.[66,133] It is the only nonhormone medication approved for VMS in the United Kingdom[134]; however, it is not as effective as other medications and is associated with AEs, including hypertension when abruptly stopped, hypotension with consistent use, lightheadedness, headaches, dry mouth, dizziness, sedation, and constipation.[133]

Oxybutynin

Oxybutynin is FDA approved for the treatment of overactive bladder. It is an anticholinergic and antimuscarinic. In an RCT, 15 mg oxybutynin extended release was efficacious in reducing VMS frequency and severity after 1 week of treatment and through the end of 12 weeks of treatment.[135] More than 50% of treated women reported dry mouth. Additional studies perhaps with lower doses may be warranted.

Neurokinin B antagonists

A newer class of agents, neurokinin B antagonists, have shown some promise in reducing VMS in healthy postmenopausal women,[65] yet these agents remain in experimental stages and are not yet available for widespread clinical use.

Nonprescription therapies

Nonprescription therapies for the treatment of VMS range from mind-body techniques, lifestyle changes, and dietary management and supplements to other therapies and approaches.

Cognitive-behavioral therapy

Cognitive-behavioral therapy is one of two mind-body techniques that has evidence for efficacy in alleviating VMS. Two rigorous RCTs showed it to be effective in helping survivors of breast cancer and perimenopausal and postmenopausal women without cancer to manage their VMS.[136,137] The intervention was effective when delivered in group as well as self-help formats. The intervention had additional benefits in mood, quality of life, and overall functioning.

Clinical hypnosis

Clinical hypnosis is another mind-body technique that has been shown to alleviate VMS. Two rigorous RCTs showed it to be effective in reducing VMS in survivors of breast cancer and in postmenopausal women.[138,139] It was shown to reduce self-reported and physiologically recorded VMS. In other work, postmenopausal women (N=71) were randomized in factorial fashion to venlafaxine plus hypnosis, placebo plus hypnosis, venlafaxine plus sham hypnosis, or placebo plus sham hypnosis.[140] Results indicated that clinical hypnosis was comparable to venlafaxine alone in terms of magnitude of effect, but the combination did not additively decrease VMS more than either treatment alone.

Mindfulness-based stress reduction

Mindfulness-based stress reduction focuses on decreasing stress through nonreactive acceptance and mindfulness of thoughts and feelings, as well as gentle yoga stretching. Evidence for managing VMS comes from one single, randomized trial in which standard mindfulness-based stress reduction training (weekly group classes, at-home practice, a daylong retreat) showed some initial efficacy in reducing the bother associated with hot flashes compared with wait-list control, yet findings from this initial study were weak, and greater research with an active control group is needed.[141] Although this intervention did improve quality of life, ratings of sleep quality, anxiety, and perceived stress, additional trials are needed to further evaluate this therapy for the management of VMS.

Weight loss

Weight loss has not yet been conclusively demonstrated to reduce VMS. Existing evidence suggesting some benefit from weight loss on VMS comes from pilot studies or trials not designed to test this question.[142-145] Some data indicate that weight loss may be most effective for managing VMS in women earlier in the menopause transition,[145] consistent with observations that higher adiposity is associated with greater VMS primarily early in the transition.[23,24] Additional trials of weight loss with VMS as a primary outcome are needed to generate evidence for or against this therapy. (See also "Body Weight" in Chapter 2.)

Physical activity/Exercise

Randomized, controlled trials have found no evidence to support use of exercise or physical activity intervention for VMS, although exercise has many other beneficial effects for health.[146,147]

Yoga

There is not robust support for the use of yoga for relieving VMS. For example, in an RCT of 249 women reporting at least 14 VMS per week, women were randomized to 12 weeks of yoga that included weekly 90-minute in-person classes (breathing exercises, 11-13 yoga poses, and 20 min of relaxation in the form of Yoga Nidra) and a recommended 20-minute home daily practice or usual activity in which they were instructed to follow their usual routine.[148] In this study, yoga did not reduce the frequency of VMS relative to the control group, yet it did reduce the number of insomnia symptoms.

Paced respiration

Paced respiration, or slow deep breathing, involves inhaling six to eight breaths per minute in through the nose and out through the mouth. Although small studies done under controlled laboratory conditions suggested that it reduced VMS,[149] larger studies do not show any benefit over other forms of breathing.[140,151]

S-equol derivatives of soy isoflavones

Soy foods and extracts, including s-equol and other derivatives and metabolites, have received a great deal of attention. However, many studies have not used robust designs and have not studied differences in efficacy between those able and not able to convert soy to s-equol (or other derivatives). Only about two-thirds of North American women are able to convert the soy isoflavone daidzein to s-equol. Products containing s-equol are one way to address the issue of conversion. Women with known allergies or intolerances to soy products should avoid this therapy. Evidence supporting the use of s-equol derivatives is mixed. A meta-analysis indicates that these studies may not have been conducted long enough because soy products may require 48 weeks (nearly a year) to reach full effect or 13 weeks to reach half effect.[152] A limitation of the meta-analysis was that it did not differentiate between different soy products or their derivatives or metabolites.[153,154]

Other over-the-counter supplements and herbal therapies

Multiple studies of therapies such as black cohosh, crinum, dioscorea, dong quai, evening primrose, flaxseed, ginseng and Siberian ginseng, hops, maca, omega-3s, pine bark, pollen extract, puerperia, and vitamin supplementation show that they are all unlikely to alleviate VMS. A Cochrane review noted that there is insufficient evidence for Chinese herbal medicine for VMS as well.[155] Other studies show that certain other vitamin and mineral supplements are no more effective than placebo in reducing VMS.[156-158] (See also Chapter 8, "Vitamins, Minerals, and Other Dietary Supplements.")

Stellate ganglion block

Stellate ganglion block, an injection of local anesthetic into the stellate ganglion sympathetic nerves typically used for pain management, can be used for treatment of VMS with caution. There is some evidence from a small randomized trial that stellate ganglion block may have some efficacy in reducing objectively measured VMS,[159] which may in turn benefit cognitive function,[160] but further data from larger randomized trials are needed to fully evaluate the utility of this approach for reducing VMS.

Acupuncture

Acupuncture has not been shown to be effective in reducing VMS when tested in RCTs with adequate controls. One review article falsely summarized evidence as positive when it was in fact equivocal,[161] and a 2016 meta-analysis of seven RCTs done in 342 survivors of breast cancer concluded that acupuncture was no more effective than sham acupuncture for VMS.[162] A notable randomized trial of 327 Australian women with seven or more moderate to severe VMS per day showed no differences between acupuncture and sham acupuncture at the end of treatment or at 3 or 6 months of follow-up.[163]

Other approaches

Women often attempt a range of techniques to manage their hot flashes, including avoiding their triggers of VMS or using cooling techniques such as dressing in layers, using breathable natural fiber clothing, and use of fans and cold packs, but these approaches do not have empirical evidence as to their efficacy. A randomized, controlled pilot study of 40 Canadian women reporting seven or more moderate to severe VMS per day were randomized to an active skin cooling device or a sham device.[164] Study results suggest that this device may merit further study in a larger, fully powered trial, but at this time, there was insufficient evidence for use of cooling techniques for VMS. Other approaches such as acupressure,[165] calibration of neural oscillations,[166] or foot reflexology[167] have received some attention for managing VMS, but evidence for their efficacy is limited, and they cannot be recommended at this time.

REFERENCES

1. World Health Organization. *Women, Ageing and Health : A Framework for Action. Focus on Gender*. Geneva, Switzerland: World Health Organization; 2007. www.who.int/ageing/publications/Women-ageing-health-lowres.pdf. Accessed February 28, 2019.

2. Kronenberg F. Hot flashes: epidemiology and physiology. *Ann N Y Acad Sci*. 1990;592:52-86.

3. Greene JG. A factor analytic study of climacteric symptoms. *J Psychosom Res*. 1976;20(5):425-430.

4. Carpenter JS, Andrykowski MA, Freedman RR, Munn R. Feasibility and psychometrics of an ambulatory hot flash monitoring device. *Menopause*. 1999;6(3):209-215.

5. Fisher WI, Thurston RC. Hot flashes: phenomenology and measurement. In: Sievert LL, Brown DE, eds. *Biological Measures of Human Experience Across the Lifespan: Making Visible the Invisible*. Switzerland: Springer;233-254.

6. Gold EB, Colvin A, Avis N, et al. Longitudinal analysis of the association between VMS and race/ethnicity across the menopausal transition: Study of Women's Health Across the Nation. *Am J Public Health.* 2006;96(7):1226-1235.

7. Thurston RC, Joffe H. Vasomotor symptoms and menopause: findings from the Study of Women's Health Across the Nation. *Obstet Gynecol Clin North Am.* 2011;38(3):489-501.

8. Gold EB, Sternfeld B, Kelsey JL, et al. Relation of demographic and lifestyle factors to symptoms in a multi-racial/ethnic population of women 40-55 years of age. *Am J Epidemiol.* 2000;152(5):463-473.

9. Thurston RC, Bromberger JT, Joffe H, et al. Beyond frequency: who is most bothered by VMS? *Menopause.* 2008;15(5):841-847.

10. Freeman EW, Sammel MD, Lin H, Liu Z, Gracia CR. Duration of menopausal hot flushes and associated risk factors. *Obstet Gynecol.* 2011;117(5):1095-1104.

11. Mishra GD, Dobson AJ. Using longitudinal profiles to characterize women's symptoms through midlife: results from a large prospective study. *Menopause.* 2012;19(5):549-555.

12. Freeman EW, Sherif K. Prevalence of hot flushes and night sweats around the world: a systematic review. *Climacteric.* 2007;10(3):197-214.

13. Politi MC, Schleinitz MD, Col NF. Revisiting the duration of VMS of menopause: a meta-analysis. *J Gen Intern Med.* 2008;23(9):1507-1513.

14. Avis NE, Crawford SL, Greendale G, et al; Study of Women's Health Across the Nation. Duration of menopausal VMS over the menopause transition. *JAMA Intern Med.* 2015;175(4):531-539.

15. Mishra GD, Kuh D. Health symptoms during midlife in relation to menopausal transition: British prospective cohort study. *BMJ.* 2012;344:e402.

16. Tepper PG, Brooks MM, Randolph JF Jr, et al. Characterizing the trajectories of VMS across the menopausal transition. *Menopause.* 2016; 23(10): 1067-1074.

17. Sievert LL, Obermeyer CM, Price K. Determinants of hot flashes and night sweats. *Ann Hum Biol.* 2006;33(1):4-16.

18. Maggio Da Fonseca A, Bagnoli V R, Souza M A, et al. Impact of age and body mass on the intensity of menopausal symptoms in 5968 Brazilian women. *Gynecol Endocrinol.* 2013;29(2):116-118.

19. Shobeiri F, Jenabi E, Poorolajal J, Hazavehei SM. The association between body mass index and hot flash in midlife women: a meta-analysis. *J Menopausal Med.* 2016;22(1):14-19.

20. Thurston RC, Sowers MR, Chang Y, et al. Adiposity and reporting of VMS among midlife women: the Study of Women's Health Across the Nation. *Am J Epidemiol.* 2008;167(1):78-85.

21. Thurston RC, Sowers MR, Sutton-Tyrrell K, et al. Abdominal adiposity and hot flashes among midlife women. *Menopause.* 2008;15(3):429-434.

22. Thurston RC, Santoro N, Matthews KA. Adiposity and hot flashes in midlife women: a modifying role of age. *J Clin Endocrinol Metab.* 2011;96(10):E1588-E1595.

23. Gold EB, Crawford SL, Shelton JF, et al. Longitudinal analysis of changes in weight and waist circumference in relation to incident VMS: the Study of Women's Health Across the Nation (SWAN). *Menopause.* 2017;24(1):9-26.

24. Thurston RC, Chang Y, Mancuso P, Matthews KA. Adipokines, adiposity, and VMS during the menopause transition: findings from the Study of Women's Health Across the Nation. *Fertil Steril.* 2013;100(3):793-800.

25. Randolph JF Jr, Sowers M, Bondarenko IV, Harlow SD, Luborsky JL, Little RJ. Change in estradiol and follicle-stimulating hormone across the early menopausal transition: effects of ethnicity and age. *J Clin Endocrinol Metab.* 2004;89(4):1555-1561.

26. Herber-Gast GC, Mishra GD, van der Schouw YT, Brown WJ, Dobson AJ. Risk factors for night sweats and hot flushes in midlife: results from a prospective cohort study. *Menopause.* 2013;20(9):953-959.

27. Jenabi E, Poorolajal J. The association between hot flushes and smoking in midlife women: a meta-analysis. *Climacteric.* 2015;18(6):797-801.

28. Staropoli CA, Flaws JA, Bush TL, Moulton AW. Predictors of menopausal hot flashes. *J Womens Health.* 1998;7(9):1149-1155.

29. Freeman EW, Sammel MD, Grisso JA, Battistini M, Garcia-Espagna B, Hollander L. Hot flashes in the late reproductive years: risk factors for African American and Caucasian women. *J Womens Health Gend Based Med.* 2001;10(1):67-76.

30. Sievert LL. Subjective and objective measures of hot flashes. *Am J Hum Biol.* 2013;25(5):573-580.

31. Gold EB, Block G, Crawford S, et al. Lifestyle and demographic factors in relation to VMS: baseline results from the Study of Women's Health Across the Nation. *Am J Epidemiol.* 2004;159(12):1189-1199.

32. Herber-Gast GC, Mishra GD. Fruit, Mediterranean-style, and high-fat and -sugar diets are associated with the risk of night sweats and hot flushes in midlife: results from a prospective cohort study. *Am J Clin Nutr.* 2013;97(5):1092-1099.

33. Daley A, Stokes-Lampard H, Thomas A, MacArthur C. Exercise for vasomotor menopausal symptoms. *Cochrane Database Syst Rev.* 2014;(11):CD006108.

34. Sarrel PM, Sullivan SD, Nelson LM. Hormone replacement therapy in young women with surgical primary ovarian insufficiency. *Fertil Steril.* 2016;106(7):1580-1587.

35. Wilson LF, Pandeya N, Byles J, Mishra GD. Hot flushes and night sweats symptom profiles over a 17-year period in mid-aged women: the role of hysterectomy with ovarian conservation. *Maturitas.* 2016;91:1-7.

36. Kravitz HM, Zhao X, Bromberger JT, et al. Sleep disturbance during the menopausal transition in a multi-ethnic community sample of women. *Sleep.* 2008;31(7):979-990.

37. Mishra GD, Chung HF, Pandeya N, et al. The InterLACE study: design, data harmonization and characteristics across 20 studies on women's health. *Maturitas.* 2016;92:176-185.

38. Chung HF, Pandeya N, Dobson AJ, et al. The role of sleep difficulties in the vasomotor menopausal symptoms and depressed mood relationships: an international pooled analysis of eight studies in the InterLACE consortium. *Psychol Med.* 2018;12:1-12.

39. Franco OH, Muka T, Colpani V, et al. Vasomotor symptoms in women and cardiovascular risk markers: systematic review and meta-analysis. *Maturitas.* 2015;81(3):353-361.

40. Thurston RC, El Khoudary SR, Sutton-Tyrrell K, et al. Vasomotor symptoms and insulin resistance in the Study of Women's Health Across the Nation. *J Clin Endocrinol Metab.* 2012;97(10):3487-3494.

41. Thurston RC, El Khoudary SR, Sutton-Tyrrell K, et al. Vasomotor symptoms and lipid profiles in women transitioning through menopause. *Obstet Gynecol.* 2012;119(4):753-761.

42. Jackson EA, El Khoudary SR, Crawford SL, et al. Hot flash frequency and blood pressure: data from the Study of Women's Health Across the Nation. *J Womens Health (Larchmt).* 2016;25(12):1204-1209.

43. Thurston RC, Sutton-Tyrrell K, Everson-Rose SA, Hess R, Matthews KA. Hot flashes and subclinical cardiovascular disease: findings from the Study of Women's Health Across the Nation Heart Study. *Circulation.* 2008;118(12):1234-1240.

44. Thurston RC, Chang Y, Barinas-Mitchell E, et al. Menopausal hot flashes and carotid intima media thickness among midlife women. *Stroke.* 2016;47(12):2910-2915.

45. Gast GC, Grobbee DE, Pop VJ, et al. Vasomotor symptoms are associated with a lower bone mineral density. *Menopause.* 2009;16(2):231-238.

46. Crandall CJ, Aragaki A, Cauley JA, et al. Associations of menopausal VMS with fracture incidence. *J Clin Endocrinol Metab.* 2015;100(2):524-534.

47. Randolph JF Jr, Sowers M, Bondarenko I, et al. The relationship of longitudinal change in reproductive hormones and VMS during the menopausal transition. *J Clin Endocrinol Metab.* 2005;90(11):6106-6112.

48. Dennerstein L, Lehert P, Burger HG, Guthrie JR. New findings from non-linear longitudinal modelling of menopausal hormone changes. *Hum Reprod Update.* 2007;13(6):551-557.

49. Freedman RR. Menopausal hot flashes, mechanisms, endocrinology, treatment. *J Steroid Biochem Mol Biol*. 2014;142:115-120.

50. Charkoudian N. Skin blood flow in adult human thermoregulation: how it works, when it does not, and why. *Mayo Clin Proc*. 2003;78(5):603-612.

51. Freedman RR, Krell W. Reduced thermoregulatory null zone in postmenopausal women with hot flashes. *Am J Obstet Gynecol*. 1999;181(1):66-70.

52. Skorupskaite K, George JT, Anderson RA. The kisspeptin-GnRH pathway in human reproductive health and disease. *Hum Reprod Update*. 2014;20(4):485-500.

53. Krajewski SJ, Burke MC, Anderson MJ, McMullen NT, Rance NE. Forebrain projections of arcuate neurokinin B neurons demonstrated by anterograde tract-tracing and monosodium glutamate lesions in the rat. *Neuroscience*. 2010;166(2):680-697.

54. Rance NE, McMullen NT, Smialek JE, Price DL, Young WS 3rd. Postmenopausal hypertrophy of neurons expressing the estrogen receptor gene in the human hypothlalmus. *J Clin Endocrinol Metab*. 1990;71(1):79-85.

55. Rometo AM, Krajewski SJ, Voytko ML, Rance NE. Hypertrophy and increased kisspeptin gene expression in the hypothalamic infundibular nucleus of postmenopausal women and ovariectomized monkeys. *J Clin Endocrinol Metab*. 2007;92(7):2744-2750.

56. Rance NE, Dacks PA, Mittelman-Smith MA, Romanovsky AA, Krajewski-Hall SJ. Modulation of body temperature and LH secretion by hypothalamic KNDy (kisspeptin, neurokinin B and dynorphin) neurons: a novel hypothesis on the mechanism of hot flashes. *Front Neuroendocrinol*. 2013;34(3):211-227.

57. Abel TW, Voytko ML, Rance NE. The effects of hormone replacement therapy on hypothalamic neuropeptide gene expression in a primate model of menopause. *J Clin Endocrinol Metab*. 1999;84(6):2111-2118.

58. Dacks PA, Rance NE. Effects of estradiol on the thermoneutral zone and core temperature in ovariectomized rats. *Endocrinology*. 2010;151(3):1187-1193.

59. Freedman RR, Blacker CM. Estrogen raises the sweating threshold in postmenopausal women with hot flashes. *Fertil Steril*. 2002;77(3):487-490.

60. Kinsey-Jones JS, Li XF, Knox AM, et al. Corticotrophin-releasing factor alters the timing of puberty in the female rat. *J Neuroendocrinol*. 2010;22(2):102-109.

61. Dacks PA, Krajewski SJ, Rance NE. Activation of neurokinin 3 receptors in the median preoptic nucleus decreases core temperature in the rat. *Endocrinology*. 2011;152(12):4894-4905.

62. Mittelman-Smith MA, Williams H, Krajewski-Hall SJ, McMullen NT, Rance NE. Role for kisspeptin/neurokinin B/dynorphin (KNDy) neurons in cutaneous vasodilatation and the estrogen modulation of body temperature. *Proc Natl Acad Sci U S A*. 2012;109(48):19846-19851.

63. Crandall CJ, Manson JE, Hohensee C, et al. Association of genetic variation in the tachykinin receptor 3 locus with hot flashes and night sweats in the Women's Health Initiative Study. *Menopause*. 2017;24(3):252-261.

64. Jayasena CN, Comninos AN, Stefanopoulou E, et al. Neurokinin B administration induces hot flashes in women. *Sci Rep*. 2015;5:8466.

65. Prague JK, Roberts RE, Comninos AN, et al. Neurokinin 3 receptor antagonism as a novel treatment for menopausal hot flushes: a phase 2, randomised, double-blind, placebo-controlled trial. *Lancet*.2017;389(10081):1809-1820.

66. Nelson HD, Vesco KK, Haney E, et al. Nonhormonal therapies for menopausal hot flashes: systematic review and meta-analysis. *JAMA*. 2006;295(17):2057-2071.

67. Feldberg W, Myers RD. A new concept of temperature regulation by amines in the hypothalamus. *Nature*. 1963;200(4913):1325.

68. Sheard MH, Aghajanian GK. Neural release of brain serotonin and body temperature. *Nature*. 1967;216(5114):495-496.

69. Hoyer D, Martin GR. Classification and nomenclature of 5-HT receptors: a comment on current issues. *Behav Brain Res*. 1996;73(1-2):263-268.

70. Blessing WW. 5-hydroxytryptamine 1a receptor activation reduces cutaneous vasoconstriction and fever associated with the acute inflammatory response in rabbits. *Neuroscience*. 2004;123(1):1-4.

71. Rusyniak DE, Zaretskaia MV, Zaretsky DV, DiMicco JA. 3,4-methylenedioxymetamphetamine- and 8-hydroxy-2-di-n-propylamino-tetralin-induced hypothermia: role and location of 5-hydroxytryptamine 1A receptors. *J Pharmacol Exp Ther*. 2007;323(2):477-487.

72. Salmi P, Ahlenius S. Evidence for functional interactions between 5-HT1A and 5-HT2A receptors in rat thermoregulatory mechanisms. *Pharmacol Toxicol*. 1998;82(3):122-127.

73. Cryan JF, Kelliher P, Kelly JP, Leonard BE. Comparative effects of serotonergic agonists with varying efficacy at the 5-HT(1A) receptor on core body temperature: modification by the selective 5-HT(1A) receptor antagonist WAY 100635. *J Psychopharmacol*. 1999;13(3):278-283.

74. Berendsen HH. The role of serotonin in hot flushes. *Maturitas*. 2000;36(3):155-164.

75. Freedman RR, Dinsay R. Clonidine raises the sweating threshold in symptomatic but not in asymptomatic postmenopausal women. *Fertil Steril*. 2000;74(1):20-23.

76. Ginsburg J, Hardiman P, O'Reilly B. Peripheral blood flow in menopausal women who have hot flushes and in those who do not. *BMJ*. 1989;298(6686):1488-1490.

77. Brincat M, de Trafford JC, Lafferty K, Studd JW. Peripheral vasomotor control and menopausal flushing—a preliminary report. *Br J Obstet Gynaecol*. 1984;91(11):1107-1110.

78. Sassarini J, Fox H, Ferrell W, Sattar N, Lumsden MA. Vascular function and cardiovascular risk factors in women with severe flushing. *Clin Endocrinol (Oxf)*. 2011;74(1):97-103.

79. Low DA, Davis SL, Keller DM, Shibasaki M, Crandall CG. Cutaneous and hemodynamic responses during hot flashes in symptomatic postmenopausal women. *Menopause*. 2008;15:290-295.

80. Thurston RC, Christie IC, Matthews KA. Hot flashes and cardiac vagal control: a link to cardiovascular risk? *Menopause*. 2010;17(3):456-461.

81. Thurston RC, Christie IC, Matthews KA. Hot flashes and cardiac vagal control during women's daily lives. *Menopause*. 2012;19(4):406-412.

82. Thurston RC, Matthews KA, Chang Y, et al. Changes in heart rate variability during VMS among midlife women. *Menopause*. 2016;23(5):499-505.

83. Freedman RR, Benton MD, Genik RJ 2nd, Graydon FX. Cortical activation during menopausal hot flashes. *Fertil Steril*. 2006;85(3):674-678.

84. Diwadkar VA, Murphy ER, Freedman RR. Temporal sequencing of brain activations during naturally occurring thermoregulatory events. *Cereb Cortex*. 2014;24(11):3006-3013.

85. Thurston RC, Maki PM, Derby CA, Sejdić E, Aizenstein HJ. Menopausal hot flashes and the default mode network. *Fertil Steril*. 2015;103(6):1572-1578 e1.

86. Thurston RC, Aizenstein HJ, Derby CA, Sejdić E, Maki PM. Menopausal hot flashes and white matter hyperintensities. *Menopause*. 2016;23(1):27-32.

87. Debette S, Markus HS. The clinical importance of white matter hyperintensities on brain magnetic resonance imaging: systematic review and meta-analysis. *BMJ*. 2010;341:c3666.

88. Woods NF, Carr MC, Tao EY, Taylor HJ, Mitchell ES. Increased urinary cortisol levels during the menopausal transition. *Menopause*. 2006;13(2):212-221.

89. Cignarelli M, Cicinelli E, Corso M, et al. Biophysical and endocrine-metabolic changes during menopausal hot flashes: increase in plasma free fatty acid and norepinephrine levels. *Gynecol Obstet Invest*. 1989;27(1):34-37.

90. Gibson CJ, Thurston RC, Matthews KA. Cortisol dysregulation is associated with daily diary-reported hot flashes among midlife women. *Clin Endocrinol (Oxf)*. 2016;85(4):645-651.

91. Gerber LM, Sievert LL, Schwartz JE. Hot flashes and midlife symptoms in relation to levels of salivary cortisol. *Maturitas*. 2017;96:26-32.

92. Widlansky ME, Gokce N, Keaney JF Jr, Vita JA. The clinical implications of endothelial dysfunction. *J Am Coll Cardiol*. 2003;42(7):1149-1160.

93. Bechlioulis A, Kalantaridou SN, Naka KK, et al. Endothelial function, but not carotid intima-media thickness, is affected early in menopause and is associated with severity of hot flushes. *J Clin Endocrinol Metab*. 2010;95(3):1199-1206.

94. Gambacciani M, Pepe A. Vasomotor symptoms and cardiovascular risk. *Climacteric*. 2009;12(supp 1):32-35.

95. Thurston RC, Chang Y, Barinas-Mitchell E, Jennings JR, von Känel R, Landsittel DP, Matthews KA. Physiologically assessed hot flashes and endothelial function among midlife women. *Menopause*. 2017;24(8):886-893.

96. Thurston RC, Johnson BD, Shufelt CL, et al. Menopausal symptoms and cardiovascular disease mortality in the Women's Ischemia Syndrome Evaluation (WISE). *Menopause*. 2017;24(2):126-132.

97. Yasui T, Uemura H, Tomita J, et al. Association of interleukin-8 with hot flashes in premenopausal, perimenopausal, and postmenopausal women and bilateral oophorectomized women. *J Clin Endocrinol Metab*. 2006;91(12):4805-4808.

98. Huang WY, Hsin IL, Chen D-R, et al. Circulating interleukin-8 and tumor necrosis factor-⊠ are associated with hot flashes in healthy postmenopausal women. *PLoS One*. 2017;12(8):e0184011.

99. Thurston RC, Sutton-Tyrrell K, Everson-Rose SA, Hess R, Powell LH, Matthews KA. Hot flashes and carotid intima media thickness among midlife women. *Menopause*. 2011;18(4):352-358.

100. Karaoulanis SE, Daponte A, Rizouli KA, et al. The role of cytokines and hot flashes in perimenopausal depression. *Ann Gen Psychiatry*. 2012;11:9.

101. Chedraui P, Jaramillo W, Pérez-López FR, Escobar GS, Morocho N, Hidalgo L. Pro-inflammatory cytokine levels in postmenopausal women with the metabolic syndrome. *Gynecol Endocrinol*. 2011; 27(9):685-691.

102. Pinkerton JV, Zion AS. Vasomotor symptoms in menopause: where we've been and where we're going. *J Womens Health (Larchmt)*. 2006;15(2):135-145.

103. Duffy O, Iversen L, Hannaford PC. The menopause "It's somewhere between a taboo and a joke": a focus group study. *Climacteric*. 2011;14(4):497-505.

104. Molnar GW. Investigation of hot flashes by ambulatory monitoring. *Am J Physiol*. 1979;237(5):R306-R310.

105. Rossouw JE, Anderson GL, Prentice RL, et al; Writing Group for the Women's Health Initiative Investigators. Risks and benefits of estrogen plus progestin in healthy postmenopausal women: principal results from the Women's Health Initiative randomized controlled trial. *JAMA*. 2002;288(3):321-333.

106. The NAMS 2017 Hormone Therapy Position Statement Advisory Panel. The 2017 hormone therapy position statement of The North American Menopause Society. *Menopause*. 2017;24(7):728-753.

107. Islam RM, Bell RJ, Billah B, Hossain MB, Davis SR. Prevalence and severity of VMS and joint pain in women at midlife in Bangladesh: a population-based survey. *Menopause*. 2016;23(7):731-739.

108. Cumming GP, Currie H, Morris E, Moncur R, Lee AJ. The need to do better—are we still letting our patients down and at what cost? *Post Reprod Health*. 2015;21(2):56-62.

109. Carpenter JS, Groves D, Chen CX, Otte JL, Miller WR. Menopause and big data: Word Adjacency Graph modeling of menopause-related ChaCha data. *Menopause*. 2017;24(7):783-788.

110. Charbonneau DH. Readability of menopause web sites: a cross-sectional study. *J Women Aging*. 2012;24(4):280-291.

111. Hsieh E, Nunez-Smith M, Henrich JB. Needs and priorities in women's health training: perspectives from an internal medicine residency program. *J Womens Health (Larchmt)*. 2013;22(8):667-672.

112. Peng W, Adams J, Sibbritt DW, Frawley JE. Critical review of complementary and alternative medicine use in menopause: focus on prevalence, motivation, decision-making, and communication. *Menopause*. 2014;21(5):536-548.

113. Singh B, Liu XD, Der-Martirosian C, et al. A national probability survey of American Medical Association gynecologists and primary care physicians concerning menopause. *Am J Obstet Gynecol*. 2005;193(3 pt 1):693-700.

114. Hitchcock CL, Prior JC. Oral micronized progesterone for vasomotor symptoms—a placebo-controlled randomized trial in healthy postmenopausal women. *Menopause*. 2012;19(8):886-893.

115. Prior JC, Elliott TG, Norman E, Stajic V, Hitchcock CL. Progesterone therapy, endothelial function and cardiovascular risk factors: a 3-month randomized, placebo-controlled trial in healthy early postmenopausal women. *PLoS One*. 2014;9(1):e84698.

116. Carroll DG, Lisenby KM, Carter TL. Critical appraisal of paroxetine for the treatment of VMS. *Int J Womens Health*. 2015;7:615-624.

117. Simon JA, Portman DJ, Kaunitz AM, et al. Low-dose paroxetine 7.5 mg for menopausal VMS: two randomized controlled trials. *Menopause*. 2013;20(10):1027-1035.

118. Stearns V, Beebe KL, Iyengar M, Dube E. Paroxetine controlled release in the treatment of menopausal hot flashes: a randomized controlled trial. *JAMA*. 2003;289(21):2827-2834.

119. Pinkerton JV, Joffe H, Kazempour K, Mekonnen H, Bhaskar S, Lippman J. Low-dose paroxetine (7.5 mg) improves sleep in women with VMS associated with menopause. *Menopause*. 2015;22(1):50-58.

120. Capriglione S, Plotti F, Montera R, et al. Role of paroxetine in the management of hot flashes in gynecological cancer survivors: results of the first randomized single-center controlled trial. *Gynecol Oncol*. 2016;143(3):584-588.

121. Slaton RM, Champion MN, Palmore KB. A review of paroxetine for the treatment of VMS. *J Pharm Pract*. 2015;28(3):266-274.

122. Kalay AE, Demir B, Haberal A, Kalay M, Kandemir O. Efficacy of citalopram on climacteric symptoms. *Menopause*. 2007;14(2):223-229.

123. Freeman EW, Guthrie KA, Caan B, et al. Efficacy of escitalopram for hot flashes in healthy menopausal women: a randomized controlled trial. *JAMA* 2011;305:267-274.

124. Sun Z, Hao Y, Zhang M. Efficacy and safety of desvenlafaxine treatment for hot flashes associated with menopause: a meta-analysis of randomized controlled trials. *Gynecol Obstet Invest*. 2013;75(4):255-262.

125. Joffe H, Guthrie KA, LaCroix AZ, et al. Low-dose estradiol and the serotonin-norepinephrine reuptake inhibitor venlafaxine for VMS: a randomized clinical trial. *JAMA Intern Med* 2014;174:1058-1066.

126. Guthrie KA, LaCroix AZ, Ensrud KE, et al. Pooled analysis of six pharmacologic and nonpharmacologic interventions for VMS. *Obstet Gynecol*. 2015;126(2):413-422.

127. Hicks JK, Bishop JR, Sangkuhl K, et al; Clinical Pharmacogenetics Implementation Consortium. Clinical Pharmacogenetics Implementation Consortium (CPIC) guideline for CYP2D6 and CYP2C19 genotypes and dosing of selective serotonin reuptake inhibitors. *Clin Pharmacol Ther*. 2015;98(2):127-134.

128. Reddy SY, Warner H, Guttuso T Jr, et al. Gabapentin, estrogen, and placebo for treating hot flushes: a randomized controlled trial. *Obstet Gynecol* 2006;108:41-48.

129. Brown JN, Wright JR. Use of gabapentin in patients experiencing hot flashes. *Pharmacotherapy*. 2009;29(1):74-81.

130. Aguirre W. Chedraui P, Mendoza J, Ruilova I. Gabepentin vs. low-dose transdermal estradiol for treating post-menopausal women with moderat to very severe hot flushes. *Gynecol Endocrinol*. 2010;26(5):333-337.

131. Hayes LP, Carroll DG, Kelley KW. Use of gabapentin for the management of natural or surgical menopausal hot flashes. *Ann Pharmacother*. 2011;45(3):388-394.

132. Rahmanian M, Mohseni A, Ghorbani R. A crossover study comparing gabapentin and fluoxetine for the treatment of VMS among postmenopausal women. *Int J Gynaecol Obstet*. 2015;131(1):87-90.

133. Rada G, Capurro D, Pantoja T, et al. Non-hormonal interventions for hot flushes in women with a history of breast cancer. *Cochrane Database Syst Rev*. 2010;CD004923.

134. Woyka J. Consensus statement for non-hormonal-based treatments for menopausal symptoms. *Post Reprod Health.* 2017;23(2):71-75.

135. Simon JA, Gaines T, LaGuardia KD; Extended-Release Oxybutynin Therapy for VMS Study Group. Extended-release oxybutynin therapy for vasomotor symptoms in women: a randomized clinical trial. *Menopause.* 2016;23(11):1214-1221.

136. Mann E, Smith M, Hellier J, Hunter MS. A randomised controlled trial of cognitive behavioural intervention for women who have menopausal symptoms following breast cancer treatment (MENOS1): trial protocol. *BMC Cancer.* 2011;11:44.

137. Ayers B, Smith M, Hellier J, Mann E, Hunter MS. Effectiveness of group and self-help cognitive behavior therapy in reducing problematic menopausal hot flushes and night sweats (MENOS 2): a ramdomized controlled trial. *Menopause.* 2012;19(7):749-759.

138. Elkins G, Marcus J, Stearns V, et al. Randomized trial of a hypnosis intervention for treatment of hot flashes among breast cancer survivors. *J Clin Oncol.* 2008;26(31):5022-5026.

139. Elkins GR, Fisher WI, Johnson AK, Carpenter JS, Keith TZ. Clinical hypnosis in the treatment of postmenopausal hot flashes: a randomized controlled trial. *Menopause.* 2013;20(3):291-298.

140. Barton DL, Schroeder KCF, Banerjee T, Wolf S, Keith TZ, Elkins G. Efficacy of a biobehavioral intervention for hot flashes: a randomized controlled pilot study. *Menopause.* 2017;24(7):774-782.

141. Carmody JF, Crawford S, Salmoirago-Blotcher E, Leung K, Churchill L, Olendzki N. Mindfulness training for coping with hot flashes: results of a reandomized trial. *Menopause.* 2011;18(6):611-620.

142. Huang AJ, Subak LL, Wing R, et al. An intensive behavioral weight loss intervention and hot flushes in women. *Arch Intern Med* 2010;170:1161-1167.

143. Kroenke CH, Caan BJ, Stefanick ML, et al. Effects of a dietary intervention and weight change on VMS in the Women's Health Initiative. *Menopause* 2012;19:980-988.

144. Caan BJ, Emond JA, Su HI, et al. Effect of postdiagnosis weight change on hot flash status among early-stage breast cancer survivors. *J Clin Oncol.* 2012;30(13):1492-1497.

145. Thurston RC, Ewing LJ, Low CA, Christie AJ, Levine MD. Behavioral weight loss for the management of menopausal hot flashes: a pilot study. *Menopause.* 2015;22(1):59-65.

146. Daley AJ, Stokes-Lampard HJ, Macarthur C. Exercise to reduce vasomotor and other menopausal symptoms: a review. *Maturitas.* 2009;63(3):176-180.

147. Sternfeld B, Guthrie KA, Ensrud KE, et al. Efficacy of exercise for menopausal symptoms: a randomized controlled trial. *Menopause.*2014;21(4)330-338.

148. Newton KM, Reed SD, Guthrie KA. Efficacy of yoga for VMS: a randomized controlled trial. *Menopause.* 2014;21(4):339-346.

149. Freedman RR, Woodward S. Behavioral treatment of menopausal hot flushes: evaluation by ambulatory monitoring. *Am J Obstet Gynecol.* 1992;167(2):436-439.

150. Huang AJ, Phillips S, Schembri M, Vittinghoff E, Grady D. Device-guided slow-paced respiration for menopausal hot flushes: a randomized controlled trial. *Obstet Gynecol.* 2015;125(5):1130-1138.

151. Carpenter JS, Burns DS, Wu J, Otte JL, et al. Paced respiration for vasomotor and other menopausal symptoms: a randomized, controlled trial. *J Gen Intern Med.* 2013;28(2):193-200.

152. Li L, Lv Y, Xu L, Zheng Q. Quantitative efficacy of soy isoflavones on menopausal hot flashes. *Br J Clin Pharmacol.* 2015;79(4):593-604.

153. Perna S, Peroni G, Miccono A, et al. Multidimensional effects of soy isoflavone by food or supplements in menopause women: a systematic review and bibliometric analysis. *Nat Prod Comm.* 2016;11(11):1733-1740.

154. Schmidt M, Arjomand-Wölkart K, Birkhäuser MH, et al. Consensus: soy isoflavones as a first-line approach to the treatment of menopausal vasomotor complaints. *Gynecol Endocrinol.* 2016;32(6):427-430.

155. Zhu X, Liew Y, Liu ZL. Chinese herbal medicine for menopausal symptoms. *Cochrane Database Syst Rev.* 2016;3:CD009023.

156. Park H, Qin R, Smith TJ, et al. North Central Cancer Treatment Group N10C2 (Alliance): a double-blind placebo-controlled study of magnesium supplements to reduce menopausal hot flashes. *Menopause.* 2015;22(6):627-632.

157. LeBlanc ES, Hedlin H, Qin F, et al. Calcium and vitamin D supplementation do not influence menopause-related symptoms: results of the Women's Health Initiative Trial. *Maturitas.* 2015;81(3):377-383.

158. Tokmak A, Öztürkkan D, Güzel Aİ, Çinar M, Çelik F, Uğur M. Evaluation of dietary intake of various vitamins in menopausal women with hot flashes. *J Clin Analytical Med.* 2016;7(6):781-785.

159. Walega DR, Rubin LH, Banuvar S, Shulman LP, Maki PM. Effects of stellate ganglion block on VMS: findings from a randomized controlled clinical trial in postmenopausal women. *Menopause.* 2014;21(8):807-814.

160. Maki PM, Rubin LH, Savarese A, et al. Stellate ganglion blockade and verbal memory in midlife women: evidence from a randomized trial. *Maturitas.* 2016;92:123-129.

161. Lopes-Júnior LC, Prado da Cruz LA, Leopoldo VC, de Campos FR, de Almeida AM, de Campos Pereira Silveira RC. Effectiveness of traditional Chinese acupuncture versus sham acupuncture: a systematic review. *Rev Lat Am Enfermagem.* 2016;24:e2762.

162. Chiu HY, Shyu YK, Chang PC, Tsai PS. Effects of acupuncture on menopause-related symptoms in breast cancer survivors: a meta-analysis of randomized controlled trials. *Cancer Nurs.* 2016;39(3):228-237.

163. Ee C, Xue C, Chondros P, et al. Acupuncture for menopausal hot flashes: a randomized trial. *Ann Intern Med.* 2016;164(3):146-154.

164. Reid RL, Magee B, Trueman J, Hahn PM, Pudwell J. Randomized clinical trial of a handheld cooling device (Menopod®) for relief of menopausal VMS. *Climacteric.* 2015;18(5):743-749.

165. Armand M, Ozgoli G, Giti RH, Majd HA. Effect of acupressure on early complications of menopause in women referring to selected health care centers. *Iran J Nurs Midwifery Res.* 2017;22(3):237-242.

166. Tegeler CH, Tegeler CL, Cook JF, Lee SW, Pajewski NM. Reduction in menopause-related symptoms associated with use of a noninvasive neurotechnology for autocalibration of neural oscillations. *Menopause.* 2015;22(6):650-655.

167. Gozuyesil E, Baser M. The effect of foot reflexology applied to women aged between 40 and 60 on vasomotor complaints and quality of life. *Complement Ther Clin Pract.* 2016;24:78-85.

4

Common Genitourinary Symptoms in Midlife Women

The Genitourinary Syndrome of Menopause

The *genitourinary syndrome of menopause* (GSM) is defined as a collection of signs and symptoms associated with estrogen deficiency that can involve changes to the labia, introitus, vagina, clitoris, bladder, and urethra.[1] The syndrome includes genital symptoms of dryness, irritation, and burning; urinary symptoms of dysuria, urgency, and recurrent urinary tract infections (UTIs); and sexual symptoms of dryness and pain. Menopausal women may experience some or all symptoms and signs, which must be bothersome for the syndrome to be diagnosed. Symptoms should not be caused by another diagnosis such as a vulvar dystrophy or infection.

Although the most common reason for vulvar and vaginal complaints in postmenopausal women is GSM, women can have other conditions responsible for their symptoms. A careful history and examination are essential for making the correct diagnosis.

Vulvovaginal assessment

A complete medical history should precede the vulvovaginal examination. In women with vulvovaginal complaints, the history should include onset, duration, predominant symptom, and prior treatment, including over-the-counter (OTC) remedies. Any vaginal discharge should be described. Timing of symptoms in relation to menopause and sexual activity can help guide diagnosis. Medical conditions, prior surgeries, and medications, including prior cancer or cancer treatment, should be reviewed. A sexual history, including current level of activity, partner status, and sexual concerns, can provide important information for an accurate diagnosis and may help to guide treatment. Prior or current sexual abuse may alert the clinician to the need for additional evaluation and care. Extragenital lesions or symptoms should be sought, because the vulvovaginal problem may be part of a systemic condition. Special attention should be paid to any possible vulvar irritants such as vaginal lubricants and moisturizers, soaps, detergents, and colored or scented toilet paper.

A complete physical examination includes evaluation for concomitant disease and a close evaluation for generalized skin lesions. The external genitalia, introitus, and perineum should all be evaluated. Any plaques, skin thickening, discoloration, or lesions should be noted. Architectural changes or scars, fissures or erythema, and masses or inflamed or infected glands should be noted. A cotton swab is used to check for vulvar pain. Bleeding or discomfort with speculum insertion should be noted. Vaginal atrophy is assessed by the presence of vaginal pallor, friability, petechiae, and loss of rugae. Vaginal pH, wet preps, and cultures are obtained as appropriate. Bimanual examination is performed to identify any tenderness, nodularity, or mass.

Biopsy of any white, pigmented, or thickened vulvar lesion is necessary not only for accurate diagnosis but also to rule out a premalignant or malignant condition. Any vulvar lesion that does not respond to treatment also should be biopsied. Referral to a specialist with expertise in vulvar complaints may be necessary in cases where symptoms do not respond to treatment or recur.

Vulvovaginal atrophy

Vulvovaginal atrophy (VVA) is a component of GSM.[2,3] Vulvovaginal atrophy is highly prevalent, affecting approximately 20% to 84% of menopausal women, although the

57

exact incidence is unknown.[4-6] In the Menopause Epidemiology (MEPI) study, a cross-sectional, population-based study of US women aged 40 to 65 years, symptoms consistent with VVA occurred in 57% of sexually active women.[7]

Bothersome VVA symptoms have a significant adverse effect on women's lives. In the MEPI study, women with female sexual dysfunction were approximately four times more likely to have VVA symptoms than women without sexual dysfunction.[7] In the Vaginal Health: Insights, Views & Attitudes (VIVA) survey, 48% of menopausal women experienced vaginal discomfort, most commonly vaginal dryness (85%) and pain during intercourse (52%).[8] For most women, vaginal discomfort negatively affected their lives, especially with regard to sexual intimacy and quality of life (QOL).

Women of any age who have low estrogen levels, such as from primary ovarian insufficiency, hypothalamic amenorrhea, prolonged lactation, or treatment with gonadotropin-releasing hormone agonists, also may present with bothersome vaginal symptoms associated with atrophic changes that require management.[9]

Women receiving treatment for cancer are at increased risk for symptomatic VVA. Chemotherapy, ovarian surgery, and pelvic radiation may result in long-duration estrogen deficiency or early menopause. Aromatase inhibitors (AIs) commonly used in the treatment of breast cancer in menopausal women induce profound estrogen deficiency, often with distressing vaginal dryness and sexual symptoms, including dyspareunia.[10]

Treatment

Given the potential for significant effect on health, sexual function, and QOL, all menopausal women should be screened for GSM, and treatment options should be discussed. Women should be informed that although vasomotor symptoms (VMS) typically improve over time, signs and symptoms associated with GSM generally worsen with prolonged estrogen deficiency beyond menopause. Before initiating treatment, a careful history should assess symptom duration, frequency, severity, and the effect on activities of daily living and sexual function. For example, dryness, pain, and irritation associated with GSM may limit exercise and choice of clothing (eg, women are no longer able to bicycle comfortably or wear tight pants). Discomfort or pain with sexual activity because of GSM may severely affect sexual interest and pleasure. Women may engage in more nonpenetrative sexual activities or stop having sex altogether. The degree of personal distress resulting from GSM also should be assessed. A pelvic examination should be performed, with careful documentation of findings. A woman's individual goals for treatment should be discussed.

Vaginal and pelvic floor activity

Regular stimulation and activity involving the vulva and vagina promote blood flow to the genital area and natural secretions that help maintain vaginal health. Penetrative sexual activity, with or without a partner, helps to maintain vaginal width, length, and tone. Self or mutual masturbation or use of a vibrator maximizes stimulation and should be encouraged as appropriate. Nonpenetrative sexual activity, such as massage or oral stimulation, may increase a couple's intimacy in place of intercourse or other penetrative activity while a treatment plan is initiated. Books, movies, or fantasy may increase arousal and also may be incorporated into sexual activity.

Pelvic floor physical therapy (PT) and the regular use of vaginal dilators (often under the guidance of a physical therapist) can be very beneficial in treating severe GSM. Vaginal dilators are available in a wide range of materials, shapes, and sizes and may be purchased without a prescription. Women are advised to start with a small lubricated dilator that enters the vagina comfortably and to slowly increase the dilator size over time. An increase in pelvic floor muscle tone, especially in response to vaginal penetration (provoked pelvic floor hypertonus), can result in persistent discomfort and dyspareunia, effectively treated by pelvic floor PT.[11] In cases of severe GSM of menopause, pharmacologic interventions to treat atrophic epithelial changes, together with pelvic floor PT to treat provoked pelvic floor hypertonus, may be required for optimal outcomes. (See also "Pelvic Floor Function" in Chapter 5.)

Nonhormone over-the-counter products

Nonhormone OTC products, including vaginal moisturizers and lubricants, are often effective initial treatment for women with GSM. Vaginal lubricants are intended for use during sexual activity, reducing friction and increasing lubrication and comfort. They are water, silicone, or oil based (Table 1).[9] Effects are short acting, so lubricants are applied to the vagina and vulva immediately before sex. They also may be applied to a device, "toy," or penis, if desired. Vaginal moisturizers are designed to adhere to the vaginal mucosa, allowing cells to retain moisture. They are longer acting and applied to the vagina and vulva on a regular basis, typically every 1 to 3 days, depending on the degree of atrophy and symptoms. Several studies have confirmed the efficacy of long-acting vaginal mois-turizers compared with placebo[12,13] and low-dose vaginal estrogen therapy (ET).[14]

Table 1. Nonhormone Therapeutic Options for Vaginal Atrophy

- **Lubricants**
  - Water based
    - Astroglide Liquid
    - Astroglide Gel Liquid
    - Astroglide
    - Just Like Me
    - K-Y Jelly
    - Pre-Seed
    - Slippery Stuff
    - Liquid Silk
    - Good Clean Love
    - YES Personal Lubricant
  - Silicone based
    - Astroglide X
    - ID Millennium
    - K-Y Intrigue
    - Pink
    - Pjur Eros
  - Oil based
    - Elégance Women's Lubricants
    - Oils (olive, coconut, mineral, baby)

- **Moisturizers**
  - Replens, RepHresh
  - Vagisil Feminease
  - K-Y SILK-E
  - Luvena
  - Silken Secret
- **Topical lidocaine**
- **Vaginal activity**
- **Pelvic floor PT**
- **Penetrative sexual activity**
- **Vaginal dilator therapy**

Abbreviation: PT, physical therapy.
Adapted from Management of Symptomatic Vulvovaginal Atrophy: 2013 Position Statement of The North American Menopause Society.[9]

Lubricants and moisturizers contain water, with other components added to act as emollients and preservatives and to prevent bacterial contamination. Other additives may include perfumes, flavors, spermicides, dyes, and warming agents, which can be irritating to sensitive, atrophic postmenopausal vaginal and vulvar tissues. Vulvar irritation or contact dermatitis might occur if a woman is allergic or sensitive to a component of the lubricant or moisturizer. Women may need to try different formulations to identify a well-tolerated, effective product. A simple, low-cost option is the use of natural oils (including coconut, mineral, or olive) for regular moisturizing and for sexual activity. In premenopausal women, the need for contraception and desired fertility should be discussed because certain lubricants may reduce the efficacy of condoms or impair sperm motility and viability.[15]

Another nonhormone option for women with severe penetrative dyspareunia is the use of topical lidocaine. In one study, 4% aqueous lidocaine applied to the vulvar vestibule before vaginal penetration resulted in significant improvements in dyspareunia and sexual function.[16]

Low-dose vaginal estrogen therapy

If symptoms do not improve with nonhormone interventions, low-dose vaginal ET is highly effective.[17] Estrogen restores vaginal blood flow, decreases vaginal pH, and improves the thickness and elasticity of vulvovaginal tissues. Many different formulations are available, including a vaginal ring, tablets, and creams (Table 2).[9,18-25] Serum estrogen levels with the use of these products typically fall within the postmenopause range.[26-29] Because low doses of vaginal ET are minimally absorbed, they might be an option for almost all women with GSM, including those with a history of cardiovascular disease (CVD) or estrogen-responsive cancers. In a large observational study, no increased risk of endometrial cancer, breast cancer, or CVD was seen with vaginal ET use.[30]

Improvements in vulvovaginal health usually occur within a few weeks of starting low-dose vaginal ET, although full efficacy may not be achieved for 2 to 3 months. All approved formulations (ring, tablets, creams) have been shown to be effective for the treatment of VVA. The choice of formulation should be based on patient preference (Table 2).[9,18-25]

Even women using systemic hormone therapy (HT) for the treatment of VMS may benefit from the addition of low-dose vaginal ET for complete relief of VVA symptoms. Alternatively, systemic ET may be provided by a vaginal ring that releases higher doses of estradiol (0.05 mg, 0.1 mg), treating both VMS and vaginal symptoms.

The 17β-estradiol vaginal ring delivers 7.5 μg estradiol per day.[21] The ring is placed into the vagina and should be changed every 3 months. The ring can be removed on a temporary basis, such as during intercourse, depending on the couple's preferences. The estradiol ring also is FDA approved for treatment of urinary urgency.

Estradiol tablets are another formulation of low-dose vaginal ET. Estradiol hemihydrate inserts (10 μg) are

Table 2. Prescription Therapies for Symptomatic Vaginal Atrophy

Composition	Product Name	FDA-Approved Dosage
Vaginal creams		
17β-estradiol	Estrace Vaginal Cream[a]	*Initial:* 2-4 g/d for 1-2 wk *Maintenance:* 1 g/1-3 × wk[b] (0.1 mg active ingredient/g)
Conjugated estrogens	Premarin Vaginal Cream	For VVA: 0.5-2 g/d for 21 d then off 7 d[b] For dyspareunia: 0.5 g/d for 21 d then off 7 d, or 2 × wk[b] (0.625 mg active ingredient/g)
Estrone	Estragyn Vaginal Cream[c]	2-4 g/d (1 mg active ingredient/g) Intended for short-term use; progestogen recommended
Vaginal rings		
17β-estradiol	Estring	Device containing 2 mg releases approximately 7.5 µg/d for 90 d (for VVA)
Estradiol acetate	Femring[a]	Device containing 12.4 mg or 24.8 mg estradiol acetate releases 0.05 mg/d or 0.10 mg/d estradiol for 90 d (both doses release systemic levels for treatment of VVA and VMS)
Vaginal tablet		
Estradiol hemihydrate	Vagifem	Initial: 1 tablet/d for 2 wk Maintenance: 1 tablet 2 × wk (tablet containing 10.3 µg of estradiol hemihydrates, equivalent to 10 µg of estradiol)
Ospemifene	Osphena	60 mg daily oral
Dehydroepiandrosterone sulfate	Intrarosa	6.5 mg nightly

Abbreviations: FDA, US Food and Drug Administration; VMS, vasomotor symptoms; VVA, vulvovaginal atrophy.
Products not noted are available in the United States and Canada.
[a]Available in the United States but not Canada
[b]Some FDA-approved dosages of conjugated estrogen and estradiol creams are greater than those currently used in clinical practice proven to be effective. Doses of 0.5-1 g of estrogen vaginal cream, used 1-2 × wk, may be adequate for many women.
[c]Available in Canada but not the United States
Management of Symptomatic Vulvovaginal Atrophy: 2013 Position Statement of The North American Menopause Society[9]; Estrace[18]; Premarin[19]; Estragyn[20]; Estring[21]; Femring[22]; Vagifem[23]; Osphena[24]; Intrarosa.[25]

placed in the vagina twice weekly after an initial nightly use of 2 weeks' duration.[23] Estradiol vaginal tablets may be less messy and more convenient for some women than estrogen vaginal creams. A generic formulation of the estradiol tablets has been approved.

Vaginal cream containing conjugated estrogens (CE) and estradiol are both approved for the treatment of VVA and dyspareunia. The approved dose for treatment of VVA with CE cream is 0.5 g to 2 g per day (21 d on, 7 d off) and for dyspareunia is 0.5 g twice weekly or 0.5 g per day (21 d on, 7 d off).[19] The approved dose of 17β-estradiol cream for VVA is 2 g to 4 g per day for 1 to 2 weeks, then 1 g one to three times a week. Lower doses of estrogen cream (0.5-1 g/d) used two to three times weekly are effective for both VVA and dyspareunia and are typical doses used in clinical practice. Because systemic absorption is dose dependent, women should be advised to use the lowest dose necessary to treat symptoms. In women for whom systemic HT is contraindicated, use of the estradiol vaginal tablet or low-dose estradiol vaginal ring generally is preferred to the use of estrogen creams because of their fixed-dosing and well-documented lack of significant systemic absorption.

Given minimal systemic absorption, women with a history of CVD or estrogen-responsive cancers may be candidates for low-dose vaginal ET if nonhormone options are ineffective.[9,31] Discussion with a woman's cardiologist or oncologist before initiating treatment is advised.[32] Special consideration is required in women with breast cancer using an AI because these agents derive their efficacy from reducing circulating estrogen to levels significantly below those typically seen in menopausal women. In studies of low-dose vaginal ET in postmenopausal survivors of breast cancer taking an AI or a selective estrogen-receptor modulator (SERM), elevations in circulating estrogen levels were seen.[33,34] (See also "Selective Estrogen-Receptor Modulators" in Chapter 9.)

Systemic absorption of vaginal ET depends on dose, frequency of administration, and delivery method.[35] Although there is a theoretical risk of endometrial hyperplasia from local absorption of low-dose vaginal ET, the addition of a progestogen generally is not indicated. Endometrial biopsy data confirming safety are available for only 1 year, whereas long-term use of these products typically is needed. Women using low-dose vaginal ET should be informed to report any vaginal bleeding, even spotting or bleeding associated with sexual activity. Any postmenopausal bleeding should be thoroughly evaluated with a pelvic examination, transvaginal ultrasound, uterine cavity evaluation, and endometrial sampling, if indicated. In women at increased risk for endometrial cancer because of obesity or the use of higher doses of vaginal ET than typically recommended, endometrial surveillance using transvaginal ultrasound or intermittent progestogen withdrawal might be considered.

Intravaginal dehydroepiandrosterone

In addition to low-dose vaginal ET, intravaginal use of the hormone dehydroepiandrosterone (DHEA) is approved for the treatment of moderate to severe dyspareunia secondary to VVA in menopausal women. In a phase 3, randomized, clinical trial (RCT), daily use of intravaginal DHEA 0.5% for 12 weeks significantly improved the vaginal maturation index (VMI), vaginal pH, signs of atrophy on examination,

and reports of vaginal dryness and dyspareunia compared with placebo.[36] Serum steroid levels remained within the normal postmenopause range, including DHEA and its metabolites DHEA sulfate, testosterone, estradiol, and estrone. Vaginal discharge because of melting of the vehicle was the only adverse event related to treatment. Endometrial safety was confirmed at 1 year.[37]

Oral ospemifene

For women who prefer an oral agent to treat GSM, ospemifene, a SERM (an estrogen agonist/antagonist) is approved for the treatment of women with moderate to severe dyspareunia associated with VVA. Daily oral administration (60 mg) improves VMI, vaginal pH, and symptoms of VVA.[38,39] Similar to other SERMs, ospemifene can increase VMS and may increase the risk of venous thromboembolism. Studies up to 52 weeks showed no endometrial hyperplasia or cancer.[40] Although ospemifene appears to have antiestrogenic effects on the breast, it is not approved for use in women with breast cancer. Similar to other SERMs, it has favorable effects on bone.[41] (See also "Selective Estrogen-Receptor Modulators" in Chapter 9.)

Laser therapy

The use of laser therapy for the treatment of GSM, vaginal laxity, and incontinence remains controversial.[42] Several small studies have shown efficacy of fractional CO_2 laser treatments for GSM. In an open-label study, 30 women with GSM received three vaginal laser treatments spaced 6 weeks apart.[43] Vaginal symptom and sexual function scores increased significantly compared with baseline at 3 months. At the 1-year follow-up, 21 women available for study noted continued symptom improvement.[44] Trials comparing laser therapy to low-dose vaginal ET are ongoing. A randomized, blinded, sham-controlled trial of laser therapy for GSM has not yet been performed but is needed before widespread use of this very costly technology with unknown long-term effects.

Supplements

Insufficient data are available to evaluate the effects of herbal supplements and isoflavone-containing foods and supplements on GSM.

Why women remain untreated

Despite the availability of many safe and effective treatments for GSM, most menopausal women remain untreated.[8,45] Data from the VIVA survey showed that most women were not aware that VVA is a medical condition, and most untreated women had never discussed their symptoms with a healthcare provider.[46] The sensitive nature of GSM, embarrassment, and safety concerns may limit many women from discussing their symptoms with a clinician.[47,48] Other potential reasons for women not seeking treatment for GSM include limited knowledge of the cause and progressive course of symptoms, knowledge that effective and safe treatments are available, and the inconvenience and cost of treatment. Potential reasons for clinicians not discussing GSM with women include an incomplete understanding of the syndrome and its effect on women's lives, inadequate knowledge about the efficacy and safety of available treatment options, embarrassment, and limited time during patient visits. (See also "Sexual Function and Dysfunction in Midlife Women" in Chapter 5.)

Other Vulvar and Vaginal Conditions

Other clinical conditions besides GSM cause vulvovaginal symptoms in postmenopausal women, including vulvodynia, vulvovaginitis, inflammatory conditions, and neoplasia. A careful history and examination are required for complete evaluation of vulvovaginal symptoms.

Persistent vulvar pain and vulvodynia

A 2015 consensus conference convened to revise vulvar pain terminology to reflect the emerging evidence about its complex varied clinical presentation and pathophysiology.[49,50] The terminology differentiates between vulvar pain caused by a specific disorder and idiopathic vulvar pain, now called *vulvodynia*. Vulvodynia is defined as vulvar pain of at least 3 months' duration without a clear identifiable cause and that may have potential associated factors (Table 3).[49]

Vulvodynia is classified on the basis of the site of pain; whether it is generalized, localized, or mixed; whether it is provoked, spontaneous, or mixed; whether the onset is primary or secondary; and the temporal pattern.[49]

Some women can have vulvar pain from a specific etiology but also can have vulvodynia. Observational studies have shown vulvodynia to be associated with other factors such as genetics, hormones, and inflammation; musculoskeletal, neurologic, and structural abnormalities; and psychosocial issues.[49] Research also has shown an association between vulvodynia and other comorbidities and common pain syndromes such as fibromyalgia, interstitial cystitis, and irritable bowel syndrome.[51] Vulvar pain can result from a specific disorder,[49] but the etiology often is multifactorial. GSM is a common cause of vulvar pain in postmenopausal women.

Table 3. 2015 Consensus Terminology and Classification of Persistent Vulvar Pain and Vulvodynia

Vulvar pain caused by a specific disorder[a]

- Infectious (eg, candidiasis, herpes)
- Inflammatory (eg, lichen sclerosis, lichen planus)
- Neoplastic (eg, Paget disease, SCC)
- Neurologic (eg, nerve compression or injury, neuroma)
- Trauma (eg, female genital cutting, obstetric)
- Iatrogenic (eg, postoperative, chemotherapy, radiation)
- Hormone deficiencies (eg, GSM)

Vulvodynia (vulvar pain of at least 3 months' duration, without clear identifiable cause)

- Localized (eg, vestibulodynia, clitorodynia) or generalized or mixed
- Provoked (eg, insertional, contact) or spontaneous or mixed
- Onset (primary or secondary)
- Temporal pattern (intermittent, persistent, constant, immediate, delayed)

Abbreviations: GSM, genitourinary syndrome of menopause; SCC, squamous-cell carcinoma.
[a]Women may have both a specific disorder (eg, lichen sclerosus) and vulvodynia.
Adapted from Bornstein J, et al.[49]

The actual incidence and prevalence of vulvar pain and vulvodynia is unknown because of the changes in diagnostic criteria, but the prevalence of chronic vulvar pain of all types ranges from 3% to 15% of women from diverse backgrounds.[52] In a self-administered survey of 2,542 women, the prevalence of vulvodynia was 8.3%, and of the women meeting vulvodynia criteria, only 48.6% had sought treatment and only 1.4% had been diagnosed with vulvodynia, which highlights the difficulty with diagnosing and treating this condition.[53]

Vulvodynia is often made as a diagnosis of exclusion. A careful history and physical examination are essential in making the diagnosis of a specific etiology for vulvar pain and before making the diagnosis of vulvodynia. Infections should be identified with the appropriate wet smear, vaginal pH, or culture if indicated. Cotton swab testing is helpful in differentiating localized versus generalized pain.

Rarely is vulvoscopy needed, and the use of concomitant 3% to 5% acetic acid can cause further pain and distress. Suspicious lesions or skin changes should be biopsied to make a specific diagnosis and rule out malignancy. Vulvar pain might be referred pain from another musculoskeletal disorder, therefore a careful evaluation

Table 4. Care Measures to Minimize Vulvar Irritation

- Wear 100% cotton underwear (no underwear at night)
- Switch to 100% cotton menstrual pads (if regular pads are irritating)
- Clean the vulva with water only
- Use mild soaps for bathing, without applying it to the vulva
- Pat the vulva dry after bathing and apply a preservative-free emollient (eg, vegetable oil or plain petrolatum) topically to retain moisture and improve barrier functions
- Use adequate lubrication for intercourse
- Apply cool gel packs to the vulvar area
- Rinse the vulva with cool water after urination and pat dry
- Avoid vulvar irritants (perfumes, dyes, shampoos, detergents) and douching

Adapted from American College of Obstetricians and Gynecologists' Committee on Gynecologic Practice; American Society for Colposcopy and Cervical Pathology (ASCCP).[50]

or assistance from a pelvic floor physical therapist can aid in the diagnosis. There are limited RCTs for the treatment of vulvodynia, and most recommendations are based on clinical experience, observational studies, and expert consensus. Before considering pharmacologic therapies, vulvar care measures to minimize vulvar irritation should be encouraged (Table 4).[50]

Some success for individual women has been reported with topical (anesthetics, estrogen, testosterone), oral (antidepressants, anticonvulsants), and injectable medications (trigger-point injections of corticosteroids with bupivacaine).[50,54] Biofeedback, vaginal dilators, pelvic floor PT, cognitive-behavioral therapy, and more recently botulism toxin and transcutaneous electric nerve stimulation have been recommended with varying efficacy.

Topical corticosteroids have not been shown to treat vulvodynia. Medical therapies should be tried one at a time for at least 3 to 6 weeks before reassessment. If all medical options are unsuccessful and a woman has pain localized to the vestibule that is associated with distress affecting her QOL, then referral to an experienced surgeon for a vestibulectomy can be considered.[50]

Vulvovaginitis

Vulvovaginitis is most commonly caused by candida, bacterial vaginosis (BV), or a sexually transmitted infection such as trichomoniasis, gonorrhea, or chlamydia. Discharge characteristics including color, odor, pH, and findings on wet prep guide diagnosis (Table 5).[55] Wet preps with saline and potassium hydroxide are helpful in identifying most yeast, trichomonads, and BV. Amines can help differentiate between BV and other etiologies. Saline microscopy that can assess for increased white blood cells and parabasal cells is helpful in making a diagnosis of atrophic and desquamative inflammatory vaginitis. Cultures should be performed for unclear, recurrent cases or to screen for sexually transmitted infections (STIs). Gonorrhea and chlamydia testing should be considered. The use of condoms for protection against STIs should always be discussed with menopausal women, who may feel that barriers are not necessary because pregnancy is no longer a medical concern. (See also "Sexually Transmitted Infections" in Chapter 6.)

Yeast vaginitis

Yeast vaginitis is most commonly caused by *Candida albicans*. Approximately 75% of women will develop symptomatic vulvovaginal candidiasis at least once in their lives, 50% will have periodic recurrences, and 8% to 10% will suffer from four or more episodes per year, the definition of recurrent disease.[56] In postmenopause, an increase in candida infection has been associated with the use of HT and systemic diseases such as diabetes mellitus (DM) and immunodeficiency states. Yeast vaginitis typically presents with itching and a thick, clumpy, white discharge, often with vulvar erythema and excoriations from itching. The discharge will be adherent to the vaginal sidewalls and has a normal pH and no odor. Wet prep shows yeast buds, spores, or hyphae, and white blood cells may be present. Yeast vaginitis is classified as complicated if the infection is present in an immune-compromised host, is caused by a nonalbicans species, or when it is considered recurrent.

Treatment includes topical, most often OTC, or systemic antifungals. For nonalbicans species resistant to azoles, boric acid suppositories (600 mg in gelatin capsules) may be prescribed for 14 nights. Careful patient instruction is necessary, because boric acid can be fatal if swallowed. Complicated yeast vaginitis may need prolonged or suppressive treatment. For recurring vulvovaginal candidiasis, 10 to 14 days of induction therapy with a topical agent or oral fluconazole followed by fluconazole 150 mg weekly for 6 months is recommended.[57]

Bacterial vaginosis

Bacterial vaginosis (BV) is considered the most common form of vaginitis and affects approximately 30%

Table 5. Typical Presentation of Vaginitis

Diagnosis	Discharge	pH	Odor	Wet prep	Treatment
Candida infection	White, thick, clumpy	4-5	No	Hyphae/Spores Moderate WBCs	Topical/ Oral antifungals
Bacterial vaginosis	Gray-yellow	>5	Yes (+) Whiff	Clue cells Few to no WBCs	Oral/Topical metronidazole
Trichomonas infection	Yellow-green Frothy or bubbly Copious	6-7	Yes	Motile Trichomonads Many WBCs	Metronidazole, Tindazole
Irritant/Allergy	Clear	<4.5	No	Epithelial cells	Removal of irritant, Topical corticosteroids, Oral antihistamines

Abbreviation: WBCs, white blood cells.
Farage MA, et al.[55]

of women.[56] It is caused by an imbalance in the vaginal microflora, with the lack of normal hydrogen peroxide-producing lactobacilli and an overgrowth of primarily anaerobic organisms. Although at least 50% of infected women have no symptoms, it usually presents with complaints of a gray-yellow discharge that has a fishy odor. Symptoms include irritation or burning; pruritus is generally absent or mild. Bacterial vaginosis is diagnosed on finding three of four Amsel criteria: abnormal thin gray discharge; vaginal pH greater than 4.5; fishy amine odor with the addition of 10% hydrogen peroxide ("whiff" test); and greater than 20% clue cells on saline microscopy. Although commercial labs now offer polymerase chain reaction-based modalities for making this diagnosis, there is no evidence that these expensive tests are better than the Amsel criteria. Bacterial vaginosis is treated with oral or vaginal metronidazole or clindamycin.

Recurrent BV may need prolonged or suppressive treatment. Treatment with intravaginal metronidazole gel 0.75% for a 7- to 10-day course (induction) followed by twice weekly intravaginal application for 4 to 6 months (suppression) has been shown to be superior to placebo.[58] Clindamycin is not recommended as suppressive therapy because of potential toxicity and has not been shown to increase cure rates.

Trichomoniasis

Trichomoniasis is the third most common cause of vaginitis, but up to 50% of infected women may be asymptomatic.[56] It is an STI caused by *Trichomonas vaginalis*.

Patients will present with copious frothy, yellow to green discharge, often with dyspareunia and vulvovaginal soreness. Bladder symptoms such as dysuria or frequency may also be present. Wet prep of the vaginal secretions will reveal the causative organism, seen as a motile round or oval protozoa with an obvious flagellum. Vaginal pH will be 5.5 to 6.0, and white blood cells are often seen. Treatment with oral or vaginal metronidazole or oral tindazole is recommended for the woman and for her sexual contacts. Nonresponders are often recurrent rather than resistant cases, but if resistance is suspected, tindazole or oral metronidazole at a prolonged high dosage should be considered. If no response is obtained, cultures for sensitivity can be sent to the Centers for Disease Control and Prevention by special arrangement. (See also "Sexually Transmitted Infections" in Chapter 6.)

Desquamative inflammatory vaginitis

Desquamative inflammatory vaginitis is found in up to 8% of women with persistent vaginitis, yet most clinicians are not familiar with this condition.[56,59] It was previously thought to be caused by a variant of lichen planus or bacterial overgrowth of an atrophic vagina, but the etiology remains unknown. A small subgroup is thought to be the result of a local toxin-induced inflammatory reaction to *Staphylococcus aureus* infection or group A streptococcal infection. The typical patient is often hypoestrogenic (postpartum, perimenopausal, or postmenopausal) and complains of burning with a profuse yellow or brown discharge with severe dyspareunia.[56] It is often associated with severe introital and vaginal erythema, in excess of what is usual for atrophic vaginitis. The lack of response to vaginal ET often leads to diagnosis. If desquamative inflammatory vaginitis is suspected, vaginal bacterial cultures often help in the diagnosis. There are no RCTs, but either clindamycin vaginal cream or 10% hydrocortisone compounded vaginal cream for 4 to 6 weeks is often used, together with vaginal ET to prevent recurrences.

Vulvar disorders

Lichenoid vulvar diseases

Lichen sclerosis, lichen planus, and lichen simplex chronicus are chronic inflammatory conditions that often present with vulvar pruritus and pain. They can all negatively affect a woman's QOL, but lichen sclerosis and lichen planus are also associated with vulvar squamous cell carcinoma; therefore, it is important for menopause clinicians to be able to recognize these dermatoses.[60]

Lichen sclerosis. Lichen sclerosis is a vulvar inflammatory disease of unknown etiology but thought to be an immune-mediated disorder. Exact prevalence is unknown, most likely because of underreporting and because many women are asymptomatic. A recent study reported the incidence to be 14.6 per 100,000 woman-years.[61] Although it can occur at any age, it is more common in prepubertal and postmenopausal women and is most frequently diagnosed after menopause. It is often associated with other autoimmune disorders and a familial predisposition has been suggested. Clinically, it appears as white papules and plaques often with purpura, hyperkeratosis, fissures, and even ulcerations from scratching. Lichen sclerosis is a chronic relapsing condition that can result in the loss of vulvar architecture and cause severe debilitating symptoms. The hallmark is severe pruritus, but pain, burning, and severe dyspareunia are common complaints. The diagnosis can be made clinically, but a biopsy should be done to confirm the diagnosis. Topical therapy with potent corticosteroids effectively treats this disorder. The risk of developing squamous cell carcinoma has been reported to be approximately 5%.[62]

Lichen planus. Lichen planus is a chronic autoimmune disorder thought to be a T-cell mediated disease that can affect skin and mucous membranes, including the vulva and vagina as well as oral gingival mucous membranes.[60] It often affects women aged in their 50s and 60s. Large population studies are lacking, therefore the actual incidence of lichen planus is unknown. There are three variants of lichen planus that can affect the vulva: classic (papulosquamous), hypertrophic (can mimic squamous cell carcinoma), and erosive (can occur with oral lichen planus). Erosive lichen planus is the most common type to affect the vulva and vagina. Biopsy is recommended to confirm the diagnosis and differentiate it from lichen sclerosis, squamous cell carcinoma, and other erosive lesions such as pemphigoid. Erosive lichen planus can cause scarring, adhesions, and stenosis of the vagina and vulva and can cause pain, dyspareunia, and vaginal discharge. Some women are asymptomatic and require no therapy, and some have spontaneous remissions. Erosive lichen planus is difficult to treat. It usually requires the use of ultrapotent topical steroid ointments, although oral corticosteroids might be necessary. There are studies reporting an incidence of squamous cell carcinoma of up to 3% in women with erosive lichen planus. The classic and hypertrophic types of lichen planus usually respond to topical steroids and do not cause scarring.

Lichen simplex chronicus. Lichen simplex chronicus is a common chronic inflammatory condition of the vulva and has been reported to be the cause of up to 35% of patient visits to vulvar specialty clinics.[63] It can be either a primary condition or secondary to another dermatologic disorder. Some women have this as part of an atopic dermatitis. Women with lichen simplex chronicus have intense pruritis that can disturb sleep,[64] often with severe skin irritation that further enhances the itch-scratch cycle.[63] Lichenoid plaques of the vulva can be seen on examination, often with excoriations and changes in skin pigmentation. There can also be a secondary infection because of these excoriations. Patient education is of most importance in the long-term management of this condition. Treatment of any underlying disorders and the elimination of possible irritants can help. Emollients can help repair the skin, and in severe cases, topical corticosteroids are necessary to reduce the inflammation. Antihistamines, especially at night, can aid in reducing the itch-scratch cycle.

Vulvar psoriasis

Vulvar psoriasis usually coexists with systemic disease. Unlike extragenital manifestations of psoriasis that are typically dry with a silvery-gray scale, vulvar plaques tend to be pink, smooth, and glossy and located in intertriginous areas. The vestibule and vagina are not involved. Symptoms of itching and pain are relapsing and remitting.

Diagnosis is helped by the presence of extragenital disease, and treatment is with topical corticosteroids, with attention to the possibility of secondary infection.

Dermatitis

Contact dermatitis. Contact dermatitis is a vulvar skin reaction to an irritant that may be nonimmunologic or of truly immunologic origin (allergic dermatitis). Contact dermatitis occurs when an irritative substance is in fleeting or chronic contact with the vulva, resulting in an immediate reaction such as stinging or pruritus. Common irritants include soap, laundry detergent, toilet paper, vaginal moisturizers and lubricants, and sanitary and incontinence pads. Scented or colored products should be avoided. Products that are hypoallergenic or formulated for sensitive skin are often less irritating. Resolution usually occurs within a short time of removal of the irritant.

Allergic dermatitis. Allergic dermatitis, by contrast, occurs 36 to 48 hours after exposure to the allergen and may persist for several days. Identification and removal of the offending irritant resolves the problem. Topical lubricating agents and protective barriers such as petroleum jelly may lessen symptoms. Topical corticosteroids can be offered to relieve more distressing symptoms.

Seborrheic dermatitis. Seborrheic dermatitis is a chronic skin condition that manifests in areas where sebaceous glands are concentrated. Lesions are pale to yellow-red and covered with an oily scale. Plaques may be seasonal or stress related and respond to topical corticosteroids or ketoconazole.

Vulvovaginal cancer

Epithelial neoplasia

In 2015, the International Society for the Study of Vulvovaginal Disease introduced a new classification and nomenclature for vulvar intraepithelial neoplasia (VIN).[65] The rationale for this change was to unify and clarify human papillomavirus (HPV) squamous cell lesions, which now include external genital condyloma and vulvar low-grade squamous intraepithelial lesions (associated with genotypes 6 and 11) and high-grade squamous intraepithelial lesions (associated with oncogenic genotypes 16, 18, and 31).[66] Vulvar low-grade squamous intraepithelial lesions are not precancerous, whereas vulvar high-grade squamous intraepithelial lesions are a precancerous condition. Vulvar high-grade squamous

intraepithelial lesions are often multifocal and are more likely to occur in women who smoke, are immunocompromised, or have other HPV high-risk conditions, including cervical disease.[67] Occult invasion has been reported as 3%. Vulvar high-grade squamous intraepithelial lesions occur more commonly in premenopausal women and require definitive treatment.

Vulvar intraepithelial neoplasia differentiated type is not associated with the usual risk factors but more often with other dermatologic disorders such as lichen sclerosis.[65] Only 5% of VIN is of the differentiated type, but this typically occurs in postmenopausal women.[68]

Wide, local excision is recommended for the treatment of differentiated VIN because it is associated with a high risk of invasive carcinoma. Diagnosis of all VIN is made by physical examination and biopsy of any suspicious lesions or skin changes. The most common complaint is pruritus, but approximately 40% of women with VIN are asymptomatic, and lesions are found on routine examination. Colposcopy or other magnification after applying 3% to 5% acetic acid to the vulva is recommended for symptomatic women without an obvious lesion, if a woman has abnormal cytology with no cervical intraepithelial lesion noted on biopsy, or to assess the extent of a lesion and if multifocal.[66] Treatment options for VIN include excisional, ablative, and topical modalities, depending on the histology and patient preference. Close surveillance is recommended because recurrence rates have been reported from 9% to 50% with all treatment regimens.

Vulvar cancer

Vulvar cancer is the fourth most common gynecologic malignancy in the United States.[69] Women have a 0.3% lifetime risk of being diagnosed, and the average age of diagnosis is 68 years. Most women present with a unifocal plaque, ulcer, or mass, although 5% of lesions are multifocal.

Squamous-cell carcinoma. Squamous-cell carcinoma is the most common type of vulvar cancer and makes up 75% to 80% of cancers.[70,71] There are two subtypes. The keratinizing, differentiated or simple type is associated with vulvar dystrophies such as lichen sclerosis, and the Bowenoid type is associated with HPV 16, 18, and 33.

Basal-cell carcinoma. Vulvar basal-cell carcinoma often presents as a dark lesion, which can be locally invasive but is usually nonmetastatic. It accounts for approximately 8%

of vulvar cancers and most commonly affects postmenopausal women (median age, 68 y).[71] Melanomas account for 6% of vulvar cancers. All vulvar cancers present with skin changes or a lesion. The diagnosis is made by office or outpatient biopsy.

Paget disease. Extramammary Paget disease is an intraepithelial adenocarcinoma of the vulva and accounts for 1% to 2% of all vulvar malignancies.[72] Most patients are white and aged in their 60s and 70s. It may be diagnosed by biopsy of an itchy, well-demarcated erythematous lesion, most commonly seen on the labia majora, although any vulvar or perineal area may be affected. The lesion will not resolve with corticosteroid treatment. A coexisting adenocarcinoma of the breast, gastrointestinal (GI) tract, or genitourinary tract is present 20% to 30% of the time,[73] and appropriate evaluation should be undertaken. Treatment is by excision, but recurrence is common. Referral to appropriate specialists who handle this condition is recommended.

Vulvar masses
Vulvar masses in postmenopausal women share the same differential as in younger women.

Epidermal inclusion cysts
Epidermal inclusion cysts are subcutaneous, smooth, mobile, and nontender. Size varies, but growth is generally slow. No treatment is necessary, but if the patient is experiencing discomfort or requests treatment, excision or incision and drainage is recommended. Needle aspiration is not recommended because it may introduce bacteria, causing a local abscess or cellulitis, and lesions tend to recur.

Bartholin gland cysts and abscesses
Bartholin glands (greater vestibular glands) are located at both sides of the introitus and provide vaginal lubrication. Bartholin cysts present as swelling in the posterior labia minora, deep to the perineal body. Noninfected cysts are nontender, whereas infected cysts (Bartholin gland abscesses) are extremely tender. Although nontender cysts in young women require no treatment, biopsy is recommended if they develop in postmenopause or if a preexisting cyst exhibits growth after menopause. Bartholin abscesses need to be incised, drained, or marsupialized. In postmenopausal women, the cyst wall, including any solid region, should be biopsied. Recurrent Bartholin cysts should be excised or marsupialized, and concern

for malignancy should be raised when these occur in a postmenopausal woman.

Condylomata acuminatum (genital warts)
Genital warts are caused by the HPV. Genital warts can be asymptomatic or cause itching and irritation. Treatment includes clinician-applied topical agents such as trichloracetic acid or podophyllum or patient-applied therapies such as imiquimod or podofilox. Diffuse or recurrent warts may require laser or surgical removal. Sexual contacts also should receive treatment if they have visible lesions.

Other vulvar masses
Other types of vulvar masses include hidradenomas, fibromas, and lipomas. Rare tumors such as syringomas or schwannomas also may be seen. Larger masses require surgical excision for therapeutic and diagnostic purposes. Referral to gynecologic oncologists is advised for wide local excision of masses of undetermined etiology.

Lower Urinary Tract and Pelvic Floor Disorders

In addition to vulvovaginal disorders, postmenopausal women often experience disorders of the lower urinary tract and pelvic floor, including recurrent UTIs, urinary incontinence, overactive bladder (OAB) syndrome, pelvic organ prolapse, anal incontinence, and defecatory dysfunction. Identifying and treating these disorders results in significant improvements in QOL for postmenopausal women.

Urinary tract infections
A small percentage of postmenopausal women experience recurrent lower UTIs. After menopause, a number of physiological changes occur that may contribute to UTI susceptibility. For example, with an increase in the vaginal pH and changes in the vaginal microbiome, there is greater vulvovaginal colonization of bacteria that can act as bladder pathogens.[74] The urine microbiome may also contribute to this condition.[75] In a study comparing postmenopausal women with and without recurrent UTIs, the strongest associated factors were the presence of incontinence, cystocele, elevated postvoid residual, history of premenopausal UTI, and type 2 DM.[76]

For women with symptomatic UTIs, the goal after initial antibiotic treatment is to help prevent recurring infections. Clinicians should first emphasize the importance

Table 6. Nonpharmacologic Strategies for Preventing Urinary Tract Infections

- Void after intercourse
- Wipe from front to back after a bowel movement to prevent spreading bacteria
- Do not use soaps or perfumed feminine hygiene products that can irritate the urethra or change the normal vaginal bacterial environment of the vagina
- Consuming cranberry extract or pure unsweetened cranberry juice may decrease the rate of urinary tract infection recurrences in healthy women[77,78]

McMurdo ME, et al[77]; Wang CH, et al.[78]

of nonpharmacologic approaches (Table 6).[77,78] Although voiding, hygiene, and dietary measures have not been conclusively proven to prevent UTIs, they involve little risk or cost and may be beneficial to many women. Consuming cranberry extract or pure unsweetened cranberry juice may decrease the rate of UTI recurrences in healthy women.

In postmenopausal women with recurrent, symptomatic UTIs caused by common pathogens such as *Escherichia coli*, therapeutic options include vaginal ET or prophylactic antibiotics. The use of low-dose vaginal ET may help reduce the risk of recurrent UTI in a number of ways. Estrogen therapy restores a lactobacillus-predominant flora and more acid environment of the vagina, thus discouraging colonization of the vagina by UTI-associated pathogens. Additionally, ET may improve the local immune response by increasing antimicrobial peptides and strengthening intracellular barriers.[79] Clinically, only ET administered by the vaginal route has been shown in studies to be effective in reducing the risk of recurrent UTIs.[76] Oral HT is not effective for this indication.[80]

Women who present with unusual bacterial pathogens or whose infection cannot be cleared may require further urologic evaluation for conditions such as incomplete bladder emptying, renal stones, and structural abnormalities of the upper urinary tract. Asymptomatic bacteriuria most often requires no treatment.

Pelvic floor disorders

Pelvic floor disorder complaints, including urinary incontinence and urgency and frequency symptoms, pelvic organ prolapse, anal incontinence, and defecatory dysfunction, become more common during perimenopause

and postmenopause. These disorders are not an inevitable result of menopause or aging and should not be considered normal.

Urinary incontinence

Urinary incontinence is a common, socially restricting, and costly problem, particularly in middle-aged and older women. Prevalence estimates in midlife women range from about 5% for severe incontinence to 60% for mild incontinence.[81] Cross-sectional epidemiologic studies have reported an increase in the prevalence of incontinence in women aged 45 to 55 years, an age range that coincides with the menopause transition.[81,82] However, longitudinal studies have shown that the development or worsening of incontinence is not associated with advancing menopause stages. Although women are more likely to report mild incontinence symptoms in early perimenopause, incontinence symptoms decline in the first 5 years after menopause.[83,84]

In the past, incontinence had been considered a symptom of urogenital atrophy related to the reduction in endogenous estrogens during menopause; however, studies do not support this.[85] Estradiol levels and short-term (year-to-year) reductions in estradiol levels have not been shown to be associated with developing incontinence during the menopause transition.[86] Over the entire menopause transition, women who have steeper declines in their endogenous estrogen levels appear less likely to complain of incontinence symptoms.[87] Postmenopause systemic ET has been shown to worsen incontinence.[88,89]

Some factors that have been associated with incontinence include age, DM, obesity, weight gain, parity, depression, and hysterectomy.[90-92]

Urinary incontinence is classified into different types:

Stress incontinence. Stress incontinence is defined as involuntary loss of urine that occurs with an activity such as coughing or sneezing that increases intra-abdominal pressure. Leakage is usually in drops, unless it is severe. Stress incontinence is thought to be related to poor urethral support (urethral hypermobility), urethral sphincter weakness (intrinsic sphincter deficiency), or dysfunction of the pelvic floor (levator ani) muscles.

Urgency incontinence. Urgency incontinence is defined as involuntary loss of urine preceded by a sensation of urgency to urinate. It is generally associated with losses of larger volumes of urine that soak through pads and clothing. Leakage results from detrusor (bladder) overactivity—uninhibited contractions of the detrusor muscle (smooth muscle of the bladder wall). Urgency incontinence can be categorized as a symptom of OAB syndrome.

Mixed incontinence. Mixed incontinence includes stress and urgency incontinence symptoms.

Extraurethral incontinence. Extraurethral incontinence is the result of an abnormal opening from the bladder such as a vesicovaginal fistula that might occur as a complication of bladder injury during a hysterectomy. It is the least common type of incontinence.

Although up to half of midlife and older women report having urinary incontinence, less than 50% seek evaluation and treatment.[93] Embarrassment, the misconception that incontinence is a normal part of childbirth or aging, lack of awareness about effective treatment options, and healthcare providers not asking about urinary incontinence are some of the most common reasons women from different ethnic backgrounds cite for not seeking care.[94,95] Even if a cure is not possible, clinicians can offer treatments or advice that can significantly improve incontinence symptoms. Asking about urinary incontinence symptoms should be part of the review of systems

in midlife and older women. Determining the causes, types, and effects of a woman's urinary incontinence is important for individualizing treatment.

Evaluation of urinary disorders starts with obtaining a good patient history (Table 7). One of the best tools to evaluate a woman's complaint of urinary incontinence is a 3-day urinary diary (Table 8). The diary can help the clinician determine the frequency and type of incontinence symptoms, associated urinary complaints such as urinary frequency, and exacerbating factors such as excessive consumption of fluids or caffeine. A complete physical examination to assess urinary disorders should be performed (Table 9).

Table 8. Information to Include in a Urinary Diary

- Type and amount of fluid intake and time of day
- Circumstances of each leakage episode (urgency on the way to the toilet or leakage with coughing, sneezing, or exercise) and time of day
- Amount of urine leaked (a few drops, wet underwear, soaked clothing) with each episode
- Use of external protection (pads), including quantity and how wet the pad is when changed
- Amount of urine voided and time of day can be helpful in some situations (normal total 24-h urine volume is 1-1.5 L)

Table 7. Evaluating Urinary Symptoms (Incontinence and OAB Syndrome)

- Ask specific questions that characterize urinary symptoms and habits.
- Assess how urinary symptoms affect each woman's life.
- Calculate the daily amount, type, and timing of fluid consumed.
- Review medical history (including medications), surgical history, and sexual history.
- Assess for a variety of pelvic floor disorders (urinary incontinence, urinary urgency or frequency, pelvic organ prolapse, and defecatory dysfunction such as constipation, fecal urgency, and anal incontinence) that commonly coexist in midlife and older women.
- Ask women about bladder pain, which can help to distinguish OAB syndrome from painful bladder syndrome. Women with painful bladder syndrome generally have chronic midline pelvic pain or pain with a full bladder.
- Ask about other important information, such as effects on sleep and proximity of toilet facilities during the day and at night for frail elderly women who may be at risk of falling.

Abbreviation: OAB, overactive bladder.

Table 9. Physical Examination for Urinary Disorders

- Assessing mental status
- Assessing mobility (immobility may contribute to a woman's ability to reach the toilet)
- Neurologic screening examination focusing on the sacral nerves, including perineal sensation and assessing anal sphincter tone (to rule out rare neurologic causes of incontinence)
- Inspection and palpation of the anterior vaginal wall and urethra to screen for urethral abnormalities such as a diverticulum, masses, and urethritis (eg, pain on palpation of the anterior vaginal wall/bladder is suggestive of interstitial cystitis)
- Inspecting the vulva and vagina for infection, discharge, and pelvic organ prolapse
- Bimanual examination to rule out pelvic masses
- Assessing pelvic floor muscles for tenderness, strength, and ability to isolate the levator ani muscles (ability to do a Kegel exercise)
- Assessing urine leakage with provocation, such as coughing or sneezing

To evaluate for incomplete bladder emptying, measuring a postvoid residual urine volume (by bladder scan or straight catheterization) within 15 minutes of voiding is recommended, in particular with concomitant pelvic organ prolapse, complaints of voiding dysfunction, or abnormal neurologic signs and symptoms. A postvoid residual of 100 mL or less is considered normal, whereas 200 mL is considered abnormal.[96] For postvoid volumes between 100 mL and 200 mL, repeating the test on a different day and clinical correlation is recommended.

Initial laboratory testing should include a urinalysis that can screen for potential medical causes of incontinence.[97] For example, the presence of hematuria may suggest bladder pathology (bladder stone or bladder cancer) that should be investigated. A urine culture can identify the presence of a UTI, which can cause or worsen incontinence symptoms.

Chronic dampness of underwear is sometimes mistaken for incontinence when the cause is an increase or change in vaginal secretions or perineal perspiration. A trial of phenazopyridine HCl, 100 mg or 200 mg given once, will color the urine orange and may help differentiate urine from watery vaginal secretions.

Additional specialized studies such as urodynamic testing or cystoscopy may be indicated in specific situations such as failure of nonsurgical treatments, inability to determine type of incontinence before planning incontinence or prolapse surgery, and a history of prior incontinence or prolapse surgery.

Management of urinary incontinence

Most incontinence can be successfully treated or managed on the basis of the clinician's impression of incontinence type from an initial history and physical examination and without the need for any specialized testing such as urodynamic testing.

After neurologic and intrinsic bladder etiologies for urinary incontinence have been ruled out by a screening neurologic examination and urinalysis, and after any UTI has been addressed, treatment can be targeted to type of incontinence.

For women with mixed incontinence (both urgency and stress), the most troublesome or dominant symptom should be addressed first. Treatment of incontinence is individualized and depends on each woman's perceived effect of incontinence on her QOL, not necessarily on how often she leaks or whether she needs to wear pads for protection. Modifiable factors that cause or worsen incontinence (excessive fluid intake, obesity, uncontrolled cough) should be considered and addressed first or at least early in treatment.[98,99] Strategies for stress and urgency incontinence include:

Incontinence pads. Women with severe incontinence should be encouraged to use incontinence pads, not menstrual pads. They provide better absorbency and better skin protection.

Fluid restriction. For women who consume large volumes of fluid, limiting total fluid intake to about 64 oz per day can significantly reduce the number of leakage episodes. However, there is a theoretical risk that concentrated urine is irritating to the bladder, so overrestriction should be discouraged.

Weight loss. For women who are overweight or obese, weight loss has been shown to reduce the frequency of incontinence episodes by up to 70%.[100]

Timed voiding. A woman is instructed to void at regular intervals by the clock rather than waiting for the physical sensation of the urge to urinate. This can avoid the urgency incontinence episodes and reduce the amount of urine in the bladder, which may decrease the frequency of stress incontinence episodes. This technique is especially useful for women who void infrequently or who have dementia.

Strategies and treatments for stress incontinence include:

Cough suppression. Smokers should be encouraged to quit smoking, and women with poorly controlled asthma or allergies should have these conditions optimally treated.

Incontinence pessaries. Although the evidence for symptom improvement in RCTs is inconclusive,[101] many clinicians find that some women have excellent results from being fitted with incontinence pessaries. Thus, a trial of an incontinence pessary is reasonable in motivated women. These can be worn at all times or just during the activities that induce incontinence (running or aerobics).

Pelvic floor exercises. Levator ani-strengthening exercises, commonly called Kegels, can improve stress incontinence by increasing the strength, bulk, and coordination of the levator ani.[102] Women have reported up to 70% improvement in incontinence episodes when doing these exercises. For Kegel instruction, women should not be asked to stop their urine flow but rather to contract the muscles they would use to delay a bowel movement. Women should also be taught to coordinate a pelvic floor muscle contraction at the time of a cough or sneeze. This maneuver can also prevent stress incontinence episodes.[103] Women can be referred to trained clinicians (physical therapists, nurse continence advisors, or nurse practitioners) for pelvic floor PT.[105,105] Pelvic floor PT includes a full assessment of motor control, strength, and endurance of the pelvic floor and core support muscles and then development of individualized and supervised exercise treatment plans that may include modalities such as biofeedback, electrical stimulation, or vaginal weighted cones. (See also "Pelvic Floor Function" in Chapter 5.)

Medications. There are no FDA-approved medications for the treatment of stress incontinence. Duloxetine, a serotonin and noradrenaline reuptake inhibitor, is approved in Canada and European countries for this use but has been used off-label in the United States; the effectiveness of this medication is limited.[106] Systemic HT or local ET does not help stress incontinence and may exacerbate it by uncertain mechanisms, including uterine weight or remodeling of suburethral collagen.[107]

Surgery. For women who have the diagnosed sign of stress incontinence and have failed more conservative treatments, surgery is an option.[108] Several effective outpatient, minimally invasive surgical procedures are currently available, such as the midurethral slings (tension-free vaginal tape and the transobturator tape).[109] These surgical treatments have a 62% to 98% success rate (either subjectively cured or significantly improved) and good safety records. The long-term outcomes (>5 y) of these stress incontinence surgeries have not been as well studied but may range from 43% to 92% subjectively cured.

Strategies and treatments for urgency incontinence include:

Avoiding caffeine. Beverages high in caffeine (coffee, cola soft drinks) can contribute to urgency incontinence by their diuretic effect and possibly by irritating the bladder mucosa.

Improving mobility or toilet access. In frail elderly persons, urgency incontinence has been associated with falls and fractures.[110] Working to either improve mobility or providing a bedside commode may help reduce leaking accidents and prevent other morbidity.

Bladder retraining. First, women must be able to isolate and contract their pelvic floor muscles, so training in Kegel exercises is required. Women are then taught to contract these muscles at the first sensation of urge. Because a levator ani contraction sends negative feedback to the detrusor muscle, this technique can suppress the detrusor contraction and prevent leakage. Women who have urinary frequency can also suppress the urge to urinate, thus extending the intervals between voids. Bladder retraining has been found to be the most effective method for treating urgency incontinence.[104]

Medications. The most effective medications to treat urgency incontinence are antimuscarinic agents, all government approved for this indication (Table 10).[111] These agents, which work to decrease the frequency and intensity of detrusor contractions, reduce urge incontinence episodes by about 60%.[112] The main adverse events of these medications are dry mouth and constipation. Imipramine HCl (10-25 mg 1-3 times/d) is a medication used off-label to control nocturnal urgency incontinence but should be used with caution in older women because of possible drowsiness and dizziness (which could be concerning if getting up in the middle of the night), as well as mental cloudiness and confusion. Local vaginal ET may be effective in postmenopausal women with urinary urgency symptoms,[113] but improvement in urge incontinence is unlikely.

Table 10. Medications Approved in North America for the Treatment of Urge Urinary Incontinence

Medication	Dosage
Darifenacin	7.5-15 mg/d
Fesoterodine fumarate	4-8 mg/d
Oxybutynin chloride	2.5-5 mg 1-3 times/d
Extended release	5-15 mg/d
Patch	Change twice weekly
Gel 10%	1 sachet or pump/d
Solifenacin	5-10 mg/d
Tolterodine tartrate	1-2 mg 1-2 times/d
Extended release	2-4 mg/d
Trospium chloride	20 mg 2 times/d
Extended release	60 mg/d

Sacral neuromodulation stimulation. For women whose urgency incontinence does not respond to other treatments, sacral neuromodulation stimulation (InterStim)

is another option.[114] This system stimulates the sacral nerve root to modulate neural reflexes influencing bladder storage and emptying. An impulse generator is surgically implanted under the skin in the upper buttock area and attached to four leads placed into the sacral nerve space at S3. Therapeutic success can be as high as 83%, depending on the definition of improvement.[115] For example, leaking episodes were reduced from 8.8 to 2.3 per day.[114]

Botulinum A injections. Another option for women whose urge incontinence does not respond to basic treatments is injection of botulinum A via cystoscopy.[116] Improvement is noted in about 60% of women, which is comparable to anticholinergic medications.

Referral to a urologist or urogynecologist is appropriate for women with complex problems, such as neurologic conditions, pelvic organ prolapse, or a history of previous incontinence surgery; combined incontinence and recurrent bladder infections; extreme personal distress secondary to incontinence; or failure of nonsurgical treatments.

Overactive bladder syndrome/Urinary urgency and frequency

Overactive bladder syndrome is a term used to describe idiopathic urinary urgency (with or without incontinence) with urinary frequency (>8 voids/24 h) and sometimes nocturia (awakening to urinate >2 times/night). Because OAB syndrome is a diagnosis based on patient-reported symptoms and exclusion of other etiologies, the evaluation includes ruling out specific causes of urgency, frequency, and nocturia symptoms.[117,118] For example, OAB syndrome symptoms may result from behaviors or a number of medical conditions (Table 11).

The estimated prevalence of these symptoms in population-based studies of men and women is about 12%.[119] The incidence increases with age and is associated with urinary incontinence and other pelvic floor disorders. For example, about 80% of women with OAB syndrome or stress incontinence reported at least one other pelvic floor symptom.[120] These symptoms have a negative effect on a woman's QOL and lead to coping behaviors such as avoidance of activities outside the home, always knowing the location of a toilet (toilet mapping), and decreased fluid intake.

Evaluation for OAB syndrome is similar to the evaluation for urinary incontinence because of the overlap between urgency incontinence and urgency or frequency symptoms.

A urinary diary that details the type and amount of fluid intake and the number of voids during the day and night can help diagnose urgency and frequency symptoms related to behavior, such as excessive fluid and/or caffeine intake (Table 8). Providing a toilet hat to measure the amount of urine produced in a 24-hour period may provide additional objective information to diagnose polyuria (>2.5 liters urine/d) or nocturnal polyuria.

Similar to the evaluation of incontinence, a complete physical examination should be performed to evaluate OAB syndrome (Table 9).

As with incontinence, the assessment of incomplete bladder emptying by measuring a postvoid residual within 15 minutes of voiding is recommended, especially with concomitant pelvic organ prolapse or abnormal neurologic signs and symptoms. A urinalysis can help identify potential medical causes, for example, the presence of hematuria may suggest bladder pathology (a stone or bladder cancer) and should be investigated. A urine culture can identify the presence of infection, which can be a cause of urgency and frequency symptoms or can worsen OAB syndrome. Other investigations, such as cystoscopy or urodynamics, may be used in some women who do not respond to treatment or who have unusual symptoms or signs such as hematuria.

Management of overactive bladder syndrome

Once a woman has been screened for behavioral and medical causes of urinary urgency, frequency, and nocturia symptoms, treatment of OAB syndrome can be initiated. Strategies and treatments for OAB syndrome include:

Restricting fluids. For women who consume large volumes of fluid, limiting total fluid intake to about 64 oz per day can significantly reduce the number of voids. Additionally, restricting fluid for a few hours before bedtime can reduce the number of nocturnal voids. There is a theoretical risk that concentrated urine is irritating to the bladder, so overrestriction should be discouraged.

Avoiding caffeine. Beverages high in caffeine (coffee, cola soft drinks) can contribute to urgency symptoms by their diuretic effect and possibly by irritating the bladder mucosa.

Improving mobility or toilet access. In frail elderly persons, working to either improve mobility or providing a bedside commode may help prevent falls and fractures.

Table 11. Differential Diagnosis for Urinary Incontinence, Urgency, Frequency, and Nocturia Symptoms

Behavioral	Excessive fluid (often associated with dieting) or caffeine intake. Caffeine is a diuretic and may increase detrusor muscle excitability. Drinking fluids just before bedtime can lead to nocturia.
Neuromuscular disorders	Women with OAB syndrome symptoms respond to pelvic floor PT, which suggests a musculoskeletal etiology. Rarely, neurologic diseases such as multiple sclerosis can present with urgency and frequency symptoms.
UTI	Recurrent UTIs or bladder infections or infectious cystitis is a common diagnosis.
Painful bladder syndrome (interstitial cystitis)	Characterized by bladder pain in conjunction with urgency and frequency symptoms. More common in women aged 30-40 y.
Urethral causes	Urethral diverticulum, isolated urethritis, urethral syndrome, urethral obstruction.
Polyuria	Causes of excessive urine production include diuretic use, uncontrolled type 2 DM, psychogenic polydipsia, diabetes insipidus, and hypercalcemia.
Increased bladder sensation	Desire to void during bladder filling at low volumes but distinguished from urgency in that urination can be postponed.
Other bladder causes	Bladder stones, intrinsic bladder tumors, or extrinsic pelvic masses (uterine fibroids, ovarian tumors) that may be causing compression of the bladder.

Abbreviations: DM, diabetes mellitus; OAB, overactive bladder; PT, physical therapy; UTI, urinary tract infection.

Pelvic floor exercises and bladder retraining. As with urge urinary incontinence, pelvic floor exercise and behavioral modification such as bladder retraining are effective treatments for OAB syndrome symptoms without incontinence.[121]

Medications. Medications most commonly used to treat OAB syndrome (with and without incontinence) are anticholinergic agents[122] (Table 10). The main adverse events of these medications are dry mouth and constipation. Caution should be used when prescribing anticholinergic drugs to older women, because these drugs have been shown to increase cognitive and thermoregulatory impairment. Vaginal ET appears to be effective in at least a subset of postmenopausal women with urinary urgency symptoms.[113]

Acupuncture. Bladder-specific treatments showed significant improvement in bladder capacity, urgency, frequency, and QOL.[123]

Sacral neuromodulation stimulation. For women whose urgency or frequency does not respond to other treatments, sacral neuromodulation stimulation (InterStim) is another option.[124] Over 2 years of treatment, InterStim reduces urgency or frequency episodes by about 50%.

Nocturia

Nocturia is a symptom that is often associated with OAB syndrome. Nocturia is frequently defined as voiding more than two times per night, because it is at this frequency that the symptom becomes most bothersome to women, affecting sleep, QOL, and mood.[125-127] Causes of nocturia can be related to low-volume bladder voids (such as with overactive bladder syndrome), nocturnal polyuria, or sleep disorders. Initial evaluation and treatment of nocturia is similar to that for OAB syndrome; however, clinicians should also be aware of age-related changes that can lead to nocturnal polyuria, such as diminished renal concentrating capacity[128] and should also assess for and treat sleep disorders such as obstructive sleep apnea.

Pelvic organ prolapse

The prevalence of pelvic organ prolapse, the herniation of the vaginal walls or uterus into the vagina or beyond the vaginal opening, increases with age. Overall, between 3% and 8% of women report symptoms or signs of prolapse, which include sensation of a vaginal protrusion or a palpable or visible bulge.[129,130] Approximately 12% of women will undergo a surgery for prolapse in their lifetimes.[131] Risk factors for prolapse include aging, parity, obesity, and hysterectomy. Many women with prolapse experience symptoms that negatively affect their daily activities, sexual function, and body image.[132]

In midlife and older women, evaluation of prolapse includes assessment of specific symptoms and their effects on life. Clinicians should ask about associated pelvic floor disorders, including urinary symptoms such as incontinence; urinary urgency, frequency, and hesitancy and defecatory dysfunction such as functional constipation and anal incontinence. A physical examination assesses for the presence and degree of prolapse and any consequences of prolapse such as skin or mucosal ulceration.

Treatment for pelvic organ prolapse depends on the level of bother and life effect women report or whether the prolapse is causing specific problems such as ulcers or incomplete bladder emptying. For women not bothered by their symptoms and who have no health consequences of their prolapse, no treatment is indicated. For mild prolapse, pelvic floor exercises may improve bulge and pressure symptoms.[133] Pessaries should always be offered to women with bothersome prolapse because they can resolve symptoms with minimal risk; up to 86% of women who desire and are successfully fitted with a pessary will continue to use it.[134] For women with bothersome prolapse beyond the vaginal opening who decline or fail conservative treatment options, surgery is an option.[135] There are many different surgeries for prolapse by vaginal, abdominal, and laparoscopic or robot-assisted approaches; however, success of prolapse surgery is variable, with estimates of prolapse recurrence of up to 30%, and depends on degree of prolapse, patient expectations, and surgeon experience.

Anal incontinence

Approximately 9% of community-dwelling women report anal incontinence—defined as the loss of anal sphincter control leading to involuntary leakage of gas or solid or liquid stool sufficient to impair QOL.[136] Up to 48% of midlife women with anal incontinence report other pelvic floor disorders, such as urinary incontinence.[120] Structural causes of anal incontinence include incompletely healed anal sphincter tears, usually from third- or fourth-degree obstetric lacerations, or denervation of the anal sphincter from childbirth, aging, or chronic straining. Functional causes of anal incontinence include constipation or diarrhea. Loss of solid or liquid stool may arise from intrinsic bowel problems such as inflammatory bowel disease, malabsorption syndromes, colonic polyps, and hemorrhoids.

Evaluation of anal incontinence in midlife women starts with a history that includes review of bowel function and related symptoms, including stool consistency; toileting habits; fecal urgency; a careful diet review; medical, obstetric, and surgical history; and review of medications. Physical examination may include a neurologic survey, evaluation of the anal sphincter by inspection and digital examination, and assessment of levator ani function. Colonoscopy, endoanal ultrasonography, or evaluation for anal sphincter denervation or function may be indicated in women who do not respond to conservative treatment or who present with symptoms or physical examination findings concerning for conditions such as inflammatory bowel disease, fecal impaction, or central nervous system disorders.

Most women will respond to conservative treatment for anal incontinence (Table 12).[137] Refractory fecal incontinence related to denervation or anal sphincter injury may require sacral nerve stimulation[138] or anal sphincter repair.[139]

Table 12. Conservative Treatment for Anal Incontinence

- Dietary changes such as bulking stool with fiber or addressing dietary causes (eg, lactose intolerance)
- Medications, including fiber supplements or antidiarrheal agents (loperamide, diphenoxylate/atropine)
- Pelvic floor physical therapy

Costilla VC, et al.[137]

Defecatory dysfunction or functional constipation

Defecatory dysfunction or functional constipation are general terms used to describe common problems of defecation including straining to defecate, a sense of incomplete rectal evacuation after defecation, and constipation. The prevalence of functional constipation in North America ranges from 2% to 27% of adults and is more common in women and older adults.[140] The etiology for functional constipation symptoms includes slow bowel motility, outlet obstruction, dyssenergic defecation, or idiopathic.

Evaluation of defecatory dysfunction or functional constipation includes a careful history: clarification of specific defecatory symptoms, dietary assessment, medical history, medication use (eg, opiates, antidepressants, or anticholinergics), and any related GI symptoms (eg, anal pain, rectal bleeding). A physical examination should include evaluation for pelvic organ prolapse and common consequences of constipation such as anal fissures or hemorrhoids. Diagnostic testing for defecatory dysfunction or functional constipation is usually reserved for women who do not respond to initial dietary, medical, and behavioral treatment or who have symptoms or physical examination findings concerning for systemic, neurologic, or local obstructive (eg, tumors) etiologies. Empiric treatment for functional constipation and the common sequelae of anal fissures and hemorrhoids is usually the first approach to management.

Anal fissures. Most anal fissures in midlife and older women are caused by local trauma related to functional constipation, and thus the most common presenting symptom is tearing pain with passage of hard bowel movements. On physical exam, clinicians will find evidence of a superficial tear, most commonly seen posteriorly and midline. The primary management of fissures is treatment for constipation (Table 13). Warm sitz baths are also useful to soothe the anal pain and to relax the anal sphincter. Additional treatments can include topical analgesics (eg, lidocaine jelly 2%) and topical vasodilators (eg, compounded nifedipine 0.2% or 0.3%) ointment.[141]

Hemorrhoids. The prevalence of symptomatic hemorrhoids in women, outside of pregnancy, peaks around midlife and is estimated to be about 4.4%.[142] About 16% of patients who present to their primary care physician report anal symptoms such as itching, burning, and pain; one-quarter of those who reported these symptoms to their healthcare providers were diagnosed with hemorrhoids.[143] The cardinal symptoms of hemorrhoids are rectal bleeding associated with defecation, anal pruritis, and anal pain. On physical examination, hemorrhoids can be external (distal to the dentate line), internal (proximal to the dentate line), or mixed. Internal hemorrhoids are also graded from I to IV by the degree to which they prolapse into or though the anal canal. The primary management of hemorrhoids, after assessment for other causes

of rectal bleeding and anal pruritis/pain, is treatment of the inciting cause, most often constipation (Table 12). Additional treatments include topical analgesic and anti-inflammatory agents (eg, lidocaine/hydrocortisone cream). For women with hemorrhoids that do not respond to conservative treatment, severely painful thrombosed hemorrhoids, or irreducible internal hemorrhoids, referral for surgical treatment may be indicated.

Table 13. Initial Treatment of Functional Constipation and Sequelae of Anal Fissures and Hemorrhoids

Medication	Dosage
Dietary	• Ensure adequate fluid intake • Ensure adequate fiber intake (20-35 g/d)
Medications	• Bulk-forming laxatives such as psyllium, methylcellulose, wheat dextrin • Surfactants/Stool softeners such as docusate sodium • Osmotic agents such as polyethylene glycol, lactulose, or magnesium citrate • Stimulant laxatives such as bisacodyl or senna are best used to relieve acute constipation
Pelvic floor PT	• When levator ani spasm or poor coordination of the pelvic floor may be contributing to the defecation problem

Abbreviation: PT, physical therapy

REFERENCES

1. Portman DJ, Gass ML; Vulvovaginal Atrophy Terminology Consensus Conference Panel.Genitourinary syndrome of menopause: new terminology fo vulvovaginal atrophy from the International Society for the Study of Women's Sexual Health and the North American Menopause Society. *Menopause.* 2014;21(10):1063-1068.

2. Mac Bride MB, Rhodes DJ, Shuster LT. Vulvovaginal atrophy. *Mayo Clin Proc.* 2010;85(1):87-94.

3. Gandhi J, Chen A, Dagur G, et al. Genitourinary syndrome of menopause: an overview of clinical manifestations, pathophysiology, etiology, evaluation, and management. *Am J Obstet Gynecol.* 2016;215(6):704-711.

4. Gold E, Sternfeld B, Kelsey J, et al. Relation of demographic and lifestyle factors to symptoms in a multi-racial/ethnic population of women 40-55 years of age. *Am J Epidemiol.* 2000;152(5):463-473.

5. Santoro N, Komi J. Prevalence and impact of vaginal symptoms among postmenopausal women. *J Sex Med.* 2009;6(8):2133-2142.

6. Palma F, Volpe A, Villa P, Cagnacci A; Writing group of AGATA study. Vaginal atrophy of women in postmenopause. Results from a multicentric observational study: The AGATA study. *Maturitas*. 2016;83:40-44.

7. Levine KB, Williams RE, Hartmann KE. Vulvovaginal atrophy is strongly associated with female sexual dysfunction among sexually active postmenopausal women. *Menopause*. 2008;15(4):661-666.

8. Simon JA, Kokot-Kierepa M, Goldstein J, Nappi RE. Vaginal health in the United States: results from the Vaginal Health: Insights, Views & Attitudes survey. *Menopause*. 2013;20(10):1043-1048.

9. Management of symptomatic vulvovaginal atrophy: 2013 position statement of The North American Menopause Society. *Menopause*. 2013;20(9):888-902.

10. Baumgart J, Nilsson K, Evers AS, Kallak TK, Poromaa IS. Sexual dysfunction in women on adjuvant endocrine therapy after breast cancer. *Menopause*. 2013;20(2):162-168.

11. Yang EJ, Lim JY, Rah UW, Kim YB. Effect of a pelvic floor muscle training program on gynecologic cancer survivors with pelvic floor dysfunction: a randomized controlled trial. *Gynecol Oncol*. 2012;125(3):705-711.

12. Loprinzi CL, Abu-Ghazaleh S, Sloan JA, et al. Phase III randomized double-blind study to evaluate the efficacy of a polycarbophil-based vaginal moisturizer in women with breast cancer. *J Clin Oncol*. 1997;15(3):969-973.

13. Lee YK, Chung HH, Kim JW, Park NH, Song YS, Kang SB. Vaginal pH-balanced gel for the control of atrophic vaginitis among breast cancer survivors: a randomized controlled trial. *Obstet Gynecol*. 2011;117(4):922-927.

14. Nachtigall LE. Comparative study: Replens versus local estrogen in menopausal women. *Fertil Steril*. 1994;61(1):178-180.

15. Stika CS. Atrophic vaginitis. *Dermatol Ther*. 2010;23(5):514-522.

16. Goetsch MF, Lim JY, Caughey AB. A practical solution for dyspareunia in breast cancer survivors: a randomized controlled trial. *J Clin Oncol*. 2015;33(30):3394-3400.

17. Rahn DD, Carberry C, Sanses TV, et al; Society of Gynecologic Surgeons Systematic Review Group. Vaginal estrogen for genitourinary syndrome of menopause: a systematic review. *Obstet Gynecol*. 2014;124(6):1147-1156.

18. Estrace [package insert]. Irvine, CA: Allergan; 2017.

19. Premarin vaginal cream [package insert]. Philadelphia, PA: Wyeth; 2011.

20. Estragyn vaginal cream [product monograph]. Montréal, Québec, Canada: Searchlight Pharma; 2016.

21. Estring [package insert]. New York: Pharmacia & Upjohn Co; 2015.

22. Femring [package insert]. Rockaway, NJ: Warner Chilcott; 2009.

23. Vagifem [package insert]. Bagsvaerd, Denmark: Novo Nordisk; 2012.

24. Osphena [package insert]. Florham Park, NJ: Shionogi; 2013.

25. Intrarosa [package insert]. Quebec City, Canada: Endoceutics; 2016.

26. Schmidt G, Andersson SB, Nordle O, Johansson CJ, Gunnarsson PO. Release of 17-beta-oestradiol from a vaginal ring in postmenopausal women: pharmacokinetic evaluation. *Gynecol Obstet Invest*. 1994;38(4):253-260.

27. Eugster-Hausmann M, Waitzinger J, Lehnick D. Minimized estradiol absorption with ultra-low-dose 10 microg 17beta-estradiol vaginal tablets. *Climacteric*. 2010;13(3):219-227.

28. Handa VL, Bachus KE, Johnston WW, Robboy SJ, Hammond CB. Vaginal administration of low-dose conjugated estrogens: systemic absorption and effects on the endometrium. *Obstet Gynecol*. 1994;84(2):215-218.

29. Santen RJ. Vaginal administration of estradiol: effects of dose, preparation and timing on plasma estradiol levels. *Climacteric*. 2015;18(2):121-134.

30. Crandall C, Hovey K, Andrews C, et al. Breast cancer, endometrial cancer, and cardiovascular events in participants who used vaginal estrogen in the Women's Health Initiative Observational Study. *Menopause*. 2018;25(1):11-20.

31. American College of Obstetricians and Gynecologists' Committee on Gynecologic Practice, Farrell R. ACOG Committee Opinion No. 659 summary: the use of vaginal estrogen in women with a history of estrogen-dependent breast cancer. *Obstet Gynecol*. 2016;127(3):618-619.

32. Le Ray I, Dell'Aniello S, Bonnetain F, Azoulay L, Suissa S. Local estrogen therapy and risk of breast cancer recurrence among hormone-treated patients: a nested case-control study. *Breast Cancer Res Treat*. 2012;135(2):603-609.

33. Kendall A, Dowsett M, Folkerd E, Smith I. Caution: vaginal estradiol appears to be contraindicated in postmenopausal women on adjuvant aromatase inhibitors. *Ann Oncol*. 2006;17(4):584-587.

34. Wills S, Ravipati A, Venuturumilli P, et al. Effects of vaginal estrogens on serum estradiol levels in postmenopausal breast cancer survivors and women at risk of breast cancer taking an aromatase inhibitor or a selective estrogen receptor modulator. *J Oncol Pract*. 2012;8(3):144-148.

35. Lethaby A, Ayeleke RO, Roberts H. Local oestrogen for vaginal atrophy in postmenopausal women. *Cochrane Database Syst Rev*. 2016;(8):CD001500.

36. Labrie F, Archer DF, Koltun W, et al; VVA Prasterone Research Group. Efficacy of intravaginal dehydroepiandrosterone (DHEA) on moderate to severe dyspareunia and vaginal dryness, symptoms of vulvovaginal atrophy, and of the genitourinary syndrome of menopause. *Menopause*. 2016;23(3):243-256.

37. Portman DJ, Labrie F, Archer DF, et al; other participating members of VVA Prasterone Group. Lack of effect of intravaginal dehydroepiandrosterone (DHEA, prasterone) on the endometrium in postmenopausal women. *Menopause*. 2015;22(12):1289-1295.

38. Portman DJ, Bachmann GA, Simon JA; Ospemifene Study Group. Ospemifene, a novel selective estrogen receptor modulator for treating dyspareunia associated with postmenopausal vulvar and vaginal atrophy. *Menopause*. 2013;20(6):623-630.

39. Bachmann GA, Komi JO; Ospemifene Study Group. Ospemifene effectively treats vulvovaginal atrophy in postmenopausal women: results from a pivotal phase 3 study. *Menopause*. 2010;17(3):480-486.

40. Simon J, Portman D, Mabey RG Jr; Ospemifene Study Group. Long-term safety of ospemifene (52-week extension) in the treatment of vulvar and vaginal atrophy in hysterectomized postmenopausal women. *Maturitas*. 2014;77(3):274-281.

41. Soe LH, Wurz GT, Kao CJ, Degregorio MW. Ospemifene for the treatment of dyspareunia associated with vulvar and vaginal atrophy: potential benefits in bone and breast. *Int J Womens Health*. 2013;5:605-611.

42. Hutchinson-Colas J, Segal S. Genitourinary syndrome of menopause and the use of laser therapy. *Maturitas*. 2015;82(4):342-345.

43. Sokol ER, Karram MM. An assessment of the safety and efficacy of a fractional CO2 laser system for the treatment of vulvovaginal atrophy. *Menopause*. 2016;23(10):1102-1107.

44. Sokol ER, Karram MM. Use of a novel fractional CO2 laser for the treatment of genitourinary syndrome of menopause: 1-year outcomes. *Menopause*. 2017;24(7):810-814.

45. Kingsberg SA, Krychman M, Graham S, Bernick B, Mirkin S. The Women's EMPOWER Survey: identifying women's perceptions on vulvar and vaginal atrophy and its treatment. *J Sex Med*. 2017;14(3):413-424.

46. Nappi RE, Kokot-Kierepa M. Vaginal health: Insights, Views & Attitudes (VIVA)—results from an international survey. *Climacteric*. 2012;15(1):36-44.

47. Kingsberg SA, Krychman ML. Resistance and barriers to local estrogen therapy in women with atrophic vaginitis. *J Sex Med*. 2013;10(6):1567-1574.

48. Krychman M, Graham S, Bernick B, Mirkin S, Kingsberg SA. The women's EMPOWER survey: women's knowledge and awareness of treatment options for vulvar and vaginal atrophy remains inadequate. *J Sex Med*. 2017;14(3):425-433.

49. Bornstein J, Goldstein AT, Stockdale CK, et al; Consensus Vulvar Pain Committee of the International Society for the Study of Vulvovaginal Disease (ISSVD), the International Society for the Study of Women's sexual Health (ISSWSH) and the International Pelvic Pain society (IPPS). 2015 ISSVD, ISSWSH and IPPS Consensus Terminology and Classification of Persistent Vulvar Pain and Vulvodynia. *Obstet Gynecol*. 2016;127(4):745-751.

50. American College of Obstetricians and Gynecologists' Committee on Gynecologic Practice; American Society for Colposcopy and Cervical Pathology (ASCCP). Committee Opinion No 673: Persistent vulvar pain. *Obstet Gynecol*. 2016;128(3):e78-e84.

51. Reed BD, Harlow SD, Sen A, Edwards RM, Chen D, Haefner HK. Relationship between vulvodynia and chronic comorbid pain conditions. *Obstet Gynecol.* 2012;120(1):145-151.

52. Gunter J. Vulvodynia: new thoughts on a devastating condition. *Obstet Gynecol Surv.* 2007;62(12):812-819.

53. Reed BD, Harlow SD, Sen A, et al. Prevalence and demographic characteristics of vulvodynia in a population-based sample. *Am J Obstet Gynecol.* 2012;206(2):170.e1-e9.

54. Haefner HK, Collins ME, Davis GD, et al. The vulvodynia guideline. *J Low Genit Tract Dis.* 2005;9(1):40-51.

55. Farage MA, Miller KW, Ledger WJ. Determining the cause of vulvovaginal symptoms. *Obstet Gynecol Surv.* 2008;63(7):445-464.

56. Nyirjesy P. Management of persistent vaginitis. *Obstet Gynecol.* 2014;124(6):1135-1146.

57. Pappas PG, Kauffman CA, Andes DR, et al. Clinical Practice Guideline for the Management of Candidiasis: 2016 Update by the Infectious Diseases Society of America. *Clin Infect Dis.* 2016;62(4):e1-e50.

58. Sobel JD, Ferris D, Schwebke J, et al. Suppressive antibacterial therapy with 0.75% metronidazole vaginal gel to prevent recurrent bacterial vaginosis. *Am J Obstet Gynecol.* 2006;194(5):1283-1289.

59. Pereira N, Edlind TD, Schlievert PM, Nyirjesy P. Vaginal toxic shock reaction triggering desquamative inflammatory vaginitis. *J Low Genit Tract Dis.* 2013;17:88-91.

60. Fruchter R, Melnick L, Pomeranz MK. Lichenoid vulvar disease: A review. *Int J Womens Dermatol.* 2017;3(1):58-64.

61. Bleeker MC, Visser PJ, Overbeek LI, van Beurden M, Berkhof J. Lichen sclerosus: incidence and risk of vulvar squamous cell carcinoma. *Cancer Epidemiol Biomarkers Prev.* 2016;25(8):1224-1230.

62. Neil SM, Lewis FM, Tatnall FM, Cox NH: British Association of Dermatologists. British Association of Dermatologists' guidelines for the management of lichen sclerosus 2010. *Br J Dermatol.* 2010;163(4):672-682.

63. Thorstensen KA, Birenbaum DL. Recognition and management of vulvar dermatologic conditions: lichen sclerosus, lichen planus, and lichen simplex chronicus. *J Midwifery Womens Health.* 2012;57(3):260-275.

64. ACOG Practice Bulletin No 93: diagnosis and management of vulvar skin disorders. *Obstet Gynecol.* 2008;111(5):1243-1253.

65. Bornstein J, Bogliatto F, Haefner HK, et al.; ISSVD Terminology Committee The 2015 International Society for the Study of Vulvovaginal Disease (ISSVD) terminology of vulvar squamous intraepithelial lesions. *J Low Genit Tract Dis.* 2016;20(1):11-14.

66. American College of Obstetricians and Gynecologists' Committee on Gyncologic Practice; American Society for Colposcopy and Cervical Pathology (ASCCP). Committee Opinion No. 675: management of vulvar intraepithelial neoplasia. *Obstet Gynecol.* 2016;128(4):e178-e182. Erratum in: Committee Opinion No. 675: management of vulvar intraepithelial neoplasia: correction. *Obstet Gynecol.* 2017;129(1):209.

67. Brinton LA, Thistle JE, Liao LM, Trabert B. Epidemiology of vulvar neoplasia in the NIH-AARP Study. *Gynecol Oncol.* 2017; 45(2):298-304.

68. Hoang LN, Park KJ, Soslow RA, Murali R. Squamous precursor lesions of the vulva: current classification and diagnostic challenges. *Pathology.* 2016;48(4):291-302.

69. Siegel RL, Miller KD, Jemal A. Cancer statistics, 2017. *CA Cancer J Clin.* 2017;67(1):7-30.

70. Alkatout I, Schubert M, Garbrecht N, et al. Vulvar cancer: epidemiology, clinical presentation, and management options. *Int J Women's Health.* 2015;7:305-313.

71. Schuurman MS, van den Einden LC, Massuger LF, Kiemeney LA, van der Aa MA, de Hullu JA. Trends in incidence and survival of Dutch women with vulvar squamous cell carcinoma. *Eur J Cancer.* 2013;49(18):3872-3880.

72. Parker LP, Parker JR, Bodurka-Bevers D, et al. Paget's disease of the vulva: pathology, pattern of involvement, and prognosis. *Gynecol Oncol.* 2000;77(1):183-189.

73. Feuer GA, Shevchuk M, Calanog A. Vulvar Paget's disease: the need to exclude an invasive lesion. *Gynecol Oncol.* 1990;38(1):81-89.

74. Stapleton AE. The vaginal microbiota and urinary tract infection. *Microbiol Spectr.* 2016;4(6): doi:10.1128/microbiolspec.UTI-0025-2016.

75. Brubaker L, Wolfe A. The urinary microbiota: a paradigm shift for bladder disorders? *Curr Opin Obstet Gynecol.* 2016;28(5):407-412.

76. Raz R, Gennesin Y, Wasser J, et al. Recurrent urinary tract infections in postmenopausal women. *Clin Infect Dis.* 2000;30(1):152-156.

77. McMurdo ME, Argo I, Phillips G, Daly F, Davey P. Cranberry or trimethoprim for the prevention of recurrent urinary tract infections? A randomized controlled trial in older women. *J Antimicrob Chemother.* 2009;63(2):389-395.

78. Wang CH, Fang CC, Chen NC, et al. Cranberry-containing products for prevention of urinary tract infections in susceptible populations: a systematic review and meta-analysis of randomized controlled trials. *Arch Intern* Med. 2012;172(13):988-996.

79. Lüthje P, Brauner H, Ramos NL, et al. Estrogen supports urothelial defense mechanisms. *Sci Transl Med.* 2013;5(190):190ra80.

80. Perrotta C, Aznar M, Mejia R, Albert X, Ng CW. Oestrogens for preventing recurrent urinary tract infection in postmenopausal women. *Cochrane Database Syst Rev.* 2008;(2):CD005131.

81. Hunskaar S, Arnold EP, Burgio K, Diokno AC, Herzog AR, Mallett VT. Epidemiology and natural history of urinary incontinence. *Int Urogynecol J Pelvic Floor Dysfunct.* 2000;11(5):301-319.

82. Hannestad YS, Rortveit G, Sandvik H Hunskaar S; Norwegian EPINCONT study. Epidemiology of Incontinence in the County of Nord-Trøndelag. A community-based epidemiological survey of female urinary incontinence: the Norwegian EPINCONT study. Epidemiology of Incontinence in the County of Nord-Trøndelag. *J Clin Epidemiol.* 2000;53(11):1150-1157.

83. Waetjen LE, Feng WY, Ye J, et al; Study of Women's Health Across the Nation. Factors associated with worsening and improving urinary incontinence across the menopausal transition. *Obstet Gynecol.* 2008;111(3):667-677.

84. Waetjen LE, Ye J, Feng WY, et al; Study of Women's Health Across the Nation. Association between menopausal transition and the development of urinary incontinence. *Obstet Gynecol.* 2009;114(5):989-998.

85. Grodstein F, Lifford K, Resnick NM, Curhan GC. Postmenopausal hormone therapy and risk of developing urinary incontinence. *Obstet Gynecol.* 2004;103(2):254-260.

86. Waetjen LE, Johnson WO, Xing G, Feng WY, Greendale GA, Gold EB; Study of Women's Health Across the Nation. Serum estradiol levels are not associated with urinary incontinence in midlife women transitioning through menopause. *Menopause.* 2011;18(12):1283-1290

87. Gopal M, Sammel MD, Arya LA, Freeman EW, Lin H, Gracia C. Association of change in estradiol to lower urinary tract symptoms during the menopausal transition. *Obstet Gynecol.* 2008;112(5):1045-1052.

88. Grady D, Brown JS, Vittinghoff E, Applegate W, Varner E, Snyder T; HERS Research Group. Postmenopausal hormones and incontinence: the Heart and Estrogen/Progestin Replacement Study. *Obstet Gynecol.* 2001;97(1):116-120.

89. Hendrix SL, Cochrane BB, Nygaard IE, et al. Effects of estrogen with and without progestin on urinary incontinence. *JAMA.* 2005;293(8):935-948.

90. Melville JL, Fan MY, Rau H, Nygaard IE, Katon WJ. Major depression and urinary incontinence in women: temporal associations in an epidemiologic sample. *Am J Obstet Gynecol.* 2009;201(5):490.e1-e7.

91. Danforth KN, Townsend MK, Lifford K, Curhan GC, Resnick NM, Grodstein F. Risk factors for urinary incontinence among middle-aged women. *Am J Obstet Gynecol.* 2006;194(2):339-345.

92. Sampselle CM, Harlow SD, Skurnick J, Brubaker L, Bondarenko I. Urinary incontinence predictors and life impact in ethnically diverse perimenopausal women. *Obstet Gynecol.* 2002;100(6):1230-1238.

93. Waetjen LE, Xing G, Johnson WO, Melnikow, J, Gold EB; Study of Women's Health Across the Nation (SWAN). Factors associated with seeking treatment for urinary incontinence across the menopausal transition. *Obstet Gynecol.* 2015;125(5):1071-1079.

94. Siddique NY, Ammarell N, Wu JM, Sandoval JS, Bosworth HB. Urinary incontinence and health-seeking behavior among white, black, and Latina women. *Female Pelvic Med Reconstr Surg.* 2016;22(5):340-345.

95. Waetjen LE, Xing G, Johnson WO, Melnikow J, Gold EB; Study of Women's Health Across the Nation (SWAN). Factors associated with reasons incontinent midlife women report for not seeking urinary incontinence treatment over 9 years across the menopausal transition. [published online ahead of print July 31, 2017]. *Menopause. 2018;25(1):29-37.*

96. Fantl JA, Newman DK, Colling J. *Urinary Incontinence in Adults: Acute and Chronic Management.* Clinical Practice Guideline No. 2, 1996 update. AHCPR Publication No 96-0682. Rockville, MD: Agency for Health Care Policy and Research, Department of Health and Human Services; 1996.

97. Moore EE, Jackson SL, Boyko EJ, Scholes D, Fihn SD. Urinary incontinence and urinary tract infection: temporal relationships in postmenopausal women. *Obstet Gynecol.* 2008;111(2 pt 1):317-323.

98. Holroyd-Leduc JM, Straus S. Management of urinary incontinence in women: scientific review. *JAMA.* 2004;291(8):986-995.

99. Shamliyan TA, Kane RL, Wyman J, Wilt TJ. Systematic review: randomized controlled trials of nonsurgical treatments for urinary incontinence in women. *Ann Intern Med.* 2008;148(6):459-473. Erratum in: *Ann Intern Med.* 2011;155(11):796.

100. Subak LL, Wing RW, West DS, et al; PRIDE Investigators. Weight loss to treat urinary incontinence in overweight and obese women. *N Engl J Med.* 2009;360(5):481-490.

101. Lipp A, Shaw C, Glavind K. Mechanical devices for urinary incontinence in women. *Cochrane Database Syst Rev.* 2014;(12):CD001756.

102. Dumoulin C, Hay-Smith EJ, Mac Habée-Séguin G. Pelvic floor muscle training versus no treatment, or inactive control treatments, for urinary incontinence in women. *Cochrane Database Syst Rev.* 2014;(5):CD005654.

103. Miller JM, Ashton-Miller JA, DeLancey JO. A pelvic muscle precontraction can reduce cough-related urine loss in selected women with mild SUI. *J Am Geriatr Soc.* 1998;46(7):870-874.

104. Burgio KL, Goode PS, Locher JL, et al. Behavioral training with and without biofeedback in the treatment of urge incontinence in older women: a randomized controlled trial. *JAMA.* 2002;288(18):2293-2299.

105. Herbison GP, Dean N. Weighted vaginal cones for urinary incontinence, *Cochrane Database Syst Rev.* 2013; (7):CD002114.

106. Mariappan P, Alhasso A, Ballantyne Z, Grant A, N⬚Dow J. Duloxetine, a serotonin and noradrenaline reuptake inhibitor (SNRI) for the treatment of stress urinary incontinence: a systematic review. *Eur Urol.* 2007;51(1):67-74.

107. Cody JD, Jacobs ML, Richardson K, Moehrer B, Hextall A. Oestrogen therapy for urinary incontinence in post-menopausal women. *Cochrane Database Syst Rev.* 2012;10:CD001405.

108. Dmochowski RR, Blaivas JM, Gormley EA, et al; Female Stress Urinary Incontinence Update Panel of the American Urological Association Education and Research, Inc, Whetter LE. Update of AUA guideline on the surgical management of female stress urinary incontinence. *J Urol.* 2010;183(5):1906-1914.

109. Ford AA, Rogerson L, Cody JD, Aluko P, Ogah J. Mid-urethra sling operations for stress urinary incontinence. *Cochrane Database Syst Rev.* 2017;7:CD006375.

110. Brown JS, Vittinghoff E, Wyman JF, et al. Urinary incontinence: does it increase risk for falls and fractures? Study of Osteoporotic Fractures Research Group. *J Am Geriatr Soc.* 2000;48(7):721-725.

111. Nabi G, Cody JD, Ellis G, Herbison P, Hay-Smith J. Anticholinergic drugs versus placebo for overactive bladder syndrome in adults. *Cochrane Database Syst Rev.* 2006;(4):CD003781.

112. Reynolds WS, McPheeters M, Blume J, et al. Comparative effectiveness of anticholinergic therapy for overactive bladder in women: a systematic review and meta-analysis. *Obstet Gynecol.* 2015;125(6):1423-1432.

113. Robinson D, Cardozo L, Milsom I, et al. Oestrogens and overactive bladder. *Neurourol Urodyn.* 2014;33(7):1086-1091.

114. Latini JM, Alipour M, Kreder KJ Jr. Efficacy of sacral neuromodulation for symptomatic treatment of refractory urinary urge incontinence. *Urology.* 2006;67(3):550-554.

115. Siegel S, Noblett K, Mangel J, et al. Three-year follow-up results of a prospective, multicenter study in overactive bladder subjects treated with sacral neuromodulation. *Urology.* 2016;94:57-63.

116. Visco AG, Brubaker L, Richter HE, et al; Pelvic Floor Disorders Network. Anticholinergic therapy vs. onabotulinumtoxina for urgency urinary incontinence. *N Engl J Med.* 2012;367(19):1803-1813.

117. Tyagi S, Thomas CA, Hayashi Y, Chancellor MB. The overactive bladder: epidemiology and morbidity. *Urol Clin North Am.* 2006;33(4):433-438.

118. Brubaker L. Urinary urgency and frequency: what should a clinician do? *Obstet Gynecol.* 2005;105(3):661-667.

119. Irwin DE, Milsom I, Hunskaar S, et al. Population-based survey of urinary incontinence, overactive bladder, and other lower urinary tract symptoms in five countries: results of the EPIC study. *Eur Urol.* 2006;50(6):1306-1314.

120. Lawrence JM, Lukacz ES, Nager CW, Hsu JW, Luber KM. Prevalence and co-occurrence of pelvic floor disorders in community-dwelling women. *Obstet Gynecol.* 2008;111(3):678-685.

121. Burgio KL. Update on behavioral and physical therapies for incontinence and overactive bladder: the role of pelvic floor muscle training. *Curr Urol Rep.* 2013;14(5):457-464.

122. Chapple CR, Kullar V, Gabriel Z, Muston D, Bitoun CE, Weinstein D. The effects of antimuscarinic treatment in overactive bladder: an update of a systematic review and meta-analysis. *Eur Urol.* 2008;54(3):543-562.

123. Emmons SL, Otto L. Acupuncture for overactive bladder: a randomized controlled trial. *Obstet Gynecol.* 2005;106(1):138-143.

124. Siegel SW, Catanzaro F, Dijkema HE, et al. Long-term results of a multicenter study on sacral nerve stimulation for treatment of urinary urge incontinence, urinary-frequency, and retention. *Urology.* 2000;56(6 suppl 1):87-91.

125. Van der Vaart CH, Roovers JP, de Leeuw JR, Heintz AP. Association between urogenital symptoms and depression in community-dwelling women aged 20 to 70 years. *Urology.* 2007;69(4):691-696.

126. Madhu C, Coyne K, Hashim H, Chapple C, Milsom I, Kopp Z. Nocturia: risk factors and associated comorbidities; findings from the EpiLUTs study. *Int J Clin Pract.* 2015;69(12):1508-1516.

127. Kupelian V, Wei JT, O'Leary MP, Norgaard JP, Rosen RC, McKinlay JB. Nocturia and quality of life: results from the Boston area community health survey. *Eur Urol.* 2012;61(1):78-84.

128. Miller M. Nocturnal polyuria in older people: pathophysiology and clinical implications. *J Am Geriatr Soc.* 2000;48(10):1321-1329.

129. Nygaard I, Barber MD, Burgio KL; Pelvic Floor Disorders Network. Prevalence of symptomatic pelvic floor disorders in US women. *JAMA.* 2008;300(11):1311-1316.

130. Rortveit G, Brown JS, Thom DH, Van Den Eeden SK, Creaseman JM, Subak LL. Symptomatic pelvic organ prolapse: prevalence and risk factors in a population-based, racially diverse cohort. *Obstet Gynecol.* 2007;109(6):1396-1403.

131. Wu JM, Matthews CA, Conover MM, Pate V, Jonsson Funk M. Lifetime risk of stress urinary incontinence or pelvic organ prolapse surgery. *Obstet Gynecol.* 2014;123(6):1201-1206.

132. Lowder JL, Ghetti C, Nikolajski C, Oliphant SS, Zyczynski HM. Body image perceptions in women with pelvic organ prolapse: a qualitative study. *Am J Obstet Gynecol.* 2011;204(5):441.e1-441.e5.

133. Hagen S, Stark D. Conservative prevention and management of pelvic organ prolapse in women. *Cochrane Database Syst Rev.* 2011;(12):CD003882.

134. Lone F, Thakar R, Sultan AH, Karamalis G. A 5-year prospective study of vaginal pessary use for pelvic organ prolapse. *Int J Gynaecol Obstet.* 2011;114(1):56-59.

135. Olsen AL, Smith VJ, Bergstrom JO, Colling JC, Clark AL. Epidemiology of surgically managed pelvic organ prolapse and urinary incontinence. *Obstet Gynecol.* 1997;89(4):501-506.

136. Whitehead WE, Borrud L, Goode PS, et al; Pelvic Floor Disorders Network. Fecal incontinence in US adults. *Gastroenterology.* 2009;137(2):512-517.

137. Costilla VC, Foxx-Orenstein AE, Mayer AP, Crowell MD. Office-based management of fecal incontinence. *Gastroenterol Hepatol (N Y).* 2013;9(7):423-433.

138. Mowatt G, Glazener C, Jarrett M. Sacral nerve stimulation for fecal incontinence and constipation in adults: a short version Cochrane review. *Neurourol Urodyn*. 2008;27(3):155-161.

139. Glasgow SC, Lowry AC. Long-term outcomes of anal sphincter repair for fecal incontinence: a systematic review. *Dis Colon Rectum*. 2012;55(4):482-490.

140. Suares NC, Ford AC. Prevalence of, and risk factors for, chronic idiopathic constipation in the community: a systematic review and meta-analysis. *Am J Gastroenterol*. 2011;106(9):1528-1591.

141. Ezri T, Susmallian S. Topical nifedipine vs. topical glyceryl trinitrate for treatment of chronic anal fissure. *Dis Colon Rectum*. 2003;46(6):805-808.

142. Johanson JF, Sonnenberg A. The prevalence of hemorrhoids and chronic constipation. An epidemiologic study. *Gastroenterology*. 1990;98(2):380-386.

143. Tournu, G, Abramowitz L, Couffignal C, et al; GREP study group; MG-PREVAPROCT study group. Prevalence of anal symptoms in general practice: a prospective study. *BMC Fam Pract*. 2017;18(1):78.

5

Other Common Symptoms in Midlife Women

Decline in Fertility
With Reproductive Aging

Before any signs of the menopause transition, women undergo a profound decline in fertility. Research conducted on populations around the world living in many different socioeconomic and cultural circumstances reveals a strikingly similar pattern: there is a decline in fertility with advancing age that accelerates after the age of 35 years. Data from population studies indicate that fertility becomes rare, about 1 in 1,000, after age 44 years.[1] This pattern is unusual in the animal kingdom. Although the females of many species become infertile near the end of their lifespans, among vertebrates, only killer whales and short-finned pilot whales have been observed to routinely cease fertility many years before the end of their lives.[2] Why this pattern evolved from an evolutionary perspective is a subject of speculation.

Proposed mechanisms for fertility loss with aging

Ovarian aging and loss of follicles begins in fetal life. The number of ovarian follicles falls throughout childhood and early adulthood. Follicular loss accelerates when women reach their late 30s. The number of ovarian follicles decreases from 1,000,000 at birth to less than 10,000 by the age of 50 years.[3]

Because many women in their late 40s still have ovarian follicles and menstruate regularly, why do they almost never successfully complete pregnancy? Evidence suggests that aging of the oocyte is the primary cause, because in clinical studies, women aged 40 years and older complete successful pregnancies at rates similar to younger women when donor oocytes from young women are used.[4]

The "production theory" of oocyte maturation posits that the oocytes that entered meiosis I first in development are the ones that activate first in life, with the later, and presumably less well-endowed, oocytes progressively moving through the production line with aging. This theory would predict that oocytes that ovulate in older women would be more likely to be meiotically defective and that the hormone profiles of the menstrual cycles of aging women could be compromised because of poorer oocyte-granulosa cooperativity. Although it is clear that older oocytes are more likely to harbor chromosomal defects,[5] it is less apparent that hormone elaboration from the follicles containing these oocytes is compromised concurrent with the drop in fertility.[6]

It is also possible that the pattern of follicle maturation drives oocyte abnormalities and thus the fertility compromise associated with reproductive aging. The "compromised microcirculation" hypothesis posits that abnormal oocytes arise from poor development of the microvasculature that may be because of a number of factors, including oxidative stress.[7] Oocyte mitochondria accrue point mutations and deletions and are reduced in number with aging.[8] Because ovarian follicles exist behind a basement membrane that forms a blood-follicle barrier, they have no blood supply until the corpus luteum is formed. The fertilized oocyte then matures for 5 to 7 days before it undergoes implantation and begins to derive a blood supply. For these reasons, the importance of adequate oocyte mitochondrial function is a topic of intense investigation and likely importance.

Prediction of fertility potential in reproductively aging women

Chronologic age is a strong predictor of fertility, but it is a relatively crude predictor for any particular woman.

Population-based studies of common ovarian markers such as follicle-stimulating hormone (FSH) and antimüllerian hormone (AMH) do not support a role for these markers in predicting pregnancy, at least in midreproductive-aged women. Testing these measures to predict fertility potential is not recommended. However, once a woman presents with infertility, her ovarian reserve becomes a critical determinant of her potential for a live birth.[6] This is because most clinical treatments to enhance fertility rely on inducing multiple follicles to ovulate. Antral follicle counts, assessed by transvaginal ultrasound (TVU), AMH, estradiol, and FSH measurements have all been proposed to be predictive of response to stimulation, but not necessarily live birth, with assisted reproductive technology, both alone and in combination. Despite the significant limitations of testing for ovarian reserve, there is a market driven by reproductive anxiety in women or their family members that promotes testing and, if testing is unfavorable, oocyte freezing.

A common problem in menopause medicine occurs when the clinician is asked to help a perimenopausal woman make critical choices about when to stop using contraception. Despite the clear-cut decline in fertility with aging, hormone patterns indicate that relatively normal, ovulatory cycles can occur up to the final menstrual period.[9] Theoretically, these cycles could be fertile; however, that the oocyte that is ovulated will be genetically normal and lead to a clinically recognized pregnancy is unlikely.

The decision to stop contraception is even more fraught with unknowns when the woman has been using hormone contraception. Because there is no opportunity to observe endogenous hormone production in this setting, it can be difficult to predict that reproduction is impossible. For the most part, the standard clinical definition of menopause (12 mo of amenorrhea in a woman aged ≥45 y) appears to work well in a real-life setting. When women are using contraceptive methods that do not allow the assessment of her natural menstrual cycles, such as oral contraceptives or a progestin intrauterine device, shared decision-making should be undertaken, taking into account the woman's perspective on the possible consequences of an unintended pregnancy.

Sexual Function and Dysfunction in Midlife Women

Although most healthcare professionals likely consider sexuality to be an important component of perceived quality of life (QOL), the sexual concerns of midlife women remain underevaluated and undertreated. Data support the notion that sexual health is important to a woman's overall sense of self and well-being, whereas sexual dysfunction can be a major and disruptive force for a woman. Sexual dysfunction has been associated with a decrease in emotional health, energy, and social function and is positively correlated with relationship conflict and nonspecific medical conditions.[10,11]

Models of sexual response

Female sexual function and dysfunction are best understood using a biopsychosocial model, an integrative model of sexual function that evolves over time reflecting a woman's fluctuations in health status, neurochemical balance, psychological issues, interpersonal concerns, and sociocultural beliefs and values.[12-14]

In order to identify female sexual dysfunction, it is important to understand healthy sexual function, which usually includes sexual desire, genital and subjective arousal, orgasmic ability, and pain-free sexual activity. Therefore, healthcare professionals can organize their assessments of sexual concerns around problems with desire, arousal, orgasm, or pain with the recognition that there often is an overlap of symptoms. The diagnosis of a sexual disorder is made if a woman is distressed or bothered by any of these problems and whether these problems are persistent or recurrent (most classification systems require symptoms to be present for a minimum of 6 mo).[15]

A few commonly referenced models have been proposed to describe normal sexual response. Masters and Johnson provided the "sexual response cycle."[16,17] This model was based on their direct observations of anatomic and physiologic changes experienced by women and men in a laboratory setting and consisted of a four-stage linear progression that they labeled "excitement," "plateau," "orgasm," and "resolution." In this model, sexual response is a natural, biologic phenomenon. The essential components of sexual response depend on adequate functioning and interplay of the hormone milieu, nerves, veins, arteries, and genitopelvic muscles. This model was modified to a triphasic model that included the concept of desire as the first stage of the sexual response along with arousal and orgasm.[18]

A third model is a nonlinear, intimacy-based model.[19] This model emphasizes that many women may be sexually neutral at the time they consider engaging in sexual activity and that the goals of sexual activity (the decision to move forward) are complex and not simply for internal satisfaction of an "innate" sexual hunger. This model introduces the concept of receptive/responsive desire that harkens back to a woman's sexual neutrality and emphasizes the effect of complex biologic and nonbiologic factors, including motivation, interpersonal issues, cultural and religious beliefs, partner health, relationship quality, past sexual abuse, and cognitive distractions, on a woman's sexual response.

Female sexual disorders

The Diagnostic and Statistical Manual of Mental Disorders, fourth edition, classifies female sexual disorders (FSD) into dysfunctions of sexual desire (hypoactive sexual desire disorder [HSDD]), sexual arousal (female sexual arousal disorder [FSAD]), orgasm (delayed or absent), and sexual pain (dyspareunia or vaginismus).[20] Although these classifications might appear to be distinct, there is evidence that they are frequently overlapping comorbidities. For example, a woman presenting with no sexual desire may also experience difficulty with arousal or have difficulties with orgasm. To attempt to address the overlap, *The Diagnostic and Statistical Manual of Mental Disorders,* fifth edition, combined HSDD and FSAD into a single dysfunction, female sexual interest/arousal disorder.[21] However, an evidenced-based nomenclature conference convened by the 2013 International Society for the Study of Women's Sexual Health (ISSWSH) that included experts experienced in diagnosis, evaluation, treatment, and research in sexual medicine and the 2015 Fourth International Conference on Sexual Medicine have endorsed maintaining HSDD and FSAD as separate entities based on clinical principles (Table 1).[15,22,23]

Neurobiology, hormones, and sexual function

The neurobiology of the sexual response is modulated by a complex interaction between sex steroids and neurotransmitters and is influenced by psychosocial factors.[24] Excitatory neurotransmitters and neuropeptides include norepinephrine and oxytocin (stimulate arousal) and melanocortins and dopamine (stimulate desire and attention). Inhibitory pathways are regulated by 5-hydroxytryptamine or serotonin (signal satiety), opioids (sexual rewards), and endocannabinoids (cause sedation). The brain, specifically the hypothalamus and limbic system, with inhibitory influences from the cortex and the midbrain, regulates sexual function through integration of input from motivational, attentional, sensory, and motor systems.[25] The pathophysiology of HSDD is thought to relate to an imbalance of the excitatory and inhibitory systems, such that there is greater inhibition, less excitation, or a combination of the two.[26]

Sex steroids also influence sexual function in women. There is some evidence that circulating androgen levels are associated with sexual desire in women.[27] Androgen levels do not change significantly with the menopause transition but instead decline gradually with age, such that for women aged in their late 40s or early 50s, testosterone levels are approximately half of what they were in their early 20s.[28] However, in contrast to natural menopause, women who have undergone bilateral oophorectomy experience an abrupt and persistent decline in circulating androgen levels.

Androgen levels were associated with sexual interest and arousal in women in several studies.[29-31] However, there is no androgen level that defines sexual dysfunction or that will distinguish between women with low sexual desire and women with normal sexual function. Therefore, androgen levels are not useful for diagnosing sexual dysfunction in women.[32]

Existing data are consistent in demonstrating that testosterone therapy improves multiple aspects of sexual functioning in naturally and surgically menopausal women with or without concomitant estrogen therapy (ET).[33-40] However, there is no testosterone product approved by FDA for the treatment of HSDD.

There are several testosterone therapy options being used off-label by US clinicians. Transdermal testosterone gels, which are FDA approved for men, are used sometimes for women by reducing the amount applied. These women are monitored for adverse events (AEs) and therapeutic delivery to avoid supraphysiologic dosing. Alternatively, some practitioners are using compounding pharmacies to formulate testosterone ointments or creams (typically 1%), pellets inserted subcutaneously, or sublingual and buccal formulations.[27] Using compounded products is not ideal given the lack of FDA regulation and concerns regarding quality, purity, potency, and consistency, with significant variability between formulations and between batches of the same formulation.

The data are not as compelling for estrogen's role in sexual desire. Observational studies suggest that relationship factors and physical and mental health are more important than estrogen levels or menopause status for sexual health.[41] Although existing data do not support the use of systemic ET for the management of FSD, local vaginal ET positively affects sexual function

Table 1. ISSWSH Sexual Disorders Nomenclature and Definitions

Hypoactive sexual desire disorder

- Lack of motivation for sexual activity as manifested by
    - Decreased or absent spontaneous desire (sexual thoughts or fantasies)
    - Decreased or absent responsive desire to erotic cues and stimulation or inability to maintain desire or interest through sexual activity
- Loss of desire to initiate or participate in sexual activity, including behavioral responses such as avoidance of situations that could lead to sexual activity, that is not secondary to sexual pain disorders and is combined with clinically significant personal distress that includes frustration, grief, incompetence, loss, sadness, sorrow or worry

Female genital arousal disorder

- The inability to maintain adequate genital response for ≥6 months, including
    - Vulvovaginal lubrication
    - Engorgement of genitals
    - Sensitivity of genitalia associated with sexual activity
- Disorders related to
    - Vascular injury or dysfunction and/or
    - Neurologic injury or dysfunction

Persistent genital arousal disorder

- Characterized by persistent or recurrent, unwanted or intrusive, distressing feelings of genital arousal, or being on the verge of orgasm (genital dysesthesia), not associated with concomitant sexual interest, thoughts, or fantasies for ≥6 months. Could be associated with
    - Limited resolution, no resolution, or aggravation of sexual symptoms by sexual activity with or without aversive and/or compromised orgasm
    - Aggravation of genital symptoms by certain circumstances
    - Despair, emotional lability, catastrophizing, and/or suicidality
    - Inconsistent evidence of genital arousal during symptoms

Female orgasm disorder

- Characterized by a persistent or recurrent distressing compromise of orgasm frequency, intensity, timing and/or pleasure associated with sexual activity for ≥6 months:
    - Frequency: Orgasm occurs with decreased frequency (diminished frequency of orgasm) or is absent (anorgasmia)
    - Intensity: Orgasm occurs with less intensity (muted orgasm)
    - Timing: Orgasm occurs too late (delayed orgasm) or too soon (spontaneous or premature orgasm) than desired by the woman
    - Pleasure: Orgasm occurs with absent or decreased pleasure (anhedonic orgasm, pleasure dissociative orgasm disorder)

Female orgasmic illness syndrome

- Characterized by peripheral and/or central aversive symptoms that occur before, during, or after orgasm, not related, per se, to a compromise of orgasm quality

---

Abbreviation: ISSWSH, International Society for the Study of Women's Sexual Health.
Adapted from Parish S, et al.[15]

by restoring vulvar and vaginal tissues and improving arousal, lubrication, and sexual comfort in postmenopausal women with the genitourinary syndrome of menopause (GSM).

Epidemiology

The prevalence of FSD varies, depending on the methodologies used, populations and age ranges studied, and the classification/nomenclature of conditions evaluated. Overall, there is a reasonable consensus that the prevalence of women who report at least one sexual dysfunction is approximately 40% to 50%, irrespective of age, although the percentage of women who report distress with sexual dysfunction is consistently lower.[22,42,43]

In the Prevalence of Female Sexual Problems Associated With Distress and Determinants of Treatment Seeking study, a widely cited, large population-based survey of 50,002 US adult women (completers, 31,581; 63% response rate; age range, 18-102 y), low desire was the most common sexual problem, reported in 37.7% of participants.[42] Low desire with distress (ie, HSDD) was present in approximately 10% of women overall and 12.3% in women aged 45 to 64 years (Table 2).[42,43] If women with comorbid depression are excluded, the prevalence is just under 7%. In the 45- to 64-year age group, the rate of arousal disorders associated with distress was 7.5%, and the rate of distressing orgasmic dysfunction was 5.7%.

Dyspareunia (pain with sexual activity) related to GSM is experienced by at least 44% of postmenopausal women, likely an underestimation.[44] Nevertheless, most midlife and older women want to remain sexually active and have good sexual health (and pain-free sexual activity). The Midlife in the United States II survey reported that having a romantic partner was the best predictor of whether a woman was sexually active, even for women aged in their 70s and 80s.[45]

Screening

There are a number of screening tools to assess for FSD, including several validated screening tools that focus on HSDD, the most common sexual dysfunction in women of all ages. The usefulness of these screening tools varies, depending on the clinical setting:

Decreased Sexual Desire Screener. Five questions, self-administered; assesses for generalized acquired HSDD.[46]

Female Sexual Function Index. Nineteen questions, self-administered; includes all domains of sexual function (desire, arousal, orgasm, and pain and includes sexual satisfaction).[47]

Female Sexual Distress Scale–Revised. Thirteen questions, self-administered. Evaluates for distress associated with FSD.[48]

Brief Sexual Symptom Checklist. Five questions that can be incorporated into a patient intake form and used as a preconsultation screening tool (Table 3).[49]

Assessment

Although a physical examination is not necessary to diagnose some sexual dysfunctions (eg, low sexual desire), it may be helpful to rule out contributing factors such as GSM.[50] A pelvic examination is indicated in women with concerns regarding sexual pain and in addition to inspection of the external genitalia and speculum examination should include assessment of the pelvic floor muscles. (See also "Pelvic Floor Function" in this chapter.) Laboratory investigations are not required for the diagnosis of any sexual dysfunction, but some testing (eg, thyroid hormone, prolactin) may be useful to rule out medical conditions that may be contributing to sexual dysfunction; testosterone levels are recommended if testosterone therapy is being considered.

With regard to sexual pain, clinicians should determine whether it occurs with initial penetration, with deeper penetration, or with both and whether there is lingering pain after sexual activity. Frequently, there is overlap between sexual disorders (eg, sexual pain related to GSM may cause low sexual desire and difficulty with arousal). (See also "Genitourinary Syndrome of Menopause" in Chapter 4.) The sexual history is often key in

Table 2.	Prevalence of Sexual Problems Associated With Distress (PRESIDE Study)			
	Desire	**Arousal**	**Orgasm**	**Any**
Valid responses	28,447	28,461	27,854	28,403
With distressing problem	2,868	1,556	1,315	3,456
Age-stratified prevalence, y				
18-44	8.9%	3.3%	3.4%	10.8%
45-64	12.3%	7.5%	5.7%	14.8%
≥65	7.4%	6.0%	5.8%	8.9%

Shifren JL, et al.[42]

Table 3. Brief Sexual Symptom Checklist

Please answer these questions about your overall sexual function in the past ≥3 mo

1. Are you satisfied with your sexual function? Yes/No. If No, please continue.

2. How long have you been dissatisfied with your sexual function? _____

3. The problem(s) with your sexual function is (mark one or more)
   a. Problem with little or no interest in sex
   b. Problem with decreased genital sensation (feeling)
   c. Problem with decreased vaginal lubrication (dryness)
   d. Problem reaching orgasm
   e. Problem with pain during sex
   f. Other _____

4. Which problem (in question 3) is most bothersome? (Circle a, b, c, d, e, or f)

5. Would you like to talk about it with your healthcare provider? Yes/No

Adapted from Hatzichristou D, et al.[49]

Table 4. Questions to Assess Sexual Concerns

- Are you currently in a sexual relationship? With men, women, or both?
- How satisfied are you with the quality and the frequency of your sexual activity?
- Most women experience sexual difficulties at some time in their lives. What concerns or questions do you have?
- How would you like your sexual life to be different or improved? What would successful treatment of concerns look like?
- Are you experiencing any changes in your sexual life that are bothering you?
- How often, if at all, do you engage in sexual activity?
- Are you satisfied with your current sexual relations?
- Do you have difficulty with sexual desire, genital arousal, or orgasm?
- Do you experience pain during sexual activity?

Additional questions once a problem has been identified

- How long have you been experiencing this problem?
- Are there any factors you can identify that contributed to the onset (and was the onset gradual or sudden)?
- Was there a time before you had the problem when you were satisfied with your sex life? (Is the condition acquired or lifelong?)
- Are you experiencing any difficulties in your relationship with your partner that could be causing your sexual problem?
- Do you experience this problem all the time or only at certain times or in certain circumstances?

Hatzichristou D, et al.[51]

determining the primary problem and thus in guiding treatment (Table 4).[51]

A complete evaluation of FSD also includes assessment of biological, psychological, relationship, and sociocultural factors that may be affecting a woman's sexual function. A detailed account of the sexual health concern is needed and includes a description of the problem onset, duration, and severity of symptoms; situations in which the problem occurs (with one sexual partner or situation or generalized to all sexual partners or all situations); and the level of bother or distress associated with the problem.

Biological factors. Assessment of biological factors includes assessment of current health, medical history (with particular attention to endocrinologic, neuromuscular, and cardiovascular disorders), surgical history, reproductive history, and a review of current medications (Table 5).[52] Some of the medications that commonly adversely affect sexual function include antidepressants, narcotics, antihypertensives, oral contraceptives, tamoxifen, aromatase inhibitors (AIs), antihistamines, anticholinergics, and others (Table 6).[53]

Psychological factors. Psychological factors can have a significant effect on women's sexual functioning. Factors such as anxiety, depression, personality variables, a history of

sexual abuse or trauma, alcohol or substance abuse issues, poor self-image, stress, and even distraction may affect sexual function.[54] There appears to be a bidirectional relationship between sexual dysfunction and depression in that depression increases the odds of sexual dysfunction and sexual dysfunction increases the odd of depression.[55]

Women with depression who are not treated with antidepressants are more likely to experience sexual distress associated with low sexual desire[56]; however, antidepressants may also be associated with sexual dysfunction, and women may experience the sexual AEs associated with antidepressant therapy before they experience the treatment effect for depression.[57]

Sociocultural factors. Factors such as limited sexual health education, religious or cultural mores or values, and societal factors such as age discrimination can negatively affect sexual functioning in women.[54] Understanding the context in which a woman presents with sexual concerns is important.

Partner and relationship factors. The presence or absence of a partner, the quality of the relationship and communication within the relationship, and partner sexual function are factors that need to be taken into account when evaluating sexual dysfunction in women.[54] For example, a chronic sexual dysfunction (eg, dyspareunia or HSDD) may lead to relationship conflict. When sexual problems are the result of a conflicted relationship (eg, no interest in being sexual with a partner who is not liked), addressing the underlying conflict would be the appropriate treatment approach rather than focusing on the sexual consequence.

Treatment of female sexual disorders

Hypoactive sexual desire disorder

Hypoactive sexual desire disorder is defined by ISSWSH nomenclature to include reduced or absent spontaneous or responsive desire causing distress.[15] Etiology can include biological, psychological, sociocultural, and interpersonal factors. Combining medical and psychotherapeutic interventions is often the logical extension of the biopsychosocial model because more than one factor may be contributing to HSDD. Individualized therapy should focus on the primary factors(s) affecting sexual function and on those most distressing to the woman.[26] For busy menopause practitioners, the Permission, Limited Information, Specific Suggestions, and Intensive Therapy (PLISSIT) model can be used to review sexual health concerns and to direct office-based counseling for HSDD or any of the other sexual disorders (Table 7).

Psychotherapy. Psychotherapy focuses primarily on the psychological and sociocultural factors contributing to distressing low desire. Interventions generally consists of psychoeducation; couples exercises, including sensate focus; and individual and group psychotherapeutic approaches including cognitive-behavioral therapy (CBT) and mindfulness CBT.

Cognitive-behavioral therapy and other psychotherapeutic interventions focus on modifying thoughts, behaviors, expectations, beliefs, and emotions; improving relationship communication; and reducing cognitive distraction.[26,59] Each sexual dysfunction (eg, HSDD, arousal disorder, orgasmic disorder, dyspareunia) can

Table 5. Medical Conditions That May Affect Sexual Function

Urogynecologic problems	Urinary tract infections, pelvic organ prolapse, urinary and fecal incontinence
Gynecologic problems	Pelvic pain, fibroids, unpredictable bleeding, genitourinary syndrome of menopause, postpartum period, breast feeding, sexually transmitted infections
Endocrine	Diabetes mellitus, thyroid disorders, hyperprolactinemia, adrenal insufficiency
Chronic illness	Back pain, cancer, psoriasis, rheumatoid arthritis, degenerative arthritis, hypertension, coronary artery disease, neurologic conditions, renal failure
Psychiatric conditions	Mood disorders (major depression, bipolar depression, adjustment disorder), anxiety disorders, psychotic illness

Adapted from Faubion SS, et al.[52]

be addressed at least in part with various psychological interventions (individual, couples, CBT, sensate focus, mindfulness). Psychotherapy may be sufficient for some sexual problems depending on the etiology and contributing factors but may not be sufficient for others.

Pharmacologic treatments. *Flibanserin* is a centrally acting nonhormone agent that acts as a multifunction postsynaptic serotonin 1A receptor agonist and a serotonin 2A receptor antagonist and shifts the balance of neurotransmitters by reducing serotonin activity and increasing dopamine and norepinephrine activity.[60] It is currently the only approved treatment for acquired, generalized HSDD in premenopausal US and Canadian women. In the United States, prescribers and pharmacists are required to certify through a risk evaluation and mitigation program because of the risk of hypotension or syncope when combined with alcohol. In 2019, on the basis of results of postmarketing studies, FDA determined that there is still a concern about consuming alcohol close in time to taking flibanserin but that it does not have to be avoided completely.[61] A "black box warning" about risks remains.

Table 6. Medications Associated With Female Sexual Dysfunction

	Desire disorder	Arousal disorder	Orgasm disorders
Psychotropics			
Antipsychotics	+		+
Barbiturates	+	+	+
Benzodiazepines	+	+	
Lithium	+	+	+
SSRIs	+	+	+
TCA	+	+	+
MAO inhibitors			+
Trazodone	+		
Venlafaxine	+		
Cardiovascular and antihypertensive medications			
Antilipids	+		
Beta-blockers	+		
Clonidine	+	+	
Digoxin	+		+
Spironolactone	+		
Methyldopa	+		
Hormone preparations			
Danazol	+		
GnRH agonists	+		
Contraceptives	+		
Antiandrogens	+	+	+
Tamoxifen	+	+	
GnRH analogs	+	+	
Ultralight contraceptive pills	+	+	
Other			
Histamine 2 receptor blockers and promotility agents	+		
Indomethacin	+		
Ketoconazole	+		
Phenytoin sodium	+		
Aromatase inhibitors	+	+	
Chemotherapeutic agents	+	+	
Anticholinergics		+	
Antihistamines		+	
Amphetamines & related anorexic drugs			+
Narcotics			+

Abbreviations: GnRH, gonadotropin-releasing hormone; MAO, monoamine oxidase; SSRIs, selective serotonin-reuptake inhibitors; TCA, tricyclic antidepressant.
Adapted from Buster JE.[53]

Flibanserin is dosed at 100 mg at bedtime, with a recommendation to discontinue use after 8 weeks if there is no improvement in symptoms.[62] Efficacy has been established in three trials involving premenopausal women with HSDD, with increases in sexual desire, increases in sexually satisfying events, and decreases in sexual distress.[63-65] Although clinical trials have shown that flibanserin is also effective in postmenopausal women,[66,67] it is not FDA approved for use in that population.

There is evidence for the efficacy of testosterone for HSDD in perimenopausal and postmenopausal women, with acne and hirsutism as the most common short-term AEs.[40] Studies of long-term cardiovascular and breast cancer risk are limited to observational studies.[68-71]

Bremelanotide is a melanocortin-receptor agonist that is theorized to increase sexual desire. Two phase 3 multicenter trials consisting of a 4-week screening period and a core phase (4-wk at-home placebo period to establish baseline, followed by a 24-wk randomized, double-blind treatment period).[72] Participants self-administered bremelanotide (1.75 mg) or placebo subcutaneously using an autoinjector, as desired, before sexual activity. The coprimary endpoints were change in the desire domain of the Female Sexual Function Index and the Female Sexual Distress Scale—Desire/Arousal/Orgasm. Results indicate that treatment with bremelanotide is associated with improvement in desire and a decrease in distress. Bremelanotide is pending review by FDA.

Female genital arousal disorder
Female genital arousal disorder (FGAD) is defined as an inability to develop or maintain genital arousal.[15] Creating a treatment plan for a woman with difficulty becoming aroused or maintaining arousal requires a careful assessment of possible causal factors (Table 8).

A promising approach to improving women's sexual arousal is to incorporate mindfulness techniques into more traditional cognitive-behavioral sex therapy treatment.[12] This approach may help women learn to focus on pleasurable sensations while becoming less distracted by negative thoughts and feelings during sex. Mindfulness meditation may also help women to manage acute or chronic stress, both of which may interfere with sexual arousal.

Pharmacotherapy treatments
Testosterone. High-quality randomized, controlled clinical trials (RCTs) demonstrated that transdermal

testosterone patch therapy can improve arousal as well as sexual desire.[73] Testosterone may have a direct effect on the vagina and genital structures independent from the effects of estrogen.[74]

Phosphodiesterase inhibitors. The data for phosphodiesterase inhibitors from RCTs for FGAD has been reviewed and has been found to be contradictory and ultimately lacking in efficacy.[75,76] In specific populations of women suffering from medical conditions interfering with genital neurovascular substrates, there may be a potential therapeutic role for these vasoactive agents.[77] A topical sildenafil cream is in development, and clinical trials are under way in women with FSAD.

Other nonhormone pharmacotherapies that may improve arousal include L-arginine, topical alprostadil (prostaglandin E1), dopaminergic drugs (eg, bupropion), and oxytocin.[12]

Devices. In addition to pharmacotherapies, some devices have been designed to treat or improve arousal, including the Eros therapy device. The Eros therapy device is the only FDA-cleared-to-market device available by prescription to treat FGAD. It is a small, battery-powered appliance that creates a direct vacuum over the clitoris causing the clitoral erectile chambers and labia to fill with blood. The vibration from the suction pump may also aid in stimulation.

Female orgasmic disorder

Female orgasmic disorder (FOD) refers to a distressing absence of orgasm, difficulty experiencing orgasm, or reduced intensity of orgasm during all or most occasions of sexual activity.[15] The symptoms may be lifelong or acquired. Difficulty reaching orgasm may be isolated to specific sexual activities, situations, or partners. Some medications, such as selective serotonin-reuptake inhibitors (SSRIs), also can delay orgasm.[78]

Psychoeducation is the primary intervention found in all evidence-based psychological interventions for FOD and is therapeutic in itself.[12] Content is typically information about sexual anatomy and physiology, variations in sexual response, and common forms of stimulation used to reach orgasm.

Directed masturbation is the most researched behavioral treatment for FOD.[12] It consists of a series of self-awareness and exploration exercises that are intended to help a woman become more familiar and comfortable with her genitals and other areas of the body that are experienced as erotic. In a progressive fashion, the

Table 7.	PLISSIT Model
P	Give the patient **PERMISSION** to talk about her sexual concerns by asking open-ended questions.
LI	Provide the patient with **LIMITED INFORMATION**, such as education about female anatomy and physiology and basic changes in sexual function throughout the aging process. Not all information must be provided at one encounter. Patients should be encouraged to make follow-up appointments for continued discussion and management as needed.
S	Make **SPECIFIC SUGGESTIONS** in response to the problem (ie, suggest lubricant use for vaginal dryness).
IT	Referral to a specialist for **INTENSIVE THERAPY** may be more appropriate after basic education and suggestions. It is best if the clinician explains this collaborative multidisciplinary approach so that the patient does not feel abandoned.

Abbreviation: PLISSIT, Permission, Limited Information, Specific Suggestions, and Intensive Therapy.
Adapted from Annon J.[58]

woman is asked to complete a series of exercises between therapy sessions to explore her body and genitals, become more aware of sexually arousing stimuli, and eventually use her self-knowledge to masturbate to orgasm.[79]

Sensate focus techniques can be used to treat FOD.[12] Vibrators, other arousal devices, and erotic media (books, video) may be used to enhance physical and psychological sexual stimulation and can override anxiety and other inhibiting thoughts.

Sexual pain disorders

Sexual pain can be a result of a number of different conditions, and identifying the condition causing the pain is critical in order to determine appropriate treatment. If the sexual pain is the result of GSM, treatments include the use of nonhormone therapies such as moisturizers to help maintain moisture and lubricants to reduce friction and enhance pleasure during sexual activity. Hormone therapies include low-dose vaginal estrogen (cream, ring, tablet) and intravaginal dehydroepiandrosterone (DHEA) used nightly.[80] Intravaginal DHEA may also

Table 8   Possible Causes of Female Genital Arousal Disorder

- Cultural or religious factors causing guilt and inhibition
- Partner conflicts
- Distracting cognitions during sex (insecurity about attractiveness or ability to please the partner sexually, memories of past sexual trauma)
- High stress
- A sexual partner whose ill health or sexual dysfunction limits sexual activity and pleasure

have beneficial effects on sexual function separate from the effect on GSM.[81]

Ospemifene is a selective estrogen-receptor modulator that is administered orally on a daily basis for management of dyspareunia in postmenopausal women.[82] If a woman has experienced sexual pain related to GSM or other skin conditions (eg, vulvar dermatoses) for a period of time, she may also experience sexual pain related to tight pelvic floor muscles (also called nonrelaxing or high-tone pelvic floor muscle dysfunction).[83] Pelvic floor physical therapy provided by a physical therapist with special training in the management of pelvic floor disorders may be helpful. (See also "Pelvic Floor Function" in this chapter.)

The *carbon dioxide laser* has been cleared by FDA for "incision, excision, ablation, vaporization, and coagulation of body soft tissues in medical specialties, including aesthetic (dermatology and plastic surgery), podiatry, otolaryngology, gynecology" and other specialties, and the YAG laser has been cleared for "incision, excision, ablation, vaporization of soft tissue for general dermatology, dermatologic, and general surgical procedures for coagulation and hemostasis." GSM is not identified as a specific indication for treatment.[84] Although small, uncontrolled clinical trials demonstrate improvements in self-reported symptoms (vaginal dryness, burning, itching, dyspareunia, and dysuria) and in Vaginal Health Index scores, longer-term safety and efficacy studies with sham control are needed.[85,86]

Pelvic Floor Function

The hormone decline associated with menopause can have a profound effect on sexual comfort because of changes in the vulvar and vaginal tissues as well as on the musculature of the pelvic floor. Although vulvovaginal atrophic issues are often appropriately addressed with local ET when a

postmenopausal woman complains of pain with intercourse, too often pelvic floor dysfunction (the true cause of prohibitive pain) is overlooked and left untreated.

Physiology

The pelvic floor muscles, known collectively as the *levator ani* muscles, consist of the superficial (transverse perineal, bulbospongiosus, and ischiocavernosus) muscles and the deep (pubococcygeus, iliococcygeus, obturator internus, and coccygeus) muscles. Their function is to provide direct support to the viscera of the urinary, genital, and rectal compartments of the pelvis and to provide secondary postural stabilization to the bony pelvis. Normal function of the pelvic floor musculature is essential in maintaining appropriate function of the pelvic organs and contributes to adequate urination, defecation, and sexual response. Abnormal function of this musculature and abnormal muscle are found in at least 25% of postmenopausal women with genitourinary, bowel, or sexual pain syndrome.[87]

Pelvic floor dysfunction

Pelvic floor dysfunction (PFD) refers to conditions in which the pelvic floor muscular support system is functioning abnormally.[88] Traditionally, the term PFD has been used synonymously with *low-tone pelvic floor dysfunction* (LTPFD) to denote weak, underactive, and hypotonic muscles that cannot attain or maintain adequate contraction, leading to symptoms of incontinence, heaviness, pressure, altered sexual sensation, and pelvic organ prolapse.[89]

Another type of PFD is when weak pelvic floor muscles cannot attain or maintain adequate relaxation and are overactive, hypertonic, spastic, and shortened. The term *high-tone pelvic floor dysfunction* (HTPFD) describes this phenomenon. Although the concept of HTPFD is infrequently seen in the menopause literature, it has been used extensively in the colorectal literature in which HTPFD is referred to as *tension myalgia of the pelvic floor*.[90] This type of dysfunction is prevalent as a source of prohibitive sexual pain in women.[89]

High-tone PFD can result from several etiologies, including muscle or nerve trauma during childbirth; urinary, vaginal, or uterine infections; adhesions and surgical trauma; instability in the sacroiliac joint, hip, or spine; accidental fall or injury; and postural stressors. High-tone pelvic floor dysfunction presents with symptoms of frequency, urgency, dysuria, urinary retention, fecal retention/constipation, penetrative dyspareunia, and/or vaginismus.[89,90]

A characteristic of HTPFD is the occurrence of myofascial trigger points (MTrPs) within the muscle.[90] Active MTrPs elicit local or referred pain similar to that of the patient's complaints, and a localized muscle twitch can be felt by the examiner on palpation. For instance, a trigger point within the pubococcygeus muscle can create a tender area with direct palpation of the muscle or it could refer pain to the introitus (creating sensations of burning that could be mistaken for a vaginal infection).

If left untreated, MTrPs and progressive muscle hypertonicity can result in compression of deeper neural structures (eg, pudendal nerve) and cause neuropathic symptoms that completely prohibit sexual activity.[90]

Risk of pelvic floor dysfunction in postmenopausal women

Although menopause does not directly cause PFD, the hormone changes associated with menopause can provide the ideal environment for the development of hypertonus. Both testosterone and estrogen receptors are present in the musculature of the pelvic floor. Hormone deficiency causes a reduction in the collagen, hyaluronic acid, elastin, and alterations in myosin filaments. These changes can decrease muscle strength, increase connective tissue density, and decrease circulation contributing to the development of stiff and weak muscles with restricted range of motion.[91]

In addition, a postmenopausal woman's PFD can be related to inflammation of surrounding visceral structures in the pelvis because of common innervations that develop during embryologic development. Chronic irritation of visceral structures can cause trophic changes within muscular and connective tissue, and a primary muscle skeletal disorder (eg, lumbopelvic or sacroiliac joint dysfunction) can affect the surrounding viscera resulting in bladder, bowel, and sexual dysfunction.[90] For example, a postmenopausal woman who has hypersensitivity associated with urogenital conditions such as chronic bacterial cystitis, chronic yeast infections, endometriosis, urethritis, provoked vestibulodynia, or interstitial cystitis may be at risk for comorbid HTPFD. Treatment directed at all conditions and all pain generators is key for a successful outcome when treating pelvic floor muscle spasm.

Last, HTPFD can occur after an injury or accident affecting the hip or back—types of injuries for which postmenopausal women are particularly vulnerable. With injury to the upper pelvic stabilizers, there is increased metabolic activity within the pelvic floor muscles causing the muscle to spasm. Over time, the muscle become fibrotic, with decreased flexibility and impaired relaxation. The increased muscle tension triggers pain and more reflex tightening, and the vicious cycle of pelvic floor hypertonus begins.[92]

Pelvic floor muscle examination

A thorough evaluation of the pelvic floor muscles begins with a detailed pain assessment and medical history. The woman's posture, alignment, gait patterns, movement of the spine, and hip are evaluated for dysfunction. Next, a systematic "front-to-back" palpation of the pelvic floor muscles is performed, noting presence of sensitive areas, shortened muscles, local tender areas, or muscle twitch as well as referred pain patterns. Pelvic floor muscle coordination can be assessed by asking the woman to contract her muscles around the examiner's gloved fingers, hold for a count of five, and then relax the muscles and produce a "bulge" movement. When the woman is unable to contract, relax, or bulge and demonstrates poor coordination in the pelvic floor muscles, she should be triaged for further evaluation. This is generally accomplished by a referral to an experienced manual physical therapist with familiarity or specialty in the pelvic floor.

Pelvic floor physical therapy

Physical therapists specializing in PFD identify and treat musculoskeletal impairments that generate or contribute to pain syndromes. Addressing impairments in the muscles, ligaments, joints, and connective tissue/fascia can significantly reduce or eliminate sexual pain. The typical woman who presents with pelvic floor pain also has weakness of the core muscles, sacroiliac joint dysfunction, or gait abnormalities. Abnormalities can be identified by testing range of motion, mobility, and muscle strength and length. The physical therapist assesses connective tissue and fascia of the upper pelvis, low back, abdominals, and lower extremities in addition to evaluating the muscles of the pelvic floor. The goals of treatment are to improve connective tissue mobility, strengthen the core muscles, normalize pelvic tone, deactivate myofascial trigger points, and improve motor control of the pelvic floor.

After working with the woman to strengthen upper pelvis core postural stabilizers via closed kinetic chain exercises and myofascial release techniques, the physical therapist directly addresses pelvic floor muscle trigger points via internal massage techniques. The sequence and combination of methods used is based on patient history, evaluation, and tolerance (Table 9). Physical therapy treatment sessions are typically 30 to 60 minutes in length and occur one or two times a week. Duration of treatment typically ranges from 12 weeks to 1 year, depending on severity of symptoms, patient tolerance, response to treatment, and compliance.

Myofascial pelvic floor physical therapy has been the source of several clinical research investigations and has been found to be superior to external therapeutic massage in relieving symptoms of pelvic pain.[93,94]

On completion of pelvic floor physical therapy, the patient is encouraged to maintain pelvic stability by performing a home exercise program that involves daily performance of gentle stretches to open the hip capsule and extend the low back. Simple yoga poses including: "downward dog," "child's pose," and "happy baby" are often employed because they can be easily performed by women at various skill levels.

Muscle relaxants

In consultation with the physical therapist, the clinician may choose to augment muscle relaxation for the woman by prescribing oral or compounded topical or transvaginal muscle relaxants.[95] Low-dose options include diazepam, baclofen, cyclobenzaprine, or methocarbamol.[90]

Vaginal dilator therapy

Vaginal dilators are used to stretch the pelvic floor muscles and restore vaginal capacity and can be a useful adjuvant to pelvic floor physical therapy. Vaginal dilators are smooth plastic, rubber or glass cylinder-shaped objects that come in a variety of widths and weights. Dilators stretch the vagina in both width and depth to improve elasticity in the tissues while building confidence in the user that she will not have pain with sexual activity. As a woman uses larger and larger diameter dilators to stretch the pelvic floor muscles, it demonstrates observable progress toward resumption of sexual activity and gives the woman a sense of participation in her care. The final goal is to achieve comfort with using a dilator that has a similar girth to partner size.

It is important that the clinician provides clear instructions to a woman before starting vaginal dilation. To begin, a dilator size that does not cause pain with insertion but does not go in too easily is chosen. Using a mirror in the exam room to show a woman exactly where and how to insert a dilator is often helpful. The woman should be instructed to use a water-based lubricant and leave the dilator in place for 5 to 10 minutes once to twice daily. Each dilator size is used for 2 to 4 weeks before progressing to the next size.[96]

Botulinum toxin A injection

In clinical practice, botulinum toxin A injection has been used to inactivate hypertonic pelvic floor muscles that do not completely resolve with pelvic floor muscle physical therapy or the use of dilators or muscle relaxants.[97] Although its use for HTPFD is considered off label, a number of clinical investigations have underscored its use for this condition.

In one pilot prospective cohort study, botulinum toxin A was injected into the levator ani muscles of 12 women with pelvic floor muscle hypertonicity who had a 2-year history of chronic pelvic pain.[98] Forty units of botulinum toxin A were injected into each of the puborectalis and pubococcygeus muscles. Median visual analog scale pain scores were significantly improved for dyspareunia (P=.01) and dysmenorrhea (P=.03). Pelvic floor muscle manometric measurements showed a 25% reduction in tension initially that was maintained at week 12 (P<.0001). Sexual activity scores were markedly improved, with a significant reduction in discomfort (P=.02).

In a similar trial, botulinum toxin A injections were more effective than placebo in reducing pain and pelvic floor pressure in 30 women with chronic pelvic pain and pelvic floor muscle spasm.[99] Participants had a total of 80 units of botulinum toxin A injected into the pelvic

Table 9.	Physical Therapy Techniques for Treating Pelvic Floor Dysfunction
Connective tissue/ Fascial mobilization	A manual technique using the finger pads to manipulate vulvar tissue externally and vaginal or rectal tissue internally to improve circulation and fascial mobility
Strain/ Counter strain	A manual therapy technique that passively shortens a muscle in order to reduce muscle tone
Ischemic compression	A manual therapy technique that applies direct pressure to a trigger point in order to elicit relaxation
Neuromuscular reeducation	A therapeutic technique used to improve coordination and kinesthetic and proprioception awareness of the pelvic floor via palpation or biofeedback

floor muscles. The change from baseline in the treatment group was significant for dyspareunia (*P*<.001) and pelvic pain (*P*=.009).

Another study reported on 29 women who received 100 to 300 units of botulinum toxin A to the pelvic floor muscles.[100] Before treatment, more than 89% of the study cohort reported severe pain with palpation of the levator ani muscles. After injection, 51.7% reported no pain, and 20.7% reported only mild pain.

In a prospective study of 37 women with pelvic pain, 100 units of botulinum toxin A delivered in split doses to the puborectalis and pubococcygeus muscles provided significant relief of dyspareunia and pelvic pain.[101]

Patient counseling

Preprocedure counseling is key to providing realistic patient expectations before botulinum toxin A is injected.[90] The woman is counseled about the drug's mechanism of action, efficacy, and duration and the fact that it is being used off label for the indication of pelvic floor muscle hypertonus. In highly anxious women or those with severe pain, administration of a sedative or an analgesic before pelvic floor injections may be offered but is usually not required. The woman also should be informed that rare complications such as local minimal bleeding, hematoma formation, nausea, vomiting, diplopia, dysphagia, temporary stress urinary incontinence, muscle weakness, and/or urinary retention can arise from botulinum toxin A injections.

Injection technique

With the patient lying supine with her legs in stirrups, a digital examination is performed to identify specific pelvic hypertonic floor muscles and MTrPs (knowledge of pelvic floor muscle anatomy is key for a successful injection).[97] The injection can be accomplished by either transperineal or transvaginal injection. The botulinum toxin A is prepared per package insert using sterile saline solution and administered in doses of 30 to 50 units to the most pain-producing hypertonic muscles, generally not exceeding 100 to 200 total units. After receiving the injections, the woman returns to the care of her pelvic floor physical therapist. Reassessment in the clinician's office is done at 2 to 3 weeks and 3 months postinjection. If hypertonus returns, reinjection may be necessary.

Care should be taken to avoid an oversimplified approach to symptoms of chronic pelvic pain and dyspareunia in a postmenopausal woman. A comprehensive approach to care dictates that if her genitourinary pain persists after estrogen deprivation issues have been

addressed, she should be carefully evaluated for PFD and triaged for appropriate interdisciplinary care.

Abnormal Uterine Bleeding

Perimenopause is defined as "the period around the onset of menopause that is often marked by various physical signs such as hot flashes and *menstrual irregularities*" (italics added). Perhaps another way to think of this is that perimenopause is the mirror image of adolescence, which is the coming on to the reproductive years, whereas perimenopause is the coming off of the reproductive years. Although the median age of menopause, at least in North America, is 52 years, perimenopause is often highly variable as to age of onset, how long it lasts, and the bleeding patterns in which it results. To women, any vaginal bleeding is considered their "period," but to clinicians, a menses implies a bleed that is preceded by ovulation and the production of progesterone.

Anovulatory cycles can be highly variable in the bleeding patterns they produce, whereas ovulatory cycles tend to be more predictable in their character. The definition of abnormal uterine bleeding (AUB) is flow outside of normal volume, duration, regularity, or frequency.[102] One-third of patient visits to the gynecologist are for AUB, and that accounts for more than 70% of all gynecologic consults in the perimenopause and postmenopause years. It should be obvious that the evaluation of women is important for two main reasons: 1) to exclude serious pathology such as carcinoma or complex atypical hyperplasia, and 2) to identify the cause of bleeding so proper therapy (which, in some cases, may be expectant management) can be instituted.

Diagnosis

Abnormal uterine bleeding is an umbrella term that encompasses heavy menstrual bleeding (previously referred to as *menorrhagia*) and intermenstrual bleeding (previously referred to as *metrorrhagia*). There has been inconsistency in the terminology used to describe AUB, and there are a number of potential causes. A classification system based on the causes of AUB, the PALM-COEIN (polyp; adenomyosis; leiomyoma; malignancy and hyperplasia; coagulopathy; ovulatory dysfunction; endometrial; iatrogenic; and not yet classified) system has been developed and approved by the International Federation of Gynecology and Obstetrics to aid clinicians and patients with communication and with clinical care (Table 10).[103]

The COEIN portion of the PALM-COEIN system covers nonstructural, hormone, or systemic causes of

AUB. Top among these causes is AUB associated with ovulatory dysfunction, or *anovulatory uterine bleeding*, defined as menstrual bleeding arising without ovulation or oligoovulation (infrequent ovulation). Anovulatory uterine bleeding presents as noncyclic menstrual blood flow ranging from spotting to heavy. The timing of the bleeding episodes and the amount of blood loss is erratic.

During an anovulatory cycle, the corpus luteum does not form.[104] If the normal cyclic secretion of progesterone does not occur, estrogen stimulates the endometrium unopposed, and it becomes proliferative and eventually outgrows its blood supply. It may slough and bleed irregularly, heavily, or longer than normal. With prolonged anovulation and unopposed estrogen exposure, the endometrium can become hyperplastic and develop atypical or even malignant cells.

New cases of endometrial cancer are estimated at 61,880 in 2019 and 12,160 deaths.[105] In one large health plan's study, endometrial hyperplasia peak incidence was: for simple, 142 per 100,000 woman-years and for complex, 213 per 100,000 woman-years, both occurring in women aged in their early 50s; and for atypical, 56 per 100,000 woman-years, occurring in women aged in their early 60s.[106] (See also "Endometrial Cancer" in Chapter 9.)

The PALM portion of the PALM-COEIN classification of causes of AUB refers to structural causes such

---

Table 10. FIGO PALM-COEIN Classification System for Causes of AUB

Structural causes (PALM)

Polyps	Includes endometrial and endocervical polyps comprised of variable vascular, glandular, and fibromuscular and connective tissue components. Often asymptomatic but at least some contribute to the genesis of AUB. Lesions are usually benign but a small minority may have atypical or malignant features. Polyps are categorized as being either present or absent, as defined by 1 or a combination of ultrasound and hysteroscopic imaging with or without histopathology.
Adenomyosis	Relationship between adenomyosis and AUB is unclear, thus extensive additional research is required. Because there exist sonographic- and MRI-based diagnostic criteria, adenomyosis has been included in the PALM part of the classification system.
Leiomyoma	Benign fibromuscular tumors of the myometrium known by several names, including *leiomyoma*, *myoma*, and the frequently used *fibroid*. Leiomyoma is generally accepted as the more accurate term. Like polyps and adenomyosis, many leiomyomas are asymptomatic, and frequently their presence is not the cause of AUB.
Malignancy and hyperplasia	Proposed that malignant or premalignant lesions (eg, atypical endometrial hyperplasia, endometrial carcinoma, and leiomyosarcoma) be categorized within this major category but further dealt with using existent WHO and FIGO classification and staging systems.

Nonstructural causes (COEIN)

Coagulopathy	Encompasses the spectrum of systemic disorders of hemostasis that may be associated with AUB. It is important to consider such disorders because they probably do contribute to some cases of AUB and because evidence indicates that relatively few clinicians consider systemic disorders of hemostasis in the differential diagnosis of women with HMB.
Ovulatory dysfunction	Disorders of ovulation may present as amenorrhea, through extremely light and infrequent bleeding, to episodes of unpredictable and extreme HMB requiring medical or surgical intervention. Ovulatory disorders can be traced to endocrinopathies (POS, hypothyroidism, hyperprolactinemia, mental stress, obesity, anorexia, weight loss, or extreme exercise such as that associated with elite athletic training).
Endometrial	When AUB occurs in the context of predictable and cyclic menstrual bleeding, typical of ovulatory cycles, and particularly when no other definable causes are identified, the mechanism is probably a primary disorder of the endometrium.
Iatrogenic	Associated with the use of exogenous gonad steroids, intrauterine systems or devices, or other systemic or local agents.
Not yet classified	Entities that are rarely encountered or are ill-defined.

Abbreviations: AUB, abnormal uterine bleeding; FIGO, International Federation of Gynecology and Obstetrics; HMB, heavy menstrual bleeding; MRI, magnetic resonance imaging; POS, polycystic ovary syndrome; WHO, World Health Organization.
Munro MG, et al.[103]

as polyps, adenomyosis, leiomyomas, and malignancies that often can be detected by physical examination, imaging, or tissue sampling.[103]

Benign uterine fibroid tumors are commonly associated with AUB. Although most fibroids are asymptomatic, others produce dramatic changes in menstrual periods (eg, heavier and prolonged periods) as well as a range of other symptoms such as excessive menstrual cramps, back pain, dyspareunia, and difficulties with bowel movements or urination. Although the cause of fibroids is unknown, hormones can stimulate their growth. Because fibroids are estrogen and progesterone sensitive, they often shrink after menopause, when ovarian production of hormones diminishes. Rarely, systemic ET may cause fibroids to resume growth. Fibroids do not usually cause acute pain, but in some cases they can undergo torsion, degenerate, or become necrotic with accompanying pain.

Endometrial or endocervical polyps can result in AUB.[107] A small percentage of cases of AUB is caused by cancer of the uterus or cervix.

Evaluation

As with all good medical practice, diagnosis begins with a thorough history and physical examination followed by appropriate laboratory and imaging tests as indicated. History should query any family history of AUB, any suspicion of underlying bleeding disorder, and use of any medications or herbal preparations such as ginseng, gingko, motherwort, contraceptives, nonsteroidal anti-inflammatory drugs (NSAIDs), and warfarin or heparin or their derivatives that might affect bleeding in general.[108,109] Physical examination should include assessment of body mass index (BMI), thyroid examination, and a pelvic examination consisting of speculum findings to rule out cervical or vaginal etiologies of bleeding as well as bimanual assessment of size and contour of the uterus.

Laboratory assessment should include a complete blood count to ascertain whether anemia is present, as well as assessment of any bleeding disorder if suspected or indicated. Pregnancy testing and thyroid screening also may be appropriate.

One of the most important aspects will be careful assessment of the bleeding pattern, although, admittedly, many women will not be aware of exactly how often or how long they bleed. For example, very cyclic, heavy, menstrual bleeding without any intermenstrual bleeding, although heavy, would be unlikely to be a sign of carcinoma or hyperplasia.

Most often, an irregular bleeding pattern is associated with no endometrial pathology. One study of 433 women used TVU and saline infusion sonohysterography (SIS) as the first step in triage and reported 79% of women aged between 35 years and menopause with irregular bleeding had no anatomic pathology,[110] presumably secondary to anovulatory bleeding, which represents normal physiology in response to declining ovarian function. Some, whose bleeding pattern is heavy menstrual bleeding, may have an enlarged cavity with increased surface area because of increasing parity, uterine hypertrophy secondary to leiomyoma with no submucous component, or adenomyosis without endometrial abnormality. In that study, endometrial abnormalities included hyperplasia, polyps, and submucous myomas.

Endometrial evaluation will be essential in triaging patients to no anatomic pathology or anatomic pathology and then whether such pathology is focal in nature and needs to be distinguished from more global processes.[111] Historically, this used to use dilatation and curettage as the primary diagnostic test. In fact, it was the most common surgical procedure in women during much of the 20th century. More recently, endometrial biopsy in an outpatient setting has gained great regularity.

Shortcomings of endometrial biopsy

After one single study, blind endometrial sampling with disposable suction piston devices became a standard approach in women with AUB.[112] An outpatient biopsy was performed on 40 women with known carcinoma in the week before their hysterectomies, and endometrial carcinoma was obtained in 39 of the 40 samples, thus a 97.5% accuracy. This was widely publicized, marketed, and promoted and was rapidly accepted as the standard of care.

In a similar study, a blind endometrial sampling was performed in 65 women with known carcinoma in the operating room just before their hysterectomies.[113] Eleven of 65 cancers were missed (sensitivity, 83%), but on opening all those uteri, when the cancers occupied 50% or more of the endometrial surface, the biopsy was 100% accurate.

Others did similar studies. In women with known carcinomas, the sensitivity of blind sampling was only 84%[114] and 68%[115] in those studies, yielding a false-negative rate of 16% and 32%, respectively. These were blind biopsies done on women with *known* carcinoma. In trying to understand why such biopsies failed in non-global pathology, one needs to look no further than a prehysterectomy study in which the Pipelle brand sampled an average of 4% of the endometrial surface area (range, 0-12%).[116]

In 2012, the American College of Obstetricians and Gynecologists (ACOG) acknowledged that the primary role of endometrial sampling in women with AUB was to determine whether carcinoma or premalignant lesions are present and that endometrial biopsy has "high overall accuracy in diagnosing endometrial cancer when an adequate specimen is obtained and when the endometrial process is global. If the cancer occupies less than 50% of the surface area of the endometrial cavity, the cancer can be missed by blind endometrial biopsy. Therefore, these tests are only an endpoint when they reveal cancer or atypical complex hyperplasia."[102,113]

This has tremendous ramifications for clinical practice. Certainly, healthcare providers, especially in low-resource areas, can begin the evaluation with a blind biopsy, but if the results do not indicate cancer or atypical hyperplasia, the evaluation is not adequate, especially if bleeding persists. Thus, the concept of distinguishing global from focal pathologies is becoming increasingly understood and important.

Imaging techniques

Clearly, the primary imaging test of the uterus for the evaluation of AUB is TVU. However, not all uteri lend themselves to a meaningful ultrasound examination, such as in cases of coexisting myomas, previous surgery, marked obesity, axial uterus, or adenomyosis. In such cases, another alternative is SIS (the installation of fluid or gel into the endometrial cavity to further delineate endometrial anatomy). This can virtually always distinguish the presence or absence of actual anatomic pathology. Furthermore, when anatomic pathology is present, such an approach can distinguish the changes that are global, allowing for blind endometrial sampling versus focal abnormalities, which should be sampled under direct vision at the time of hysteroscopy.

Hysteroscopy as a diagnostic tool also may be employed, although it is more expensive, requires more anesthesia, and if performed, is preferably done in an office setting.[102] Disposable hysteroscopes make this recommendation easier to follow.

Transvaginal ultrasonography

The vaginal probe provides a degree of image magnification as if the ultrasound was performed through a low power microscope and can be considered a form of "sonomicroscopy."[117] Things can be seen with the vaginal probe that could not be seen with the naked eye, if the structure could be held at arm's length and squinted at. This is because these are high-frequency transducers in closer proximity to the structure being studied, providing this degree of image magnification.

Early observational studies and then subsequent large multicenter trials, mostly from western Europe, clearly established the fact that, in postmenopausal women with bleeding, a distinct endometrial echo is indicative of a lack of significant tissue and has higher negative predictive value for endometrial cancer than blind endometrial sampling.[117] This caused ACOG to state in a committee opinion that when an endometrial echo less than or equal to 4 mm on TVU is obtained, an endometrial biopsy is not required.[118]

There are less data collected on perimenopausal women with AUB. One potential pitfall is that such women will have cycling of the endometrium based on erratic estrogen production of perimenopausal ovaries. Thus, the use of TVU in such patients must be timed to the end of a bleeding episode when the endometrial echo will be as thin as one would expect throughout the whole month. In addition, this prevents misinterpretation of endometrial moguls, which can occur because of the heterogeneity of the topography of the functional is as it proliferates. In addition, not all uteri lend themselves to meaningful ultrasound examination.

In the study of 433 perimenopausal women aged 37 to 54 years, 10.2% required sonohysterography because the unenhanced TVU done at the end of a bleeding cycle was inadequate to effectively characterize and measure the endometrium.[110] In that study, 64.7% of women had an endometrial thickness of 5 mm or less, and 25.1% had an endometrial thickness greater than 5 mm and, therefore, underwent SIS to characterize global versus focal changes. Final diagnosis of all women in this study revealed that 79% had dysfunctional anovulatory bleeding; 13% had polyps; 3.5% had hyperplasia; and 5.3% had submucous myomas (although 33% had sonographic evidence of myomas, only the 5.3% were submucous).

Hysteroscopy is certainly an alternative approach, although issues of operator dependence, cost, analgesia/anesthesia concerns, and availability of the resource must be taken into account.

The diagnostic evaluation is paramount to successful therapeutic decision making and will have important ramifications for triage for appropriate therapies, particularly surgical versus medical versus expectant management.

Management

Therapy will be directed by proper diagnosis. Further, the concept of "no anatomic abnormality," as in bleeding related to ovulatory dysfunction, use of contraceptives, adenomyosis, or simply an enlarged cavity surface area related to increased size, may be approached in a variety of ways. After pregnancy and malignancy have been excluded, treatment goals for patients with AUB include regulation of menstrual cycles, minimization of blood loss, and improvement in QOL. For heavy menstrual periods, the treatment goals are to prevent further worsening of anemia and reduce the need for blood transfusion. For many patients who are not anemic, the bleeding is more of a QOL issue rather than of medical significance. Thus, for some, the knowledge that there is no serious problem and, especially for women with dysfunctional anovulatory bleeding, the knowledge that this is a normal part of the transition from the reproductive to the nonreproductive years may be sufficiently reassuring to manage them expectantly.

Pharmacologic therapy

Hormone treatments. According to a recent survey conducted among members of ACOG, the most commonly selected first-line choice for AUB treatment in the United States was combined oral contraceptives (COCs).[119] The levonorgestrel intrauterine system (LNG-IUS) was the next most-frequently selected option. Combined oral contraceptives can correct menstrual irregularities resulting from oligo-ovulation or anovulation and make menstruation more predictable. They can also reduce excessive menstrual bleeding in most affected women and are considered a reasonable option for initial management of menorrhagia. (See also "Contraceptives" in Chapter 11.)

The COC is less effective for the treatment of heavy menstrual periods in women with organic pathology, although the response can be variable. Menstrual blood loss is reduced by about 50% in women using COCs, and the reduction is most apparent during the first 2 days of the menstrual flow. Extended cycle or continuous-combined oral contraceptives with the 20 µg ethinylestradiol/100 µg LNG formulation, either 84/7 regimens that shorten the hormone-free interval and decrease the number of days of bleeding per year or the 365-day regimen designed to eliminate bleeding altogether, is associated with significant reduced bleeding compared with cyclic use. Shortening of the hormone-free interval from 7 to 4 days significantly decreases the number of withdrawal bleeding days in each cycle and increases the amenorrhea rate.

Obviously, all clinicians have treated patients who are already on COCs who experience what is referred to as breakthrough bleeding. Usually, adjustment of the dose or type of pill can overcome this, although persistent bleeding of such a nature should trigger further diagnostic evaluation in case some coexisting organic pathology also is present.

The LNG-IUS is another effective therapy. Because of the effect of LNG on the endometrium, the duration and amount of menstrual bleeding are reduced. There is evidence that LNG-IUS improves QOL to a greater extent than usual medical therapies, including COCs. This effect may begin during the first menstrual cycle after the placement of the device, and bleeding becomes progressively less over time. Women should be counseled about the inconvenience of breakthrough bleeding observed during the initial months of treatment.[120] (See also "Contraceptives" in Chapter 11.)

Nonsteroidal anti-inflammatory drugs. Nonsteroidal anti-inflammatory drugs reduce prostaglandin synthesis. Prostaglandins may have a role in aberrant neovascularization leading to dysfunctional uterine bleeding. Oral NSAIDs are an excellent treatment to reduce heavy menstrual bleeding. Compared with placebo, they decrease menstrual cramping and reduce menstrual blood loss by 33%.[121] There is no evidence of a difference between the individual NSAIDs (naproxen and mefenamic acid) in reducing heavy menstrual bleeding. Mefenamic acid 500 mg three times a day for 5 days and ibuprofen 600 mg every 6 hours or 800 mg every 8 hours are commonly prescribed during the first 3 days of the menstrual cycle to reduce blood loss and menstrual cramping.

Tranexamic acid. The pharmacologic mechanism of tranexamic acid (TXA) involves reversibly blocking lysine-binding sites on plasminogen, preventing plasmin and fibrin polymer interaction resulting in fibrin degradation, the stabilization of clots, and reduction of bleeding. It is contraindicated in women with increased risk for thromboembolism. It has been routinely used for many years to reduce blood loss and the need for blood transfusion during and after surgical procedures.

Tranexamic acid has been used for the treatment of heavy menstrual bleeding outside of the United States for several decades. Its therapeutic effect is superior to placebo and results in significant reduction in objective measurement of idiopathic heavy menstrual bleeding.[122] In all studies analyzed, only mild to moderate AEs were reported, mostly gastrointestinal (GI), and there were no reports of thromboembolic events with the use of TXA. FDA has approved TXA at an oral dosage of 1,300 mg (two 650-mg tablets) three times daily for 5 days each menstrual cycle.

The oral bioavailability of TXA only is about 35%, which makes frequent administrations necessary. The disadvantages of frequent administrations include decreased patient compliance and increased risk of GI AEs, most commonly nausea, vomiting, and diarrhea. The prospect of using a single antifibrinolytic medication to relieve a common gynecologic condition is certainly potentially cost saving as well as morbidity reducing if it results in a decrease in the amount of surgery for treating heavy menstrual bleeding.

Endometrial ablation

Endometrial ablation is a minimally invasive alternative for the treatment of heavy menstrual bleeding and is associated with a high level of patient satisfaction. It is usually reserved for patients refractory to medical treatment and who wish to avoid definitive treatment with hysterectomy. Although endometrial ablation is a less invasive surgical alternative to hysterectomy, it does not eliminate surgical risk and is followed by further surgery within 4 years in up to 38% of the women who undergo this treatment.[123] Endometrial ablation should be considered as an alternative to hysterectomy, especially in older women who have opted to retain their uterus and not in women with a desire for future fertility.

Patient age is an important predictor of treatment success. In contrast to the original resectoscopic endometrial ablation, several ablation devices offer the advantage of being performed in an office setting. Careful patient selection seems to be the key to decrease the occurrence of endometrial cancer after ablation. In a systematic review of studies in which 22 postablation endometrial cancer cases were reviewed, time to diagnosis of endometrial cancer ranged from 2 weeks to 10 years after endometrial ablation.[124] Most women had symptoms of persistent bleeding or pain after the procedure. Eighty-six percent of the women with cancer presented with risk factors for endometrial cancer such as obesity, complex atypical endometrial hyperplasia, diabetes mellitus (DM), hypertension, and postmenopausal status. Thus, endometrial ablation should be restricted to premenopausal women who have low risk factors for endometrial cancer and who have documented normal endometrial histopathologic features at preablation evaluation.

Uterine fibroids

Uterine fibroids occur in 25% of women of reproductive age and often are associated with AUB, particularly irregular and/or heavy bleeding. Although hysterectomy is still widely offered as a treatment for uterine fibroids, there are different treatment options to discuss as well, in order that women are able to make an informed choice.

A combination of presenting clinical symptoms, fibroid size and location, and the woman's desire for fertility all influence the choice of therapeutic modality that can be offered and will be accepted by a woman to treat her symptomatic fibroids.

Nonsurgical treatments

There is no medical treatment that can cure fibroids, but a number of treatments are available that provide symptom relief, although there are relatively few studies that include only those with fibroids. Clearly, in perimenopausal women, such therapies are employed with the goal of sufficient symptom control until menopause, at which time the AUB will cease, and definitive surgery (ie, hysterectomy) will not be necessary.

Tranexamic acid and mefenamic acid. These are two common nonhormone options. Tranexamic acid has been used as first-line treatment for heavy menstrual bleeding and is frequently used for those with small fibroids despite there being little evidence of efficacy.[125] However, compared with placebo, the safety and efficacy of the modified-release variant have been proven in women with fibroids.

Mefenamic acid is an NSAID that is commonly used for dysmenorrhea and also leads to a modest reduction in heavy menstrual bleeding in women without fibroids, although it is less effective than TXA. However, there have been no trials to date to show the benefits of NSAIDs in women with fibroids.[121]

Levonorgestrel-releasing intrauterine system. The LNG-IUS is used for treatment of heavy menstrual bleeding.[126,127] Studies have demonstrated relief of menstrual symptoms and a nonsignificant effect on volume. The overall incidence of spontaneous expulsion of the LNG-IUS is 9.6% over a 3-year period. This is increased to 15.8% in the presence of fibroids.

Gonadotropin-releasing hormone agonists. Gonadotropin-releasing hormone (GnRH) agonists may be used before fibroid surgery because they reduce both uterine volume and fibroid size.[128] They correct preoperative iron-deficiency anemia, if present, and reduce intraoperative blood loss. If uterine size is such that a midline incision is planned, this can be avoided in many women with the use of GnRH agonists. Some argue that they render myomectomy more difficult because they destroy tissue planes and increase the risk of recurrence and are associated with AEs in situations in which they confer no benefit or in which alternative, cheaper drugs with fewer AEs are available. Add-back therapy may be initiated at the same time as the treatment with a GnRH agonist to reduce hypoestrogenic AEs such as vasomotor symptoms (VMS) and loss of bone mineral density, if use for more than 6 months is anticipated in those who do not desire surgery.

Selective progesterone-receptor modulators. The only selective progesterone-receptor modulator clinically available in some countries is ulipristal acetate (UPA). Ulipristal acetate controlled menstrual bleeding in 90% of participants when taken as 5 mg per day and in 98%, when taken as 10 mg per day.[129] Ulipristal acetate also has some effect on fibroid size, although less than GnRH agonists.

The potential long-term effects of UPA on the endometrium are under study because of an unusual histologic pattern of benign, nonphysiologic, endometrial changes that occurred in many of the women treated with UPA. Common AEs for its use are headaches, nasopharyngitis, abdominal pain, and hot flashes.

The antiprogesterone properties of mifepristone have been used for the treatment of fibroids and have been shown to be effective in reducing heavy menstrual bleeding and improving QOL at low doses.[130]

Other medical treatments

Other medical treatments can be used, although frequently they are less effective in the presence of fibroids. Those that induce amenorrhea such as the oral contraceptive pill and norethisterone acetate may be valuable, and studies have been undertaken with AIs, although the AE profile of the latter may diminish long-term use for this indication.

Uterine artery embolization

Uterine artery embolization, performed by an appropriately trained interventional radiologist, is a minimally invasive treatment option for uterine fibroids. A catheter is inserted through the femoral artery in the groin under local anesthetic and directed toward the uterine arteries using fluoroscopy. The uterine artery is blocked on each side using an appropriate embolic agent. The objective of uterine artery embolization is to infarct completely all the fibroid tissue while preserving the uterus, ovaries, and surrounding pelvic structures.

Uterine artery embolization was used initially for massive obstetric hemorrhage. It is indicated for symptomatic fibroids and is an alternative to myomectomy because it allows conservation of the uterus and involves only a short hospital stay. The most common problem associated with uterine artery embolization is postprocedure pain that can usually be controlled by analgesics. Expulsion of a necrotic fibroid, chronic vaginal discharge, and primary ovarian insufficiency are less common effects associated with uterine artery embolization.

Uterine artery embolization has been shown to be a safe and effective treatment for menstrual disorders.[131,132] Major complications were rare and reported not to be more common than after surgery. Because the effects on fertility and pregnancy are still unclear, this treatment is generally reserved for perimenopausal women.

Uterine artery embolization is associated with some decrease in ovarian function in women aged older than 45 years, which may lead to menopause.[133]

Surgical treatments

Hysterectomy. Hysterectomy is the established surgical treatment for women who have completed their families and no longer plan to give birth. Although hysterectomy is a major surgical procedure, for women with fibroids it results in resolution of most symptoms, particularly when related to menstrual disorders, and has a high satisfaction rate.[134]

Myomectomy. Myomectomy is a surgical procedure to remove uterine fibroids and reconstruct the uterus. It is used as a fertility-sparing option. Myomectomy can be associated with considerable bleeding, risk of hysterectomy, prolonged postoperative stay, postoperative adhesion formation, and recurrence of the fibroids.[135,136]

Myomectomy can be performed as an open procedure and also by laparoscopy or hysteroscopy, depending on the position of the fibroids and the skill of the surgeon. It may also depend on the size and number of fibroids that can be treated laparoscopically, and the skills required are often only available in specialist units.[137] These constraints also apply to vaginal myomectomy. Hysteroscopic myomectomy is most suitable for fibroids smaller than 5 cm in diameter and in which most of the fibroid is within the uterine cavity.[138,139] Submucosal or pedunculated fibroids distort the endometrial cavity and may be covered with vessels that break down, leading to irregular bleeding. Those smaller than about 5 cm in diameter can be removed hysteroscopically, a procedure facilitated by the development of instrumentation that has increased the safety and ease of the procedure. If larger, then a two-step procedure might be used with prior administration of a drug such as a GnRH agonist that will shrink the fibroid.

Malignant and premalignant disease

Although a wide range of benign gynecologic problems present with AUB, it is also a common presenting symptom of endometrial cancer, endometrial hyperplasia, cervical cancer, and less commonly, cancer of the vagina or even vulva. (See also "Endometrial Cancer" and "Cervical Cancer" in Chapter 9).

Endometrial polyps

Endometrial polyps are usually removed because their malignant potential is uncertain and they may cause irregular bleeding in particular. Removal can often be carried out under local anesthetic.

Endometrial hyperplasia of low malignant potential

Often cases of endometrial hyperplasia of low malignant potential may be handled with conservative management and appropriately timed endometrial resampling to check for regression. More often, however, progestogens, administered either orally or by a LNG-IUS, are employed. A systematic review of progestogens for treatment of hyperplasia concluded that the LNG-IUS is a good treatment for nonatypical hyperplasia, with both high success and high compliance rates.[140] Definitive therapy in selected cases may use hysterectomy.

Atypical hyperplasia

Cases of atypical hyperplasia are usually treated with total hysterectomy and bilateral salpingo-oophorectomy. In selected cases, especially fertility-sparing, high-dose progestogens are used.

Gynecologic malignancies

Most often, gynecologic malignancies will involve referral to appropriate specialists and consultants.

Memory Impairment

The term *cognition* describes the group of mental processes by which knowledge is acquired and used. It encompasses mental skills such as attention and concentration, learning and memory, language, spatial abilities, judgment, problem solving, and reasoning.

Sex hormones—estrogens, progesterone, and testosterone—modulate aspects of brain function through a number of mechanistic pathways that are initiated after hormones bind to receptors on neurons and glia, the two types of brain cells in the central nervous system. Hormones influence neurotransmitter systems, including acetylcholine, serotonin, norepinephrine, glutamate, gamma-aminobutyric acid (GABA), and dopamine. They can exert anti-inflammatory effects, enhance blood flow to the brain, promote the expression of growth factors that sustain neural function, and stimulate the formation of synapses to facilitate neuronal communication. In clinical studies, hormones have been shown to influence neural networks involved in attention, memory, and other cognitive functions. Especially relevant for menopause is the influence of estrogens on the function and structure of two brain regions—the hippocampus and the prefrontal cortex. These brain areas are rich in estrogen receptors and modulate aspects of learning, memory, and higher-order cognitive functions. Estradiol in animal models has also been shown to protect against the neuropathology of Alzheimer disease (AD).

Dementia refers to the loss of memory and other intellectual abilities severe enough to interfere substantially with the ability to function independently in daily life. It is perhaps the most-feared consequence of aging. Alzheimer disease, the most common cause of dementia, accounts for well over half of cases.[141] Alzheimer disease is more frequent in women than men, primarily because women generally live longer. However, other factors appear to contribute to the greater burden of the disease in women, including women's greater vulnerability to genetic risk factors[142] and a higher prevalence of modifiable risk factors for AD, such as high BMI and low physical activity. Alzheimer disease and other forms of dementia may be preceded by a period of moderate difficulty with memory or other cognitive abilities. The term *mild cognitive impairment* is sometimes used to refer to excessive difficulty with memory or other aspects of cognition that fall short of dementia but may presage its development.[143]

Menopause and cognitive changes

Complaints of difficulty concentrating and remembering are common during the menopause transition and early postmenopause[144] and can influence work and relationship quality.[145] However, cognitive changes attributable to menopause are more subtle than those attributable to dementia. Obvious changes in cognitive ability should be fully investigated to rule out concomitant medical or neurologic disorders.

Both menopause stage and menopause symptoms appear to influence cognitive function at midlife. Some cross-sectional studies found that memory and other cognitive abilities were worse after the natural menopause transition than before.[146,147] Two longitudinal studies examined these effects, specifically examining how cognition changed across the menopause transition after accounting for age and other factors that also influence cognition. In the Study of Women's Health Across the Nation (SWAN), the expected rate of improvement on tests of processing speed over time was significantly lower in late perimenopause than in premenopause, but learning after the transition was as good as it was before.[148] A similar analysis of memory showed only a trend. Age, depression, anxiety, sleep disturbance, and VMS did not account for the transient decrement in cognitive performance observed during late perimenopause.[149] In the Penn Ovarian Aging Study, memory declined significantly from the premenopause stage to the postmenopause stage.[150]

Memory for verbal information also can be compromised in the immediate period after surgical menopause and in the longer term in women who undergo surgical menopause before the typical age of menopause.[151,152] In contrast, oophorectomy after natural menopause generally is not associated with a decline in cognitive performance.[152] Small trials show that ET can prevent declines in memory after surgical menopause in younger women.[151,153] Those trials, as well as studies of pharmacologic suppression of estradiol, demonstrate that estrogen contributes to memory function in younger women.[154]

As with menopause stage, menopause symptoms can contribute to cognitive difficulties. Anxiety symptoms are associated with slower processing speed and memory performance, whereas depression is associated with lower processing speed.[148] Sleep difficulties also are associated with poorer memory and attention.[155] Although reported hot flashes are generally unrelated to cognitive performance, there appears to be an association between physiologic hot flashes measured with ambulatory skin conductance monitors and memory performance.[155,156]

Serum estradiol concentrations in midlife are not reliably associated with scores on memory tests.[147,157] More research is needed to determine whether hormone and/or nonhormone treatment of hot flashes during the menopause transition improves memory.

Lifestyle and cognition

Observational data indicate that some activities and lifestyle choices may benefit memory or help protect against dementia. These include maintaining an extensive social network, remaining physically and mentally active, increasing dietary intake of omega-3 fatty acids and certain vitamins from natural foods, following a Mediterranean diet, not smoking, consuming alcohol only in moderation, and reducing cardiovascular risk factors such as hypertension, DM, and high cholesterol.[158] Evidence is perhaps strongest for a role of regular exercise in preventing cognitive decline.[159] Meta-analyses of RCTs suggested a small benefit of the Mediterranean diet supplemented by olive oil and tai chi exercise on global cognition and the Mediterranean diet plus olive oil and soy isoflavone supplements on memory.[158] Cognitive training may also have benefit, although there is limited evidence to support commercially available memory programs. Trials of dietary supplements with vitamin E, B vitamins, gingko biloba, DHEA, and omega-3 fatty acids have generally failed to show significant cognitive benefit.

Hormone therapy and cognition

In older women in late postmenopause, research suggests that hormone therapy (HT) has a small or no overall effect on cognition. In the ancillary Women's Health Initiative (WHI) Study of Cognitive Aging and in other large trials involving older postmenopausal women, HT had no consistent effect on cognition.[157,160,161] In the WHI Study of Cognitive Aging, there was a small negative effect on verbal memory and a small positive effect on figural (nonverbal) memory in women with a uterus using estrogen-progestin therapy (EPT).[160] In women without a uterus who were assigned to ET, there was a small negative effect on a visual task (the ability to identify rotation in space).[161] Long-term follow-up of these women showed very small sustained negative effects on cognition.[162]

Three large RCTs focused on early postmenopausal women: the Kronos Early Estrogen Prevention Study (KEEPS), the Women's Health Initiative Memory Study of Younger Women (WHIMSY), and the Early Versus Late Intervention Trial With Estradiol (ELITE). KEEPS found no cognitive benefit or harm of oral or transdermal estrogens.[163] WHIMSY found no sustained cognitive benefit or risk from oral estrogen in women from the WHI aged 50 to 55 years at the time of randomization.[164] ELITE found no cognitive benefit or risk of oral estradiol when given to women close to or more remote from menopause.[165] The cognitive effects of HT on women with moderate to severe VMS are unknown, although a small clinical trial showed cognitive benefits.[166] (See also "Estrogen Therapy and Estrogen-Progestogen Therapy" in Chapter 11.)

On the basis of trial evidence, HT should not be recommended to improve cognition in women, recognizing the lack of clinical trial evidence for women with moderate to severe VMS and the possibility that the cognitive effects may differ between symptomatic and asymptomatic women. Concerns about the negative effects of EPT on dementia and cognition in older postmenopausal women do not appear to apply to younger postmenopausal women. Women with primary ovarian insufficiency have not yet been adequately studied but may be vulnerable to cognitive decline.[167]

Cognitive consequences of induced menopause may differ from those of natural menopause. For women undergoing surgical menopause, there is limited clinical trial evidence that hormone therapy begun soon after surgery may benefit cognitive skills such as verbal memory, at least in the short term.[151] Hysterectomy (with or without oophorectomy) is linked to early onset dementia in women aged younger than 50 years[168]; fortunately, the absolute risk of dementia before age 65 is rare. Some studies have shown that oophorectomy in women aged younger than 46 years is also associated with increased risk of cognitive decline or dementia in late life,[152,169] although other research has not observed long-term cognitive sequelae of hysterectomy or oophorectomy.[170]

Alzheimer disease and vascular dementia

It is estimated that up to half of the cases of AD in the United States and worldwide are attributable to seven modifiable risk factors—DM, midlife hypertension, midlife obesity, smoking, depression, cognitive inactivity or low educational attainment, and physical inactivity.[171-174] For many factors, the optimal time for effective intervention is likely to be during midlife rather than during old age.

In the Women's Health Initiative Memory Study (WHIMS), an RCT conducted in relatively healthy postmenopausal women aged 65 years and older, the risk of dementia was doubled for women using EPT.[175] The increase in risk for women without a uterus who used ET was not significant.[176] On the basis of this evidence, initiating HT after a women reaches age 65 years is not recommended for primary prevention of dementia.[177-178] (See also "Estrogen Therapy and Estrogen-Progestogen Therapy" in Chapter 11.)

Three lines of evidence nevertheless suggest a possible benefit of HT in preventing AD and dementia. First, observational studies imply potential reductions in AD risk when HT is used at younger ages.[179-182] Second, clinical trial findings show transdermal estradiol during the early postmenopause stage is associated with reductions in AD pathology.[183] Third, analysis of 18-year cumulative

follow-up data from the WHI revealed that women randomized to ET had a significantly lower risk of dying from AD or dementia compared with women randomized to receive placebo.[184] This effect was not observed in women randomized to EPT, and the effect was not dependent on timing of initiation. However, given the inconsistencies in the WHI and WHIMSY regarding HT and AD, the evidence is insufficient to conclude that HT helps prevent late-life dementia, regardless of timing.

Few studies have focused on HT and vascular dementia, which is most often caused by multiple ischemic strokes. A nationwide study of Finnish women found a decreased risk of vascular dementia in women who had used HT.[185] However, consistent evidence from clinical trials (including the WHI) and observational research (including the Nurses' Health Study) indicates that standard-dose oral HT increases the risk of ischemic stroke for postmenopausal women by about one-third.[186-188] This risk is not modified by age or timing with respect to menopause.[188] For younger postmenopausal women, the absolute risk of stroke from standard-dose oral HT is rare, but risk is more substantial for older women. Although evidence is limited, low doses of transdermal estradiol (≤50 μg/d) appear not to alter stroke risk.[189]

Sleep Disturbance

Menopause-specific factors; aging; stress and other psychological factors; and coexisting health conditions can each contribute to sleep problems and poor sleep health. Sleep disturbances typically seen by healthcare providers in their care of midlife women include insomnia, obstructive sleep apnea (OSA), restless legs syndrome (RLS), and periodic limb movement disorder (PLMD). These are not mutually exclusive conditions, and OSA as well as RLS and PLMD commonly coexist with insomnia and difficult sleep.

Insomnia

Difficulty sleeping (the symptom)/insomnia (the disorder) is one of the most common complaints of women going through the menopause transition and the most common sleep disorder in the general population.

Insomnia disorder is defined by the American Psychiatric Association as a sleep complaint that occurs at least three times per week for at least 3 months and is associated with distress or impaired daytime personal functioning.[21] Cross-sectional data from the National Institutes of Health indicate that the prevalence of sleep disturbances is high and widely variable in midlife women.[190]

A report that focused on midlife sleep health in women aged 40 to 59 years using data from the 2015 National Health Interview Survey indicated that perimenopausal women were more likely than premenopausal and postmenopausal women to sleep fewer than 7 hours, on average, in a 24-hour period.[191] Postmenopausal women were more likely to report poor sleep quality (defined as waking not feeling well rested). A greater percentage of postmenopausal women had trouble falling asleep (27.1%) as well as staying asleep (35.9%) at least four times in the past week compared with the percentages of premenopausal (16.8% and 23.7%, respectively) and perimenopausal (24.7% and 30.8%, respectively) women. Thus, the most prevalent and consistently observed sleep complaints continue to be those related to wakefulness during sleep episodes (sleep maintenance), even after adjusting for age and other risk factors.[192,193]

Etiology

During midlife, sleep can be disrupted by age-related physiologic changes as well as by medical conditions. Menopause is associated with changes in behavior and other biologic functions such as mood swings, anxiety or depression, stress—and sleep disturbances—therefore, symptoms that are truly associated with menopause may be difficult to differentiate from those associated with aging.[194]

Four major categories of possible causes of insomnia in midlife women have been described: menopause-related insomnia (often related to VMS and continues to be underdiagnosed or misdiagnosed); primary insomnia (psychophysiologic); secondary insomnia (associated with sleep disorders, mental or medical disorders, or aging); and insomnia induced by behavioral, environmental, or psychosocial factors. In longitudinal analyses conducted in both SWAN and the Penn Ovarian Aging Study, VMS were strongly associated with sleep problems, but reproductive hormone concentrations (estradiol, FSH) were not.[195,196]

Midlife women who have VMS compared with those who do not have more sleep complaints and are at higher risk for depression. Longitudinal studies have demonstrated that depressive symptoms increase during the menopause transition,[197] and depressive symptoms are strongly associated with VMS.[198,199] Moreover, anxiety, which has been identified as the strongest predictor of poor sleep quality,[196,200,201] commonly coexists with depressed mood and VMS in midlife women.[202] Lack or loss of sleep can be considered a life stressor with the potential to affect physiological resilience, psychosocial

functioning, and the aging process.[202,203] Therefore, the multifaceted associations among depressed mood, anxiety, VMS, and sleep disturbances across the menopause transition likely involve complex and bidirectional interrelationships.

Diagnosis

Perceptions of sleep do not necessarily accord with objectively recorded sleep changes, which creates complexity for clinical practice. When self-reported sleep quality and recorded sleep patterns are assessed in midlife women, there is little concordance between them.[204] Objectively assessed sleep quality using polysomnography as well as collected self-reports in a population-based sample of midlife women demonstrated that menopause was not related to diminished sleep quality as indicated by polysomnography; however, both perimenopausal and postmenopausal women were twice as likely to be dissatisfied with their sleep compared with premenopausal women.[205]

In most clinical practice settings, an insomnia assessment does not include polysomnography or actigraphy. In the office setting, it is relatively straightforward to simply ask your patient whether she has trouble or difficulty sleeping.[206] A more detailed clinical sleep interview or referral to a sleep specialist should follow (Table 11).[207-210] Clinicians should ask patients to complete a sleep diary for 1 to 2 weeks. Sleep diaries provide a prospective record of sleep timing and duration to describe day-to-day variability and time in bed and to corroborate self-reports of sleep difficulty.[211] One example is the Consensus Sleep Diary, developed in collaboration with insomnia experts and potential users.[212] A number of self-report questionnaires are available to complement these data. The Pittsburgh Sleep Quality Index[213] and the Insomnia Severity Index[214] are two widely used global screening measures that provide an index of sleep quality and severity, respectively, and have validated standard scoring cutoffs.

Treatment

A key consideration in developing an appropriate treatment plan is to recognize that the poor sleep quality about which some midlife women complain could be attributed to important etiologic factors experienced during the menopause transition. In particular, emotional distress or VMS, as well as nonmenopause-related factors including primary sleep disorders (OSA and PLMD or RLS) and comorbid medical or psychiatric conditions should be

Table 11. Subjective Assessment of Insomnia in Menopausal Women: Clinical Interview

- Type of insomnia symptoms
- Other sleep problems (loud snoring, sleep apnea, restless legs) and circadian rhythm disturbances (shift work and delayed sleep-wake phase disorder)
- Effect on functioning
- Timing (onset, duration)
- Predisposing, precipitating, perpetuating, and alleviating factors
- Associated symptoms, including menopause complaints
- Other medical and psychiatric conditions, including use of prescription medications, nonprescription (over-the-counter) medications, and supplements
- Social context (lifestyle or work change)
- Sleep-wake schedule and environment (including pets)
- Alcohol and caffeine use, particularly use of alcohol close to bed (can cause light, disrupted sleep), caffeine use later in the day, other substances
- Previous treatments, effectiveness of treatments

Include patient and bed partner, if possible.
Tal JZ, et al[207]; Brewster GS, et al[208]; Ong JC, et al[209]; Saaresranta T, et al.[210]

Table 12. Elements of Sleep Hygiene Education: DOs and DON'Ts

DO	DON'T
Awaken same time each morning	Nap (unless a shiftworker)
Increase daytime bright light exposure	Drink alcohol
Establish daily activity routine	Use stimulants (caffeine, nicotine)
Exercise regularly	Expose yourself to bright light at night
Set aside a worry time	Exercise within 3 h before bedtime
Comfortable sleep environment	Eat a heavy meal or drink within 3 h before bed
Do something relaxing before bedtime	Expose yourself to noise/noisy sleep environment
Try a warm bath	Try to sleep in an excessively warm or cold bedroom
Develop regular presleep rituals and a regular bedtime	Use the bed for things other than sleep or sex
	Be a clock-watcher
	Try to sleep (a paradox: the harder you try the more difficult it will be to fall asleep)

Hauri PJ, et al[215]; Posner D, et al[216]; Stepanski et al.[217]

considered. Symptoms and signs of sleep abnormalities in midlife women should not be attributed primarily to menopause before ruling out underlying sleep disorders and other contributing factors and deserve a thorough evaluation.

Nonpharmacologic and behavioral approaches to managing insomnia symptoms and disorders begin with sleep hygiene. The aim is to develop good sleep habits by avoiding or eliminating behaviors that can interfere with sleep and replacing them with behaviors that will promote sleep (Table 12).[215-217] However, although the clinical guidelines for the management of chronic insomnia from the American Academy of Sleep Medicine (AASM) recommend that all patients with chronic insomnia should adhere to rules of good sleep hygiene, the guideline acknowledges that there is insufficient evidence to indicate that sleep hygiene alone is effective in the treatment of chronic insomnia.[218] An analysis of data from the SWAN Sleep Study suggests that insomnia is not associated with poor sleep hygiene in midlife women.[219] Initial interventions should include at least one behavioral treatment, such as stimulus-control therapy or relaxation therapy, or a combination of cognitive therapy, stimulus-control therapy, and sleep-restriction therapy with or without relaxation therapy (Table 13).[220,221]

Although in aggregate the available data do seem to support the benefits of HT on sleep quality for midlife and older women, independent of hot flashes, it is not indicated for the treatment of primary sleep disorders.[222,223] Hormone treatments for menopause symptoms may be prescribed as first-line therapy for hot flash-related sleep disturbance because of their effectiveness in improving perceived sleep quality.[177,224] (See also "Estrogen Therapy and Estrogen-Progestogen Therapy" in Chapter 11.) Nonhormone therapies that are typically prescribed for patients with hot-flash related sleep disturbance include SSRIs (escitalopram, paroxetine), serotonin-norepinephrine reuptake inhibitors (venlafaxine), and GABA agents (gabapentin).[225,226]

Selective GABA agents, which are marketed as hypnotics, include the "Z-drugs" zolpidem, zaleplon, and zopiclone (not commercially available in the United States)/eszopiclone. Z-drugs are short-acting nonbenzodiazepine hypnotic sleeping aids that improve sleep quality by shortening time to sleep onset and reducing wake time after sleep onset. Compared with benzodiazepines, Z-drugs have shown improved pharmacokinetic profiles and demonstrated fewer withdrawal effects, less tolerance or addictive concerns, and less loss of effectiveness over time; nevertheless, their AEs, neuropsychiatric sequelae, and incidence of poisoning and death may prove to be similar to older hypnotics.[227] This may be a particular problem with zolpidem, for which FDA has required a dose reduction and a recommendation that women should not drive or engage in other activities that require complete mental alertness the day after taking the drug because they eliminate zolpidem slower than men do.[228]

Ramelteon is a melatonin receptor agonist with no affinity for GABA receptors or for receptors that bind neuropeptides, cytokines, serotonin, dopamine, noradrenaline, acetylcholine, and opiates. It has a rapid onset of action and may be useful for treating insomnia characterized by sleep-onset difficulty.[207]

Another available hypnotic is suvorexant, with a novel mechanism of action. It is a dual orexin (hypocretin) receptor antagonist that promotes sleep by reducing arousal and wakefulness. Its list of potential AEs includes daytime sleepiness and suicidal ideation. It is a schedule IV drug because, according to the US Drug Enforcement Agency, of its potential to produce physical and, similar to zolpidem, psychological dependence (including abuse potential).[229]

Sleep-disordered breathing

Sleep-disordered breathing (SDB) is a term that comprises a range of sleep-related breathing disorders listed in the *International Classification of Sleep Disorders,* of which OSA is considered the most prevalent, being diagnosed in 2% to 5% of adult women compared with 3% to 7% of adult men and occurring in all ethnic groups.[230] In a community-based random sample of 1,000 women, an OSA prevalence of 0.6% in premenopausal and 1.9% in postmenopausal women was found, the latter being very similar to the prevalence in age-matched men.[231] Other estimates indicate that the prevalence of moderate to severe OSA is markedly higher in midlife women. In one study, the OSA prevalence estimates were 4%, 17%, and

Table 13. Rules for Stimulus-Control and Sleep-Restriction Therapies

Stimulus control	Sleep restriction
1. Go to bed only when sleepy	1. Determine average total sleep time from 1-2 wk of sleep diary recording
2. Use bed only for sleep or sex	2. Time in bed should not be <5 h
3. If not asleep within 15-20 min, leave the bedroom—do not watch the clock	3. Determine average sleep efficiency (total sleep time divided by time in bed) over a 5-d period
4. Return to bed only when sleepy	• If 90% or more, increase time in bed by 15-20 min
5. Repeat steps 3 and 4 as needed	• If <85%, decrease time in bed by 15-20 min (but not to <5 h)
6. Regardless of the amount of time spent sleeping, always wake up at the same time	• If 85-89%, no change in time in bed
7. Avoid daytime naps	4. Keep a regular wake time
	5. No napping

Morganthaler T, et al[220]; Yang CM, et al.[221]

43% in women who were aged 20 to 44 years, 45 to 54 years, and 55 to 70 years, respectively.[232]

Etiology

The etiology of SDB is multifactorial. Obesity is considered the major predisposing risk factor. In midlife women, narrowing of the gender disparity in SDB has been attributed to menopause.[233] In a longitudinal analysis of participants in the Sleep in Midlife Women Study, a long-term (1989-2007) follow-up assessment that included polysomnography, showed that the transition from premenopause to postmenopause (later menopause stage and time in menopause) was associated with increased SDB severity.[234] This finding was not entirely explained by chronologic aging or by changes in body habitus. However, there was evidence of an exposure-response relationship between progression through menopause and SDB. Thus, further research with prospective cohorts followed from premenopause thru the menopause transition and into postmenopause is needed to clarify the risk factors and mechanisms that contribute to SDB in general and OSA in particular in midlife women.

Diagnosis

Clinically, midlife women with SDB tend to present differently than men do.[235] Most persons with OSA will awaken in the morning feeling tired and unrefreshed regardless of how much they have slept. However, women tend to report fatigue, lack of energy, or tiredness rather than daytime sleepiness, as well as experience morning headaches, more often than men do. In both men and women, sleep-disrupting body movements may be observed. Obstructive sleep apnea commonly co-occurs with insomnia, with PLMD movements in sleep, and with depressive symptoms and disorders; these coexisting disorders may be more common in women than in men.[236-238]

Diagnosis requires patient and bed partner history, a physical examination, and an all-night polysomnogram.[239,240] Questionnaires have been developed to screen for OSA (eg, Berlin Questionnaire[241] and STOP-Bang[242]) but do not replace polysomnography for making a diagnosis and implementing treatment.

Treatment

The severity of OSA is sensitive to weight loss, and even modest weight loss with behavioral and/or medical therapies may produce significant benefit. Surgical weight loss (bariatric surgery) for patients who are obese may produce more immediate and dramatic results, but those with OSA most likely to benefit from this intervention have yet to be defined. Nasal continuous positive-airway pressure (with adjunctive supplemental oxygen if indicated) therefore remains the mainstay of treatment for most persons with OSA, especially if it is moderate to severe. Studies on the effect of HT on OSA have been mixed, with positive studies showing only minor effects, and some studies demonstrating no improvement.[207]

Restless legs and periodic limb movements in sleep

Survey data revealed that 69% of women with RLS experienced symptom worsening after menopause.[243] Rather than menopause being directly correlated with RLS, sleep disruption in menopause can exacerbate other preexisting sleep disorders, including RLS.[244]

Periodic limb movement disorder is thought to be rare, and the exact prevalence is not known. No sex difference has been described for either periodic limb movements

in sleep or PLMD; however, it has been reported that periodic limb movements are common after menopause, and clinically significant periodic limb movements (>5 events/h of sleep) occur frequently.[245] The prevalence increases with advancing age.[246]

Etiology

Common etiologic factors for RLS include iron deficiency (iron plays a role in dopamine function) and dopamine dysfunctional states that include dopamine antagonists as well as most antidepressants and a number of other pharmacologic agents (SSRIs, tricyclic antidepressants [TCAs], monoamine oxidase inhibitors, glucocorticoids, antipsychotics, antihistamines, and calcium channel blockers).[246,247] Among antidepressants, bupropion is an exception because it does not exacerbate the symptoms of RLS, likely because of its dopamine-promoting activity.[248] Symptoms of RLS increase during pregnancy and occur in persons with renal disease (chronic renal failure/ uremia) and iron deficiency (decreased brain iron stores; serum ferritin <50 µg/L).[246,247] Prolonged immobility also is a contributing factor.

A strong association between RLS and VMS has been reported, but no association has been found between HT use and RLS.[243,249] The increasing prevalence of RLS with age may confound potential menopause-hormone associations.[250] Evidence from some studies do not support a strong link between PLMD and hormone changes in menopause, based on both estradiol or FSH concentrations as well as on response to HT.[245] Moreover, despite PLMD's known association with RLS, a shared pathophysiology involving dopaminergic dysfunction and low brain iron has not been established.[251]

Diagnosis

Restless legs syndrome is a clinical diagnosis that is confirmed by history and physical examination. Four essential diagnostic criteria must be met for a diagnosis of RLS; polysomnography is not routinely indicated in its evaluation (Table 14).[252] Many normal sleepers are unaware of their episodes of periodic limb movements. Periodic limb movement disorder diagnosis requires polysomnography to demonstrate the electromyogram finding and confirm the clinical history.[253]

Treatment

The AASM RLS treatment recommendations include removing potential aggravators such as sleep deprivation, alcohol, exercise (too much or too little), caffeine, and smoking.[254] Nonpharmacologic interventions include a variety of options, such as sleep hygiene, regular bedtime/wake time, appropriate time in bed (≤8 h), moderate daytime and reduced nighttime exercise, relaxation exercises, warm baths/thermal biofeedback, leg vibration/massage, acupuncture, enhanced external counter pulsation, passive stretching exercises, and referral to the Restless Legs Syndrome Foundation. There is insufficient evidence to evaluate the use of nonpharmacologic therapy for RLS, including accommodative strategies, sleep hygiene, behavioral and stimulation therapies, compression devices, exercise, and nutritional considerations.

Based on the strength of the evidence for efficacy, the AASM recommends standard (highest)-level pharmacotherapies that include two specific dopaminergic agents, pramipexole and ropinirole.[254]Therapies with a guideline level of recommendation (second level) included levodopa (with a dopa decarboxylase inhibitor), opioids, gabapentin enacarbil, cabergoline, and rotigotine.[255] Gabapentin, pregabalin, carbamazepine, and clonidine were recommended as third-level options. If serum ferritin is low (<50 μg/L), iron treatment could be beneficial. The AASM provided no recommendations for PLMD because of insufficient evidence to evaluate the use of pharmacologic therapy for persons diagnosed with periodic leg movement disorder alone. Although estrogen may have antidopaminergic activity, a role for estrogen (alone or in combination with progesterone) for treating postmenopausal women with either PLMD or RLS awaits supporting safety and efficacy data.

Headache

Headache is a common symptom of a wide variety of medical disorders. Approximately one-half of the adult population worldwide is affected by a headache disorder.[256]

The first step in treating a patient who presents with a complaint of headache is to distinguish whether there is a primary (no underlying cause) or secondary (an underlying cause such as aneurysm or tumor) headache disorder. Fortunately, primary headache disorders are the most common causes of headache, with migraine being the most common cause of presentation to healthcare providers for "bad" headache(s).

The most common primary headache disorders can be divided into these categories: 1) migraine; 2) tension-type headache (TTH); 3) trigeminal autonomic cephalgias (TACs; cluster headache being the most common type); and 4) "other" primary headache disorders (includes

Table 14. Diagnostic Criteria for Restless Legs Syndrome

1. An urge to move
2. Urge to move is accompanied or caused by uncomfortable and unpleasant sensations in the legs that begin or worsen during periods of rest or inactivity, such as lying and sitting
3. Symptoms are partially or totally relieved by movement such as walking or stretching, at least as long as activity continues
4. Symptoms are worse in the evening or night than during the day or occur only in the evening or night

The occurrence of these criteria is not solely accounted for as symptoms primary to another medical or a behavioral condition (eg, myalgia, venous stasis, leg edema, arthritis, leg cramps, positional discomfort, habitual foot tapping). International Restless Legs Study Group.[252]

cough-, exercise-, cold-, or sex-induced headaches, thunderclap headaches, and primary stabbing headaches).[257] In addition, headache disorders can present in their chronic variant, which is defined as primarily based on the number of headache days per month into episodic (<15 headache d/m) and chronic (≥15 headache d/mo for >3 mo).

Most patients who present to an outpatient clinic with a chief complaint of headache meet the criteria for migraines. Although TTHs are much more common, the adult population rarely seeks help for episodic tension headaches because they are self-limited and easily alleviated. Unfortunately, although headache is one of the most common neurologic disorders, about half of those who request treatment for TTH or migraine either do not receive appropriate treatment or are dissatisfied with their treatment.[258]

Although most primary headaches are not life threatening, some characteristics (Table 15)[259] may be an indication of a more serious problem in which headache is a symptom of another underlying cause, such as a brain tumor (secondary headache).

Migraine headache

Migraine is the prototypical "bad" headache that has a significantly higher prevalence in women than in men.[260] Although it often starts at the time of menarche, migraine reaches peak prevalence during midlife, with about a third of women aged in their 30s fulfilling criteria for migraine diagnoses.

Migraine is manifested by a headache of moderate to severe throbbing or pulsating pain that is worse on one side of the head and usually aggravated by physical activity. The International Headache Society's (IHS) diagnostic criteria for migraine includes a history of at least five attacks of this nature, each lasting 4 to 72 hours (can be shorter if treated), with at least one of these symptoms: phonophobia, photophobia, and nausea and/or vomiting.[257]

Table 15. Red Flags for Secondary Headache

- Systemic symptoms (fever, weight loss, rash)
- Systemic illness (malignancy, immunosuppression)
- Neurologic symptoms and/or signs (alterations in consciousness, abnormal neurologic exam)
- Sudden/Abrupt onset
- New onset or progressive headache
- Headache different from previous headache history

Katz M.[259]

Migraine and aura

There are two types of migraine headaches: those with aura and those without aura. Migraines without aura are much more common than migraines with aura. Both types of migraines may have accompanying premonitory symptoms such as fatigue, difficulty concentrating, neck stiffness, sensitivity to light and/or sound, nausea, blurred vision, yawning, and pallor. These symptoms may occur hours or several days before a headache. Research indicates that migraines also may be accompanied by cutaneous allodynia or excessive skin sensitivity (eg, pain when brushing the hair or touching the scalp).[257,261] Patients with cutaneous allodynia should be treated as early as possible in the course of the migraine because their headaches may be less responsive to medication if treatment is delayed.

An aura is a neurologic symptom that occurs just before or at the onset of a migraine. Aura symptoms are typically visual, lasting about 20 minutes, characterized by flashing lights or wavy lines or even temporary loss of vision (scotomata), often in the peripheral visual fields. A person also may have speech problems or experience numbness, tingling, or weakness in an extremity, although this is rare. Such sensory deficits occur gradually over 5 or more minutes and should last less than 1 hour, at which point they should revert to baseline. Several different symptoms or deficits can occur in succession.[262] Only two episodes of aura are sufficient for the diagnoses of migraine with aura, according to the IHS.[263] It is important to keep in mind that most patients who experience migraine with aura also experience migraine without aura. In fact, in patients who report migraine with aura, the aura occurs on average in only 20% of headache attacks.[264]

Migraine triggers

Most presumed migraine triggers have not been well studied. There are several common factors that may be migraine triggers for susceptible patients (Table 16).[265]

Studies have clearly established a connection between headaches and menstrual periods (called *menstrual migraines*) in susceptible women, with 60% of women with migraines reporting some association with their menstrual cycles.[266,267] Two subtypes of migraine are defined by the IHS in relation to menstrual migraine attacks.[263] Migraine attacks that occur only perimenstrually are categorized as *pure menstrual migraine*, a relatively rare condition that affects less than 10% of premenopausal women with migraine. In contrast with pure menstrual migraine, most women with migraine experience both attacks associated with menses and at other times of the cycle, known as *menstrually related migraine*.

In most women with migraine, headaches tend to improve during pregnancy when estrogen levels are more stable. Women with migraine without aura often see a decrease in migraines with natural menopause, whereas women who experienced only menstrual migraines often experience complete resolution of migraine.[268,269]

It remains unclear whether a true association between migraine and menopause symptoms exists, although a common link between migraine and VMS has been postulated.[268,269] Most work in hormone regulation of migraine has focused on estrogen, with data from SWAN suggesting a two-hit hypothesis of menstrual migraine triggering by showing a faster decline in urinary estradiol in women with migraine than in controls, suggesting that faster estrogen decline is an inherent trait of women with migraine.[270] Although progesterone also influences neuronal activity, less is known about the exact role of progestogens in migraine.

Treatment

Abortive therapy. Migraine therapy is traditionally divided into abortive therapy for acute pain and preventive therapy to decrease recurrences. Using a headache diary to identify (and avoid) triggers can be very helpful in headache management.[263] Data that should be recorded include the time a headache was experienced, the symptoms, and the potential triggers (particular foods, menses, or stress). For rare attacks, nonprescription

Table 16. Migraine Triggers

- Stress
- Specific foods, skipping meals, alcohol
- Hormone factors (eg, menstrual migraine)
- Sleep: Sleep disturbance/sleeping late
- Environmental factors: Lights, smoke, perfume/odors, weather, heat
- Activity: Exercise, sexual activity

Kelman L.[265]

pharmacologics such as aspirin or acetaminophen combinations with caffeine can be effective as abortive agents. Paradoxically, caffeine can be a migraine trigger for some patients and also can increase withdrawal headaches and lead to medication-overuse headache, thus usually is not favored.[271] Antiemetics (chlorpromazine, metoclopramide, prochlorperazine) can benefit headache and nausea.[272] Older medications such as butalbital and isometheptene mucate-dichloralphenazone-acetaminophen are no longer recommended for migraine therapy because of the lack of clear evidence of effect and also their risk of habituation and abuse.

The advent of the triptan prescription medications (almotriptan, frovatriptan, rizatriptan, sumatriptan, eletriptan, naratriptan, and zolmitriptan) has greatly improved abortive migraine therapy. The triptans are extremely effective and safe, although they are contraindicated in patients with cardiovascular disease. Nonsteroidal anti-inflammatory drugs are often recommended in combination with a triptan.

Preventive therapy. For women with menstrual migraines who have regular menstrual cycles, an NSAID or a triptan may be used preventively, beginning about 2 days before the expected onset of symptoms for the usual length of symptoms (typically 5-7 d), with twice-daily treatment.[273] Although these mini-prevention strategies are often very appealing to patients, they are not feasible in women with irregular periods, creating a need for the use of daily migraine preventives.

Daily preventive medication is in general considered when a patient has headaches more than 2 days per week or if headache severity and disability affects QOL. Any preventive medication is about 50% likely to be effective for any given patient. Prescription drugs found to be effective in preventing migraines include beta-blockers such as propranolol, metoprolol, nadolol, and timolol; the angiotensin II receptor blocker candesartan; TCAs

such as nortriptyline and amitriptyline; and anticonvulsants such as topiramate and divalproex.[272]

With a preventive drug, starting doses should be low and increased slowly. Drugs should be taken for at least 2 months before the full effects can be assessed. Because there are no pretests that can determine the potential effectiveness of a particular migraine preventive in a specific migraine patient, the choice of a particular preventive, if generally made on the basis of the AE profile, should be avoided (ie, avoid beta blockers in asthma) or used (somnolence with TCAs in patients with comorbid sleep problems).

In addition to first-line agents, second-line agents such as SSRIs, selective norepinephrine reuptake inhibitors, and gabapentinoids can be safely used in midlife women with migraine.

Nutraceuticals such as magnesium, riboflavin, butterbur, feverfew, and coenzyme Q10 are nonprescription preventive medications that, when taken daily, may be effective and safe for many migraine sufferers.[274] They can be used as baseline preventive treatment that may diminish the need for other preventive medications. Botulinum toxins delivered by subcutaneous injections to multiple sites also can be effective.[272] Nonpharmacologic migraine interventions, including greater occipital nerve blocks and neurostimulation, are gathering evidence.[275,276] Finally, a class of specific migraine treatment targets calcitonin gene-related peptide, a neuropeptide vasodilator involved in migraine, with monoclonal antibodies to the ligand and receptor.[277] Because these medications are injected and more expensive than other preventive options, they are generally prescribed by specialists after failure of other preventive therapies. In clinical trials, they reduce migraine days by 1 to 2 days per month compared with placebo.[278]

Hormone therapy. Hormone therapy can be used in premenopausal and perimenopausal women to mitigate falling estrogen levels.[269,279] No hormone product is FDA approved to prevent or treat headaches. Benefit is more likely if falling estrogen levels can be avoided (eg, adding a low-dose estrogen supplement during the withdrawal phase of oral contraceptives; using continuous HT; using continuous-release transdermal estrogen).[280] Some evidence suggests that progestogens can prevent or aggravate headaches.[266] If headaches are worsened by a progestogen such as medroxyprogesterone acetate (MPA), switching to micronized progesterone may help. (See also "Estrogen Therapy and Estrogen-Progestogen Therapy" in Chapter 11.)

Caution should be used when prescribing estrogen-containing oral contraceptives for a woman who has migraine with aura, because studies suggest that these women have a small increased risk of ischemic stroke, especially in those who also smoke.[268,281,282] (See also "Contraceptives" in Chapter 11.) However, studies have been variable because such risk is confounded by numerous risk factors that are likely synergistic, such as smoking, hypertension, DM, and hyperlipidemia, as well as the dose of estrogen.[283] Additionally, migraine alone has been variably reported to be an independent risk factor for stroke. Evidence is inconsistent linking migraine and stroke in older women and in men, with the highest risk present in younger women smokers on high doses of exogenous estrogen.[282,283-285] Despite this increased risk, the absolute risk to any one person remains fairly low.[284] It remains unclear whether treating migraines and preventing attacks can affect potential ischemic stroke risk.[286]

Centers for Disease Control and Prevention (CDC) and World Health Organization (WHO) guidelines recommend that women with migraine with aura not use combined hormone contraception and advise caution when prescribing combined hormone contraception to women with migraine without aura.[287,288] A similar contraindication has *not* been identified for those with migraine who need HT doses for treatment of symptoms of menopause and/or their headaches.[279,283,289]

For some women with menstrual migraines, stabilization of hormone levels is a necessity to control their symptoms, and an understanding of the related risks and associated discussion with the woman is critical. Additional reassurance is provided by the observation that AEs in migraine with aura appear to be related primarily to high doses of estrogen that were used in older versions of oral contraceptives and are less likely to occur with newer hormone contraceptives that contain lower doses of estrogen.[290]

Tension-type headache

Tension-type headache (TTH) is the most common headache type in the general population.[291] The term TTH replaces previous terms such as *stress* or *tension headache*, *muscle-contraction headache*, and *psychogenic headache*.[282] It has a lifetime prevalence of nearly 90%, suggesting that almost all people will experience this type of headache at some point in their lives.[293]

The typical presentation of a TTH attack is a bilateral, mild to moderate intensity, nonthrobbing (often described as a steady squeezing or pressing pain in the head or neck) headache that can last between 30 minutes and 7 days. In contrast to migraine, which is defined by the presence of specific symptoms (nausea; sensitivity to light and sound), TTH is characterized by the *absence* of these features. Additionally, there should be no worsening of the headache with normal physical activity and no aura associated with it.

Tension-type headache can be acute (frequent or infrequent) or chronic (>15 d/mo). The current pathophysiologic model of TTH suggests that pericranial myofascial pain-receptor sensitivity causes episodic TTH, whereas central sensitization of pain caused by prolonged nociceptive stimuli from pericranial myofascial tissues seems to be responsible for chronic TTH.[294]

Genetic factors may play a role in the development of chronic TTH, and women have a slightly higher prevalence of TTH than do men. Stress and mental tension are reported to be the most common precipitants for TTH.[295] Although TTHs are not thought to be hormonally regulated (in contrast with migraine), and the association between TTH and the changes associated with the menopause transition has been identified in several studies, most women either report stability or mild worsening of TTH with menopause.[296]

Diagnosis

The diagnosis of TTH is based on clinical impression, and there are no diagnostic tests specific for TTH. Routine imaging is not recommended for cases without worrying signs. The potential diagnostic difficulty arises in distinguishing between TTH and probable migraine. Although TTH attacks are generally bilateral and featureless, in up to a quarter of patients, they can be unilateral and described as throbbing and sometimes associated with light or sound sensitivity or nausea.[297,298] If present, these symptoms should always be mild to moderate and never moderate to severe as in migraine. Furthermore, TTH attacks should not be aggravated by routine physical activity, as is typically true for migraine.[299]

Treatment

Most TTHs can be effectively treated with nonprescription analgesics. Low-dose NSAIDs such as naproxen 375 mg to 550 mg or ibuprofen 200 mg to 400 mg are the first-line treatment. Additionally, anti-inflammatory drugs such as aspirin 500 mg or acetaminophen 500 mg to 1,000 mg can be used. Evidence for efficacy of muscle relaxants (aside from tizanidine) is weak, and these, as well as combination medications (ie, those containing caffeine or codeine), should be avoided because of risk of habituation and development of chronic daily headaches or medication-overuse headaches.[271,300] Opiates may be helpful in some patients, but their use should not be necessary given the mild to moderate nature of pain, and they should be avoided given the associated risks.

Nonpharmacologic therapies, including physical therapy, stress management, relaxation therapy, and biofeedback, can be very helpful and are frequently underused.[301] For those who need prophylactic treatment (>2 attacks/wk on average), evidence suggests that TCAs are probably the most effective. Other medications that may be useful include the antidepressants mirtazapine and venlafaxine, the anticonvulsants topiramate and gabapentin, and the muscle relaxant tizanidine. In contrast, the available evidence suggests that SSRIs are not effective for TTH prophylaxis.[292]

Trigeminal autonomic cephalgias

Trigeminal autonomic cephalgias (TACs) are characterized by unilateral head pain in the distribution of the trigeminal nerve with ipsilateral autonomic features (ptosis, miosis, lacrimation, rhinorrhea, and nasal congestion).[257] This group of rare primary headache disorders occurs primarily in men. Included in this group are *cluster headaches*, characterized by disabling attacks of severe pain (≥8 attacks/d) lasting 15 minutes to 3 hours, frequently grouped in "clusters" that last weeks or months and often followed by periods of remission. Similar in quality to cluster attacks but much more brief, short-lasting unilateral neuralgiform headache attacks with conjunctival injection and tearing (SUNCT) and short-lasting unilateral neuralgiform headache attacks with cranial autonomic symptoms (SUNA) headaches can occur up to 200 times per day and last seconds or minutes.

Paroxysmal hemicranias and its chronic version, hemicrania continua, although rare, are more frequently found in women.[302] In addition to having TACs features, the exacerbations can often be migrainous in nature, leading to common misdiagnosis of this syndrome. The diagnosis is confirmed by its response to indomethacin, a brief trial of which should be considered in diagnostically challenging cases. Because of the short duration of symptoms, indomethacin is most effectively used prophylactically.[303]

In addition to their differences in duration and frequency, TACs also differ in their response to treatment. Cluster headaches respond to oxygen therapy as well as subcutaneous sumatriptan for abortive therapy, and verapamil is first line for preventive therapy.[304] SUNCT and SUNA headaches are responsive acutely to treatment with intravenous lidocaine and lamotrigine,

whereas topiramate and gabapentin are the most effective medications available for prevention.[305]

Other primary headache disorders

Other primary headache disorders are relatively uncommon and include new daily persistent headache; primary stabbing headache (icepick headache); headache precipitated by cough, exertion, or sexual intercourse; thunderclap headache; and hypnic headache. The pathogenesis of these headache disorders is poorly understood, and treatment is suggested on the basis of anecdotal reports and uncontrolled trials.

Ongoing treatment

Frequent occurrence of all the primary headache syndromes can lead to chronic headache (chronic tension headache, chronic cluster, chronic migraine), defined by its frequency as 15 or more headache days per month for 3 or more months. Additionally, over-the-counter and prescription drugs used for acute treatment of all these primary headaches can contribute to more frequent headaches (medication-overuse headache). Care should be taken to monitor the use of acute headache drugs, and if headaches occur more than twice a week, consider preventive medications. For many midlife women, headaches are debilitating and frustrating, greatly interfering with QOL at a time when career and family responsibilities are already stressful.[306] A supportive relationship between the headache sufferer and her healthcare professional can be extremely effective in determining the appropriate individual interventions.

Arthralgia

Chronic musculoskeletal pain is very common, affecting approximately 50% of adult populations.[307] It is always more common in women, although the reasons for this are not fully understood.[308] The most common sources of pain are the lower back, neck, knee, hand, hip, and shoulder.

Musculoskeletal pain is present in more than half of women around the time of the menopause.[309,310] Joint pain has been shown to be maximal in women aged between 45 and 55 years.[311] Although this appears to implicate menopause and estrogen deficiency, direct causal evidence for a link is lacking, perhaps because musculoskeletal pain is so common in populations in the first place. In the Melbourne Women's Midlife Health Project, with an 8-year follow-up, postmenopausal women were twice as likely to have joint pain and stiffness.[312] However, these population studies often do not delineate joint or other musculoskeletal pain from arthritis.

Arthralgia is a subjective term, used to refer to pain in a joint or joints. The implication is that this does not cause harm to the joints and is considered separately from arthritis, in which there are clinical signs in keeping with an underlying pathological abnormality of a joint. In patients presenting with arthralgia, it is important to assess and exclude the possibility of early arthritis or another underlying inflammatory rheumatic disorder. Many women who experience arthralgia during menopause will not have an associated joint disorder, and the pain may be associated with hormone changes during this time.[309] However, this is a diagnosis of exclusion—there are a number of other conditions that can also commonly cause arthralgia in this setting, and it is important that the clinician approaches this symptom in a systematic way so as not to miss a reversible alternative cause (Table 17).

Taking the history

Patient-reported joint pain does not always emanate from the joint, and this should not be referred to as arthralgia. A careful history is vital when this symptom is first volunteered. Ask the patient to describe the nature of the pain and to point to the sites of pain. Do they feel pain away from the joints? Is it over bone, muscles, bursae, or entheses (points of insertion of ligaments or tendons into bone)? Pain over the shoulders may relate to a rotator cuff tendinopathy, which is common in midlife women. Or is it far more generalized, with nonspecific pain in all four quadrants of the body, suggestive of fibromyalgia? Here pain is felt away from joints.

Polymyalgia rheumatica is the most common form of vasculitis. It can be associated with joint pain, but the predominant symptom tends to be myalgia and associated inflammatory stiffness. Are there any red flags, such as weight loss, fevers, or night pain to suggest polymyalgia rheumatica, neoplasia, or even infection?

In those with arthralgia, it is important to be clear about the pattern and nature of joint involvement, mainly to exclude prearthritis, early arthritis, or other soft-tissue abnormality and to detect pointers to a secondary (potentially treatable) cause. Ask the patient whether there is any swelling or early morning stiffness of more than 30 minutes (which might suggest an inflammatory arthritis). How related were the onset of symptoms to menopause? Was there a history of injury or other relevant preceding condition such as rash or fever and sudden-onset arthralgia, suggesting a viral illness? Does the patient have symptoms suggestive of thyroid disease or risk factors for vitamin D deficiency (these latter can present with arthralgia but also often proximal muscle symptoms)? A myopathy may be present.

Examination

It is important to briefly examine, palpate, and ask the patient to move painful joints: a diagnosis can usually be made on the basis of the history and the examination (Table 18).

If arthritis is suspected, it is important that a likely diagnosis of type of arthritis is made because management and treatment options for different types of arthritis vary widely. If in any doubt, and particularly when

Table 17. Causes of Musculoskeletal Pain That Are Not Arthralgia

Condition	Possible causes
Myalgia	• Drug induced (statins, fibrates) • Endocrine (vitamin D deficiency, thyroid, Cushing disease) • Menopause • Polymyalgia rheumatica
Entheseal/Tendon/Bursitis pain	• Injury • Asymmetric gait; obesity; biomechanical • Drug induced (quinolones)
Bone pain	• Metabolic (Paget disease) • Neoplasia (multiple myeloma, metastatic) • Infection (brucellosis, tuberculosis) • Fracture (trauma, osteoporotic fracture)
Fibromyalgia	• Associated with fatigue, sleep disturbance, anxiety or depression, catastrophizing, other pain syndromes (migraine, irritable bowel syndrome, atypical chest pain)

certain symptoms or signs suggest that an inflammatory arthritis is present, an early review by a rheumatologist should be requested. Inflammatory arthritis and secondary causes often can be excluded on further blood testing (Table 19). There are useful tests for those with a true polyarthralgia (pain affecting many joints; Table 20). (See also "Arthritis" in Chapter 6.)

General management

If a secondary cause(s) or exacerbating factor is found, this should be investigated as appropriate and treated and the symptoms monitored. It can take several months for arthralgia from vitamin D deficiency or hypothyroidism, for example, to fully resolve.

Identification of a drug as a possible cause of arthralgia needs careful, measured discussion among the patient, healthcare provider, and other relevant caregivers, taking into account the effects on QOL and the relative risks and benefits of staying on the drug versus reducing drug dose, switching to another drug within the same or different class, or simple cessation. In some instances for which there is diagnostic doubt, a drug holiday may be agreed on to assess whether arthralgia is truly associated (during which time no other treatments should change, including pharmacologic and nonpharmacologic therapies). Objective measures (pain visual analog scale or numerical rating scale for average or worst joint pain) should be used to give objective measures of pain.

Statins and bisphosphonates are commonly implicated by patients and providers as causes of myalgia and/or arthralgia. Statin-induced myalgia or arthralgia is actually very uncommon (those on statins usually have another cause of pain, and this should be actively sought); if suspected strongly on temporal grounds, the risk-benefit of reducing or stopping the drug should be carefully discussed and documented before trial of cessation or class switching (in the case of a statin, assuming liver function and creatinine kinase are normal, there is no safety requirement to withdraw the drug). For bisphosphonates, there may be therapeutic alternatives such as denosumab that can be tried.

Aromatase inhibitors are a particularly common cause of arthralgia and may be seen in as many as 50% of users.[313] If medically required, and there are no reasonable alternatives, management of arthralgia symptoms can be implemented to maintain necessary therapy, per recommendations.[314] Mild arthralgia should be treated symptomatically with lifestyle change, including exercise and weight loss, and the response documented. For more

> **Table 18.** Patient Questions for Arthralgia Diagnosis
>
> - Site: Is it one, a few, or many joints?
> - Symmetry: Are the symptoms symmetrical or just in small joints?
> - Swelling: Is there any objective abnormality of the joint such as redness, joint deformity, joint swelling, warmth, or restriction of movement to suggest an arthritis? Tenderness is often present in arthritis but not always in arthralgia (although can be present in the absence of arthritis).

severe symptoms, treatment with an oral analgesic such as acetaminophen or an NSAID to enable continuation of therapy should be offered (risk-benefit of NSAIDs or cox-2 inhibitors should be carefully considered). Any decision to modulate, switch, or change drugs should be overseen by the treating oncologist. Switching to an alternative agent within or between classes may lead to an improvement in symptoms (for example, anastrozole to letrozole). There is no clinical trial evidence to support the use of omega-3 fatty acids to treat this type of arthralgia.[315]

Menopause-associated arthralgia

Arthralgia is part of the syndrome of symptoms at the time of menopause in at least 50% of women (musculoskeletal pain is frequently found to be one of the most commonly reported symptoms in international populations).[310,316-318] In this situation, it is typically transient and self-limiting and often not the predominant symptom. However, in 21% of women, it is the most troublesome symptom.[310] Arthralgia and muscle pain are often associated with fatigue, mood change, sleep disturbance, raised BMI, anxiety, or stress independently of menopause. All these symptoms may be associated with menopause in addition.

Natural history

Menopause-associated arthralgia is typically transient and self-limiting and may not present to a clinician. However, it may be a source of persistent pain for a minority of women or be associated with evolution into more chronic widespread pain or fibromyalgia in susceptible women. Arthralgia may also precede forms of arthritis—this may simply be because osteoarthritis and rheumatoid arthritis are relatively common conditions in perimenopausal and postmenopausal women. However, in some women, true arthritis is misdiagnosed as arthralgia, or arthralgia precedes evolution of true arthritis. For these reasons,

Table 19. Causes of Arthralgia in Perimenopause

Primary

Idiopathic	• Timing and presence of other estrogen deficiency symptoms (absence of identifiable secondary causes)

Secondary

	Cause	Features
Endocrine	• Hypothyroidism • Hyperparathyroidism (primary or secondary) • Vitamin D deficiency • Anemia	• Fatigue, weight gain, hyporeflexia, proximal myopathy • Abdominal pains, high calcium • Fatigue, proximal myopathy • Fatigue, shortness of breath
Drug related	• Statins and other lipid-lowering drugs • AIs • SERMs • Bisphosphonates (particularly intravenous • Thiazide diuretics	• Relevant temporal history • Response, if appropriate, to drug holiday/cessation (AIs should not be stopped without oncology guidance)
Metabolic	• Liver disease • Renal disease	• Appropriate history or abnormality on blood testing
Rheumatic	• Connective tissue disease (lupus[a]; scleroderm[a]; Sjorgren disease[a]) • Sarcoidosis[a] • Vasculitis • Hyperuricemia • Hypermobility	• Rashes, oral ulcers, other clinical features of the disease • Other blood test abnormalities (positive ANA or ANCA, raised serum ACE, raised serum urate • Evidence on examination
Infection	• Parvovirus • Hepatitis B[a]; hepatitis C; HIV[a] • Ross River virus • Brucellosis[a] • Whipple disease[a] • Lyme disease[a]	• Relevant rash, viral symptoms • Relevant travel or other risk history • History of insect bite
Malignancy	• Disseminated bony malignancy • Paraneoplastic syndrome	• Red flags (weight loss, bone pain, fever) • Other clinical features of malignancy

Abbreviations: ACE, angiotensin-converting enzyme; AIs, aromatase inhibitors; ANA, antinuclear antibody; ANCA, antineutrophil cytoplasmic antibody; HIV, human immunodeficiency virus; SERMs, selective estrogen-receptor modulators.
[a]May be associated with arthralgia or a frank arthritis.

persisting arthralgia should be reviewed intermittently to ensure no change in the diagnosis.

Management

There is little evidence for the management of perimenopausal arthralgia. General advice for musculoskeletal pain is always to control weight (and lose weight where BMI is raised) and to exercise regularly. Both aerobic exercise and exercise aimed to improve muscle strength and range of motion of specific joints may be beneficial. There is some evidence that moderate levels of physical activity can improve perimenopausal arthralgia.[319] If there is deconditioning evident, a graded and gradual increase in exercise should be planned, avoiding sudden overloading of painful joints, which may exacerbate pain and cause patients to lose confidence in this approach. This includes avoidance of heavy manual handling or repetitive hand use in cases of hand arthralgia.

Dietary measures to treat menopause symptoms and regulate estrogen levels may be helpful in managing arthralgia. One clinical trial of a complex intervention that included dietary and exercise supervision demonstrated that adopting a diet low in carbohydrates, meats, and fats reduced arthralgia.[320] The use of supplements such as phytoestrogens, evening primrose oil, starflower oil, fish oils, or ginseng are reportedly used for non-VMS, including arthralgia, by 32% of postmenopausal women in Australia.[321] However, there is no clinical trial evidence for the effects of these agents on arthralgia in isolation.

Supportive treatment likely to help chronic arthralgia includes strategies to improve associated symptoms of stress, anxiety, or depression and to improve sleep quality if sleep disturbance is present.[322,323] (See also "Sleep Disturbance" in this chapter.)

Where pain is persistent and moderate to severe (rating as ≥3-4/10), a regular simple analgesic such as acetaminophen may be required. It should only be continued if it is found to be effective because of the low risk of GI AEs with long-term use. NSAIDs should be used sparingly because of other undesirable AEs and only in low-risk patients. They may be helpful in managing persistent symptoms unresponsive to acetaminophen.

Current indications for systemic HT focus on menopause symptoms such as VMS and gynecologic symptoms not responding to local therapy. In the WHI, a US study of more than 10,000 postmenopausal women, after 12 months' time, joint pain and stiffness were reduced in the estrogen-only arm of the study compared with the placebo group, but the effects were not marked (76.3%

vs 79.2%; *P*=.001).[324] There was also noted to be reduced incidence of new joint pain in those randomized to conjugated estrogens and MPA compared with those on placebo.[325] Joint ache or myalgia reduced from 63% to 57% in another study of 2,130 postmenopausal women randomized to this same combination, and this was significantly different to those taking placebo.[326] If menopausal arthralgia is severe and persisting, impairing QOL, and it has not responded to other measures, it may be reasonable to discuss whether HT may be tried, particularly in the presence of other incapacitating menopause symptoms.

Fibromyalgia

Among the most common sources of chronic arthralgia and myalgia in adult women is fibromyalgia (previously known as *myofascial pain syndrome).* The cause of this condition is not fully understood. Women with fibromyalgia have heightened pain sensitivity and a tendency toward other chronic pain syndromes.[323]

History and examination

Pain from fibromyalgia tends to be found in all four quadrants: primarily axial, with diffuse aching in the neck; shoulders; back; and pelvis. A history of poor sleep (either sleep disturbance or seemingly adequate sleep but feeling routinely unrefreshed in the morning) and persistent unexplained fatigue are typical and should be sought. Arthralgia and myalgia in these patients are typically accompanied by multiple other symptoms that may include tingling, burning, or swelling of limbs. A number of factors have been shown to be predictive (being female, catastrophizing, and high depression and anxiety scores).[323] There is no detectable joint swelling or synovitis (although peripheral puffiness can be seen), and muscle strength is normal. Characteristic tender trigger points may be found although are not necessary for a diagnosis of fibromyalgia.[327] Patients with fibromyalgia also tend to display heightened pain sensitivity at other nonjoint, nonspinal sites (eg, forearm squeeze may be painful). A history of pain affecting other systems often may be present (eg, migraine, irritable bowel or bladder, premenstrual syndrome or pelvic pain, nonspecific chest pain).[328] It is likely that there is a common pathogenesis to these different manifestations of chronic pain. Many of these conditions are seen to be more common at the time of menopause. The relationship of the symptoms to menopause should be noted and appropriate advice given as above.

Table 20. Possible Useful Investigations for Polyarthralgias

- Full blood count
  - Biochemistry profile including urea and electrolytes
  - Liver function tests
  - Calcium
- Acute-phase proteins
  - C-reactive protein
  - Erythrocyte sedimentation rate
- Serum urate
- Creatinine kinase
- Thyroid function
  - Parathyroid hormone
- Hematinic (if anemia suspected)
  - Iron studies
  - B$_{12}$
  - Folate (if anemia is suspected)
- Vitamin D
- Autoantibodies (if clinically indicated)
  - Antinuclear antibody
  - Rheumatoid factor
  - Cyclic citrullinated peptide antibodies
- Viral or other serologic testing (if clinically indicated)
  - Parvovirus B19
  - Hepatitis B
  - Hepatitis C
  - HIV

Abbreviation: PT, physical therapy.
Adapted from Management of Symptomatic Vulvovaginal Atrophy: 2013 Position Statement of The North American Menopause Society.[9]

Management

Fibromyalgia is again a diagnosis of exclusion. After appropriate clinical assessment and investigation, giving a clear diagnosis and full explanation (to prevent ongoing, fruitless medical investigation and overmedicalization) is then essential. Sleep hygiene is important.[323] Institution of an aerobic conditioning program with graded exercise can be helpful.[329] A careful approach to analgesia is important, starting with standard analgesics such as acetaminophen and anti-inflammatory medications such as ibuprofen when indicated. Opiates are often ineffective in the treatment of this form of pain. Consistent with the concept that the pain of fibromyalgia is related to aberrant neurotransmission and/or pain processing, other FDA-approved neuroactive neuropathic medications for the treatment of fibromyalgia include pregabalin, gabapentin, duloxetine, and milnacipran. Tricyclic antidepressants such as low-dose amitriptyline as well as later-generation SSRIs are often used, the latter particularly when there is associated depression.

Treatment of fibromyalgia may be challenging. Some cases, particularly when established and resistant to therapy, may benefit from a chronic multidisciplinary pain program or from other specialist pain management. Addressing any identifiable biopsychosocial aspects to the presentation and ongoing pain is often essential if treatment is to be successful.

Intimate Partner Violence

Intimate partner violence (IPV) is a serious and increasing health problem affecting many vulnerable populations of women. Several organizations (ie, the Institute of Medicine; ACOG) recommend the routine screening of all women for IPV.[330,331]

WHO affirms that violence against women is a violation of human rights.[332] Worldwide, most of this violence is because of IPV. Globally, 38% of all reported female murders are committed by male intimate partners. Abused women have increased risks of low-birthweight babies, abortion, depression, and HIV.

Much of the emphasis in research on IPV has been on reproductive-aged women; menopausal and postmenopausal women are recognized as an often-invisible population who are at risk of being abused, neglected, and exploited. Most abused women do not seek care, and older women, in particular, are rarely screened. In one study, only 3% of women aged 65 years or older were asked about IPV.[333,334]

Definition

Intimate partner violence is defined as coercive control in a deliberate manner by someone who is currently, or was previously, in an intimate relationship with another person, regardless of duration or significance of the relationship.[335]

With relational violence, the term *intimate partner* is preferred to *domestic* because intimate partner is more inclusive—it does not imply a shared residence between the two people. Intimate partner violence is not limited to situations that include physical assault. Intimate partner violence covers a spectrum of assaultive and coercive behaviors (Table 21).[335] These behaviors can occur in any combination, in sporadic episodes, or chronically, spanning from days to even decades.

Although most IPV takes the form of relational violence against women, it occurs in any type of relationship

(same or opposite sex, familial, etc). Both survivors and perpetrators of abuse may self-identify as male, female, transgender, gender nonconforming, or as a member of another gender or sexual minority. The bulk of violence occurs against women in heterosexual relationships.

Incidence and prevalence

Surveillance data from the CDC found an increasing incidence of IPV.[336] More than one-third of US women experienced contact sexual violence, physical violence, and/or stalking victimization by an intimate partner during her lifetime (Table 22). Almost one in three women (32.4%) has experienced physical violence, and one in six women (16.4%) reported contact sexual violence by an intimate partner in her lifetime. Within the past 12 months, 5.6 million women reported experiencing IPV. In the same time frame, 4% (physical) and 2% (sexual) of women report violence and its effects.

The prevalence of psychological aggression by an intimate partner is even more common. This is sometimes excluded in discussions on IPV. Rates for psychological aggression reveal that almost half (47.1%) had lifetime exposure and 14% had experienced psychological aggression in the last 12 months (Table 23).[336]

Adverse childhood experiences are associated with an increased likelihood of IPV. This is evident in the increased presence of various psychosocial characteristics such as depression, anxiety, impulsivity, and problem drinking in affected persons.[337] The presence of past abuse, especially in childhood, has a significant

---

Table 21. Assaultive and Coercive Behaviors in IPV

- Actual or threatened physical assault
- Sexual violence, including forced sexual intercourse and other forms of sexual coercion or exploitation
- Psychological/Emotional abuse such as insults, belittling, constant humiliation, intimidation, threats of harm, or threats to take away children
- Controlling behaviors, including isolation from family/friends, monitoring movements, or restricting access to finances, employment, education, or medical care
- Destruction of property or personal possessions
- Sustained social isolation
- Spiritual abuse
- Maltreatment of dependents including children, other family members, or animals/pets

Abbreviation: IPV, intimate partner violence.
Alpert E, et al.[335]

influence for women to experience abuse and violence in the future.

Clinical presentation

Abusive acts are rarely isolated events. Violence usually recurs and often increases in frequency and severity over time. Abused persons may sustain life-threatening injuries, or they can suffer less-obvious effects that are just as debilitating. Unaddressed or treatment-nonresponsive health conditions may be because of current or previous IPV.

ACOG notes that women can present with a myriad of complaints, including acute injuries to the head, face, breasts, abdomen, genitalia, or reproductive system, or with nonacute presentations such as chronic headaches, sleep and appetite disturbances, palpitations, chronic pelvic pain, urinary frequency or urgency, irritable bowel syndrome, sexual dysfunction, abdominal symptoms, and recurrent vaginal infections.[331] Internalized stress, or somatization, contributes to clinical manifestations of nonacute symptoms, and posttraumatic stress disorder can result. This is often linked to depression, anxiety,

substance abuse, and suicide. Some women may exhibit red flag indicators (Table 24).[335]

The medical community can play a vital role in identifying women who are experiencing IPV and halting the cycle of abuse through screening, offering ongoing support, and reviewing available prevention and referral options.[331]

Menopausal women

Limited research exists in menopausal women and their experiences with IPV. In one sample of older women, there was a prevalence of 26.5% of lifetime partner violence, encompassing physical, sexual, and threats and controlling behavior.[334] Violence in the past 5 years was reported by 3.5% of women; 2.2% of women reported violence in the past year. More than 20 episodes of violence in their lifetimes was reported by some women.

A validated questionnaire designed to measure violence during the climacterium found abuse negatively affected QOL and behavior for 90% of affected women.[333] Abused women had increased comorbidities:

Table 22. Lifetime Prevalence of Contact Sexual Violence, Physical Violence, and/or Stalking Victimization by an Intimate Partner — US Women, 2010-2012 Average Annual Estimates

	Lifetime			12 mo		
	Weighted %	**95% CI**	**Victims, no[a]**	**Weighted %**	**95% CI**	**Victims, no[d]**
Any contact sexual violence, physical violence, and/or stalking	37.3	36.3-38.3	44,981,000	6.6	6.0-7.1	7,919,000
Contact sexual violence[b]	16.4	15.6-17.1	19,743,000	2.1	1.8-2.4	2,542,000
Physical violence	32.4	31.5-33.4	39,111,000	3.9	3.5-4.4	4,730.000
Slapped, pushed, shoved	30.3	29.3-31.2	36,517,000	3.6	3.2-4.0	4,330,000
Any severe physical violence[c]	23.2	22.3-24.1	27,999,000	2.5	2.2-2.8	2,991,000
Stalking	9.7	9.1-10.3	11,740,000	2.5	2.2-2.9	3,027,000
Any contact sexual violence, physical violence, and/or stalking with IPV-related impact[d]	27.4	26.5-28.3	33,034,000	4.7	4.2-5.1	5,617,000

Abbreviations: CI, confidence interval; IPV, intimate partner violence.
[a]Rounded to the nearest thousand.
[b]Contact sexual violence by an intimate partner includes rape, being made to penetrate someone else, sexual coercion, and/or unwanted sexual contact perpetrated by an intimate partner.
[c]Severe physical violence includes hit with a fist or something hard, kicked, hurt by pulling hair, slammed against something, tried to hurt by choking or suffocating, beaten, burned on purpose, used a knife or gun.
[d]IPV-related impact includes experiencing any of the following: being fearful, concerned for safety, any posttraumatic stress disorder symptoms, injury, need for medical care, need for housing services, need for victim advocate services, need for legal services, missed at least one day of work or school, and contacting a crisis hotline. For those who experienced rape or made to penetrate, it also includes having contracted a sexually transmitted infection or having become pregnant. IPV-related impact questions were assessed in relation to specific perpetrators, without regard to the time period in which they occurred, and asked in relation to any form of IPV experienced (contact sexual violence, physical violence, stalking, psychological aggression, and reproductive/sexual control) in that relationship. By definition, all stalking victimizations result in impact because the definition of stalking requires the experience of fear or concern for safety.
Adapted from Smith SG, et al.[336]

Table 23. Lifetime and 12-Month Prevalence of Psychological Aggression by an Intimate Partner —US Women, NISVS 2010-2012 Average Annual Estimates

	Lifetime			12 mo		
	Weighted %	95% CI	Victims, no[a]	Weighted %	95% CI	Victims, no[d]
Any psychological aggression	47.1	46.1-48.2	56,892,000	14.1	13.4-14.9	17,022,000
Any expressive aggression	39.3	38.3-40.3	47,461,000	10.1	9.4-10.7	12,133,000
Any coercive control	39.7	38.7-40.7	47,940,000	10.4	9.8-11.1	12,571,000

Abbreviation: CI, confidence interval.
[a]Rounded to the nearest thousand.
Adapted from Smith SG, et al.[336]

depression/psychological disorders (approximately 70%), hypertension (54%), or uterine/ovarian/breast cancer (approximately 14%).

Although findings vary in the literature, studies suggest that women who have experienced previous and current abuse report menopause symptoms more frequently. Increased reports of VMS have been found in women aged 42 to 52 years with a history of childhood abuse or neglect.[338]

Using the Data Registry on Experiences in Aging, Menopause, and Sexuality database, 3,740 women aged 40 years and older (most postmenopausal) showed an association between recent abuse (1 y) and bothersome menopause symptoms.[339] In this study, most women reporting abuse characterized it as verbal/emotional. Vasomotor symptoms were not increased overall, but severity scores for total mean menopause symptoms and scores in five of the other categories were significantly higher in abused women. Symptoms were grouped into six categories: vasomotor, sleep, neurocognitive, bowel or bladder function, sexual function, and general items.

Postmenopausal women suffering IPV may have specific needs (Table 25).[340]

Who's at greatest risk?

Intimate partner violence affects women of all age, ethnic, religious, educational, and socioeconomic strata. However, available research indicates higher prevalence in certain groups.[341,342] Using the social-ecologic model as a framework,[343,344] four major risk-factor categories for IPV include individual risk, relationship risk, community risk, and societal and population risk (Table 26).

Gender and sexual minorities

Abuse in gender and sexual minorities, including lesbian, bisexual, transgender, or gender nonconforming, is just as common as in heterosexual relationships, yet unique

barriers exist.[345] These persons may not feel comfortable disclosing their sexual orientation to healthcare providers and often are even more reluctant to disclose abuse (Table 27).[346] Transgender women are at highest risk for

Table 24. Red Flag Indicators of IPV

Physical trauma	Acute injuries: lacerations, contusions, dislocations, factures, head injury, findings of strangulation (facial petechiae, laryngeal edema)
Strangulation injuries	More common than previously thought; harder to detect in darker-skinned women
Gynecologic problems	Lacerations, contusions, STIs (including HIV/AIDS), unintended pregnancy, rapid repeat pregnancies, rape/sexual assault
Somatic signs and symptoms	Headaches, chest, abdominal or pelvic pain, fatigue, eating disorders, functional gastrointestinal disorders
Neurologic findings	Altered mental status, seizures, motor or sensory deficits, memory problems
Behavioral/ Psychiatric signs	Anxiety, depression, panic, suicidal ideation/attempt, substance abuse
Social red flags	Frequent missed appointments, nonadherence to prescriptions or medical instructions, delayed presentation to care
Partner red flags	Excessively attentive or jealous partner, partner insists on accompanying a patient during exams or speaking for patient, displays inappropriate dominance

Abbreviation: IPV, intimate partner violence; STIs, sexually transmitted infections.
Alpert E, et al.[335]

> **Table 25.** Specific Needs of Postmenopausal Women Suffering IPV
>
> - Long-term abuse becomes a "way of life"
> - Attempts to cope, including substance abuse and other physical/mental health consequences
> - Blame by adult children highlights intergenerational IPV effects
> - Empowerment from within—coping with IPV requires reframing thinking because insecurities are fueled by repeated abuse
>
> Abbreviation: IPV, intimate partner violence.

> **Table 27.** Barriers for Gender and Sexual Minorities Suffering IPV
>
> 1. Limited understanding of IPV in lesbian, bisexual, transgender, and queer persons because of the paucity of research in this area. There are unique power and control tactics wherein a partner may threaten to divulge the relationship to family/friends or an employer, creating significant anxiety from being "outed," with potentially devastating and very real consequences such as fear, loss of children, employment, relationships with family/friends, or housing.
> 2. Stigma—referring to society's subtle and explicit negative regard for those who aren't heterosexual. Reluctance in seeking help occurs if others are unaware of a person's sexual orientation or gender identity. Therefore, some may remain in abusive relationships instead of seeking help.
> 3. Systemic inequalities in two key support systems: the justice system and emergency shelters. Some state policies exclude lesbian, bisexual, transgender, and queer persons from obtaining protection orders. This discourages seeking help. Emergency shelters may not provide gender and sexual minority-sensitive services. Many institutional obstacles remain for this population.
>
> Abbreviation: IPV, intimate partner violence.
> Calton JM, et al.[346]

violence, especially ethnic minorities. The "dose effect" of daily violence and discrimination takes its toll on transgender people.[347] This cumulative effect results in high rates of unemployment, substance abuse, smoking, increased risk of HIV infection, and high percentage

> **Table 26.** Major IPV Risk-Factor Categories
>
> ### Individual risk factors
> - Women who are single, separated, or divorced
> - Adolescents/Young adults
> - Pregnant women who have been previously abused
> - Ethnic minorities
> - Immigrant women
> - Gender and sexual minorities
> - Low income/Unemployed
> - Recently sought a restraining/vacate order
> - Emotional dependence/Insecurity, low self-esteem
> - Depression, antisocial/borderline personality traits
> - Abuse alcohol/drugs or partners do
> - Victim of prior physical/psychological abuse (strong predictor)
>
> ### Relationship factors
> - Marital conflict/instability
> - Excessively jealous or possessive partner
> - Partner experiencing unemployment/job instability
>
> ### Community factors
> - Poverty and associated factors
> - Low social capital: lack of institutions/relationships/norms—shape community social interactions
> - Weak community sanctions against IPV (ie, neighbors unwilling to intervene with witnessed violence)
>
> ### Societal and population factors
> - Traditional gender roles: women as domestic, submissive, not working; men as providers, family decision-makers
>
> Abbreviation: IPV, intimate partner violence.

of suicide attempts. It underscores the importance of recognizing this high-risk population when they access the healthcare system.

Elder abuse

Older persons are often the most physically and psychologically vulnerable patients, and emotional abuse is a problem. Cognitive impairment is a major risk factor for elder abuse. Depression, anxiety, and social isolation add to this risk.[348] Physical and sexual abuse, although present, occurs less frequently in this age group, and psychological and emotional abuse can be more widespread. In some circumstances, healthcare providers would be better served by shifting the lens to focus on caregivers to identify and mitigate potential and current abuse.

In a study of adults aged 60 years and older, more than 11% reported experiencing at least one of four mistreatment categories (potential neglect and emotional, physical, and sexual abuse) in the past year.[349] Low social support and previous traumatic experience were most consistently correlated with mistreatment. The effect of the legacy of abuse over the lifespan is again demonstrated.

Table 28. Tests Developed to Improve IPV Screening

- HITS (Hurt, Insult, Threaten, Scream)
- OAS/OVAT (Ongoing Abuse Screen/Ongoing Violence Assessment Tool)
- STaT (Slapped, Threatened and Throw)
- HARK (Humiliation, Afraid, Rape, Kick)
- WAST (Woman Abuse Screen Tool)
- Modified CTQ-SF (Modified Childhood Trauma Questionnaire—Short Form)

Abbreviation: IPV, intimate partner violence.
Nelson HD, et al.[351]

Intimate partner violence screening

There is no consensus on whether older women should be screened for IPV. Although some groups recommend that all women be screened, the US Preventive Services Task Force says there is benefit for screening reproductive-aged women, and WHO recommends against IPV screening.[330,348,350] No gold standard exists, but many tests have been developed to improve IPV screening (Table 28).[351] None of these has been validated in older women.[352]

Healthcare providers are concerned about time constraints, lack of knowledge, and standardized policies as barriers to providing routine IPV screening. Appropriate training for providers is necessary regardless of patient- or provider-initiated methods. Electronic medical records can help with prompts and templates to assist with documentation.

Legal issues

Safety is paramount when managing patients with IPV issues. Confidentiality must be assured and maintained. Protection orders can be obtained emergently, temporarily, or permanently. The healthcare provider should also be familiar with local and state laws regarding mandatory reporting. Familiarity with the law is usually required in suspected abuse of children, older people, and disabled persons and when criminal activity is described (sexual assault, stalking, weapon use). Discuss with the woman first whether a report is going to be made; abused women may be at risk of retaliation.

Intervention

Once IPV is identified, perform a complete assessment and document the results in the medical record. Next, evaluate safety issues, and a safety plan should be developed. Most women will not report being in immediate

danger. Those who do should urgently be referred to intimate partner violence experts. Women should be offered referral to services relevant to their situations (ie, support/advocacy groups, domestic violence agencies, shelter/housing assistance, mental health services, and assistance with children or elders).

Table 29. System-Based Approach to Improving IPV Screening and Prevention

- Provider and health professional education, a core strategy proven to have significant effect
- Patient engagement and support
- Policies/Procedures for clinical settings
- Collaboration with IPV advocates
- Reminders in the electronic medical record
- Quality incentives integrated into clinical flow

Abbreviation: IPV, intimate partner violence.

Trauma-informed system change and provider role

Effective IPV screening and prevention models in the literature use multifactorial approaches.[353,354] Implementation of IPV screening and counseling requires an integrated response within a healthcare system, with buy-in from patients, healthcare professionals, and health-system leaders and policy makers.[355] A social-ecologic model is a useful framework for this systems-based methodology. A system-based approach includes several important strategies that can affect the multiple facets of the healthcare system (Table 29).

Appropriate resources needed to triage patients at the time of screening is optimal to provide referrals for patients who want services and availability for those who may desire services in the future. A collaborative approach with community-based services is essential, having support to manage crises as they arise. Quality improvement should be evaluated continuously, so adjustments can be appropriately made.

The Kaiser-Permanente system serves as model for this integrated approach, resulting in a 10-fold intimate partner violence identification increase from 2000 to 2014.[356]

Healthcare providers can be agents of system improvement. Systems-based practices can be integrated into clinical workflow by clinicians themselves, along with assistance and training of ancillary staff who work in collaboration with community advocates who are qualified to offer IPV specialized support and services.

REFERENCES

1. Menken J, Trussell J, Larsen U. Age and infertility. *Science*. 1986;233(4771):1389-1394.

2. Croft DP, Brent LJ, Franks DW, Cant MA. The evolution of prolonged life after reproduction. *Trends Ecol Evol*. 2015;30(7):407-416.

3. te Velde ER, Scheffer GJ, Dorland M, Broekmans FJ, Fauser BC. Developmental and endocrine aspects of normal ovarian aging. *Mol Cell Endocrinol*. 1998;145(1-2):67-73.

4. Sauer MV, Paulson RJ, Lobo RA. Reversing the natural decline in human fertility. An extended clinical trial of oocyte donation to women of advanced reproductive age. *JAMA*. 199;268(10):1275-1279. Erratum in: *JAMA*. 1993;268(4):476.

5. Pellestor F, Andréo B, Arnal F, Humeau C, Demaille J. Maternal aging and chromosomal abnormalities: new data drawn from in vitro unfertilized human oocytes. *Hum Genet*. 2003;112(2):195-203.

6. Practice Committee of the American Society for Reproductive Medicine. Testing and interpreting measures of ovarian reserve: a committee opinion. *Fertil Steril*. 2015;103(3):e9-e17.

7. Gaulden ME. Maternal age effect: the enigma of Down syndrome and other trisomic conditions. *Mutat Res*. 1992;296(1-2):69-88.

8. Bentov Y, Casper RF. The aging oocyte—can mitochondrial function be improved? *Fertil Steril*. 2013;99(1):18-22.

9. Santoro N, Crawford SL, El Khoudary SR, et al. Menstrual cycle hormone changes in women traversing the menopause: Study of Women's Health Across the Nation. *J Clin Endocrinol Metab*. 2017;102(7):2218-2229.

10. Laumann EO, Paik A, Rosen RC. Sexual dysfunction in the United States: prevalence and predictors. *JAMA*. 1999;281(6):537-544. Erratum in: *JAMA*. 1999;281(13):1174.

11. Biddle AK, West SL, D'Aloisio AA, Wheeler SB, Borisov NN, Thorp J. Hypoactive sexual desire disorder in postmenopausal women: quality of life and health burden. *Value Health*. 2009;12(5):763-772.

12. Kingsberg SA, Althof S, Simon JA, et al. Female sexual dysfunction—medical and psychological treatments, committee 14. *J Sex Med*. 2017;14(12):1463-1491. Erratum in: *J Sex Med*. 2018;15(2):270.

13. Rosen RC, Barsky JL. Normal sexual response in women. *Obstet Gynecol Clin North Am*. 2006;33(4):515-526.

14. Althof SE, Lieblum SR, Chevret-Measson M, et al. Psychological and interpersonal dimensions of sexual function and dysfunction. *J Sex Med*. 2005;2(6):793-800.

15. Parish SJ, Goldstein AT, Goldstein SW, et al. Toward a more evidence-based nosology and nomenclature for female sexual dysfunctions—part II. *J Sex Med*. 2016;13(12):1888-1906.

16. Masters WH, Johnson VE. *Human Sexual Response*. Boston, MA: Little Brown; 1966.

17. Masters WH, Johnson VE. *Human Sexual Inadequacy*. Boston, MA: Little Brown; 1970.

18. Kaplan HS. *The New Sex Therapy: Active Treatment of Sexual Dysfunctions*. New York: Brunner/Mazel; 1974.

19. Basson R. Female sexual response: the role of drugs in the management of sexual dysfunction. *Obstet Gynecol*. 2001;98(2):350-353. Erratum in: *Obstet Gynecol*. 2001;98(3):522.

20. American Psychiatric Association. *Diagnostic and Statistical Manual of Medical Disorders*. 4th ed, text rev. Washington, DC: American Psychiatric Press; 2000.

21. American Psychiatric Association. *Diagnostic and Statistical Manual of Mental Disorders*. 5th ed (DSM-5). Arlington, VA: American Psychiatric Association; 2013.

22. McCabe MP, Sharlip ID, Lewis R, et al. Incidence and prevalence of sexual dysfunction in women and men: a consensus statement from the Fourth International Consultation on Sexual Medicine 2015. *J Sex Med*. 2016;13(2):144-152.

23. Derogatis LR, Sand M, Balon R, Rosen R, Parish SJ. Toward a more evidence-based nosology and nomenclature for female sexual dysfunctions—part I. *J Sex Med*. 2016;13(12):1881-1887.

24. Pfaus JG. Pathways of sexual desire. *J Sex Med*. 2009;6(6):1506-1533.

25. Kingsberg SA, Clayton AH, Pfaus JG. The female sexual response: current models, neurobiological underpinnings and agents currently approved or under investigation for the treatment of hypoactive sexual desire disorder. *CNS Drugs*. 2015;29(11):915-933.

26. Goldstein I, Kim NN, Clayton AH, et al. Hypoactive sexual desire disorder: International Society for the Study of Women's Sexual Health. (ISSWSH) expert consensus panel review. *Mayo Clin Proc*. 2017;92(1):114-128.

27. Shifren JL, Davis SR. Androgens in postmenopausal women: a review. *Menopause*. 2017;24(8):970-979.

28. Davison SL, Bell R, Donath S, Montalto JG, Davis SR. Androgen levels in adult females: changes with age, menopause, and oophorectomy. J *J Clin Endocrinol Metab*. 2005;90(7):3847-3853.

29. Davis SR, Davison SL, Donath S, Bell RJ. Circulating androgen levels and self-reported sexual function in women. *JAMA*. 2005;294(1):91-96.

30. Randolph JF Jr, Zheng H, Avis NE, Greendale GA, Harlow SD. Masturbation frequency and sexual function domains are associated with serum reproductive hormone levels across the menopausal transition. *J Clin Endocrinol Metab*. 2015;100(1):258-266.

31. Wahlin-Jacobsen S, Pedersen AT, Kristensen E, et al. Is there a correlation between androgens and sexual desire in women? *J Sex Med*. 2015;12(2):358-373.

32. Davis SR, Worsley R, Miller KK, Parish SJ, Santoro N. Androgens and female sexual function and dysfunction—findings from the Fourth International Consultation of Sexual Medicine. *J Sex Med*. 2016;13(2):168-178.

33. Buster JE, Kingsberg SA, Aguirre O, et al. Testosterone patch for low sexual desire in surgically menopausal women: a randomized trial. *Obstet Gynecol*. 2005;105(5 pt 1):944-952.

34. Braunstein GD, Sundwall DA, Katz M, et al. Safety and efficacy of a testosterone patch for the treatment of hypoactive sexual desire disorder in surgically menopausal women: a placebo-controlled trial. *Arch Intern Med*. 2005;165(14):1582-1589.

35. Shifren JL, Davis SR, Moreau M, et al. Testosterone patch for the treatment of hypoactive sexual desire disorder in naturally menopausal women: results from the INTIMATE NM1 Study. *Menopause*. 2006;13(5):770-779. Erratum in: *Menopause*. 2007;14(1):157.

36. Davis SR, van der Mooren MJ, van Lusen RH, et al. Efficacy and safety of a testosterone patch for the treatment of hypoactive sexual desire disorder in surgically menopausal women: a randomized, placebo-controlled trial. *Menopause*. 2006;13(3):387-396. Erratum in: *Menopause*. 2006;13(5):850.

37. Davis SR, Moreau M, Kroll R, et al; APHRODITE Study Team. Testosterone for low libido in postmenopausal women not taking estrogen. *N Engl J Med*. 2008;359(19):2005-2017.

38. Heard-Davison A, Heiman JR, Kuffel S. Genital and subjective measurement of the time course effects of an acute dose of testosterone vs. placebo in postmenopausal women. *J Sex Med*. 2007;4(1):209-217.

39. Panay N, Al-Azzawi F, Bouchard C, et al. Testosterone treatment of HSDD in naturally menopausal women: the ADORE study. *Climacteric*. 2010;13(2):121-131.

40. Simon J, Braunstein G, Nachtigall L, et al. Testosterone patch increases sexual activity and desire in surgically menopausal women with hypoactive sexual desire disorder. *J Clin Endocrinol Metab*. 2005;90(9):5226-5233.

41. Santoro N, Worsley R, Miller KK, Parish SJ, Davis SR. Role of estrogens and estrogen-like compounds in female sexual function and dysfunction. *J Sex Med*. 2016;13(3):305-316.

42. Shifren J, Monaz BU, Rusoo PA, Segreti A, Johannes CB. Sexual problems and distress in United States women: prevalence and correlates. *Obstet Gynecol*. 2008;112(5):970-978.

43. Johannes CB, Clayton AH, Odom DM, et al. Distressing sexual problems in United States women revisited: prevalence after accounting for depression. *J Clin Psychiatry*. 2009;70(12):1698-1706.

44. Kingsberg SA, Wysocki S, Magnus L, Krychman M. Vulvar and vaginal atrophy in postmenopausal women: findings from the REVIVE (REal Women's VIews of Treatment Options for Menopausal Vaginal ChangEs) survey. *J Sex Med.* 2013;10(7):1790-1799.

45. Thomas HN, Hess R, Thurston RC. Correlates of sexual activity and satisfaction in midlife and older women. *Ann Fam Med.* 2015;13(4):336-342.

46. Clayton AH, Goldfischer ER, Goldstein I, Derogatis L, Lewis-D'Agonstino DJ, Pyke R. Validation of the Decreased Sexual Desire Screener (DSDS): a brief diagnostic instrument for acquired hypoactive sexual desire disorder (HSDD). *J Sex Med.* 2009;6(3):730-738.

47. Rosen R, Brown C, Heiman J, et al. The Female Sexual Function Index (FSFI): a multidimensional self-report instrument for the assessment of female sexual function. *J Sex Marital Ther.* 2000;26(2):191-208.

48. Derogatis L, Clayton A, Lewis-D'Agonstino D, Wunderlich G, Fu Y. Validation of the female sexual distress scale—revised for assessing distress in women with hypoactive sexual desire disorder. *J Sex Med.* 2008;5(2):357-364.

49. Hatzichristou D, Rosen RC, Broderick G, et al. Clinical evaluation and management strategy for sexual dysfunction in men and women. *J Sex Med.* 2004;1(1):49-57.

50. Clayton AH, Goldstein I, Kim NN, et al. The International Society for the Study of Women's Sexual Health process of care for management of hypoactive sexual desire disorder in women. *Mayo Clin Proc.* 2018;93(4):467-487.

51. Hatzichristou D, Kirana PS, Banner L, et al. Diagnosing sexual dysfunction in men and women: sexual history taking and the role of symptom scales and questionnaires. *J Sex Med.* 2016;13(8):1166-1182.

52. Faubion SS, Rullo JE. Sexual dysfunction in women: a practical approach. *Am Fam Physician.* 2015;92(4):281-288.

53. Buster JE. Managing female sexual dysfunction. *Fertil Steril.* 2013;100(4):905-915.

54. Kingsberg SA, Rezaee, RL. Hypoactive sexual desire in women. *Menopause.* 2013;20(13):1284-1300.

55. Atlantis E, Sullivan T. Bidirectional association between depression and sexual dysfunction: a systematic review and meta-analysis. *J Sex Med.* 2012;9(6):1497-1507.

56. Rosen RC, Shifren JL, Monz BU, Odom DM, Russo PA, Johannes, CB. Correlates of sexually related personal distress in women with low sexual desire. *J Sex Med.* 2009;6(6):1549-1560.

57. Lorenz T, Rullo J, Faubion S. Antidepressant-induced female sexual dysfunction. *Mayo Clin Proc.* 2016;91(9):1280-1286.

58. Annon JS. Behavioral *Treatment of Sexual Problems: Brief Therapy.* Oxford, England: Harper and Row; 1976.

59. Brotto L, Atallah S, Johnson-Agbakwu C, et al. Psychological and interpersonal dimensions of sexual function and dysfunction. *J Sex Med.* 2016;13(4):538-571.

60. Stahl SM, Sommer B, Allers KA. Multifunctional pharmacology of flibanserin: possible mechanism of therapeutic action in hypoactive sexual desire disorder. *J Sex Med.* 2011;8(1):15-27.

61. US Food and Drug Administration. FDA orders important safety labeling changes for Addyi: Studies affirm need for warnings related to alcohol use with Addyi [press release]. April 11, 2019. www.fda.gov/news-events/press-announcements/fda-orders-important-safety-labeling-changes-addyi. Accessed May 21, 2019.

62. Addyi [prescribing information]. Raleigh, NC: Sprout; 2015.

63. Derogatis LR, Komer L, Katz M, et al; VIOLET Trial Investigators. Treatment of hypoactive sexual desire disorder in premenopausal women: efficacy of flibanserin in the VIOLET Study. *J Sex Med.* 2012;9(4):1074-1085.

64. Thorp J, Simon J, Dattani D, et al; DAISY trial investigators. Treatment of hypoactive sexual desire disorder in premenopausal women: efficacy of flibanserin in the DAISY study. *J Sex Med.* 2012;9(4):793-804.

65. Katz M, DeRogatis LR, Ackerman R, et al; BEGONIA trial investigators. Efficacy of flibanserin in women with hypoactive sexual desire disorder: results from the BEGONIA trial. *J Sex Med.* 2013;10(7):1807-1815.

66. Simon JA, Kingsberg SA, Shumel B, Hanes V, Garcia M Jr, Sand M. Efficacy and safety of flibanserin in postmenopausal women with hypoactive sexual desire disorder: results of the SNOWDROP trial. *Menopause.* 2014;21(6):633-640.

67. Portman DJ, Brown L, Yuan J, Kissling R, Kingsberg SA. Flibanserin in postmenopausal women with hypoactive sexual desire disorder: results of the PLUMERIA Study. *J Sex Med.* 2017;14(6):834-842.

68. Dimitrakakis C, Jones RA, Liu A, Bondy CA. Breast cancer incidence in postmenopausal women using testosterone in addition to usual hormone therapy. *Menopause.* 2004;11(5):531-535.

69. Davis SR, Wolfe R, Farrugia H, Ferdinand A, Bell RJ. The incidence of invasive breast cancer among women prescribed testosterone for low libido. *J Sex Med.* 2009;6(7):1850-1856.

70. Glaser RL, Dimitrakakis C. Reduced breast cancer incidence in women treated with subcutaneous testosterone, or testosterone with anastrozole: a prospective, observational study. *Maturitas.* 2013;76(4):342-349.

71. Spoletini I, Vitale C, Pelliccia F, Fossati C, Rosano GM. Androgens and cardiovascular disease in postmenopausal women: a systematic review. *Climacteric.* 2014;17:625-634.

72. Clayton AH, Kingsberg SA, Simon J, Jordan R, Lucas J. The investigational drug bremelanotide for hypoactive sexual desire disorder (HSDD): efficacy analyses from the RECONNECT studies [abstract]. *J Sex Med.* 2018;15(2):S7-S8. Abstract 014.

73. Davis SR, Braunstein GD. Efficacy and safety of testosterone in the management of hypoactive sexual desire disorder in postmenopausal women. *J Sex Med.* 2012;9(4):1134-1148.

74. Pessina MA, Hoyt RF Jr, Goldstein I, Traish AM. Differential effects of estradiol, progesterone, and testosterone on vaginal structural integrity. *Endocrinology.* 2006;147(1):61-69.

75. Nappi RE, Cucinella L. Advances in pharmacotherapy for treating female sexual dysfunction. *Expert Opin Pharmacother.* 2015;16(6):875-887.

76. Chivers ML, Rosen RC. Phosphodiesterase type 5 inhibitors and female sexual response: faulty protocols or paradigms? *J Sex Med.* 2010; 7(2 pt 2):858-872.

77. Schoen C, Bachmann G. Sildenafil citrate for female sexual arousal disorder: a future possibility? *Nat Rev Urol.* 2009;6(4):216-222.

78. Labbate LA, Grimes JB, Arana GW. Serotonin reuptake antidepressant effects on sexual function in patients with anxiety disorders. *Biol Psychiatry.* 1998;43(12):904-907.

79. Heiman JR, LoPiccolo J. *Becoming Orgasmic: A Sexual and Personal Growth Program for Women.* Rev and expanded ed. New York: Simon & Schuster; 1988.

80. Labrie F, Archer DF, Koltun W, et al; VVA Prasterone Research Group. Efficacy of intravaginal dehydroepiandrosterone (DHEA) on moderate to severe dyspareunia and vaginal dryness, symptoms of vulvovaginal atrophy, and of the genitourinary syndrome of menopause. *Menopause.* 2016;23(3):243-256.

81. Labrie F, Archer D, Bouchard C, et al. Lack of influence of dyspareunia on the beneficial effect of intravaginal prasterone (dehydroepiandrosterone, DHEA) on sexual dysfunction in postmenopausal women. *J Sex Med.* 2014;11(7):1766-1785

82. Portman DJ, Bachmann GA, Simon JA; Ospemifene Study Group. Ospemifene, a novel selective estrogen receptor modulator for treating dyspareunia associated with postmenopausal vulvar and vaginal atrophy. *Menopause.* 2013;20(6):623-630.

83. Faubion SS, Sood R, Kapoor E. Genitourinary syndrome of menopause: management strategies for the clinician. *Mayo Clin Proc.* 2017;92(12):1842-1849.

84. American College of Obstetricians and Gynecologists. Women's Health Care Physicians. *Fractional Laser Treatment of Vulvovaginal Atrophy and US Food and Drug Administration Clearance: Position Statement.* May 2016. www.acog.org/Resources-And-Publications/Position-Statements/Fractional-Laser-Treatment-of-Vulvovaginal-Atrophy-and-US-Food-and-Drug-Administration-Clearance. Accessed May 21, 2019.

85. Arunkalaivanan A, Kaur H, Onuma O. Laser therapy as a treatment modality for genitourinary syndrome of menopause: a critical appraisal of evidence. *Int Urogynecol J.* 2017;28(5):681-685.

86. Salvatore S, Nappi RE, Zerbinati N, et al. A 12-week treatment with fractional CO2 laser for vulvovaginal atrophy: a pilot study. *Climacteric.* 2014;17(4):363-369.

87. Wu JM, Vaughan CP, Goode PS, et al. Prevalence and trends of symptomatic pelvic floor disorders in U.S. women. *Obstet Gynecol.* 2014;123(1):141-148.

88. Butrick CW. Pathophysiology of the pelvic floor hypertonic disorders. *Obstet Gynecol Clin North Am.* 2009;36(3):699-705.

89. Faubion SS, Shuster LT, Bharucha AE. Recognition and management of nonrelaxing pelvic floor dysfunction. *Mayo Clin Proc.* 2012;87(2):187-193.

90. Moldwin RM, Fariello JY. Myofascial trigger points of the pelvic floor: associations with urological pain syndromes and treatment strategies including injection therapy. *Curr Urol Rep.* 2013;14(5):409-417.

91. Kim HK, Kang SY, Chung YJ, Kim JH, Kim MR. The recent review of the genitourinary syndrome of menopause. *J Menopausal Med.* 2015;21(2):65-71.

92. Hartmann D, Sarton J. Chronic pelvic floor dysfunction. *Best Pract Res Clin Obstet Gynaecol.* 2014;28(7):977-990.

93. FitzGerald MP, Anderson RU, Potts J, et al; Urological Pelvic Pain Collaborative Research Network. Randomized multicenter feasibility trial of myofascial physical therapy for the treatment of urological chronic pelvic pain syndromes. *J Urol.* 2009;182(2):570-580.

94. FitzGerald MP, Kotarinos R. Rehabilitation of the short pelvic floor. I: Background and patient evaluation. *Int Urogynecol J Pelvic Floor Dysfunct.* 2003;14(4):261-268.

95. Rogalski MJ, Kellogg-Spadt S, Hoffman AR, Fariello JY, Whitmore KE. Retrospective chart review of vaginal diazepam suppository use in high-tone pelvic floor dysfunction. *Int Urogynecol J.* 2010;21(17):895-899.

96. Idama TO, Pring DW. Vaginal dilator therapy—an outpatient gynecological option in the management of dyspareunia. *J Obstet Gynecol.* 2000;20(3):303-305.

97. Goldstein AT, Burrows L J, Kellogg-Spadt S. Intralevator injection of botulinum toxin for the treatment of hypertonic pelvic floor muscle dysfunction and vestibulodynia. *J Sex Med.* 2011;8(5):1287-1290.

98. Jarvis SK, Abbott JA, Lenart MB, Steensma A, Vancaillie TG. Pilot study of botulinum toxin type A in the treatment of chronic pelvic pain associated with spasm of the levator ani muscles. *Aust N Z J Obstet Gynaecol.* 2004;44(1):46-50.

99. Abbott JA, Jarvis SK, Lyons SD, Thomson A, Vancaille TG. Botulinum toxin type A for chronic pain and pelvic floor spasm in women: a randomized controlled trial. *Obstet Gynecol.* 2006;108(4):915-923.

100. Adelowo A, Hacker MR, Shapiro A, Modest AM, Elkadry E. Botox toxin type A (Botox) for refractory myofascial pelvic pain. *Female Pelvic Med Reconstr Surg.* 2013;19(5):288-292.

101. Nesbitt-Hawes EM, Won H, Jarvis SK, Lyons SD, Vancaillie TG, Abbott JA. Improvement in pelvic pain with botulinum toxin type A—single vs repeat injections. *Toxicon.* 2013;63:83-87.

102. Committee on Practice Bulletins—Gynecology. Practice bulletin no. 128: diagnosis of abnormal uterine bleeding in reproductive-aged women. *Obstet Gynecol.* 2012;120(1):197-206.

103. Munro MG, Critchley HO, Broder MS, Fraser IS; FIGO Working Group on Menstrual Disorders. FIGO classification system (PALM-COEIN) for causes of abnormal uterine bleeding in nongravid women of reproductive age. *Int J Gynaecol Obstet.* 2011;113(1):3-13.

104. Chaudhry S, Berkley C, Warren M. Perimenopausal vaginal bleeding: diagnostic evaluation and therapeutic options. *J Womens Health (Larchmt).* 2012;21(3):302-310.

105. National Cancer Institute. Surveillance, Epidemiology, and End Results Program. *Cancer Stat Facts: Uterine Cancer.* https://seer.cancer.gov/statfacts/html/corp.html. Accessed May 21, 2019.

106. Reed SD, Newton KM, Clinton WL, et al. Incidence of endometrial hyperplasia. *Am J Obstet Gynecol.* 2009;200(6):678.e1-678.e6.

107. Baak JP, Mutter GL, Robboy S, et al. The molecular genetics and morphometry-based endometrial intraepithelial neoplasia classification system predicts disease progression in endometrial hyperplasia more accurately then the 1994 World Health Organization classification system. *Cancer.* 2005;103(11):2304-2312.

108. Basila D, Yuan CS. Effects of dietary supplements on coagulation and platelet function. *Thromb Res.* 2005;117(1-2):49-53.

109. Wittkowsky AK. A systematic review and inventory of supplement effects on warfarin and other anticoagulants. *Thromb Res.* 2005;117(1-2):81-86.

110. Goldstein SR, Zeltser I, Horan CK, Snyder JR, Schwartz LB. Ultrasonography-based triage for perimenopausal patients with abnormal uterine bleeding. *Am J Obstet Gynecol.* 1997;177(1):102-108.

111. Goldstein SR. Modern evaluation of the endometrium. *Obstet Gynecol.* 2010;116(1):168-176.

112. Stovall TG, Photopulos GJ, Poston WM, Ling FW, Sandlers LG. Pipelle endometrial sampling in patients with known endometrial carcinoma. *Obstet Gynecol.* 1991;77(6):954-956.

113. Guido RS, Kanbour-Shakir A, Rulin MC, Christopherson WA. Pipelle endometrial sampling. Sensitivity in the detection of endometrial cancer. *J Reprod Med.* 1995;40(8):553-555.

114. Larson DM, Krawisz BR, Johnson KK, Broste SK. Comparison of the Z-Sampler and Novak endometrial biopsy instruments for in-office diagnosis of endometrial cancer. *Gynecol Oncol.* 1994;54(1):64-67.

115. Ferry J, Farnsworth A, Webster M, Wren B. The efficacy of the pipelle endometrial biopsy in detecting endometrial carcinoma. *Aust N Z J Obstet Gynaecol.* 1993;33(1):76-78.

116. Rodriguez MH, Platt LD, Medearis AL, Lacarra M, Lobo RA. The use of transvaginal sonography for evaluation of postmenopausal size and morphology. *Am J Obstet Gynecol.* 1988;159(4):810-814.

117. Goldstein SR. Pregnancy I: embryo. In: *Endovaginal Ultrasound.* 2nd ed. New York: Wiley-Liss; 1991:55-70.

118. ACOG Committee Opinion No. 734: the role of transvaginal ultrasonography in evaluating the endometrium of women with postmenopausal bleeding. *Obstet Gynecol.* 2018;131(5):e124-e129.

119. Matteson KA, Anderson BL, Pinto SB, Lopes V, Schulkin J, Clark MA. Practice patterns and attitudes about treating abnormal uterine bleeding: a national survey of obstetricians and gynecologists. *Am J Obstet Gynecol.* 2011;205(4):321.e1-8.

120. Gupta J, Kai J, Middleton L, Pattison H, Gray R, Daniels J; ECLIPSE Trial Collaborative Group. Levonorgestrel intrauterine system versus medical therapy for menorrhagia. *N Engl J Med.* 2013;368(2):128-137.

121. Lethaby A, Duckitt K, Farquhar C. Nonsteroidal anti-inflammatory drugs for heavy menstrual bleeding. *Cochrane Database Syst Rev.* 2013;(1):CD000400.

122. Bryant-Smith AC, Lethaby A, Farquhar C, Hickey M. Antifibrinolytics for heavy menstrual bleeding. *Cochrane Database Syst Rev.* 2018;(4):CD000249.

123. Fergusson RJ, Lethaby A, Shepperd S, Farquhar C. Endometrial resection and ablation versus hysterectomy for heavy menstrual bleeding. *Cochrane Database Syst Rev.* 2013;(11):CD000329.

124. AlHilli MM, Hopkins MR, Famuyide AO. Endometrial cancer after endometrial ablation: systematic review of medical literature. *J Minim Invasive Gynecol.* 2011;18(3):393-400.

125. Lumsden MA, Wedisinghe L. Tranexamic acid therapy for heavy menstrual bleeding. *Expert Opin Pharmacother.* 2011;12(13):2089-2095.

126. Gupta JK, Daniels JP, Middleton LJ, et al; ECLIPSE Collaborative Group. A randomised controlled trial of the clinical effectiveness and cost-effectiveness of the levonorgestrel-releasing intrauterine system in primary care against standard treatment for menorrhagia: the ECLIPSE trial. *Health Technol Assess.* 2015;19(88):i-xxv, 1-118.

127. Senol T, Kahramanoglu I, Dogan Y, Baktiroglu M, Karateke A, Suer N. Levonorgestrel-releasing intrauterine device use as an alternative to surgical therapy for uterine leiomyoma. *Clin Exp Obstet Gynecol.* 2015;42(2):224-227.

128. Lumsden MA, West CP, Thomas E, et al. Treatment with the gonadotrophin releasing hormone-agonist goserelin before hysterectomy for uterine fibroids. *Br J Obstet Gynaecol.* 1994;101(5):438-442.

129. Donnez J, Tatarchuk TF, Bouchard P, et al; PEARL I Study Group. Ulipristal acetate versus placebo for fibroid treatment before surgery. *N Engl J Med.* 2012;366(5):409-420.

130. Tristan M, Orozco LJ, Steed A, Ramirez-Morera A, Stone P. Mifepristone for uterine fibroids. *Cochrane Database Syst Rev.* 2012;(8):CD007687.

131. Gupta JK, Sinha A, Lumsden MA, Hickey M. Uterine artery embolization for symptomatic uterine fibroids. *Cochrane Database Syst Rev.* 2014;(12):CD005073.

132. Manyonda IT, Bratby M, Horst JS, Banu N, Gorti M, Belli AM. Uterine artery embolization versus myomectomy: impact on quality of life—results of the FUME (Fibroids of the Uterus: Myomectomy versus Embolization) Trial. *Cardiovasc Intervent Radiol.* 2012;35(3):530-536.

133. Rashid S, Khaund A, Murray LS, et al. The effects of uterine artery embolisation and surgical treatment on ovarian function in women with uterine fibroids. *BJOG.* 2010;117(8):985-989.

134. McPherson K, Metcalfe MA, Herbert A, et al. Severe complications of hysterectomy: the VALUE study. *BJOG.* 2004;111(7):688-694.

135. LaMote AI, Lalwani S, Diamond MP. Morbidity associated with abdominal myomectomy. *Obstet Gynecol.* 1993;82(6):897-900.

136. Kongnyuy EJ, Wiysonge CS. Interventions to reduce haemorrhage during myomectomy for fibroids. *Cochrane Database Syst Rev.* 2014;(8):CD005355.

137. Palomba S, Zupi E, Falbo A, et al. A multicenter randomized, controlled study comparing laparoscopic versus minilaparotomic myomectomy: reproductive outcomes. *Fertil Steril.* 2007;88(4):933-941.

138. Bosteels J, Kasius J, Weyers S, Broekmans FJ, Mol BW, D'Hooghe TM. Hysteroscopy for treating subfertility associated with suspected major uterine cavity abnormalities. *Cochrane Database Syst Rev.* 2015;(2):CD009461.

139. Varma R, Soneja H, Clark TJ, Gupta JK. Hysteroscopic myomectomy for menorrhagia using Versascope bipolar system: efficacy and prognostic factors at a minimum of one year follow up. *Eur J Obstet Gynecol Reprod Biol.* 2009;142(2):154-159.

140. Ørbo A, Arnes M, Hancke C, Vereide AB, Pettersen I, Larsen K. Treatment results of endometrial hyperplasia after prospective D-score classification: a follow-up study comparing effect of LNG-IUD and oral progestins versus observation only. *Gynecol Oncol.* 2008;111(1):68-73.

141. Reitz C, Brayne C, Mayeux R. Epidemiology of Alzheimer disease. *Nat Rev Neurol.* 2011;7(3):137-152.

142. Neu SC, Pa J, Kukull W, et al. Apolipoprotein E genotype and sex risk factors for Alzheimer disease: a meta-analysis. *JAMA Neurol.* 2017;74(10):1178-1189.

143. Gauthier S, Reisberg B, Zaudig M, et al; International Psychogeriatric Association Expert Conference on mild cognitive impairment. Mild cognitive impairment. *Lancet.* 2006;367(9518):1262-1270.

144. Sullivan Mitchell E, Fugate Woods N. Midlife women's attributions about perceived memory changes: observations from the Seattle Midlife Women's Health Study. *J Womens Health Gend Based Med.* 2001;10(4):351-362.

145. Woods NF, Mitchell ES. Symptom interference with work and relationships during the menopausal transition and early postmenopause: observations from the Seattle Midlife Women's Health Study. *Menopause.* 2011;18(6):654-661.

146. Weber MT, Maki PM, McDermott MP. Cognition and mood in perimenopause: a systematic review and meta-analysis. *J Steroid Biochem Mol Biol.* 2014;142:90-98.

147. Rentz DM, Weiss BK, Jacobs EG, et al. Sex differences in episodic memory in early midlife: impact of reproductive aging. *Menopause.* 2017;24(4):400-408.

148. Greendale GA, Huang MH, Wight RG, et al. Effects of the menopause transition and hormone use on cognitive performance in midlife women. *Neurology.* 2009;72(21):1850-1857.

149. Greendale GA, Wight RG, Huang MH, et al. Menopause-associated symptoms and cognitive performance: results from the Study of Women's Health Across the Nation. *Am J Epidemiol.* 2010;171(11):1214-1224.

150. Epperson CN, Sammel MD, Freeman EW. Menopause effects on verbal memory: findings from a longitudinal community cohort. *J Clin Endocrinol Metab.* 2013;98(9):3829-3838.

151. Phillips SM, Sherwin BB. Effects of estrogen on memory function in surgically menopausal women. *Psychoneuroendocrinology.* 1992;17(5):485-495.

152. Kurita K, Henderson VW, Gatz M, et al. Association of bilateral oophorectomy with cognitive function in healthy, postmenopausal women. *Fertil Steril.* 2016;106(3):749-756.

153. Sherwin BB. Estrogen and/or androgen replacement therapy and cognitive functioning in surgically menopausal women. *Psychoneuroendocrinology.* 1988;13(4):345-357.

154. Sherwin BB, Tulandi T. "Add-back" estrogen reverses cognitive deficits induced by a gonadotropin-releasing hormone agonist in women with leiomyomata uteri. *J Clin Endocrinol Metab.* 1996;81(7):2545-2549.

155. Maki PM, Drogos LL, Rubin LH, Banuvar S, Shulman LP, Geller SE. Objective hot flashes are negatively related to verbal memory performance in midlife women. *Menopause.* 2008;15(5):848-856.

156. Maki PM, Rubin LH, Savarese A, et al. Stellate ganglion blockade and verbal memory in midlife women: evidence from a randomized trial. *Maturitas.* 2016;92:123-129.

157. Henderson VW, Popat RA. Effects of endogenous and exogenous estrogen exposures in midlife and late-life women on episodic memory and executive functions. *Neuroscience.* 2011;191:129-138.

158. Lehert P, Villaseca P, Hogervorst E, Maki PM, Henderson VW. Individually modifiable risk factors to ameliorate cognitive aging: a systematic review and meta-analysis. *Climacteric.* 2015;18(5):678-689.

159. Sofi F, Valecchi D, Bacci D, et al. Physical activity and risk of cognitive decline: a meta-analysis of prospective studies. *J Intern Med.* 2011;269(1):107-117.

160. Resnick SM, Maki PM, Rapp SR, et al; Women's Health Initiative Study of Cognitive Aging Investigators. Effects of combination estrogen plus progestin hormone treatment on cognition and affect. *J Clin Endocrinol Metab.* 2006;91(5):1802-1810.

161. Resnick SM, Espeland MA, An Y, et al; Women's Health Initiative Study of Cognitive Aging Investigators. Effects of conjugated equine estrogens on cognition and affect in postmenopausal women with prior hysterectomy. *J Clin Endocrinol Metab.* 2009;94(11):4152-4161.

162. Espeland MA, Brunner RL, Hogan PE, et al; Women's Health Initiative Study of Cognitive Aging Study Group. Long-term effects of conjugated equine estrogen therapies on domain-specific cognitive function: results from the Women's Health Initiative Study of Cognitive Aging extension. *J Am Geriatr Soc.* 2010;58(7):1263-1271.

163. Gleason CE, Dowling NM, Wharton W, et al. Effects of hormone therapy on cognition and mood in recently postmenopausal women: findings from the randomized, controlled KEEPS-Cognitive and Affective Study. *PLoS Med.* 2015;12(6):e1001833.

164. Espeland MA, Shumaker SA, Leng I, et al; WHIMSY Study Group. Long-term effects on cognitive function of postmenopausal hormone therapy prescribed to women aged 50 to 55 years. *JAMA Intern Med.* 2013;1723(15):1429-1436.

165. Henderson VW, St John JA, Hodis HN, et al. Cognitive effects of estradiol after menopause: a randomized trial of the timing hypothesis. *Neurology.* 2016;87(7):699-708.

166. Joffe H, Hall JE, Gruber S, et al. Estrogen therapy selectively enhances prefrontal cognitive processes: a randomized, double-blind, placebo-controlled study with functional magnetic resonance imaging in perimenopausal and recently postmenopausal women. *Menopause.* 2006;13(3):411-422.

167. Ryan J, Scali J, Carrière I, Amieva H, et al. Impact of a premature menopause on cognitive function in later life. *BJOG.* 2014;121(13):1729-1739.

168. Phung TK, Waltoft BL, Laursen TM, et al. Hysterectomy, oophorectomy and risk of dementia: a nationwide historical cohort study. *Dement Geriatr Cogn Disord.* 2010;30(1):43-50.

169. Rocca WA, Bower JH, Maraganore DM, et al. Increased risk of cognitive impairment or dementia in women who underwent oophorectomy before menopause. *Neurology.* 2007;69(11):1074-1083.

170. Kritz-Silverstein D, Barrett-Connor E. Hysterectomy, oophorectomy, and cognitive function in older women. *J Am Geriatr Soc.* 2002;50(1):55-61.

171. Barnes DE, Yaffe K. The projected effect of risk factor reduction on Alzheimer's disease prevalence. *Lancet Neurol.* 2011;10(9):819-828.

172. Rouch L, Cestac P, Hanon O, et al. Antihypertensive drugs, prevention of cognitive decline and dementia: a systematic review of observational studies, randomized controlled trials and meta-analyses, with discussion of potential mechanisms. *CNS Drugs.* 2015;29(2):113-1130.

173. Chang-Quan H, Hui W, Chao-Min W, et al. The association of antihypertensive medication use with risk of cognitive decline and dementia: a meta-analysis of longitudinal studies. *Int J Clin Pract.* 2011;65(12):1295-1305.

174. Levi Marpillat N, Macquin-Mavier I, Tropeano AI, Bachoud-Levi AC, Maison P. Antihypertensive classes, cognitive decline and incidence of dementia: a network meta-analysis. *J Hypertens.* 2013;31(6):1073-1082.

175. Shumaker SA, Legault C, Rapp SR, et al; WHIMS Investigators. Estrogen plus progestin and the incidence of dementia and mild cognitive impairment in postmenopausal women: the Women's Health Initiative Memory Study: a randomized controlled trial. *JAMA.* 2003;289(20):2651-2662.

176. Shumaker SA, Legault C, Kuller L, et al; Women's Health Initiative Memory Study. Conjugated equine estrogens and incidence of probable dementia and mild cognitive impairment in postmenopausal women: Women's Health Initiative Memory Study. *JAMA.* 2004;291(24):2947-2985.

177. The NAMS 2017 Hormone Therapy Position Statement Advisory Panel. The 2017 hormone therapy position statement of The North American Menopause Society. *Menopause.* 2017;24(7):728-753.

178. Marjoribanks J, Farquhar C, Roberts H, Lethaby A, Lee J. Long-term hormone therapy for perimenopausal and postmenopausal women. *Cochrane Database Syst Rev.* 2017;1:CD004143.

179. Henderson VW, Benke KS, Green RC, Cupples LA, Farrer LA; MIRAGE Study Group. Postmenopausal hormone therapy and Alzheimer's disease risk: interaction with age. *J Neurol Neurosurg Psychiatry.* 2005;76(1):103-105.

180. Henderson VW, Espeland MA, Hogan PE, et al. Prior use of hormone therapy and incident Alzheimer's disease in the Women's Health Initiative Memory Study [abstract]. *Neurology.* 2007;68(suppl 1):A205.

181. Shao H, Breitner JC, Whitmer RA, et al; Cache County Investigators. Hormone therapy and Alzheimer disease dementia: new findings from the Cache County study. *Neurology.* 2012;79(18):1846-1852.

182. Whitmer RA, Quesenberry CP, Zhou J, Yaffe K. Timing of hormone therapy and dementia: the critical window theory revisited. *Ann Neurol.* 2011;69(1):163-169.

183. Kantarci K, Lowe VJ, Lesnick TG, et al. Early postmenopausal transdermal 17β-estradiol therapy and amyloid-β deposition. *J Alzheimers Dis.* 2016;53(2):547-556.

184. Manson JE, Aragaki AK, Rossouw JE, et al; WHI Investigators. Menopausal hormone therapy and long-term all-cause and cause-specific mortality: the Women's Health Initiative randomized trials. *JAMA.* 2017;318(10):927-938.

185. Mikkola TS, Savolainen-Peltonen H, Tuomikoski P, et al. Lower death risk for vascular dementia than for Alzheimer's disease with postmenopausal hormone therapy users. *J Clin Endocrinol Metab.* 2017;102(3):870-877.

186. Rossouw JE, Prentice RL, Manson JE, et al. Postmenopausal hormone therapy and risk of cardiovascular disease by age and years since menopause. *JAMA.* 2007;297(13):1465-1477. Erratum in: *JAMA.* 2008;299(12):1426.

187. Grodstein F, Manson JE, Stampfer MJ, Rexrode K. Postmenopausal hormone therapy and stroke: role of time since menopause and age at initiation of hormone therapy. *Arch Intern Med.* 2008;168(8):861-866.

188. Henderson VW, Lobo RA. Hormone therapy and the risk of stroke: perspectives 10 years after the Women's Health Initiative trials. *Climacteric.* 2012;15(3):229-234.

189. Løkkegaard E, Nielsen LH, Keiding N. Risk of stroke with various types of menopausal hormone therapies. *Stroke.* 2017;48(8):2266-2269. Erratum in: *Stroke.* 2018;49(3):e142.

190. National Institutes of Health. National Institutes of Health State-of-the-Science Conference statement: management of menopause-related symptoms. *Ann Intern Med.* 2005;142(12 pt 1):1003-1013.

191. Vahratian A. Sleep duration and quality among women aged 40-59, by menopausal status. *NCHS Data Brief.* 2017;(286):1-8.

192. Joffe H, Massler A, Sharkey KM. Evaluation and management of sleep disturbance during the menopause transition. *Semin Reprod Med.* 2010;28(5):404-421.

193. Kravitz HM, Zhao X, Bromberger JT, et al. Sleep disturbance during the menopausal transition in a multi-ethnic community sample of women. *Sleep.* 2008;31(7):979-990.

194. Jehan S, Masters-Isarilov A, Salifu I, et al. Sleep disorders in postmenopausal women. *J Sleep Disord Ther.* 2015;4(5):pii: 1000212.

195. Kravitz HM, Janssen I, Bromberger JT, et al. Sleep trajectories before and after the final menstrual period in the Study of Women's Health Across the Nation (SWAN). *Curr Sleep Med Rep.* 2017;3(3):235-250.

196. Freeman EW, Sammel MD, Gross SA, Pien GW. Poor sleep in relation to natural menopause: a population-based 14-year follow-up of midlife women. *Menopause.* 2015;22(7):719-726.

197. Bromberger JT, Kravitz HM. Mood and menopause: findings from the Study of Women's Health Across the Nation (SWAN) over 10 years. *Obstet Gynecol Clin North Am.* 2011;38(3):609-625.

198. Bromberger JT, Schott LL, Kravitz HM, et al. Longitudinal change in reproductive hormones and depressive symptoms across the menopausal transition: results from the Study of Women's Health Across the Nation (SWAN). *Arch Gen Psychiatry.* 2010;67(6):598-607.

199. Burleson MH, Todd M, Trevathan WR. Daily vasomotor symptoms, sleep problems, and mood: using daily data to evaluate the domino hypothesis in middle-aged women. *Menopause.* 2010;17(1):87-95.

200. Freedman RR, Roehrs TA. Sleep disturbance in menopause. *Menopause.* 2007;14(5):826-829.

201. Cheng MH, Hsu CY, Wang SJ, Lee SJ, Wang PH, Fuh JL. The relationship of self-reported sleep disturbance, mood, and menopause in a community study. *Menopause.* 2008;15(5):958-962.

202. Kravitz HM, Schott LL, Joffe H, Cyranowski JM, Bromberger JT. Do anxiety symptoms predict major depressive disorder in midlife women? The Study of Women's Health Across the Nation (SWAN) Mental Health Study (MHS). *Psychol Med.* 2014;44(12):2593-2602.

203. Hadley EC, Kuchel GA, Newman AB; Workshop Speakers and Participants. Report: NIA Workshop on Measures of Physiologic Resiliencies in Human Aging. *J Gerontol A Biol Sci Med Sci.* 2017;72(7):980-990.

204. Shaver JL, Woods NF. Sleep and menopause: a narrative review. *Menopause.* 2015;22(8):899-915.

205. Young T, Rabago D, Zgierska A, Austin D, Laurel F. Objective and subjective sleep quality in premenopausal, perimenopausal, and postmenopausal women in the Wisconsin Sleep Cohort Study. *Sleep.* 2003;26(6):667-672.

206. Lee KA, Anderson DJ. Screening midlife women for sleep problems: why, how, and who should get a referral? *Menopause.* 2015;22(7):783-785.

207. Tal JZ, Suh SA, Dowdle C, Nowakowski S. Treatment of insomnia, insomnia symptoms, and obstructive sleep apnea during and after menopause: therapeutic approaches. *Curr Psychiatry Rev.* 2015;11(1):63-83.

208. Brewster GS, Riegel B, Gherman PR. Insomnia in the older adult. *Sleep Med Clin.* 2018;13(1):13-19.

209. Ong JC, Arnedt JT, Gehrman PR. Insomnia diagnosis, assessment, and evaluation. In: Kryger M, Roth T, Dement WC, eds. *Principles and Practice of Sleep Medicine.* 6th ed. Philadelphia, PA: Elsevier; 2017:785-793.

210. Saaresranta T, Polo-Kantolo P, Polo O. Practical approach for the diagnosis and management of insomnia during menopause transition. In: Attarian HP, Viola-Saltzman M, eds. *Sleep Disorders in Women. A Guide to Practical Management.* 2nd ed. New York: Springer Science+Business Media; 2013:293-324.

211. Buysse DJ. Insomnia. *JAMA.* 2013;309(7):706-716.

212. Carney CE, Buysse DJ, Ancoli-Israel S, et al. The consensus sleep diary: standardizing prospective sleep self-monitoring. *Sleep.* 2012;35(2):287-302.

213. Buysse DJ, Reynolds CF 3rd, Monk TH, Berman SR, Kupfer DJ. The Pittsburgh Sleep Quality Index: a new instrument for psychiatric practice and research. *Psychiatry Res*. 1989;28(2):193-213.

214. Bastien CH, Vallieres A, Morin CM. Validation of the Insomnia Severity Index as an outcome measure for insomnia research. *Sleep Med*. 2001;2(4):297-307.

215. Hauri PJ. *The Sleep Disorders. Current Concepts*. Kalamazoo, MI: Scope, Upjohn; 1977.

216. Posner D, Gehrman PR. Sleep hygiene. In: Perlis M, Aloia M, Kuhn B, eds. *Behavioral Treatments for Sleep Disorders. A Comprehensive Primer of Behavioral Sleep Medicine Treatment Protocols*. London: Elsevier; 2011:31-43.

217. Stepanski EJ, Wyatt JK. Use of sleep hygiene in the treatment of insomnia. *Sleep Med Rev*. 2003;7(3):215-225.

218. Schutte-Rodin S, Broch L, Buysse D, Dorsey C, Sateia M. Clinical guideline for the evaluation and management of chronic insomnia in adults. *J Clin Sleep Med*. 2008;4(5):487-504.

219. Kline CE, Irish LA, Buysse DJ, et al. Sleep hygiene behaviors among midlife women with insomnia or sleep-disordered breathing: the SWAN Sleep Study. *J Womens Health (Larchmt)*. 2014;23(11):894-903.

220. Morgenthaler T, Kramer M, Alessi C, et al; American Academy of Sleep Medicine. Practice parameters for the psychological and behavioral treatment of insomnia: an update. An American Academy of Sleep Medicine report. *Sleep*. 2006;29(11):1415-1419.

221. Yang CM, Spielman AJ, Glovinsky P. Nonpharmacologic strategies in the management of insomnia. *Psychiatr Clin North Am*. 2006;29(4):895-919.

222. Attarian H, Hachul H, Guttuso T, Phillips B. Treatment of chronic insomnia disorder in menopause: evaluation of literature. *Menopause*. 2015;22(6):674-684.

223. Manson JE, Chlebowski RT, Stefanick ML, et al. Menopausal hormone therapy and health outcomes during the intervention and extended poststopping phases of the Women's Health Initiative randomized trials. *JAMA*. 2013;310(13):1353-1368.

224. Rossouw JE, Anderson GL, Prentice RL, et al; Writing Group for the Women's Health Initiative Investigators. Risks and benefits of estrogen plus progestin in healthy postmenopausal women: principal results from the Women's Health Initiative randomized controlled trial. *JAMA*. 2002;288(3):321-333.

225. Guttuso T Jr. Effective and clinically meaningful non-hormonal hot flash therapies. *Maturitas*. 2012;72(1):6-12.

226. Nelson HD, Vesco KK, Haney E, et al. Nonhormonal therapies for menopausal hot flashes: systematic review and meta-analysis. *JAMA*. 2006;295(17):2057-2071.

227. Gunja N. The clinical and forensic toxicology of Z-drugs. *J Med Toxicol*. 2013;9(2):155-162.

228. US Food and Drug Administration. Questions and answers: risk of next-morning impairment after use of insomnia drugs; FDA requires lower recommended doses for certain drugs containing zolpidem (Ambien, Ambien CR, Edluar, and Zolpimist). www.fda.gov/Drugs/DrugSafety/ucm334041.htm. Last updated February 13, 2018. Accessed May 21, 2019.

229. Drug Enforcement Administration, Department of Justice. Schedules of controlled substances: placement of suvorexant into Schedule IV. Final rule. *Fed Regist*. 2014;79(167):51243-51247.

230. American Academy of Sleep Medicine. *International Classification of Sleep Disorders*. 3rd ed. Darien, IL: American Academy of Sleep Medicine; 2014.

231. Bixler EO, Vgontzas AN, Lin HM, et al. Prevalence of sleep-disordered breathing in women: effects of gender. *Am J Respir Crit Care Med*. 2001;163(3 pt 1):608-613.

232. Hall MH, Kline CE, Nowakowski S. Insomnia and sleep apnea in midlife women: prevalence and consequences to health and functioning. *F1000Prime Rep*. 2015;7:63.

233. Lin CM, Davidson TM, Ancoli-Israel S. Gender differences in obstructive sleep apnea and treatment implications. *Sleep Med Rev*. 2008;12(6):481-496.

234. Mirer AG, Young T, Palta M, Benca RM, Rasmuson A, Peppard PE. Sleep-disordered breathing and the menopausal transition among participants in the Sleep in Midlife Women Study. *Menopause*. 2017;24(2):157-162.

235. Young T, Hutton R, Finn L, Badr S, Palta M. The gender bias in sleep apnea diagnosis—are women missed because they have different symptoms? *Arch Intern Med*. 1996;156(21):2445-2451.

236. Guilleminault C, Palombini L, Poyares D, Chowdhuri S. Chronic insomnia, postmenopausal women, and sleep disordered breathing: part 1. Frequency of sleep disordered breathing in a cohort. *J Psychosom Res*. 2002;53(1):611-615.

237. Pillar G, Lavie P. Psychiatric symptoms in sleep apnea syndrome: effects of gender and respiratory disturbance index. *Chest*. 1998;114(3):697-703.

238. Valipour A, Lothaller H, Rauscer H, Zwick H, Burghuber OC, Lavie P. Gender-related differences in symptoms of patients with suspected breathing disorders in sleep: a clinical population study using the sleep disorders questionnaire. *Sleep*. 2007;30(3):312-319.

239. Myers KA, Mrkobrada M, Simel DL. Does this patient have obstructive sleep apnea? The Rational Clinical Examination systematic review. *JAMA*. 2013;310(7):731-741.

240. Kapur VK, Auckley DH, Chowdhuri S, Kuhlmann DC, Mehra R, Ramar K, Harrod CG. Clinical practice guideline for diagnostic testing for adult obstructive sleep apnea: an American Academy of Sleep Medicine clinical practice guideline. *J Clin Sleep Med*. 2017;13(3):479-504.

241. Netzer NC, Stoohs RA, Netzer CM, Clark K, Strohl KP. Using the Berlin Questionnaire to identify patients at risk for sleep apnea syndrome. *Ann Intern Med*. 1999;131(7):485-491.

242. Chung F, Abdullah HR, Liao P. STOP-Bang questionnaire: a practical approach to screen for obstructive sleep apnea. *Chest*. 2016;149(3):631-638.

243. Ghorayeb I, Bioulac B, Scribans C, Tisan F. Perceived severity of restless legs syndrome across the female life cycle. *Sleep Med*. 2008;9(7):799-802.

244. Eichling PS, Sahni J. Menopause related sleep disorders. *J Clin Sleep Med*. 2005;1(3):291-300.

245. Polo-Kantola P, Rauhala E, Erkkola R, Irjala K, Polo O. Estrogen replacement therapy and nocturnal periodic limb movements: a randomized controlled trial. *Obstet Gynecol*. 2001;97(4):548-554.

246. Phillips B. Movement disorders: a sleep specialist's perspective. *Neurology*. 2004;62(suppl 2):S9-S16.

247. Garcia-Borreguero D, Cano-Pumarega I. New concepts in the management of restless legs syndrome. *BMJ*. 2017;356:j104.

248. Bayard M, Bailey B, Acharya D, et al. Bupropion and restless legs syndrome: a randomized controlled trial. *J Am Board Fam Med*. 2011;24(4):422-428.

249. Wesstrom J, Nilsson S, Sundstrom-Poromaa I, Ulfberg J. Restless legs syndrome among women: prevalence, co-morbidity and possible relationship to menopause. *Climacteric*. 2008;11(5):422-428.

250. Baker FC, Joffe H, Lee KA. Sleep and menopause. In: Kryger M, Roth T, Dement WC, eds. *Principles and Practice of Sleep Medicine*. 6th ed. Philadelphia, PA: Elsevier; 2017:1553-1563.

251. Jones LC, Earley CJ, Allen RP, Jones BC. Of mice and men, periodic limb movements and iron: how the human genome informs the mouse genome. *Genes Brain Behav*. 2008;7(5):513-514.

252. International Restless Legs Syndrome Study Group. 2012 Revised IRLSSG diagnostic criteria for RLS. http://irlssg.org/diagnostic-criteria/. Accessed May 21, 2019.

253. Claman DM, Redline S, Blackwell T, et al; Study of Osteoporotic Fractures Research Group. Prevalence and correlates of periodic limb movements in older women. *J Clin Sleep Med*. 2006;2(4):438-445.

254. Aurora RN, Kristo DA, Bista SR, et al; American Academy of Sleep Medicine. The treatment of restless legs syndrome and periodic limb movement disorder in adults—an update for 2012: practice parameters with an evidence-based systematic review and meta-analyses: an American Academy of Sleep Medicine Clinical Practice Guideline. *Sleep*. 2012;35(8):1039-1062.

255. Aurora RN, Kristo DA, Bista SR, et al. Update to the AASM Clinical Practice Guideline: "The treatment of restless legs syndrome and periodic limb movement disorder in adults—an update for 2012: practice parameters with an evidence-based systematic review and meta-analyses." *Sleep*. 2012;35(8):1037.

256. Hainer BL, Matheson EM. Approach to acute headaches in adults. *Am Fam Physician*. 2013;87(10):682-687.

257. Headache Classification Committee of the International Headache Society (IHS). The International Classification of Headache Disorders, 3rd edition. *Cephalalgia*. 2018;38(1):1-211.

258. Loder EW. Headache in the primary care setting. In: Loder EW, Martin VT, eds. Headache: A Guide for the Primary Care Physician. Philadelphia, PA: American College of Physicians; 2004:1-10.

259. Katz M. The cost-effective evaluation of uncomplicated headache. *Med Clin North Am*. 2016;100(5):1009-1017.

260. Stewart WF, Wood C, Reed ML, Roy J, Lipton RB; AMPP Advisory Group. Cumulative lifetime migraine incidence in women and men. *Cephalalgia*. 2008;28(11):1170-1178.

261. Quintela E, Castillo J, Muñoz P, Pascual J. Premonitory and resolution symptoms in migraine: a prospective study in 100 unselected patients. *Cephalalgia*. 2006;26(9):1051-1060.

262. Ravishankar K. The art of history-taking in a headache patient. *Ann Indian Acad Neurol*. 2012;15(suppl 1): S7-S14.

263. Headache Classification Committee of the International Headache Society (IHS). The International Classification of Headache Disorders, 3rd edition (beta version). *Cephalalgia*. 2013;33(9):629-808.

264. Kelman L. The aura: a tertiary care study of 952 migraine patients. *Cephalalgia*. 2004;24(9):728-734.

265. Kelman L. The triggers or precipitants of the acute migraine attack. *Cephalalgia*. 2007;27(5):394-402.

266. Martin VT, Behbehani M. Ovarian hormones and migraine headache: understanding mechanisms and pathogenesis—part 2. *Headache*. 2006;46(3):365-386.

267. Pavlović JM, Stewart WF, Bruce CA, et al. Burden of migraine related to menses: results from the AMPP study. *J Headache Pain*. 2015;16:24.

268. MacGregor EA. Estrogen replacement and migraine. *Maturitas*. 2009;63(1):51-55.

269. MacGregor EA. Migraine headache in perimenopausal and menopausal women. *Curr Pain Headache Rep*. 2009;13(5):399-403.

270. Pavlović JM, Allshouse AA, Santoro NF, et al. Sex hormones in women with and without migraine: evidence of migraine-specific hormone profiles. *Neurology*. 2016;87(1):49-56.

271. Peck KR, Ruland MM, Smitherman TA. Factors associated with medication-overuse headache in patients seeking treatment for primary headache. *Headache*. 2018;58(5):648-660.

272. Charles A. Migraine. *N Eng J Med*. 2017;377(6):553-561.

273. Tepper SJ. Tailoring management strategies for the patient with menstrual migraine: focus on prevention and treatment. *Headache*. 2006;46(suppl 2):S61-S68.

274. D'Onofrio F, Raimo S, Spitaleri D, Casucci G, Bussone G. Usefulness of nutraceuticals in migraine prophylaxis. *Neurol Sci*. 2017; 38(suppl 1):117-120.

275. Young WB. Blocking the greater occipital nerve: utility in headache management. *Curr Pain Headache Rep*. 2010;14(5):404-408.

276. Robbins MS, Lipton RB. Transcutaneous and percutaneous neurostimulation for headache disorders. *Headache*. 2017; 57(suppl 1):4-13.

277. Ong JJY, Wei DY, Goadsby PJ. Recent advances in pharmacotherapy for migraine prevention: from pathophysiology to new drugs. *Drugs*. 2018;78(4):411-437.

278. Avomig [package insert]. Thousand Oaks, CA: Amgen; 2019.

279. Ripa P, Ornello R, Degan D, et al. Migraine in menopausal women: a systematic review. *Int J Womens Health*. 2015;7:773-782.

280. Loder E, Rizzoli P, Golub J. Hormonal management of migraine associated with menses and the menopause: a clinical review. *Headache*. 2007;47(2):329-340.

281. Bousser MG, Welch KM. Relation between migraine and stroke. *Lancet Neurol*. 2005;4(9):533-542.

282. Sheikh HU, Pavlovic J, Loder E, Burch R. Risk of stroke associated with use of estrogen containing contraceptives in women with migraine: a systematic review. *Headache*. 2018;58(1):5-21.

283. Shuster LT, Faubion SS, Sood R, Casey PM. Hormonal manipulation strategies in the management of menstrual migraine and other hormonally related headaches. *Curr Neurol Neurosci Rep*. 2011;11(2):131-138.

284. Kurth T, Kase CS, Schürks M, Tzourio C, Buring JE. Migraine and risk of haemorrhagic stroke in women: prospective cohort study. *BMJ*. 2010;341:c3659.

285. Kurth T, Winter AC, Eliassen AH, et al. Migraine and risk of cardiovascular disease in women: prospective cohort study. *BMJ*. 2016;353:i2610. Erratum in: *BMJ*. 2016;353:i3411.

286. Mancia G, Rosei EA, Ambrosioni E, et al; MIRACLES Study Group. Hypertension and migraine comorbidity: prevalence and risk of cerebrovascular events: evidence from a large, multicenter, cross-sectional survey in Italy (MIRACLES study). *J Hypertens*. 2011;29(2):309-318.

287. Curtis KM, Tepper NK, Jatloui TC, et al. US Medical Eligibility Criteria for Contraceptive Use 2016. *MMWR Recomm Rep*. 2016;65(3):1-103.

288. World Health Organization. *Medical Eligibility Criteria for Contraceptive Use*. 5th ed. 2015. https://apps.who.int/iris/bitstream/handle/10665/181468/9789241549158_eng.pdf?sequence=1. Accessed May 21, 2019.

289. Kurth T, Gaziano JM, Cook NR, Logroscino G, Diener HC, Buring JE. Migraine and risk of cardiovascular disease in women. *JAMA*. 2006;296(3):283-291. Erratum in: JAMA. 2006;296(6):654; *JAMA*. 2006;2396(3):1 p following 291.

290. Calhoun AH. Hormonal contraceptives and migraine with aura—is there still a risk? *Headache*. 2017;57(2):184-193.

291. Stovner LJ, Hagen K, Jensen R, et al. The global burden of headache: a documentation of headache prevalence and disability worldwide. *Cephalalgia*. 2007;27(3):193-210.

292. Chowdhury D. Tension type headache. *Ann Indian Acad Neurol*. 2012;15(suppl 1):S83-S88.

293. Lyngberg AC, Rasmussen BK, Jørgensen T, Jensen R. Has the prevalence of migraine and tension-type headache changed over a 12-year period? A Danish population survey. *Eur J Epidemiol*. 2005;20(3):243-249.

294. Bezov D, Ashina S, Jensen R, Bendtsen L. Pain perception in tension-type headache. *Headache*. 2011;51(2):262-271.

295. Spierings EL, Ranke AH, Honkoop PC. Precipitating and aggravating factors of migraine versus tension-type headache. *Headache*. 2001;41(6):554-558.

296. Karlı N, Baykan B, Ertaş M, et al; Turkish Headache Prevalence Study Group, Onal AE. Impact of sex hormonal changes on tension-type headache and migraine: a cross-sectional population-based survey in 2,600 women. *J Headache Pain*. 2012;13(7):557-565.

297. Pfaffenrath V, Isler H. Evaluation of the nosology of chronic tension-type headache. *Cephalalgia*. 1993;13(suppl 12):60-62.

298. Rasmussen BK, Jensen R, Olesen J. A population-based analysis of the diagnostic criteria of the International Headache Society. *Cephalalgia*. 1991;11(3):129-134.

299. Iversen HK, Langemark M, Andersson PG, Hansen PE, Olesen J. Clinical characteristics of migraine and episodic tension-type headache in relation to old and new diagnostic criteria. *Headache*. 1990;30(8):514-519.

300. Monteith TS, Oshinsky ML. Tension-type headache with medication overuse: pathophysiology and clinical implications. *Curr Pain Headache Rep*. 2009;13(6):463-469.

301. Freitag F. Managing and treating tension-type headache. *Med Clin North Am*. 2013;97(2):281-292.

302. Prakash S, Patel P. Hemicrania continua: clinical review, diagnosis and management. *J Pain Res*. 2017;10:1493-1509.

303. Matharu MS, Cohen AS, Frackowiak RS, Goadsby PJ. Posterior hypothalamic activation in paroxysmal hemicrania. *Ann Neurol*. 2006;59(3):535-545.

304. Hoffmann J, May A. Diagnosis, pathophysiology, and management of cluster headache. *Lancet Neurol*. 2018;17(1):75-83.

305. Cohen AS. Short-acting unilateral neuralgiform headache attacks with conjunctival injection and tearing. *Cephalalgia.* 2007;27(7):824-832.

306. Moloney MF, Strickland OL, DeRossett SE, Melby MK, Dietrich AS. The experiences of midlife women with migraines. *J Nurs Scholarsh.* 2006;38(3):278-285.

307. Fayaz A, Croft P, Langford RM, Donaldson LJ, Jones GT. Prevalence of chronic pain in the UK: a systematic review and meta-analysis of population studies. *BMJ Open.* 2016;6(6):e010364.

308. Wijnhoven HA, de Vet HC, Picavet HS. Explaining sex differences in chronic musculoskeletal pain in a general population. *Pain.* 2006;124(1-2):158-166.

309. Magliano M. Menopausal arthralgia: fact or fiction. *Maturitas.* 2010;67(1):29-33.

310. Obermeyer CM, Reher D, Alcala LC, Price K. The menopause in Spain: results of the DAMES (Decisions At MEnopause) study. *Maturitas.* 2005;52(3-4):190-198.

311. Prieto-Alhambra D, Judge A, Javaid MK, Cooper C, Diez-Perez A, Arden NK. Incidence and risk factors for clinically diagnosed knee, hip and hand osteoarthrit is: influences of age, gender and osteoarthritis affecting other joints. *Ann Rheum Dis.* 2014;73(9):1659-1664.

312. Szoeke CE, Cicuttini FM, Guthrie JR, Dennerstein L. The relationship of reports of aches and joint pains to the menopausal transition: a longitudinal study. *Climacteric.* 2008;11(1):55-62.

313. Lintermans A, Neven P. Pharmacology of arthralgia with estrogen deprivation. *Steroids.* 2011;76(8):781-785.

314. Coleman RE, Bolten WW, Lansdown M, et al. Aromatase inhibitor-induced arthralgia: clinical experience and treatment recommendations. *Cancer Treat Rev.* 2008;34(3):275-282.

315. Hershman DL, Unger JM, Crew KD, et al. Randomized multicenter placebo-controlled trial of omega-3 fatty acids for the control of aromatase inhibitor-induced musculoskeletal pain: SWOG S0927. *J Clin Oncol.* 2015;33(17):1910-1917.

316. Chim H, Tan BH, Ang CC, Chew EM, Chong YS, Saw SM. The prevalence of menopausal symptoms in a community in Singapore. *Maturitas.* 2002;41(4):275-282.

317. Olaolorun FM, Lawoyin TO. Experience of menopausal symptoms by women in an urban community in Ibadan, Nigeria. *Menopause.* 2009;16(4):822-830.

318. Syed Alwi SA, Lee PY, Awi I, Mallik PS, Md Haizal MN. The menopausal experience among indigenous women of Sarawak, Malaysia. *Climacteric.* 2009;12(6):548-556.

319. Aparicio VA, Borges-Cosic M, Ruiz-Cabello P, et al. Association of objectively measured physical activity and physical fitness with menopause symptoms. The Flamenco Project. *Climacteric.* 2017;20(5):456-461.

320. Xi S, Mao L, Chen X, Bai W. Effect of health education combining diet and exercise supervision in Chinese women with perimenopausal symptoms: a randomized controlled trial. *Climacteric.* 2017;20(2):151-156.

321. Gartoulla P, Davis SR, Worsley R, Bell RJ. Use of complementary and alternative medicines for menopausal symptoms in Australian women aged 40-65 years. *Med J Aust.* 2015;203(3):146e1-146e6.

322. Vitiello MV, Rybarczyk B, Von Korff M, Stepanski EJ. Cognitive behavioral therapy for insomnia improves sleep and decreases pain in older adults with co-morbid insomnia and osteoarthritis. *J Clin Sleep Med.* 2009;5(4):355-362.

323. Rahman A, Underwood M, Carnes D. Fibromyalgia. *BMJ.* 2014; 348:g1224.

324. Chlebowski RT, Cirillo DJ, Eaton CB, et al. Estrogen alone and joint symptoms in the Women's Health Initiative randomized trial. *Menopause.* 2013;20(6):600-608.

325. Barnabei VM, Cochrane BB, Aragaki AK, et al; Women's Health Initiative Investigators. Menopausal symptoms and treatment-related effects of estrogen and progestin in the Women's Health Initiative. *Obstet Gynecol.* 2005;105(5 pt 1):1063-1073.

326. Welton AJ, Vickers MR, Kim J, et al; WISDOM team. Health related quality of life after combined hormone replacement therapy: randomised controlled trial. *BMJ.* 2008;337:a1190.

327. Ablin J, Neumann L, Buskila D. Pathogenesis of fibromyalgia—a review. *Joint Bone Spine.* 2008;75(3):273-279.

328. Vincent A, Whipple MO, McAllister SJ, Aleman KM, St Sauver JL. A cross-sectional assessment of the prevalence of multiple chronic conditions and medication use in a sample of community-dwelling adults with fibromyalgia in Olmsted County, Minnesota. *BMJ Open.* 2015;5(3):e006681.

329. Busch AJ, Barber KA, Overend TJ, Peloso PM, Schachter CL. Exercise for treating fibromyalgia syndrome. *Cochrane Database Syst Rev.* 2007;(4):CD003786.

330. Institute of Medicine. *Clinical Preventive Services for Women: Closing the Gaps.* Washington, DC: National Academy of Sciences; 2011.

331. ACOG Committee Opinion No 518: intimate partner violence. *Obstet Gynecol.* 2012;119(2 pt 1):412-417.

332. World Health Organization. *Violence Against Women.* Updated November 29, 2017. www.who.int/en/news-room/fact-sheets/detail/violence-against-women. Accessed May 21, 2019.

333. Moraes SD, da Fonseca AM, Soares JM Jr, et al. Construction and validation of an instrument that breaks the silence: the impact of domestic and/or sexual violence on women's health, as shown during climacterium. *Menopause.* 2012;19(1):16-22.

334. Bonomi AE, Anderson ML, Reid RJ, et al. Intimate partner violence in older women. *Gerontologist.* 2007;47(1):34-41.

335. Alpert E; Massachusetts Medical Society Committee on Violence Intervention and Prevention. *Intimate Partner Violence: The Clinicians Guide to Identification, Assessment, Intervention, and Prevention.* 6th ed. Waltham, MA: Massachusetts Medical Society; 2015.

336. Smith SG, Chen J, Basile KC, et al. *The National Intimate Partner and Sexual Violence Survey (NISVS): 2010-2012 State Report.* Atlanta, GA: National Center for Injury Prevention and Control, Centers for Disease Control and Prevention; 2017.

337. Mair C, Cunradi CB, Todd M. Adverse childhood experiences and intimate partner violence: testing psychosocial mediational pathways among couples. *Ann Epidemiol.* 2012;22(12):832-839.

338. Thurston RC, Bromberger J, Chang Y, et al. Childhood abuse or neglect is associated with increased vasomotor symptom reporting among midlife women. *Menopause.* 2008;15(1):16-22.

339. Vegunta S, Kuhle C, Kling, JM, et al. The association between recent abuse and menopausal symptom bother: results from the Data Registry on Experiences in Aging, Menopause, and Sexuality (DREAMS). *Menopause.* 2016;23(5):494-498.

340. Tetterton S, Farnsworth E. Older women and intimate partner violence: effective interventions. *J Interpers Violence.* 2011;26(14):2929-2942.

341. McCauley J, Kern DE, Kolodner K, et al. The "battering syndrome": prevalence and clinical characteristics of domestic violence in primary care internal medicine practices. *Ann Intern Med.* 1995;123(10):737-746.

342. Walton-Moss BJ, Manganello J, Frye V, Campbell JC. Risk factors for intimate partner violence and associated injury among urban women. *J Community Health.* 2005;30(5):377-389.

343. Centers for Disease Control. Injury Prevention & Control: Division of Violence Prevention. *Veto Violence: The Social-Ecological Model.* https://vetoviolence.cdc.gov/violence-prevention-basics-social-ecological-model. Accessed May 21, 2019.

344. Dahlberg LL, Krug EG. Violence—a global public health problem. In: Krug E, Dahlberg LL, Mercy JA, Zwi AB, Lozano R, eds. *World Report on Violence and Health.* Geneva, Switzerland: World Health Organization; 2002:1-56.

345. Ard KL, Makadon HJ. Addressing intimate partner violence in lesbian, gay, bisexual, and transgender patients. *J Gen Intern Med.* 2011;26(8):930-933.

346. Calton JM, Cattaneo LB, Gebhard KT. Barriers to help seeking for lesbian, gay, transgender, and queer survivors of intimate partner violence. *Trauma Violence Abuse.* 2016;17(5):585-600.

347. Grant JM, Mottet LA, Tanis J, Harrison J, Herman JL, Keisling M. *Injustice at Every Turn: A Report of the National Transgender Discrimination Survey.* Washington, DC: National Center for Transgender Equality and National Gay and Lesbian Task Force; 2011.

348. Committee Opinion No. 568: elder abuse and women's health. *Obstet Gynecol.* 2013;122(1):187-191.

349. Acierno R, Hernandez MA, Amstadter AB, et al. Prevalence and correlates of emotional, physical, sexual, and financial abuse and potential neglect in the United States: the National Elder Mistreatment Study. *Am J Public Health.* 2010;100(2):292-297.

350. Feder G, Wathen CN, MacMillian HL. An evidence-based response to intimate partner violence: WHO guidelines. *JAMA.* 2013;310(5):479-480.

351. Nelson HD, Bougatsos C, Blazina I. Screening women for intimate partner violence: a systematic review to update the US Preventive Services Task Force Recommendations. *Ann Intern Med.* 2012;156(11):796-808.

352. Moyer VA; US Preventive Services Task Force. Screening for intimate partner violence and abuse in elderly and vulnerable adults: US Preventive Services Task Force recommendation statement. *Ann Intern Med.* 2013;158(6): 478-486.

353. Ambuel B, Hamberger LK, Guse CE, Melzer-Lange M, Phelan MB, Kistner A. Healthcare can change from within: sustained improvement in the health care response to intimate partner violence. *J Fam Violence.* 2013;28(8):833-847.

354. Hamberger LK, Rhodes K, Brown J. Screening and intervention for intimate partner violence in healthcare settings: creating sustainable system-level programs. *J Womens Health* (Larchmt). 2015;24(1):86-91.

355. Miller E, McCaw B, Humphreys BL, Mitchell C. Integrating intimate partner violence assessment and intervention into healthcare in the United States: a systems approach. *J Womens Health (Larchmt).* 2015;24(1):92-99.

356. Kaiser Permanente Institute for Health Policy. *Kaiser Permanente Policy Story, v1, no. 10: Transforming the Health Care Response to Domestic Violence.* 2012. https://residency-scal-kaiserpermanente. org/healthpolicyelective/wp-content/uploads/sites/8/2016/02/ KP-Story-1.10-DomesticViolenceUPDATED-1-21-15.pdf. Accessed May 9, 2019.

6

Diseases Common in Midlife Women

Arthritis

Musculoskeletal disorders, including arthritis, are among the most common reason for years lived with disability in the Western world.[1] There are many causes of arthritis, but all present with joint-based pain and differing amounts of swelling and restriction of movement of joints, usually associated with some loss of function or impaired quality of life (QOL). Arthritis is generally more common with increasing age and also more common in women. It is therefore not unusual to see and manage patients with arthritis at the time of menopause. In some situations, there may be predictive variables (age, sex), meaning that symptoms of both arthritis and menopause occur together by chance.

For some forms of arthritis, there may be an interaction between menopause and either the incidence or severity of the arthritis.[2] It is particularly important to identify and refer women with inflammatory arthritis such as rheumatoid arthritis (RA), given that this form of arthritis can be rapidly progressive and associated with other morbidity and early irreversible joint damage and given that there are a wide range of established drug treatments that can slow or stop the disease and associated damage. Inflammatory spinal pain can be insidious, and it is important to differentiate it from more common mechanical back pain.

Etiology

Cartilage

Estrogen is synthesized by aromatase in connective tissues. Estrogen receptors are present in all joint tissues, including articular cartilage, subchondral bone, and synovium.[3]

Low levels of estrogen appear to promote cartilage growth or prevent its degradation.[4,5] After ovariectomy, resistance to articular cartilage compressibility is reduced but appears to be reversed by estrogen replacement.[6] Increased articular cartilage has been found on knee magnetic resonance imaging (MRI) in those taking hormone therapy (HT).[7] Studies in animal models of arthritis suggest that estrogen and selective estrogen receptor modulators (SERMs) may be protective[3,8]; however, there are far less data on the effects of HT in humans, and it must be emphasized that there is no current indication for the use of HT to treat any form of arthritis per se.

Bone

The effects of estrogen on bone turnover are well known from treatment of osteoporosis, although other forms of treatment have tended to supersede HT. Bone-targeting agents would appear beneficial in some forms of arthritis as well.[9] In a cross-sectional study, women receiving estrogen therapy (ET) had less osteoarthritis (OA)-related bony changes on knee magnetic resonance imaging (MRI) than those who were not.[10] In monkeys, estrogen replacement after ovariectomy appeared to limit the new bone formation seen in OA.[11]

Inflammation

Estrogen is known to be anti-inflammatory and mildly immunosuppressive. Its role as a steroid hormone of pregnancy requires this. Women with RA routinely note improvement or even remission during pregnancy, and much of this effect is attributed to the anti-inflammatory properties of estrogen. Joint damage in arthritis is driven by activation of inflammatory-signaling pathways inducing proteinases.[12] Hormone therapy and SERMs such as levormeloxifene and raloxifene have been reported to reduce levels of two markers of subsequent matrix degradation: cartilage oligomeric matrix protein and crosslinked C-telopeptides of type II collagen.[9,13,14]

Pain

Estrogen receptors and aromatase are present in dorsal root ganglion, hypothalamus, limbic system, neuron, and joint. Estrogen therapy has been shown to decrease synovial nerve fiber neurotrophins in an animal model of OA.[15] Estrogen and testosterone reduce pain, activating inhibitory pain pathways in the spinal cord, whereas progestins have been reported to promote pain.[16,17] During a normal menstrual cycle, drops in estrogen were associated with increased pain-reporting using objective measures of pain induction, whereas high estrogen/low progesterone was associated with activation of the endogenous opioid system and less pain.[17,18] Those with low testosterone states are more prone to pain.[17] Entering menopause may for some be like constantly being in the low estrogen part of the cycle, heightening the pain experience for any given pathology. Fatigue, poor sleep, and mood change occurring in menopause are also well known to enhance pain perception.

History and examination

A careful history and examination can support the diagnosis of the type of arthritis. Pattern recognition is important, as well as an awareness of the relative frequency of diseases. The considerations are the same as when approaching someone with arthralgia, noting the site, symmetry, and presence and severity of swelling. (See also "Arthralgia" in Chapter 5.) The presence and duration of early morning stiffness (or inactivity stiffness) should be noted: prolonged stiffness (>30 min) is suggestive of inflammatory arthritis, as is symmetrical swelling that is maximal at the metacarpophalangeal joints (Table 1; Figure 1A). If inflammatory arthritis such as RA is suspected, the patient should be referred to a rheumatologist (ideally to an early arthritis clinic) without delay (Table 2).[19] A variety of investigations such as blood tests, imaging, and ultrasound are often helpful in confirming the diagnosis if arthritis is suspected but should be arranged in a personalized way to avoid unnecessary testing (Table 3).

Common forms of arthritis occurring in perimenopause

Osteoarthritis

Osteoarthritis is the most common form of arthritis; the lifetime risk for women who are obese is 60%.[20] It is a whole-organ disease (affecting articular cartilage, bone, synovium, ligament).[12] It leads in many to progressive loss of cartilage and change in bone (leading to classical osteophytes on X-ray; Figure 1B), with associated pain and loss of function. There is usually evidence of joint swelling and tenderness. Osteoarthritis ultimately leads to joint failure for many and is the most common reason for total joint replacement, an increasingly unsustainable

Table 1. Three Simple Questions for the General Clinician Diagnosing Arthritis

	RA[a]	OA	Gout/Pseudogout[b]
1. Does the patient have joint-based pain?	Y	Y	Y
Single or multiple?	Multiple	Either	Typically single or few
Symmetrical?	Y	Y/N	N
Episodic or progressive?	Progressive[a]	Either	Episodic[b]
With activity?	Variable	Y	Sometimes
2 Is there early morning stiffness >30 min?	Y	N	Y (flares)
3. Can I see joint swelling?	Y	Y	Y
Are the joints red?	N	N	Y (flares)
Are the joints tender?	Y	Y/N	Y (flares)
Is there MCP joint swelling?	Usually	Ocasionally	Occasionally

Abbreviations: MCP, metacarpophalangeal; OA, osteoarthritis; RA, rheumatoid arthritis.
[a]Early, established disease (rarely palindromic RA can occur with episodes of flare and remission).
[b]Based on new presentation of gout. Established, tophaceous gout can give persistent pain and progressive arthritis.

financial burden (500,000 hip replacements alone are predicted for OA in the United States by 2030).[21,22] However, it is also increasingly understood that in early disease, symptoms may stabilize or improve. The disease can have many courses, with marked variation in symptoms between persons with any given structural change.[23]

Etiopathogenesis. We now know that OA is driven by excessive degradation, often in the context of inadequate or abnormal repair in a variety of connective tissues. Although the initiating factor for this process is not clear, it has been found to be an active, cellular-driven process that is guided in part by mechanical factors.[24] In animal models of OA, knock-out of critical pathways such as proteinases has been found to protect from the disease[25]; ovariectomy removes the relative protection to the disease seen in female mice, implicating a role for sex hormones. These observations are important because they suggest that OA is not simply a disease of "wear and tear" or is inevitable and that the disease process should be modifiable.

Risk factors. Important risk factors for OA include obesity, female sex, congenital joint abnormality or deformity, joint injuries, occupational factors associated with joint overuse, and family history.[12] A large number of genes exert generally low risk; approximately 50% of disease risk is estimated to be genetic.[26,27]

Clinical features. The most commonly affected sites are the knee, hip, and hand. Pain in the affected joint can be intermittent or constant, typically with use, and some swelling is not unusual. In the hand, the distal interphalangeal and proximal interphalangeal joints are most commonly affected, followed by the base of the thumb (Figure 1B). There may be apparent bony swelling (nodes) of the interphalangeal joints, which if present is highly suggestive of OA. Blood tests are typically normal, although there may be a modestly elevated C-reactive protein (CRP; Table 3). Diagnostic changes are detectable by X-ray in established disease but may be absent in early disease.

There is a female preponderance at all sites.[28] Onset of hand OA has long been noted to occur around the time of menopause.[29] Hand OA appears different from other forms of OA in its having an upsurge in incidence in women aged around 50 years; approximately 90% of patients in secondary-care clinics with erosive (more severe) hand OA are women.[30] In such cases in

Figure 1. Different Types of Arthritis

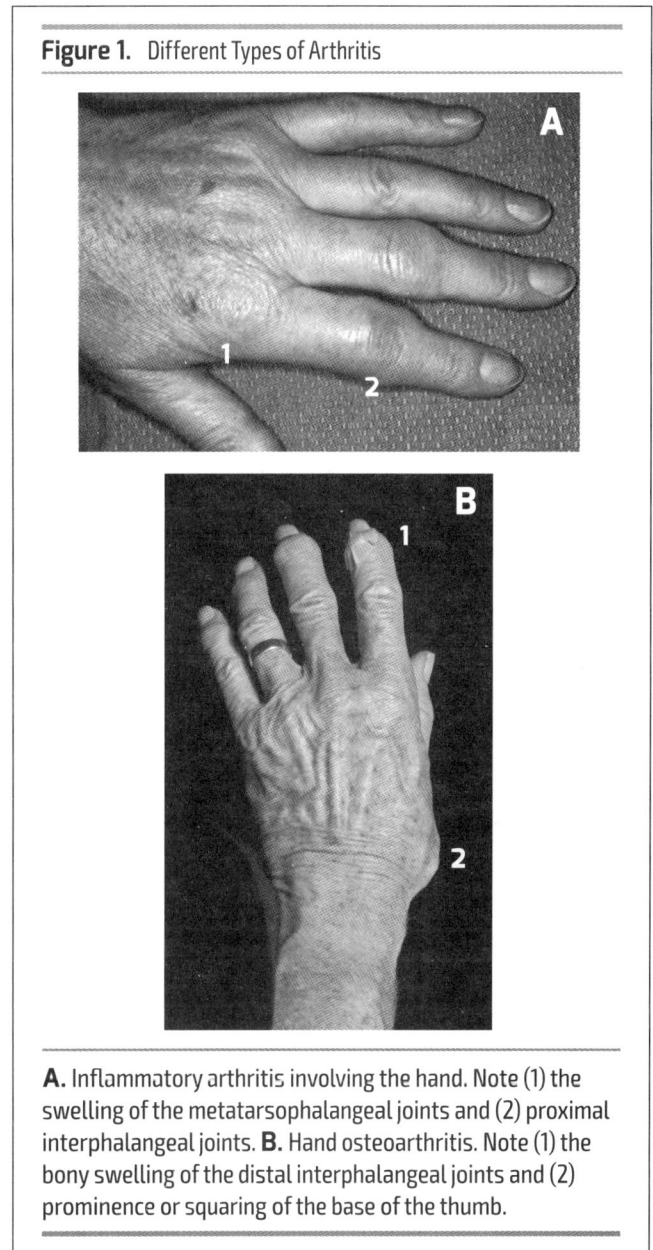

A. Inflammatory arthritis involving the hand. Note (1) the swelling of the metatarsophalangeal joints and (2) proximal interphalangeal joints. **B.** Hand osteoarthritis. Note (1) the bony swelling of the distal interphalangeal joints and (2) prominence or squaring of the base of the thumb.

perimenopause, symptoms may resolve over 2 to 5 years; however, there is no proven causal link between estrogen deficiency and OA.[2]

Management. A clear diagnosis of OA should be made and shared with the patient, avoiding alternative and confusing terminology (such as "degeneration" or "wear and tear"). Management should be focused on the woman and should include an assessment of the effect of OA on her work, leisure activities, function, and QOL. Women should be educated about their disease and given constructive messages early in the disease, including its

Table 2. Features That Suggest Rheumatoid Arthritis in Recent-Onset Inflammatory Arthritis

- Symptoms persisting more than 2 wk
- Swollen joints, especially in hands (wrists, metatarsophalangeal joints, proximal interphalangeal joints)
- Tenderness across the metatarsophalangeal joints
- Positive rheumatoid factor
- Positive anticitrullinated protein antibodies
- Elevated inflammatory markers (erythrocyte sedimentation rate, C-reactive protein)
- Number of swollen joints
- Symmetrical pattern (can start asymmetrically)
- Absence of an alternative diagnosis such as erosive osteoarthritis, crystal arthritis

Patients with these features should be referred immediately for review by a rheumatologist in an early arthritis clinic.
Burmester GR, et al.[19]

natural history and possibility of improvement with or without intervention.[31,32] All women with OA should be encouraged to remain working and to exercise.[33]

Management of OA falls into four broad areas: supportive/lifestyle measures (encouraging weight control or loss and general exercise), nonpharmacologic measures (eg, joint-specific exercises or devices that mechanically offload joints), pharmacologic measures, and ultimately, evidence-based surgical interventions, such as joint replacement (Figure 2).[33,34] There is no evidence that simple washout of the joint is helpful for those with OA, and this should be avoided. These measures are complementary and can be used in combination or in a step-wise fashion.

Nonpharmacologic measures are usually joint specific (eg, range of motion exercises and base-of-thumb splinting for hand OA or knee braces and arch supports for those with some forms of knee OA).[33] Not all those with OA will need regular oral analgesia. For those who do, acetaminophen and topical nonsteroidal anti-inflammatory drugs (NSAIDs; applied as gel or cream) are first-line treatments. Both have been shown to be effective for the treatment of the pain of OA and have preferable adverse event (AE) profiles compared with oral NSAIDs.

Stronger analgesia such as opiates or oral NSAIDs may be indicated but should be used with caution given the risks associated with these drugs; intra-articular steroid injections are often helpful in managing symptoms and flares.[34] The current incomplete understanding of this disease means that, unlike in RA, disease-modifying drugs

do not yet exist for OA. There is at present no definite evidence for the use of HT in this setting. Newer agents that improve pain control or may modify the disease, targeting relevant biologic pathways, are currently in clinical trials.[35]

Rheumatoid arthritis

Rheumatoid arthritis is a classical form of inflammatory arthritis. It is three times more common in women than men; peak age of onset is between 35 and 55 years; and it commonly affects perimenopausal and postmenopausal women.[36,37]

Etiopathogenesis. Far more is now known about important etiologic risk factors for RA than was known before. Genetic factors include the possession of the shared epitope HLA-DRB1 disease risk-associated alleles.[36] Antibodies to citrullinated (modified) proteins are strongly associated with disease development and progression: they have been shown to predate the disease by many years and are associated with actions of bacteria associated with periodontal disease.[38] Cigarette smoking interacts with both genetic factors and autoantibodies to potentiate disease.[39]

Rheumatoid arthritis often goes into remission during pregnancy, but despite this and the sex association, a causal relationship for hormones has not yet been defined (HT may reduce cyclic citrullinated peptide [CPP] antibodies in the presence of the shared epitope HLA-DRB1).[40] Synovial inflammation leads to pannus formation, a destructive, dysregulate tissue within the joint in which infiltrating immune cells (lymphocytes and macrophages) release proteinases and proinflammatory cytokines such as tumor necrosis factor (TNF)-α, leading to loss of articular cartilage and bony erosion.[41] If not stopped, this leads to progressive, irreversible joint damage, with ensuing functional impairment and disability.

Clinical features. Rheumatoid arthritis typically affects multiple peripheral joints in a symmetric pattern and progressive manner, with associated signs of inflammation: pain, swelling, warmth, loss of function, and sometimes redness (although marked erythema over joints is more typical in gout or septic arthritis). Prolonged morning stiffness is typically present in active disease, along with some systemic symptoms (fatigue, malaise, sweats/fever).[42] This systemic disease can involve other organs (lungs, pericardium, eyes, skin, nerves). Laboratory studies usually reveal elevated acute-phase proteins (erythrocyte sedimentation; CRP); rheumatoid factor is commonly found in women with RA but also may be present in other rheumatic and

Figure 2. Treatments for Osteoarthritis in Adults

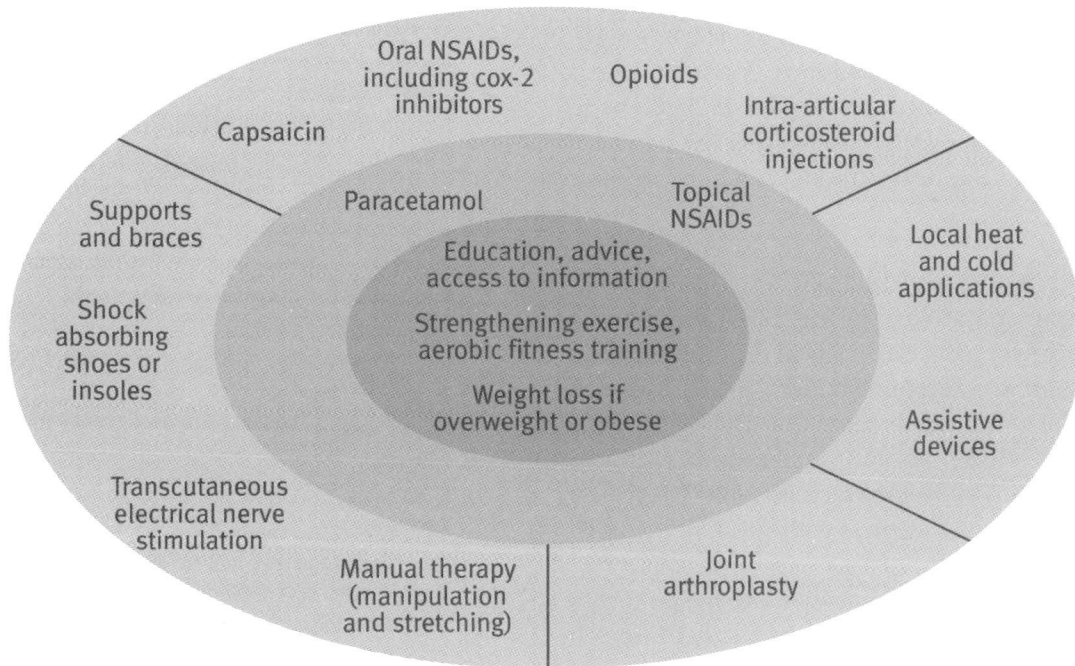

Starting at the center and working outward, the treatments are arranged in the order in which they should be considered, taking into account individual persons' different needs, risk factors, and preferences. The core treatments (center) should be considered first for every person with osteoarthritis. If further treatment is required, consider the drugs in the second circle before the drugs in the outer circle. The outer circle also shows adjunctive treatments (both nonpharmacologic and surgical), which have less well-proven efficacy, provide less symptom relief, or are of increased risk to the patient compared with those in the second circle. Abbreviation: NSAIDs, nonsteroidal anti-inflammatory drugs. Conaghan PG, et al.[33] Reproduced with permission from BMJ Publishing Group Ltd. Copyright 2008 *BMJ*.

nonrheumatic conditions and with age.[36] Antibodies to CPP when present are more specific; the possession of either antibody is associated with increased risk of erosion and joint damage, which treatment seek to prevent; this association is more marked in smokers and those with the shared epitope.[43]

Ultrasound and other imaging modalities (Table 3) are used in the assessment and monitoring of RA.[44] There may be sex differences associated with cardiovascular disease (CVD) risk, which is higher in those with RA and other inflammatory joint diseases.[45]

Management. The treatment of RA has been transformed in the last 20 years by the new biologics era. Early diagnosis (ahead of damage) is vital, with rapid, early disease modification, which is stepped up until disease remission is achieved.[19,36,46]

The mainstay of treatment is disease-modifying antirheumatic drugs such as methotrexate, often used in combination with other drugs that double the chance of achieving disease remission (eg, hydroxychloroquine or sulphasalazine), with blood-test monitoring. Modern biologic agents are typically antibodies or other large complex proteins that effectively block pathogenic targets—the main target being TNF-α as well as inhibitors of interleukin-6 and -1 and of other aspects of the immune response (such as T-cell costimulation or B cells).[46] As a result of biologic treatments, the mainstay still being anti-TNF therapy, and newer targeted disease-modifying antirheumatic drugs such as janus kinase inhibitors, it is now rare to see the previously common advanced joint deformities or women requiring joint replacement.[19] However, these treatments are controls rather than cures; patients are on drug treatment for life. Novel methods of inducing tolerance are being sought to effect a much-needed cure and to be able to predict response to the increasing numbers of treatments available.

There was no statistically significant effect in incidence or severity of RA in those taking HT in the Women's Health Initiative (WHI).[47] In small randomized, controlled trials (RCTs), it appears safe to use HT in women with RA, checking usual exclusions. Vascular risk is increased in those with RA, so this should be borne in mind when prescribing.[40] Hormone therapy has been reported to mitigate against bone loss and improve some symptoms.[48]

Seronegative spondyloarthritis

Inflammatory spondyloarthropathies present with inflammatory back pain, classically in the mid and lower spine (around the thoracolumbar junction), with or without peripheral joint involvement.[49] Restriction of spinal movements and flattening of the lumbar spine, with tenderness and sensitivity over the sacroiliac joints, is typical. A history of prolonged stiffness with inactivity is often suggestive.

Spondyloarthritis is often insidious in onset; it may be misdiagnosed for many years, particularly in women, and misattributed to mechanical back pain. It may be associated with iritis, inflammatory bowel disease, tendinopathies, and peripheral enthesitis, which is the site of pathology in the disease (the insertion of tendon to bone). Magnetic resonance imaging of the spine and sacroiliac joints is now used routinely in the diagnosis of inflammatory spinal disease, which alongside X-ray change when present aids in diagnosis by clinical criteria.[50] Nonsteroidal anti-inflammatory drugs and physiotherapy treatments are used as first-line treatments. However, as in RA, biologic treatments such as those blocking TNF and other pathogenic cytokines such as interleukin-17 are transforming the treatment of this disease.

Psoriatic arthritis is a related condition that can present with peripheral arthritis.[51] The pathogenesis is different from RA, although the inflammation and damage seen can be similar; biologics such as TNF antagonists are used as treatment in this disease.

One caveat is that there are no proven blood biomarkers for these diseases. The acute-phase response may be entirely normal in spondyloarthritis and psoriatic arthritis, and antibody testing is typically negative. If an inflammatory arthritis is suspected, the woman should be referred for further assessment by a rheumatologist.

Crystal arthropathies

The crystal-deposition diseases represent a category of inflammatory arthritis whereby crystals precipitate in the

---

Table 3. Investigation of New-Onset Arthritis

1. Blood tests for RA (no blood test for OA)
   a. Complete blood count: Anemia, leukocytosis, thrombocytosis.
   b. Acute phase reactants: ESR, CRP.
   c. Autoantibodies: Rheumatoid factor, anti-CCP antibodies (approximately 30% with RA are negative).
2. Other useful blood tests
   a. Vitamin D; thyroid function; PTH/calcium profile.
   b. Hepatitis B/C (if there are risk factors).
   c. Antinuclear antibodies (rare causes, such as connective tissue disease—in presence of rash, sicca, oral ulcers, etc).
   d. If red flags—investigate for malignancy and refer.
3. Imaging
   a. Not always necessary.
   b. X-rays.
      i. Hands and feet: look for joint space narrowing, periarticular osteopenia, or bone erosions (RA).
      ii. Affected joint: may see joint space narrowing, bone cysts, subchondral sclerosis, bone erosions, osteophytes (OA).
   c. Ultrasound
      i. May be helpful if X-rays are normal or in early disease.
      ii. Detects inflammatory arthritis, including synovitis and erosion.
      iii. Can exclude soft tissue causes of pain (eg, tendinopathies).

Abbreviations: CPP, cyclic citrullinated peptide; CRP, C-reactive protein; ESR, erythrocyte sedimentation rate; OA, osteoarthritis; PTH, parathyroid hormone; RA, rheumatoid arthritis.

---

joint, inducing an acute immune response that results in joint swelling and acute pain. Fever and joint redness may accompany these attacks, which can easily be confused with a septic arthritis if occurring for the first time. The two common forms of this disease, *gout* and *pseudogout*, can be seen in aging women, particularly when other risk factors are present.

Gout

Gout is caused by excessively high serum uric acid levels and by the subsequent precipitation of monosodium urate crystals in the joints and other tissues.[52] This may occur spontaneously or be triggered by any changes in health status, such as minor trauma or acute infections, or by alcohol ingestion.

Clinical features. Although gout is predominant in men during early life, it has significant increase in prevalence in postmenopausal women, particularly when associated with hypertension, diuretic use, and kidney disease, as well as with the metabolic syndrome and obesity.[52] A history of high ethanol intake or family history should be sought. Dose alterations of medications that influence serum uric acid levels, such as diuretics (particularly thiazides) and aspirin, can trigger gouty attacks. In addition to classical signs of inflammatory arthritis, evidence of soft-tissue tophi, masses caused by deposition of crystals in tissues other than the joints (eg, over the helix of the ear or in the olecranon bursa of the elbow), can be highly suggestive.

The diagnosis of acute gout is confirmed by detecting monosodium urate crystals in synovial fluid obtained from an involved joint, typically using polarizing microscopy.[52] An elevated serum urate (hyperuricemia) can be suggestive but is not diagnostic because it can exist without gout. Uric acid levels also drop in gouty flare, so can in theory be normal. An X-ray may show para-articular erosions suggestive of tophi.

Classically, acute gout involves the base of the great toe or another single joint (monoarthritis), but any joint can be involved, and multiple joints can be affected simultaneously (midfoot, ankle, knee, or hand are other common sites). These episodes are characterized by abrupt onset of extreme joint pain, redness, and swelling of the involved joints that lasts at most 5 to 7 days before resolving.

Management. Acute attacks may be aborted if treated early with oral colchicine or with high doses of NSAIDs, if tolerated and prescription is not contraindicated (a proton pump inhibitor should be coprescribed for gastroprotection, particularly if used at high doses). After an attack is fully established, treatment with NSAIDs is effective, although many patients with gout cannot tolerate this class of medication because of renal, cardiac, or gastrointestinal problems. In those patients, either intra-articular or systemic corticosteroid treatment such as oral prednisolone is effective. Inflammasome/interleukin-1 inhibitors can in theory also be used, although are not licensed for routine use.[53]

Chronic gout (frequent disabling attacks with or without tophi) should be treated with long-term medication that lowers the serum uric acid level to below 6 mg/dL (360 μmol/L); these include uricosurics such as allopurinol and febuxistat and pharmaceutical uricase, the enzyme that degrades uric acid.[54,55] With normalization of serum uric acid concentrations, tophi will gradually resorb over time.

Pseudogout

Calcium pyrophosphate dihydrate deposition is a common feature of aging or osteoarthritic joints and may be detected radiographically as chondrocalcinosis. Occasionally, these crystals trigger an inflammatory response similar to that seen in gout and may cause a syndrome that is clinically indistinguishable from true gout, pseudogout.

Clinical features. Pseudogout occurs most commonly in middle-aged and elderly patients with evidence of OA in the affected joints. Like gout, it may occur spontaneously or be triggered by trauma, surgery, or changes in systemic medical conditions. Unlike gout, it most commonly involves the large joints such as the knees and wrists, and acute episodes last longer, sometimes up to 20 days, before resolution. Any joint may be affected by acute pseudogout. The diagnosis can only be made definitively by detecting calcium pyrophosphate dihydrate crystals by microscopy.[56]

Management. Acute pseudogout attacks are managed in a manner similar to gout. High-dose NSAIDs are effective, if tolerated. In cases for which NSAIDs are not practical, intra-articular or systemic corticosteroids are effective. Unlike gout, there are not yet effective strategies that result in crystal resorption. For patients with frequent attacks, prophylactic use of colchicine or long-term NSAIDs, if deemed appropriate and safe for the patient, can be tried.

Joint pain in menopause

Musculoskeletal pain is more common in women and increases during and after perimenopause. It should be borne in mind that not all musculoskeletal pain is arthralgia, and not all joint pain is arthritis. Those in perimenopause have increased risk for OA (particularly hand) and RA. Definitive evidence for HT for prevention or treatment of either form of arthritis is lacking. There is some limited evidence that HT may help musculoskeletal symptoms or OA at a population level, but sufficient evidence is lacking to routinely recommend it on an individual basis. Those with symptoms and signs suggesting inflammatory arthritis, including RA, should be referred urgently to an early arthritis clinic for further assessment. If arthralgia or arthritis is seen to occur at the time of menopause with other related symptoms, it is reasonable to treat possible reversible causes and other systemic menopause symptoms and try to record as objectively as possible the response of musculoskeletal symptoms to these treatments.

Depression

The idea that women could be exposed to hormone-related mood symptoms or to *windows of vulnerability* for reproductive-related depression is not a new concept. For the past several decades, accumulated evidence ranging from epidemiologic studies to animal data and clinical observations have corroborated the concept that some (but not all) women are particularly sensitive to changes in the hormone milieu,[57,58] particularly those experienced premenstrually, during the postpartum period, or during the menopause transition.[59-61] In fact, a heightened vulnerability to hormone changes has been postulated to explain, at least in part, the fact that women are twice as likely to suffer from depression during the reproductive years compared with men, whereas this difference seems to be attenuated outside the reproductive lifespan.

The concept of a menopause-associated depression, however, has been more controversial and intensely debated. It is undeniable that the transition from reproductive years into the postmenopause period involves changes in sex hormones and metabolism; it is also well known that some women experience changes in lifestyle behaviors, sexuality, and other aspects of their health that ultimately have a compounded effect on functioning and QOL.[62]

As in any other stage in life, depression during the midlife years may be expressed or experienced in many different ways. Many factors should be taken into consideration, including cardiovascular (CV) and metabolic risk factors, the presence and severity of vasomotor symptoms (VMS) and sleep changes,[63] ethnicity, lifestyle behaviors (eg, exercise levels, smoking),[64] and stressful life events.[65]

Adding to the complexity of these cases, the characterization of psychological symptoms has not been consistent across studies; in some, clear distinctions between distress or burnout, depressive symptoms, or clinical depression were lacking. Similarly, menopause staging has not been consistently or accurately characterized across multiple studies; some have omitted key information on menstrual patterns, hormone profiles, or other reproductive-related changes and therefore limited the applicability of findings to specific groups or subgroups of midlife women.[66]

Depressive symptoms and clinical depression

Numerous cross-sectional studies indicate a higher risk for depressive symptoms in perimenopausal women (45-70%) compared with premenopausal women (25-30%). In a small, prospective study, the risk for onset of depression was 14 times higher during the 24 months surrounding the final menses compared with the 31 years preceding that time (ie, premenopause years).[67]

In the Study of Women's Health Across the Nation (SWAN), Hispanic women seemed particularly vulnerable to developing depressive symptoms compared with other racial or ethnic groups, a finding that could be partially explained by the large percentage of women with low socioeconomic status and with concomitant health problems.[65]

At least three large longitudinal cohort studies have examined the prevalence of depressive symptoms in perimenopausal women—SWAN,[68] the Penn Ovarian Aging Study,[69] and the Seattle Midlife Women's Health Study.[70] These cohort studies followed women for a significant period of time (3-15 y), and most documented an increased risk for the occurrence of depressive symptoms during the menopause transition, with estimates showing a progressive increased risk from the early transition (1.5-fold increased risk) to the late transition (1.8- to 2.8-fold increased risk).

In the Harvard Moods and Cycles study, a population-based, prospective cohort of 460 late-premenopausal women, there was a 2-fold increased risk for the development of significant depressive symptoms (defined as a Center for Epidemiologic Studies Depression Scale score ≥16) and for clinical depression (confirmed with the *Structured Clinical Interview for DSM-IV*) in women entering perimenopause compared with age-matched women who remained premenopausal.[71] A greater risk for depressive symptoms was found even in those with no prior history of depression, especially in those who experienced adverse life events or significant VMS.

A 2- to 4-fold increased risk of clinical depression during the menopause transition and early postmenopause also was found in SWAN,[68] although the greatest risk for a major depressive episode was identified in those who had previously experienced a major depressive episode during the premenopause years.[72]

The menopause transition and early postmenopause constitute for some women a window of vulnerability for the development of depressive symptoms and clinical depression. The risk for developing depressive symptoms seems increased even in those with no history of clinical depression (ie, new onset in the context of the menopause transition). However, most women experiencing depression during the midlife years had in fact suffered a prior episode of depression.

Does anxiety play a role in depression?

Anxiety is highly prevalent in women across the lifespan; for decades we have known that approximately 30% of women will experience an anxiety disorder in their lifetimes compared with 19% of men.[73] In addition, data suggest that women reporting a history of both depression and anxiety disorders may experience poorer QOL during the midlife years, independent of the presence or severity of other conditions such as VMS or sleep disturbances.[74]

Notwithstanding, anxiety has received less attention than depression from most researchers and clinicians dedicated to women's mental health. Published studies on anxiety in midlife women are sparse, and very few were prospective in nature. Anxiety disorders also constitute a heterogeneous group, with several comorbid conditions and significant symptom overlap. Possible predictors of anxiety in late-premenopausal women (aged 36-45 y) were examined during a 3-year follow-up study.[75] Similar to previous studies on depression, a history of an anxiety disorder strongly predicted the occurrence of an episode during the study; moreover, anxiety sensitivity and neuroticism (ascertained with the NEO [neuroticism, extraversion, openness] Five-Factor Inventory) were predictors of anxiety disorder—new onset or recurrent.

Data on four symptoms of anxiety—irritability, nervousness or tension, feeling fearful for no reason, and heart pounding or racing—were examined in a study to identify women with high anxiety versus low anxiety and characterize a cluster of anxiety symptoms that could be more independent of VMS, health factors, or psychosocial stressors.[76] Women without high anxiety at the beginning of the study exhibited a surge in anxiety that peaked in late perimenopause—much higher than that observed in the premenopause years. These findings suggest a window of vulnerability for increased anxiety for a subgroup of women during the menopause transition.

It is quite difficult to disentangle the somatic, physiological, and behavioral experiences associated with a hot flash or an anxiety disorder. The emergence of a hot flash, for example, may generate physiological and behavioral responses (ie, feeling awkward or embarrassed, starting to avoid social situations) that might result in a state of anxiety and further intensify the hot flash experience. More accurate clinical assessments and validated measures are needed to help clinicians better distinguish menopause-related somatic complaints from psychological symptoms.

Sleep disturbances

Overall, women are more likely to experience insomnia or sleep complaints than men; they often have more difficulties initiating or maintaining sleep and report sleep problems associated with depression or pain.[77,78]

Depressed midlife women may experience changes in sleep patterns—less time in bed, shorter total sleep time, longer sleep-onset latency, and a tendency toward lower sleep efficiency—compared with nondepressed women.[79] In one study, depressed women did not report a higher frequency of nocturnal VMS or an increased number of awakenings because of nocturnal VMS, a finding that goes against the domino hypothesis, which links the occurrence of depression to sleep disruption caused by nocturnal VMS in midlife years. It is important that clinicians carefully consider, investigate, and treat primary sleep disorders in midlife years, including obstructive sleep apnea and restless legs syndrome, while exploring the association of sleep problems with concurrent psychiatric disorders such as depression and anxiety. (See also "Sleep Disturbance" in Chapter 5.)

Estrogens and mood regulation

Evidence suggests that estrogen exerts a modulatory effect via neurotransmitter pathways and neural receptors. Estrogen modulates monoaminergic systems, namely serotonin and noradrenaline neurotransmission, that are intrinsically associated with the development and treatment of depressive symptoms.[58] Estrogen receptors are widely distributed in the brain, and estrogen activity can be found in brain regions known to be involved in mood and cognitive regulation (prefrontal cortex, hippocampus).[80] Overall, the effects of estrogen on serotonin and noradrenaline could be said to be beneficial to mood.[57] Estradiol administration limits the activity of monoamine oxidases, which are enzymes involved in serotonin degradation.[81] It also increases both isoforms of tryptophan hydroxylase, the rate-limiting enzyme of serotonin synthesis.[82,83] Thus, estradiol administration results in an overall net increase in serotonin synthesis and availability. Estrogen may also have mood-enhancing (or antidepressant-like) properties because of its stimulating effect on brain-derived neurotropic factor, an important neuroprotective agent at multiple levels.[84]

The role of estrogen for the development of depression in midlife women was examined in 56 asymptomatic postmenopausal women with a history of perimenopause depression who received transdermal estradiol (100 μg/d) for 3 weeks and were then randomized to continue on estradiol or matched placebo skin patches for 3 additional weeks in a double-blind fashion.[85] No depressive symptoms were observed during the 3-week open-label phase with estradiol. Women with a history of perimenopausal depression reported an increase in depressive symptoms when switched to placebo, whereas those who remained on estradiol therapy continued to be asymptomatic. The study demonstrated that some midlife women could be particularly susceptible to develop behavior or mood changes when exposed to changes in estrogen levels, supporting the critical window hypothesis for the role of estrogen as a contributing or mitigating factor for depression in midlife women.

Role of antidepressants in treating depression in midlife women

Women constitute most of the participants commonly included in clinical trials for depression, yet studies that focused particularly on the management of depression during perimenopause and postmenopause are scarce. Most studies on pharmacologic interventions have explored the efficacy and safety of antidepressants such as selective serotonin reuptake inhibitors (SSRIs) and selective norepinephrine reuptake inhibitors (SNRIs). Some were open trials that included a lead-in phase to exclude those with a significant response to placebo before active treatment. Satisfactory response and good tolerability has been documented with citalopram,[86] escitalopram,[87] and duloxetine.[88] Antidepressant use resulted in significant improvements in menopause-related symptoms (hot flashes, night sweats, and somatic complaints).

Mirtazapine and citalopram were tested as adjunctive treatments to ET in open studies in depressed perimenopausal and postmenopausal women, with remission rates of 87.5% with mirtazapine[89] and 91.6% with citalopram.[86] In a pooled analysis of eight clinical trials, the SNRI venlafaxine showed higher response rates (48%) compared with SSRIs (28%) in midlife women who were suffering from depression and were not receiving estrogen-based treatments.[90] However, this difference was significantly reduced in depressed women receiving ET, which could indicate a synergistic effect of estrogen when combined with SSRIs.

One could speculate that women would be more vulnerable to recurrent depressive episodes in the absence of estrogen during the postmenopause years and not receiving estrogen treatments because they would not sustain the same antidepressant response to SSRIs without the synergistic effects of estrogen. A direct comparison between an SSRI and an SNRI (escitalopram and desvenlafaxine, respectively) in midlife women, however, did not reveal significant differences, with both treatments showing good efficacy and tolerability.[91]

Other trials using SNRIs—particularly desvenlafaxine—have documented the benefits of these agents not only for the improvement of depression in perimenopausal and postmenopausal women but also for QOL improvement and better overall functioning.[92,93] Quetiapine, an agent classified as an atypical antipsychotic most commonly used for the treatment of patients with schizophrenia and unipolar and bipolar depression, also has shown some improvements in depression, sleep complaints, and VMS in an open trial.[94,95]

In a preliminary 8-week open trial with vortioxetine, symptomatic midlife women with major depressive disorder exhibited robust antidepressant response (75%) and achieved significant improvements in QOL and menopause-related symptoms—including a reduction in frequency and severity of hot flashes.[96]

Overall, midlife women with a prior history of depression and a previous satisfactory response to a particular antidepressant agent should be treated with the same medication. For those experiencing depression for the first time, evidence suggests that various SSRIs and SNRIs could be chosen with reassurance of good efficacy and tolerability at usual doses.[66] The choice of an antidepressant for midlife women could be guided by a few principles, including data on efficacy and tolerability, data on tolerability/treatment adherence with regard to AEs such as sexual dysfunction and weight changes, and data on drug safety (eg, drug-drug interactions), particularly when managing concurrent medical conditions.

Estrogen therapy for depression

Despite accumulating evidence on the antidepressant properties of estrogen—particularly in depressed, perimenopausal women—the acceptability of estrogen as an antidepressant therapy has been somewhat limited.[57] Only a small percentage of RCTs have examined the benefits of ET in clinically depressed women.

To date, four small studies—including two RCTs—have demonstrated the efficacy of estradiol for the management of depressive disorders during perimenopause.[97,100] Two of the RCTs had similar designs and used standardized tools to confirm the diagnosis of depression and characterize menopause staging.[97,98] Antidepressant effects were well documented, and significant mood improvement was observed in those suffering from new-onset or recurrent major depressive disorder in the presence or absence of concomitant VMS. Moreover, the antidepressant effects of estradiol persisted after a 4-week washout period, even after reemergence of hot flashes and night sweats.[97]

Estrogen also has been used as an augmentation strategy for women with unsatisfactory response to antidepressants. Most studies suggest that estrogen might augment clinical response to antidepressants, including SSRIs and SNRIs.[90,101]

Results have been less promising in postmenopausal women with depression. The efficacy of transdermal estradiol (0.1 mg) compared with placebo in late-postmenopausal women suffering from mild to moderate depression has been examined.[102] After 8 weeks of treatment, both groups showed similar decrease in depressive symptoms from baseline. The study suggested that a subgroup of depressed postmenopausal women (ie, those with a past history of major depression) could be particularly responsive to placebo.

In a 24-week RCT, the effects of oral HT (a continuous combination of 2 mg estradiol valerate and 2 mg dienogest daily) were examined.[103] Women were considerably younger (average age, 55 y), and the use of HT led to significant improvements in depressive scores (reduction in Hamilton Depression Rating Scale scores). These findings, however, should be examined with caution given the unusually high dropout rates observed in treatment users (32%) and placebo users (58%).

Last, in an RCT of perimenopausal and postmenopausal women who were experiencing depression and sleep disturbances, women exhibited improvements with either transdermal 17β-estradiol 0.05 mg per day, zolpidem 10 mg per day, or placebo, but the study failed to demonstrate meaningful differences between the active treatments.[104]

A pilot study of perimenopausal women who were predominantly nondepressed compared the effects of the levonorgestrel-containing intrauterine system (LNG-IUS) plus low-dose transdermal estradiol (gel 0.06% containing 0.75 mg estradiol per 1.25 g metered dose) to the LNG-IUS alone (plus inactive gel) for 50 days.[105] The study assessed depressive symptoms, fatigue, sleep, and the effect of hot flashes on functioning. Overall, the study revealed the beneficial effects of the LNG-IUS plus transdermal estradiol for the improvement of hot flashes and daytime fatigue, with minimal or nonsignificant effects on sleep and no significant changes in mood (improvement or worsening).

A double-blind RCT examining the benefits of ET (oral estradiol 2 mg/d) on cognition, mood, and QOL in postmenopausal women (average age, 73 y) found no significant changes after 20 weeks of treatment.[106]

As an overall observation, ET—particularly transdermal estradiol—has shown antidepressant properties similar to that observed with antidepressants, particularly when administered to perimenopausal, depressed women. Transdermal 17β-estradiol appears to lead to a greater antidepressant effect size (drug-placebo difference) and could therefore constitute a potential treatment for depressed mood in this population. The same hormone intervention formulation (estradiol) and route of administration (transdermal) was not effective in treating depressed postmenopausal women[102]; this particular finding suggests that the menopause transition might not only be a critical window of risk for depression but also a window of opportunity for the effective use of ET for depression in midlife years.[107]

Other benefits of estrogen therapy

One study examined whether HT could prevent the onset of depression in perimenopausal and early postmenopausal women.[108] In a double-blind RCT, perimenopausal and early postmenopausal women (aged 45-60 y) received transdermal estradiol (0.1 mg/d) or placebo for 12 months. Oral micronized progesterone or placebo pills also were given every 3 months to women receiving active treatment or placebo, respectively. Of 172 participants, 43 developed clinically significant depressive symptoms. Those assigned to placebo were more likely to develop and report depressive symptoms compared with those receiving placebo (32.3% vs 17.3%); the mood benefits were evident in women in the early menopause transition but not in postmenopausal women later in the transition. The study suggests that ET also could have a role in preventing the development of clinically significant depressive symptoms in nondepressed midlife women.

Other putative benefits of HT include effects on sleep and anxiety. Most trials comparing HT with placebo have shown an improvement in perceived sleep quality and self-reported sleeping problems; objective measures of sleep, however, have shown more modest results—essentially, a reduction in sleep fragmentation, with reduced wakefulness and arousals.[109,110] (See also "Sleep Disturbance" in Chapter 5.)

In some cases, the use of HT has led to lower anxiety scores and fewer sleep complaints in HT users than nonusers,[111] whereas other RCTs have shown little or no effect.[112,113] Low anxiety scores at study entry (a "floor effect") could in part justify the lack of more robust findings.

Midlife women and treating depression

Midlife in women may represent a window of vulnerability for the development of depressive symptoms. At the same time, this critical window also may constitute a window of opportunity for the administration of estradiol to symptomatic or asymptomatic women across different systems/domains.

Women appear to be particularly vulnerable to depression during the perimenopausal and early postmenopausal years, and the greatest risk factor is a prior history of depression. As in any given time across the lifespan, antidepressants remain the front-line treatment for those suffering from clinically significant depression.

Clinicians should carefully consider the various treatment strategies available and determine the extent to which they can be tailored to address the multiple symptom domains for each patient. It is plausible to consider the benefits of a brief trial of transdermal estradiol for perimenopausal women presenting with bothersome menopause symptoms (eg, VMS) and concurrent depressive symptoms before considering the need for antidepressant use (monotherapy or concomitant use). Women with a history of multiple depressive episodes presenting with severe depressive symptoms and/or expressing suicidal ideation should be promptly treated with antidepressant pharmacotherapies and close monitoring.

Other interventions, including evidence-based psychotherapies (particularly behavior-based interventions), should be considered as part of the treatment armamentarium for the reduction of the symptom burden and functional impairment associated with depression.

Data on exercise, balanced diet, and dietary supplements are still limited. Omega-3 fatty acids have been investigated as monotherapy[114] or in combination with antidepressants[115] and showed beneficial effects on mood and menopause-related symptoms.

Thyroid Disease

Thyroid disorders are common in women, increasing in prevalence with age. In a subset of more than 3,000 multiethnic women aged 42 to 52 years participating in SWAN, approximately 1 in 10 women had evidence of thyroid dysfunction—a thyroid-stimulating hormone (TSH) level outside of the normal range (two-thirds were higher than normal; one-third was below normal).[116] In the National Health and Nutrition Examination Survey III, the percentage of women with evidence of thyroid antibodies, a harbinger of autoimmune thyroid dysfunction, increased from 15.8% in women aged 40 to 49 years to 26.5% in those aged older than 80 years.[117] Symptoms of thyroid dysfunction (altered menstrual cycle length, change in amount of bleeding, sleep disruption, fatigue, mood swings, forgetfulness, heat intolerance, palpitations) can be confused with symptoms common to the menopause transition.

Normal physiology

The primary function of the thyroid is to regulate metabolism. Thyroid hormone is synthesized when the thyroid gland extracts iodine from the circulation, combines it with the amino acid tyrosine, and converts it to the thyroid hormones triiodothyronine (T_3) and thyroxine (T_4). The thyroid gland stores thyroid hormone until it is released into the bloodstream. Most thyroid hormones circulate bound to proteins. Thyroid hormones affect the liver, muscle, heart, bone, and central nervous system. Thyroid-stimulating hormone secreted by the pituitary gland reflects circulating thyroid hormone concentration and, via a negative feedback loop, regulates thyroid hormone release.

Screening for thyroid disease

Recommendations for screening for thyroid disease vary. The American Thyroid Association (ATA) recommends screening all adults beginning at age 35 and every 5 years thereafter.[118] The American Association of Clinical Endocrinologists (AACE) recommends screening older patients (age not specified), especially women; the American College of Physicians suggests that women aged 50 years and older with an incidental finding suggestive of symptomatic thyroid disease should be evaluated. In 2015, the US Preventive Services Task Force (USPSTF) concluded that current evidence is insufficient to assess the balance of benefits and harms of screening for thyroid dysfunction in nonpregnant, asymptomatic adults.[119]

Hypothyroidism

Hypothyroidism, a condition reflecting low production of thyroid hormone and most often caused by Hashimoto thyroiditis, is the most common thyroid disorder in women, occurring seven times more often in women than men, with an increased incidence in midlife.[120] A woman with hypothyroidism may complain of fatigue, lethargy, cold intolerance, weight gain, constipation, dry skin, and heavier, longer menstrual cycles.[121] If a woman has a family history of thyroid disorders, experienced postpartum thyroiditis, received radioactive iodine treatment for Graves disease or multinodular goiter, or reports a history of type 2 diabetes mellitus (DM), polycystic ovary syndrome, or other endocrine/autoimmune disorders, her risk of hypothyroidism increases.[122]

Diagnosis

The serum TSH level measure is the gold standard to detect hypothyroidism.[120] The normal range is defined as 0.4 mIU/L to 4.5 mIU/L, although this may differ slightly in different laboratories. If the TSH level is elevated, free T_4 (FT_4) and antithyroperoxidase antibodies should be measured; a low FT_4 value confirms the diagnosis of overt hypothyroidism. A high TSH value with an elevated FT_4 may be suggestive of a rare TSH-producing pituitary adenoma but more likely may confirm that a woman may have taken extra thyroid hormone before her appointment. If the patient has symptoms of hypothyroidism, low FT_4, and low TSH, the possibility of central hypothyroidism arises, and an evaluation of the pituitary and hypothalamus is indicated.[123,124] Slight elevations in TSH levels with normal FT_4, especially in older persons, could be consistent with subclinical hypothyroidism, often reported to increase with age.[125] The presence of antithyroperoxidase antibodies in patients with subclinical hypothyroidism predicts progression to overt hypothyroidism.[118] Alternatively, the increased incidence of TSH elevation might simply represent a normal manifestation of the aging hypothalamic pituitary-thyroid axis.[126] Age-stratified TSH norms have been suggested by some but have yet to be formally established.[118,121]

Treatment

Patients with overt hypothyroidism merit thyroid hormone replacement therapy to relieve symptoms and normalize TSH and thyroid hormone levels (without overtreating).[118,120,121,127] Levothyroxine (LT_4) is considered to be the standard of care. The usual replacement dose of LT_4 averages 1.6 µg per kg of body weight per day. In patients aged older than 50 years up to 60 years without coronary heart disease (CHD), therapy should be initiated with a LT_4 dose of 25 µg to 50 µg per day, with a progressive increase every 2 to 3 weeks until euthyroidism is reached.[120,127] In patients with known CHD, the starting dose of LT_4 is lower—12.5 µg to 25 µg per day. This can be titrated at 6- to 8-week intervals by 12.5 µg to 25 µg, depending on the TSH levels and clinical response. In treated patients, the target for TSH is within the normal range; TSH levels should be checked 4 to 6 weeks after any LT_4 dose change.

Monitoring

Once the replacement dose is established, TSH values should be monitored every 6 to 12 months.[118,120,121,127] If the patient changes thyroid hormone preparations (eg, new insurance or pharmacy change from branded to generic or a different generic preparation), TSH should be rechecked after 6 to 8 weeks because therapeutic equivalence of preparations may differ. Because concurrent administration of levothyroxine with food, vitamins, calcium, and iron may significantly interfere with absorption, patients should take LT_4 separately. Compliance may be enhanced by recommending that LT_4 be taken with water 60 minutes before breakfast; alternatively, some patients prefer taking LT_4 in the evening 3 or more hours after the last meal.

Effect of estrogen therapy

If the patient treated with thyroid hormone starts oral ET, TSH levels should be monitored 6 to 8 weeks later.[120,128] Anticipate that the dose of LT_4 may need to be increased. Oral (but not transdermal) estrogens increase thyroid-binding globulin (TBG), which in turn reduces the FT_4 values; androgen therapy induces opposite effects.[129] A normally functioning thyroid gland compensates for increased TBG with an increase of thyroid hormone production to maintain FT_4, but a hypothyroid gland with compromised thyroid reserve cannot. Conversely, when oral ET is discontinued, thyroid function should be monitored again 6 to 8 weeks later. The dose of LT_4 may need to be reduced as TBG concentrations decrease and FT_4 increases in response. Case reports suggest that an increase in the dose of LT_4 might be necessary when raloxifene or soy supplements are initiated in women with hypothyroidism.[120]

Subclinical hypothyroidism

A healthy, asymptomatic woman with no history or signs of thyroid disease with an elevated TSH level in the presence of normal thyroid hormone concentrations might qualify for a diagnosis of *subclinical hypothyroidism*.[130] The prevalence of subclinical hypothyroidism is between 4% and 8.5%, increasing to 15% in elderly populations.[131] Before making the diagnosis, the TSH test should be repeated after 3 to 6 months to confirm. Up to 60% of cases will regress to euthyroidism over 5 years, whereas 1% to 5% of cases per year, perhaps more in those with positive thyroperoxidase antibodies, will progress to overt hypothyroidism.[125]

Consequences

Some, but not all, observational studies link subclinical hypothyroidism with an increased risk for CHD, heart failure (HF), and mortality.[120,132] These events may depend on the age of the patient as well as the relative degree of thyroid failure. In one analysis, even persons whose TSH level was on the high side of the normal range had subtle increases in blood pressure and lipid levels.[131] Paradoxically, CV events and mortality appear to be increased more often in persons aged younger than 65 to 70 years with subclinical hypothyroidism rather than in the elderly.[118,125,126,133,134]

In a nested case-cohort design in the WHI observational study, subclinical hypothyroidism was not associated with an increased risk of myocardial infarction (hazard ratios [HRs] for myocardial infarction by age show an elevation in risk in women aged 50-64 y compared with older women with subclinical hypothyroidism, although the confidence intervals [CIs] were wide, and the differences were not statistically significant).[135] In an evaluation from the 55,000-participant Thyroid Studies Collaboration, subclinical hypothyroidism was associated with a 2-fold increase in CHD events and mortality but only if the TSH level was elevated above 10 mIU/L.[136]

Treatment considerations

Whether a midlife woman with subclinical hypothyroidism should be treated is a hotly debated topic and one on which the experts do not necessarily agree. When reviewed for the USPSTF in 2015, evidence for benefit of treatment of subclinical hypothyroidism was sparse and inconsistent.[137] In a 1-year RCT of 737 men and women (mean age, 74.4 y) with normal baseline FT$_4$ and TSH levels 4.6 mIU/L to 19.99 mIU/L, randomization to LT$_4$ (median dose, 50 µg) reduced TSH but did not improve hypothyroid symptoms or tiredness on standard questionnaires; no apparent benefits or serious AEs were

detected.[138] In the absence of clinical trial evidence substantiating improved clinical outcomes, recommendations for replacement therapy are largely based on observational studies and expert opinion.[118,120,125,131] In an analysis from the UK General Practitioner Research Database, treatment of subclinical hypothyroidism in patients with TSH levels of 5 mIU/L to 10 mIU/L was associated with fewer CHD events in younger patients (40-70 y), but similar benefit was not seen for persons aged older than 70 years.[139]

Clinical approach

In AACE/ATA guidelines, an individualized approach to treatment of subclinical hypothyroidism is recommended.[118] Treatment should be considered for patients whose TSH level falls between the upper limit of normal and 10 mIU/L and who have symptoms of hypothyroidism (dry skin, cold sensitivity, fatigue, muscle cramps, voice changes, constipation), positive thyroperoxidase antibodies, or evidence of atherosclerotic CVD, HF, or associated risk factors. Treatment is also recommended for patients with TSH levels higher than 10 mIU/L.[118,120,125] Patients with subclinical hypothyroidism do not necessarily require full replacement doses; treatment with 25 µg to 75 µg of LT$_4$ daily usually suffices in normalizing thyroid hormone status and might reduce the likelihood of overtreating and inducing subclinical hyperthyroidism.[118,131]

Hyperthyroidism

Symptoms of hyperthyroidism—anxiety, palpitations, lighter and less frequent menses, and heat intolerance—also mimic the menopause transition. The prevalence of overt hyperthyroidism is 0.5% (approximately 1 in 200 persons).[140] The most common etiologies include Graves disease, toxic multinodular goiter, and solitary hyperfunctioning (toxic) adenoma.

Diagnosis

The initial diagnostic test of choice for hyperthyroidism remains the TSH level. If the TSH is suppressed, FT$_4$ should be measured to assess the degree of thyroid hormone excess. If FT$_4$ is normal, total T$_3$ (TT$_3$) should also be measured and, if elevated, might point to the presence of an autonomously functioning (toxic) thyroid nodule.[140] If thyrotoxicosis is strongly suspected clinically, diagnostic accuracy improves if free T$_4$ and total T$_3$ are assessed concurrently with TSH. In a patient with a symmetrically enlarged thyroid, recent onset of orbitopathy (Graves eye changes), and moderate to severe hyperthyroidism, the diagnosis of Graves disease is likely, and further evaluation of the etiology of hyperthyroidism is unnecessary. In a patient with thyrotoxicosis with a nonnodular thyroid and no definite orbitopathy (eye changes), measurement of TSH receptor antibodies or radioactive iodine uptake can be used to distinguish Graves disease from other etiologies. Markedly increased uptake in a homogenous distribution is consistent with Graves disease, whereas a heterogeneous distribution is consistent with multinodular goiter. A solitary "hot" nodule may be responsible for hyperthyroidism, especially if the TT_3 is elevated. A lack of thyroid uptake points to the diagnosis of thyroiditis, either Hashimoto autoimmune thyroiditis or glandular destruction caused by a viral infection.

Management

Most women who have hyperthyroidism should be referred to an endocrinologist for consultation. The diagnosis should be confirmed, and the patient begun on therapeutic intervention and long-term monitoring. Initial therapy includes beta-blockers for symptomatic relief, and if the diagnosis is Graves disease or multinodular goiter, concurrent antithyroid drugs (methimazole).[140] Radioactive iodine thyroid ablation is the most definitive nonsurgical therapy for Graves disease and toxic multinodular goiter, but it is used less often for treatment of Graves disease because it can result in permanent thyroid destruction and the requirement of lifelong thyroid hormone replacement.

Subclinical hyperthyroidism

If the TSH level falls below the normal range in the presence of normal thyroid hormone levels, the patient might meet criteria for the diagnosis of *subclinical hyperthyroidism*.[125,140-142] Concerns with subclinical hyperthyroidism include increased osteoporosis risk and fractures, atrial fibrillation, HF, and possibly increased CHD and CHD mortality, especially in women of advanced age.[142]

Diagnosis

Subclinical hyperthyroidism occurs infrequently: 0.7% have TSH levels less than 0.1 mIU/L and 1.8% have low TSH levels (<0.4 mIU/L).[140] Suppressed TSH can be related to exogenous thyroid hormone use, severe nonthyroidal illness, and pituitary hypothalamic disease, as well as to advanced age and to black ethnicity because of changes in the hypothalamic-pituitary set point.[141] The course is variable: 0.5% to 7% progress to overt hyperthyroidism, and 5% to 12% revert to normal TSH levels. It is therefore reasonable to monitor an asymptomatic, healthy woman

over 2 to 3 months to document persistence of these findings. If the TSH level remains below the normal range with normal thyroid hormone concentrations, particularly if suppressed to less than 0.1 mIU/L, the specific thyroid disorder should be determined (most commonly toxic multinodular goiter, followed by Graves disease and solitary autonomous [toxic] nodules).

Treatment considerations

The 2016 ATA guidelines recommend treatments similar to those for overt hyperthyroidism when the TSH level is persistently less than 0.1 mIU/L in all persons aged 65 years and older; in patients with cardiac risk factors, heart disease, or osteoporosis; in postmenopausal women not taking estrogen or bisphosphonates (and therefore at risk of accelerated bone loss); and in persons with hyperthyroid symptoms.[140] Treatment could be considered in patients aged younger than 65 years without specified risk factors.

When TSH is persistently below the lower limit of normal but is 0.1 mIU/L and above, treatment should be considered in those aged 65 years and older and in patients with cardiac disease, osteoporosis, or symptoms of hyperthyroidism.[140] When TSH is persistently below the lower limit of normal but is 0.1 mIU/L and above, asymptomatic patients aged younger than 65 years without cardiac disease or osteoporosis can be observed without further investigation of the etiology of the subnormal TSH hormone or treatment. With treatment, hypothyroidism may result, and ultimately, thyroid replacement therapy could be required.

Bone effects

In the Study of Osteoporotic Fractures, use of thyroid hormone itself did not increase risk of fracture if the TSH level was maintained in the normal range.[143] However, in women aged older than 65 years, suppressed TSH levels (<0.1 mIU/L)—either as a result of excess endogenous thyroid hormone production or exogenous thyroid hormone use—were associated with a 3-fold increase in hip fractures and a 4-fold increase in vertebral fractures. As assessed by TSH measurements, approximately 20% of patients receiving levothyroxine therapy may be overtreated.[144] In a report from the Thyroid Studies Collaboration that included 70,298 participants, subclinical hyperthyroidism was associated with increased hip, vertebral, and any fracture.[145] In prospective cohort studies, even in adults with euthyroidism, with TSH levels within the normal range, hip fracture rates were elevated in those with the lowest versus the highest TSH values.[146,147] These reports suggest that in older persons or those with compromised bone density, maintaining TSH levels in the upper range of normal might be associated with fewer fractures. Bone mineral density should be measured, preferably at a cortical site such as the hip, in women with a long history of LT$_4$ therapy; doses used in the past were often higher than currently recommended.[148]

Thyroid nodules

A thyroid nodule is a discrete lesion within the thyroid gland that is radiologically distinct from the surrounding thyroid parenchyma. Although thyroid nodules are palpable in about 5% of women,[149] high-resolution ultrasound examination of asymptomatic patients suggests that thyroid nodules occur in as many as 19% to 68% of the US population, with higher prevalence in women and the elderly.[149,150] Thyroid nodules are of concern because they can harbor thyroid cancers.

Evaluation and management

The ATA updated its guidelines for evaluation and management of thyroid nodules and thyroid cancers in 2015[149]; in 2016, the AACE, along with the American College of Endocrinology and with Mexican experts, updated their recommendations.[150] If a thyroid nodule is detected on physical examination or reported as an incidental finding on another imaging study, TSH should be measured. If the TSH level is low, a radionucleotide thyroid scan should be obtained to determine the functional status of the nodule. Hyperfunctioning hot nodules are rarely malignant; cytology is not necessary, and therapy for hyperthyroidism should be considered.[149] A higher serum TSH level, even within the upper part of the reference range, is associated with increased risk of malignancy in a thyroid nodule, as well as more advanced-stage thyroid cancer.

The next step is a diagnostic thyroid ultrasound to define the anatomy of the gland, to accurately measure the diameter of the nodule(s), to ascertain clinical characteristics of the nodule(s), and to survey cervical lymph nodes—all important parameters for management decisions.[149] If ultrasound confirms the presence of a nodule, the patient should be referred to an endocrinologist for fine-needle aspiration (FNA). Generally, only nodules 1 cm or larger should be evaluated because they have greater potential to be clinically significant cancers. Depending on other characteristics of the nodule, FNA might be recommended for a nodule of lesser diameter.

The cytology of the cellular aspirate in conjunction with the medical history, clinical findings, and ultrasound characteristics will dictate further management. Immunocytochemistry and molecular testing may be of benefit in select cases.[150] Most benign nodules can be monitored with serial annual ultrasounds, and depending on whether the nodule has grown, a repeat of FNA may be indicated. Levothyroxine suppressive therapy is not recommended.

Thyroid cancer

Thyroid cancer can present as a large, palpable neck mass, possibly with symptoms related to mass effect, but more commonly, thyroid cancers are diagnosed as a result of thyroid nodule evaluation. Thyroid cancer occurs in 7% to 15% of cases, depending on age, sex, history of radiation exposure, family history, and other factors,[149] with an overall US thyroid cancer incidence rate of 15.3 cases per 100,000 persons.[151] Thyroid cancer is diagnosed in women three times more often than in men, with peak incidence occurring between age 40 and 50 years.

Differentiated thyroid cancer, including papillary and follicular cancers, make up most (>90%) of all thyroid cancers.[149] An apparent 2- to 3-fold increased risk in thyroid cancer rates over the past decade is hypothesized to reflect the increasing use of neck ultrasonography or other imaging (with incidental findings) and subsequently early diagnosis and treatment. Thyroid cancer treatment is managed by an endocrinologist. The 5-year survival rate for thyroid cancer overall is 98.1%.[151] In 2017, after a systematic review,[152] the USPSTF determined that the net benefit of screening for thyroid cancer is negative and recommends against screening in asymptomatic adults.[151]

Gallbladder Disease

Gallstones (cholelithiasis) are common in the United States and are estimated to affect between 10% and 15% of the adult population.[153] The Third National Health and Nutrition Examination Survey estimated that 6.3 million men and 14.2 million women in the United States aged 20 to 74 years have gallbladder disease.[154] Gallstones occur two times more frequently in women than in men; the highest incidence is seen in American Indians, followed by Mexican Americans.[155,156] Choledocholithiasis, the presence of gallstones in the common bile duct—usually from symptomatic passage of gallstones from the gallbladder—has been noted to affect approximately 5% to 19% of patients at the time of cholecystectomy, with increasing incidence with age.[157-159] Most gallstones, however, are asymptomatic.

A woman's risk of gallstones increases with obesity, increased parity, age, and hormone use. Gallstones are also seen more commonly during rapid weight loss, such as with low-calorie diets or bariatric surgery, because extra cholesterol is secreted in bile.[154] Exogenous oral estrogens, whether administered in combined hormonal contraceptives or in HT, increase the risk of developing cholesterol gallstones by increasing the hepatic secretion of biliary cholesterol, which in turn, leads to an increase in cholesterol saturation of bile. Oral estrogens also reduce gallbladder motility.[160,163] The clinical manifestations of symptomatic gallbladder disease include persistent right upper-quadrant or epigastric abdominal pain; nausea and vomiting; fever or chills, jaundice, or tea-colored urine; and light-colored stools, which may signify serious infection or inflammation of the gallbladder, liver, or pancreas.

Multiple studies have demonstrated that cholelithiasis, cholecystitis, and cholecystectomy occur more frequently in women on HT.[164-166] In the WHI, with an average participant age of 63 years, treatment with oral conjugated equine estrogens (CEEs) or oral CEEs plus medroxyprogesterone acetate (MPA) increased the risk of cholecystitis and cholelithiasis. The attributable risk in the CEE arm was 15.5 per 1,000 per 5 years of use, with similar risks seen with CEEs plus MPA.[163,167] The risk of gallbladder disease increased with duration of use. Data from the WHI and the Heart and Estrogen/Progestin Replacement Study show that the risk of gallbladder disease increased after 5.6 years of use for those using CEEs plus MPA, with an absolute risk increase of 27 per 1,000 (95% CI, 21-34), whereas the risk for those on CEEs after 7 years showed an increase in absolute risk of 45 per 1,000 (95% CI, 36-57).[164,168]

The formulation and route of HT administration appears to affect the risk of gallbladder disease, in which greater risk is seen with oral estrogens, presumably because of the first-pass hepatic effect after oral ingestion. In the Million Women Study, current estrogen users were 64% more likely (95% CI, 1.58-1.69) to experience gallbladder disease than never users (relative risk [RR], 1.64),[169] but risks were significantly lower with transdermal than with oral therapy (RR, 1.24 vs 1.74). One RCT compared the effect of transdermal and oral estrogens on gallstone formation and focused on biliary markers of gallstone formation, an intermediate outcome, compared with clinical gallstone formation.[170] The study found that both estrogen formulations altered bile comparably in ways that would be expected to form gallstones.

A large prospective cohort study of 70,928 women (64.8% reported ever using HT) over 11.5 years, designed to examine hormone and environmental factors that affect diseases in women, identified 2,819 incident cholecystectomies performed during the study period.[171] After adjustment for body mass index, parity, level of education, DM, and hypercholesterolemia, HT use was associated with an adjusted HR for cholecystectomy of 1.10 compared with nonusers (95% CI, 1.01-1.20). The increase in risk was only associated with oral unopposed estrogens (adjusted HR, 1.16; 95% CI, 1.06-1.27), which was significantly greater than the risk seen with transdermal estrogens (P=.03) or with oral preparations that combined estrogen with a progestogen (P=.03). Oral CEEs alone were associated with a significantly higher risk of cholecystectomy than oral CEEs plus a progestogen (P=.01). Over 5 years, about one excess cholecystectomy would be expected per 150 women using oral ET without a progestogen compared with women not using ET.

Minimal data are available regarding gallbladder cancer and estrogen use, with none reported in the WHI.[163] Observational and preclinical studies suggest a possible benefit of HT on liver fibrosis, specifically in the context of hepatitis C-related liver disease, and fatty liver,[172] but additional research is needed before definitive conclusions can be made.

Hormone therapy should be administered with caution to postmenopausal women who have gallstones or a history of gallbladder disease, especially when using oral estrogen alone or combination HT. Although a lower risk of gallbladder disease has been seen with transdermal HT compared with oral and oral estradiol compared with CEEs, these findings have not been confirmed in RCTs. Therefore, a thorough discussion of gallbladder-related risks should be included when counseling women on the risks and benefits of HT.

Sexually Transmitted Infections

Although postmenopausal women do not have to be concerned about the possibility of pregnancy, they are not protected against sexually transmitted infections (STIs). The risk of STIs—including *Chlamydia trachomatis*, *Neisseria gonorrhoeae*, genital herpes (herpes simplex virus [HSV]), human papillomavirus (HPV), hepatitis B and C, HIV, syphilis, and vaginal trichomoniasis—is a lifelong concern for women not in long-term, mutually monogamous relationships. Older women may not be as knowledgeable about infection risks nor accustomed to taking steps to minimize these risks compared with younger women who have lived with the threat of acquired immune deficiency syndrome for their entire sexual lives.

For that reason, safe sex guidelines should be discussed with patients who disclose that they are, or may become, sexually active (Table 4).

Epidemiologic studies show that the rates of STIs such as chlamydia and HIV are increasing in older American women and men, although the absolute number of cases remains quite low. For example, chlamydia infections reported in women aged 55 to 64 years increased from 11 to 16 cases per 100,000 population between 2012 and 2016. However, the absolute risk of a chlamydial infection for women in this age group in 2016 was about one case per 6,250 women.[173] The most important predictor of STIs in older persons is the number of sexual partners they have had in the past year, especially if two or more partners. Although there is no "epidemic" of STIs in older US adults, as is periodically reported by the media, STIs are a concern that must be addressed by clinicians.

Most STIs are more easily transmitted from a man to a woman than from a woman to man. Women are twice as likely as men to contract gonorrhea, hepatitis B, and HIV, if exposed. Moreover, STIs are less likely to produce symptoms in women and therefore may not be diagnosed until serious complications develop. Also, once infected, STI symptoms may be unrecognized or ignored, and information may be withheld during medical visits to avoid embarrassing questions posed by the history taker.

Postmenopausal women may be more or less susceptible to infection by sexually transmitted pathogens compared with younger women, depending on the pathogen. Sexually active postmenopausal women with genital atrophy may be at increased risk of acquiring HIV infection because the delicate genital tissue is prone to small tears and cuts that can act as pathways for infection.[174,175] Alternatively, postmenopausal women are less likely to acquire cervical chlamydia infection once exposed because of the loss of the target tissue for infection, the exposed columnar epithelium of the cervical ectropion, which has been replaced through squamous metaplasia. Women who have undergone total hysterectomy are no longer at risk of acquiring cervical infection with gonorrhea or chlamydia, eliminating the risk of pelvic inflammatory disease (PID), although chlamydial or gonococcal urethritis may occur after exposure.

Women having sex with women have fewer STIs than heterosexual women, but some pathogens, particularly those associated with bacterial vaginosis (BV), can be

Table 4. Safer Sex Guidelines for Women of All Ages

- Choose sex partners carefully.
- Discuss sexual histories with your partner, and don't let embarrassment compromise your health.
- Consider having both you and your partner checked for STIs before starting a sexual relationship.
- Ask to be screened for STIs if you have had more than one partner in the past 12 months, a new partner in the past 90 days, or if you have reason to suspect that your partner is having sex with other partners.
- Always insist that a male partner use a latex condom for genital, oral, and anal sex unless you are in a long-term, mutually monogamous relationship.
- Don't let a male partner's erection difficulties keep him from using a condom. Dream up some erotic or stimulating methods for putting on the condom to keep his erection going. If all else fails, get a female condom.
- If your vagina is dry, use of an intimate (sexual) lubricant can make intercourse more comfortable and possibly lessen the risk of tears in your skin. Use only water-based lubricants with latex condoms. Never use petroleum-based products like petroleum jelly, shortening, mineral oil, massage oils, body lotions, and cooking oil to lubricate condoms because they can cause condoms to break or leak
- After a confirmed diagnosis of gonorrhea, chlamydia, syphilis, HIV, pelvic inflammatory disease, or trichomoniasis, urge any sex partners within the past 6 months to be tested and treated.
- If you have possible STI symptoms such as a new vaginal discharge, a vulvar rash or sores, bleeding after sex, abdominal pain during sex, or chronic pelvic pain, discuss STI testing with your clinician.
- Hepatitis B vaccination is recommended for all unvaccinated, uninfected persons being evaluated or treated for an STI

Abbreviations: HIV, human immunodeficiency virus; STI, sexually transmitted infection.

passed horizontally from woman to woman. Clinicians can provide counseling to lower this risk.[176]

Screening and testing for sexually transmitted infections

Decisions about screening and testing for STIs must be based on strategies that maximize the likelihood of finding infections when present but avoid unnecessary testing of women at minimal risk to reduce the chances of false-positive test results. The prevalence of disease in a population affects screening test performance: in low-prevalence settings, even very good tests have poor predictive value positives.[177] The personal and social consequences of a falsely positive STI test can be devastating to a relationship, and even the possibility of this occurrence should be minimized. The categories of STI screening and testing in sexually active women of all ages are routine screening, targeted screening, contact testing, coinfection testing, and diagnostic testing (Table 5).[178]

Other than screening for HIV and hepatitis C in certain populations, there are no "routine" STI screening tests that should be performed for all sexually active postmenopausal women. Instead, STI screening decisions are based on a woman's responses to questions posed during sexual history taking. At a minimum, there are questions that should be asked of older women who are no longer at risk of pregnancy (Table 6).[179]

Specific sexually transmitted infections in older women

Chlamydia

Most *Chlamydia trachomatis* infections occur in women aged younger than 25 years; in 2015, the incidence of chlamydia infections in US women aged 40 to 44 years was about 1 case in 700 women, and for women aged 45 to 54 years, about 1 case per 1,900 women.[173] Diagnostic testing should be performed in women with purulent cervical or vaginal discharge, dysuria not attributable to a urinary tract infection, deep dyspareunia, or abnormal vaginal bleeding. Nucleic acid amplification tests are extremely sensitive and have replaced screening by chlamydia culture. A self-collected or clinician-collected vaginal swab is the preferred sample source. Urine testing is acceptable but is estimated to detect up to 10% fewer infections when compared with vaginal and endocervical swab samples.[180] The Centers for Disease Control and Prevention (CDC) recommended treatment of cervical chlamydia infection is a single dose of azithromycin 1 g orally or doxycycline 100 mg orally twice daily for 7 days.[181] Test of cure is not necessary after chlamydia treatment in most cases. However, women treated for chlamydia should be rescreened in 3 months to detect reinfection by a new partner or failure to treat their prior partner(s).

Gonorrhea

Gonorrhea infection can be found in the cervix, anus, urethra, pharynx, and eyes. In postmenopausal women who have had a hysterectomy, gonococcal cervicitis and pelvic inflammatory disease are no longer a concern. Symptoms may include pain or burning when urinating, increased vaginal discharge, and postcoital, intermenstrual, or

Table 5. Categories of Screening for STIs

- *Routine screening* is defined as screening of defined populations of asymptomatic women based on age, pregnancy status, or geographic factors, irrespective of personal behaviors or risk factors.

- *Targeted screening* is performed for women who have an increased risk of infection based on their own personal sexual behaviors. For example, if a woman has had prior chlamydia or gonorrhea infection, particularly in past 24 months; more than one sexual partner in the past year; a new partner in the past 90 days; has suspicion that a recent partner may have had concurrent partners; or has exchanged sex for drugs or money in the past year, she should be offered screening for chlamydia and gonorrhea. Other factors identified locally, including prevalence of infection in the community, are important as well.

- *Contact testing* is done when the woman's sexual partner is suspected or known to have chlamydia, gonorrhea, syphilis, HIV, or hepatitis B or C.

- *Coinfection testing* is performed after a woman is diagnosed with one STI to find coincident infection with other pathogens. Women diagnosed with chlamydia, gonorrhea, syphilis, HIV, or primary herpes should be screened for other pathogens. Coinfection testing is not necessary for women diagnosed with recurrent genital warts or recurrent herpes because these may be longstanding infections and do not necessarily reflect current sexual behaviors. Bacterial vaginosis and vaginal candidiasis are not sexually transmitted and are not a reason to perform coinfection testing.

- *Diagnostic testing* should be performed for any woman who, because of symptoms or signs of infection, is suspected of having an STI.

Abbreviations: HIV, human immunodeficiency virus; STI, sexually transmitted infection. Grimes DA, et al;[177] California STD/HIV Prevention Training Center. California Department of Public Health-STD Control Branch.[178]

postmenopausal bleeding. Screening and testing are performed by nucleic acid amplification tests obtained with a vaginal sample, as with chlamydia testing. Because drug-resistant strains of gonorrhea are a significant problem in the United States, the CDC recommends cotreatment with a cephalosporin followed by a second drug to delay the emergence of additional resistant strains.[181] The CDC-recommended regimen for the treatment of cervical, urethral, or rectal gonorrhea is intramuscular ceftriaxone 250 mg followed by azithromycin 1 g orally. If injectable ceftriaxone is not available, oral cefixime 400 mg as a single dose (given with azithromycin 1 g orally) is an alternative regimen. Quinolones are no longer recommended for treatment of gonorrhea.

Screening for chlamydia and gonorrhea. The USPSTF recommends routine screening for chlamydia and gonorrhea in sexually active women aged 24 years and younger and targeted screening in older women who are at increased risk for infection.[182] The guideline defines increased risk as having a new sex partner, more than one sex partner, a sex partner with concurrent partners, or a sex partner who has an STI; inconsistent condom use in persons who are not in mutually monogamous relationships; a previous or coexisting STI; and exchanging sex for money or drugs.

Expedited partner therapy. Expedited partner therapy is the clinical practice of treating the sex partners of women diagnosed with chlamydia, gonorrhea, or in some cases, trichomoniasis, by providing prescriptions or medications to the patient to take to her partner without a clinician evaluation of the partner.[183] This strategy has been endorsed by the CDC as way to maximize treatment of partners when women are diagnosed with gonorrhea, chlamydia, or trichomoniasis. Although evaluation and treatment of the partner or referral of the partner to his or her own clinician is preferred, the CDC recognizes that this is not always possible. The legal status of expedited partner therapy varies by state. The CDC has resources that can assist healthcare professionals in determining whether their state allows this practice (www.cdc.gov/std/ept/legal/default.htm).

Genital herpes

Genital herpes is caused by HSV type 1 and type 2. Transmission of the HSV occurs as a consequence of skin-to-skin genital contact. Most cases of genital herpes are caused by HSV2. The overall seroprevalence of HSV2 infection in the general US population is 16.2% of adults aged 14 to 49 years.[184] Most people infected with HSV2 do not have symptoms of primary infection and have not been diagnosed. Although HSV1 is the cause of an increasing proportion of genital herpes, it more commonly causes infections of the mouth and lips ("fever blisters"). Herpes simplex virus 1 infection of the genitals can be caused by oral-genital or by genital-genital contact. Anyone with a history of either type should be aware of the transmissibility of the infection through genital, oral, and anal contact, mainly when they have a herpes outbreak but through asymptomatic cervicovaginal shedding as well. Asymptomatic shedding occurs more often with HSV2 than with HSV1 infection.[185] Episodes of shedding are less common in women infected for longer than 1 year.

Genital herpes outbreaks usually start with a prodrome of burning, itching, and skin hypersensitivity. This is

| Table 6. | STI Screening Questions That Should Be Asked of Older Women |

1. *Partners:* Are you currently sexually active? In the past 12 months, how many partners have you had? Are your sex partners men, women, or both? Has your current partner(s) or any recent partners been diagnosed or treated for an STI?
2. *Practices:* What kind of sexual contact do you have, or have you had? Genital, anal, or oral contact?
3. *Protection:* Do you and your partner(s) use protection against STIs? If so, what kind of protection do you use? How often do you use this protection? If not, could you tell me the reason?
4. *Past history of sexually transmitted infections:* Have you been diagnosed with an STI in the past 2 years? When? How were you treated? Have you had any recurring symptoms?
5. *Prior screening:* Have you ever been screened for HIV? When? What was the result?

Abbreviations: HIV, human immunodeficiency virus; STI, sexually transmitted infection. US Department of Health and Human Services. Centers for Disease Control and Prevention.[179]

followed by the appearance of one or more vesicles or pustules on the vulva, perineum, or rectum. The pustules break, leaving tender ulcers that may require 2 to 3 weeks to heal with primary herpes and about 7 to 10 days with recurrent herpes. Other signs and symptoms of primary genital herpes may include flu-like symptoms, including fever, muscle aches, and inguinal lymphadenopathy.[186] Approximately 70% to 90% of those who have primary genital herpes will experience at least one recurrent outbreak, although recurrent outbreaks are less severe and of shorter duration in immunocompetent persons.[187] In some women, the first clinical episode is a recurrence because the primary infection was not recognized. Complications include an increased susceptibility to other STIs, including HIV.[188]

Diagnostic testing of suspicious lesions can be performed with a type-specific herpes culture or a polymerase chain reaction test of a sample taken from an active lesion. Based on these results, women can be counseled that recurrences are much less frequent for genital HSV1 infection than HSV22 infection. The USPSTF Force recommends against routine serologic screening for genital HSV infection in asymptomatic adolescents and adults, including those who are pregnant (D recommendation).[186] Select women who have had multiple sexual partners may benefit from serologic screening for HSV2 but only if they plan to protect themselves if seronegative (with the use of condoms) or their partners if seropositive (with daily antiviral drug suppressive therapy). Serologic testing for HSV2 also is helpful in the determination of serodiscordant couples. If one partner is known to be infected with herpes, the other can be tested. If the tested person is seronegative for HSV2 and therefore susceptible to infection, the infected partner can be given a daily suppressive dose of an antiviral medication (eg, acyclovir, valacyclovir, or famciclovir) to reduce the likelihood of horizontal transmission from the infected to the uninfected partner.[181]

There is no treatment that cures herpes, but initiation of antiviral medications during the earliest phase of an outbreak can shorten its duration. The CDC-recommended courses of antiviral drugs, including acyclovir, famciclovir, and valacyclovir, are given for 7 to 10 days for episodes of primary herpes and as 1-, 2-, 3-, or 5-day regimens for recurrent genital herpes.[181] In addition, daily suppressive regimens are suggested by the CDC to reduce the frequency of recurrences in those with six or more outbreaks a year

Hepatitis B

Hepatitis B is concentrated primarily in the blood but also is present to a lesser extent in semen, vaginal secretions, and wound exudates. In adults, the hepatitis B virus is transmitted primarily by percutaneous exposure to blood (eg, by injection-drug use) and sexual contact. Risk factors for sexual transmission in heterosexuals include having unprotected sex with an infected partner, having unprotected sex with more than one partner, and a history of another STI.[189] Although 90% of those infected at birth develop chronic hepatitis, less than 10% of those infected as adults will do so.[190] Acute hepatitis is self-limiting, whereas chronic hepatitis can result in cirrhosis and liver cancer.

The national strategy for control of hepatitis B is through vaccination, not through case finding. For this reason, routine hepatitis B serology screening of the general population or targeted screening based on sexual behaviors is not recommended. The USPSTF recommends screening for hepatitis B infection in persons at high risk for infection, defined as HIV-positive persons, injection-drug users, household contacts or sex partners of persons with hepatitis B virus infection, men who have sex with men, and immigrants from geographic regions with a hepatitis B surface antigen prevalence of 2% or higher.[191,192] Many perimenopausal and postmenopausal women may not have received the hepatitis B vaccination since its introduction in 1982 and therefore may be at risk for infection. Women with

multiple sexual partners (or who have other risk factors, such as needle sharing) who have not been vaccinated against hepatitis B should be advised to do so. Adults with diabetes and chronic liver disease should also be given the hepatitis B vaccine.

Hepatitis C

Hepatitis C is caused by a virus that attacks the liver, leading to inflammation.[193] Unlike hepatitis B, which may resolve spontaneously, most hepatitis C infections become chronic, incurring a risk of cirrhosis and liver cancer. Most people have no symptoms and do not know they are infected until liver damage is detected years later. Hepatitis C is passed mainly by blood contact and rarely through sexual contact. The most common mode of transmission is through sharing intravenous drug equipment. Routine screening of the blood supply was instituted in 1992, so women who received blood transfusions, blood products, or organ transplants or who were on kidney dialysis before 1992 may have acquired hepatitis C in this way.

Routine screening of all adults for hepatitis C is not recommended. However, "baby boomers" are at the highest risk of hepatitis C infection, with infection rates five times that of other birth cohorts.[193] In 2012, the CDC recommended that all adults born from 1945 to 1965 should receive one-time testing for hepatitis C without prior ascertainment of hepatitis C risk and that persons identified with hepatitis C infection should receive a brief alcohol screening and intervention, followed by referral to appropriate care services for hepatitis C infection.

HIV

Over the past 2 decades, new treatments for HIV infection have sharply reduced the number of AIDS cases and AIDS deaths in the United States. Because 16% of people infected with HIV don't know that they are infected, they miss opportunities for prompt treatment to delay or prevent progression to AIDS, as well as prevention of horizontal transmission of HIV to an uninfected partner.[181] For this reason, the CDC and the USPSTF recommend that adults aged between 15 and 65 years receive a one-time HIV screening, regardless of risk factors.[194] All persons who seek evaluation and treatment for STIs should be screened for HIV infection, as well as at the time of an STI diagnosis (eg, early syphilis, gonorrhea, and chlamydia) in populations at high risk for HIV infection.[181] Beyond this, targeted HIV screening is recommended for women who are past or present injection-drug users, are sex partners of injection-drug users, exchange sex for money or drugs, are sex partners of HIV-infected persons, have had sex with men who have sex with men since the most recent HIV test, and have had more than one sex partner since their most recent HIV test.[195] Persons at high risk for HIV infection should be screened for HIV at least annually.[195,196]

Little is known about HIV risk in older women; however, the potential for infection should not be underestimated. In 2015, 17% of new HIV infections in the United States occurred in persons aged 50 years and older.[175] Blacks accounted for an estimated 43% of all diagnoses in people aged 50 years and older; whites for 36%; and Hispanics/Latinos accounted for 17%. Forty percent of people aged 55 years and older were diagnosed with AIDS at the time of HIV diagnosis (ie, diagnosed late in the course of the infection).

Most labs now use fourth-generation HIV antigen/antibody combination test or a third-generation antibody immunoassay. The antigen/antibody test will become positive about 4 weeks earlier than the antibody immunoassay test and minimizes the "window period" after infection but before a positive test result. If a screen is repeatedly reactive, it is followed by a supplemental test (eg, an HIV1/HIV2 antibody differentiation assay, Western blot, or indirect immunofluorescence assay). Point-of-care rapid HIV tests (antibody only) also are available for use on saliva or blood, but their results must be confirmed with conventional methods.

Guidelines recommend antiretroviral therapy for all HIV-infected patients to reduce the risk of disease progression and transmission.[181,197,198] Given the complexities of using combinations of antiretroviral drugs, referral to an infectious-disease specialist or HIV-experienced primary care provider for management is appropriate. In combination with other proven HIV-prevention methods, preexposure prophylaxis may be a useful tool for women at the highest risk of HIV acquisition.[196]

A retrospective study performed in Brazil compared menopause symptoms in 537 women aged 40 to 60 years, 273 of whom were HIV-positive and 264 HIV-negative.[199] There was no difference in the prevalence of menopause symptoms in the seropositive and seronegative women. Another Brazilian study showed that early natural menopause was more frequent in the HIV-infected women and those with chronic hepatitis C virus infection.[200] It has been demonstrated that perimenopausal women with HIV may be at higher risk for depression; therefore, appropriate depression screening is indicated.[201]

Human papillomavirus

Human papillomavirus causes almost all cervical cancers, as well as some cancers of the vagina, vulva, penis, anus, rectum, and oropharynx. Human papillomavirus 16 and 18 are referred to as high-risk HPV, because infections with these strains are associated with long-term persistence and progression to preinvasive, and ultimately, invasive cervical lesions. By age 50, at least 80% of US women will have acquired genital HPV infection.[202] Most people with HPV will not have any symptoms and will clear the infection on their own. Low-risk HPVs (especially HPV 6 and 11) may cause genital warts or low-grade cervical lesions. Vaccination against HPV infections has been available in the United States since 2006, and CDC guidelines recommend routine vaccination of girls and women aged 9 through 26 years.[203] Although CDC guidelines have not yet changed, FDA expanded the approved use of the 9-valent vaccine (Gardasil 9) to include women and men aged 27 through 45 years.[204] (See also "Cervical Cancer" in Chapter 9.)

Syphilis

Syphilis, which is caused by the bacterium *Treponema pallidum*, is often called the "great imitator" because so many of its signs and symptoms are indistinguishable from those of other diseases. Many people infected with syphilis have no symptoms for years yet remain at risk for complications. The primary stage is usually marked by a single chancre, which heals within 3 to 6 weeks. Multiple chancres, skin rashes, and mucous membrane lesions characterize the second stage, followed by the latent stage when symptoms disappear. Untreated, death can result from progressive syphilitic infection.

Syphilis screening tests, the rapid plasma regain and Venereal Disease Research Laboratory, are nontreponemal tests used by most labs.[205] A positive screening test must be confirmed by a treponemal serum antibody test, either the microhemagglutination *Treponema pallidum* or the fluorescent treponemal antibody. Because of the possibility of false positives in the presence of certain medical conditions, women with reactive nontreponemal tests must have the diagnosis confirmed with a treponemal test.

Routine screening of women is not recommended because of the low incidence of syphilis in the general population. Targeted screening contact testing and coinfection testing all include testing for syphilis. The USPSTF recommends screening for syphilis infection in persons who are at increased risk for infection.[205] These include being HIV-positive, having a history of incarceration, a history of commercial sex work, and residing in a geographic area with high syphilis prevalence that is classified as a "hot spot." In primary, secondary, and early latent stages, syphilis can be cured with a single injection of benzathine penicillin. Three doses are needed to treat those infected for more than a year (late-latent stage) or tertiary syphilis. All patients diagnosed with syphilis should be screened for HIV infection.

Vaginal trichomoniasis

Vaginal trichomoniasis is the most common curable STI in sexually active women, and unlike other STIs, occurs equally in older and younger women.[206] Caused by the single-cell protozoan parasite *Trichomonas vaginalis*, trichomoniasis involves the vagina, the endocervix, and the urethra. Although initial transmission occurs sexually, untreated infection can last for months to years, and women should be counseled that *any* current or previous sex partner could have been the source of infection. About 5% of adult women have asymptomatic vaginal colonization. When women have symptoms, most have a yellow-green or gray vaginal discharge, vulvovaginal irritation and itching, a strong unpleasant odor, and sometimes discomfort during intercourse and urination. The diagnosis is confirmed with saline suspension, point-of-care tests, or nucleic acid testing.

CDC guidelines state that low-risk women should not be routinely screened for trichomoniasis but that periodic screening of women who are HIV positive should be considered.[181] Trichomoniasis is treated with either metronidazole or tinidazole, given by mouth as a single dose. Treatment of sex partners is important; up to 20% of patients will be reinfected within 3 months.

Bacterial vaginosis

In heterosexual relationships, BV is not sexually transmitted in the classic sense, but its acquisition is sexually associated. Although the cause is not fully understood, BV is associated with an imbalance in the vaginal bacterial flora in which the normal lactobacilli are replaced by *Gardnerella vaginalis* and other anaerobic bacteria.[181] The risk for BV increases by having a new sex partner or multiple sex partners and douching.

Symptoms of BV include a thin, white or gray vaginal discharge with a high pH and a strong fishy odor, but some women have no signs or symptoms. Complications for perimenopausal and postmenopausal women include an increased susceptibility to other STIs and PID. Bacterial vaginosis is diagnosed based on the four Amsel's criteria: a thin homogeneous white vaginal discharge that smoothly coats the vaginal walls, clue cells accounting for at least 20% of vaginal epithelial cells on microscopy of a saline suspension, vaginal fluid pH higher than 4.5,

and a positive "whiff" test (or amine test), defined as the release of a characteristic fishy odor after the addition of potassium hydroxide (10% KOH [potassium, oxygen, and hydrogen]) to a sample of the discharge.[207] Bacterial vaginosis also can also be diagnosed with point-of-care tests that use DNA probes to detect high concentrations of *G vaginalis*.

The CDC recommends treatment with vaginal or oral metronidazole or clindamycin vaginal cream.[181] Oral tinidazol and clindamycin orally or by vaginal ovules can be used as alternative regimens. No studies support the addition of any available lactobacillus formulations or probiotics as an adjunctive therapy in women with BV. Bacterial vaginosis recurs in up to 30% of cases, and repeated antibiotic courses may be required, or twice-weekly suppression metronidazole vaginal gel can be considered.[207]

REFERENCES

1. Murray CJ, Atkinson C, Bhalla K, et al; US Burden of Disease Collaborators. The state of US health, 1990-2010: burden of diseases, injuries, and risk factors. *JAMA*. 2013;310(6):591-608.

2. Watt FE. Hand osteoarthritis, menopause and menopausal hormone therapy. *Maturitas*. 2016;83:13-18.

3. Lugo L, Villalvilla A, Largo R, Herrero-Beaumont G, Roman-Blas JA. Selective estrogen receptor modulators (SERMs): new alternatives for osteoarthritis? *Maturitas*. 2014;77(4):380-384.

4. da Silva JA, Colville-Nash P, Spector TD, Scott DL, Willoughby DA. Inflammation-induced cartilage degradation in female rodents. Protective role of sex hormones. *Arthritis Rheum*. 1993;36(7):1007-1013.

5. Kavas A, Cagatay ST, Banerjee S, Keskin D, Tezcaner A. Potential of raloxifene in reversing osteoarthritis-like alterations in rat chondrocytes: an in vitro model study. *J Biosci*. 2013;38(1):135-147.

6. Turner AS, Athanasiou KA, Zhu CF, Alvis MR, Bryant HU. Biochemical effects of estrogen on articular cartilage in ovariectomized sheep. *Osteoarthritis Cartilage*. 1997;5(1):63-69.

7. Wluka AE, Davis SR, Bailey M, Stuckey SL, Cicuttini FM. Users of oestrogen replacement therapy have more knee cartilage than non-users. *Ann Rheum Dis*. 2001;60(4):332-336.

8. Sniekers YH, Weinans H, Bierma-Zeinstra SM, van Leeuwen JP, van Osch GJ. Animal models for osteoarthritis: the effect of ovariectomy and estrogen treatment—a systematic approach. *Osteoarthritis Cartilage*. 2008;16(5):533-541.

9. Karsdal MA, Bay-Jensen AC, Lories RJ, et al. The coupling of bone and cartilage turnover in osteoarthritis: opportunities for bone antiresorptives and anabolics as potential treatments? *Ann Rheum Dis*. 2014;73(2):336-348.

10. Carbone LD, Nevitt MC, Wildy K, et al; Health, Aging and Body Composition Study. The relationship of antiresorptive drug use to structural findings and symptoms of knee osteoarthritis. *Arthritis Rheum*. 2004;50(11):3516-3525.

11. Ham KD, Carlson CS. Effects of estrogen replacement therapy on bone turnover in subchondral bone and epiphyseal metaphyseal cancellous bone of ovariectomized cynomolgus monkeys. *J Bone Miner Res*. 2004;19(5):823-829.

12. Bijlsma JW, Berenbaum F, Lafeber FP. Osteoarthritis: an update with relevance for clinical practice. *Lancet*. 2011;377(9783):2115-2126.

13. Christgau S, Tankó LB, Cloos PA, et al. Suppression of elevated cartilage turnover in postmenopausal women and in ovariectomized rats by estrogen and a selective estrogen-receptor modulator (SERM). *Menopause*. 2004;11(5):508-518.

CHAPTER 6

14. Karsdal MA, Bay-Jensen AC, Henriksen K, Christiansen C. The pathogenesis of osteoarthritis involves bone, cartilage and synovial inflammation: may estrogen be a magic bullet? *Menopause Int*. 2012;18(4):139-146.

15. Yoshida A, Morihara T, Matsuda K, et al. Immunohistochemical analysis of the effects of estrogen on intraarticular neurogenic inflammation in a rat anterior cruciate ligament transection model of osteoarthritis. *Connect Tissue Res*. 2012;53(3):197-206.

16. Dawson-Basoa ME, Gintzler AR. Estrogen and progesterone activate spinal kappa-opiate receptor analgesic mechanisms. *Pain*. 1996;64(3):608-615.

17. Vincent K, Warnaby C, Stagg CJ, Moore J, Kennedy S, Tracey I. Brain imaging reveals that engagement of descending inhibitory pain pathways in healthy women in a low endogenous estradiol state varies with testosterone. *Pain*. 2013;154(4):515-524.

18. Smith YR, Stohler CS, Nichols TE, Bueller JA, Koeppe RA, Zubieta JK. Pronociceptive and antinociceptive effects of estradiol through endogenous opioid neurotransmission in women. *J Neurosci*. 2006;26(21):5777-5785.

19. Burmester GR, Pope JE. Novel treatment strategies in rheumatoid arthritis. *Lancet*. 2017;389(10086):2338-2348.

20. Murphy L, Schwartz TA, Helmick CG, et al. Lifetime risk of symptomatic knee osteoarthritis. *Arthritis Rheum*. 2008;59(9):1207-1213.

21. Losina E, Paltiel AD, Weinstein AM, et al. Lifetime medical costs of knee osteoarthritis management in the United States: impact of extending indications for total knee arthroplasty. *Arthritis Care Res*. 2015;67(2):203-215.

22. Kurtz S, Ong K, Lau E, Mowat F, Halpern M. Projections of primary and revision hip and knee arthroplasty in the United States from 2005 to 2030. *J Bone Joint Surg Am*. 2007;89(4):780-785.

23. Nicholls E, Thomas E, van der Windt DA, Croft PR, Peat G. Pain trajectory groups in persons with, or at high risk of, knee osteoarthritis: findings from the Knee Clinical Assessment Study and the Osteoarthritis Initiative. *Osteoarthritis Cartilage*. 2014;22(12):2041-2050.

24. Glyn-Jones S, Palmer AJ, Agricola R, et al. Osteoarthritis. *Lancet*. 2015;386(9991):376-387.

25. Ma HL, Blanchet TJ, Peluso D, Hopkins B, Morris EA, Glasson SS. Osteoarthritis severity is sex dependent in a surgical mouse model. *Osteoarthritis Cartilage*. 2007;15(6):695-700.

26. Spector TD, MacGregor AJ. Risk factors for osteoarthritis: genetics. *Osteoarthritis Cartilage*. 2004;12(suppl A):39-44.

27. Loughlin J. Genetic contribution to osteoarthritis development: current state of evidence. *Current Opin Rheumatol*. 2015;27(3):284-288.

28. Prieto-Alhambra D, Judge A, Javaid MK, Cooper C, Diez-Perez A, Arden NK. Incidence and risk factors for clinically diagnosed knee, hip and hand osteoarthritis: influences of age, gender and osteoarthritis affecting other joints. *Ann Rheum Dis*. 2014;73(9):1659-1664.

29. Cecil RL, Archer BH. Arthritis of the menopause: a study of fifty cases. *JAMA*. 1925;84(2):75-79.

30. Punzi L, Ramonda R, Sfriso P. Erosive osteoarthritis. *Best Pract Research Clin Rheumatol*. 2004;18(5):739-758.

31. Zhang W, Moskowitz RW, Nuki G, et al. OARSI recommendations for the management of hip and knee osteoarthritis, Part II: OARSI evidence-based, expert consensus guidelines. *Osteoarthritis Cartilage*. 2008;16(2):137-162.

32. Zhang W, Nuki G, Moskowitz RW, et al. OARSI recommendations for the management of hip and knee osteoarthritis: part III: Changes in evidence following systematic cumulative update of research published through January 2009. *Osteoarthritis Cartilage*. 2010;18(4):476-499.

33. Conaghan PG, Dickson J, Grant RL; Guideline Development Group. Care and management of osteoarthritis in adults: summary of NICE guidance. *BMJ*. 2008;336(7642):502-503.

34. Fernandes L, Hagen KB, Bijlsma JW, et al; European League Against Rheumatism (EULAR). EULAR recommendations for the non-pharmacological core management of hip and knee osteoarthritis. *Ann Rheum Dis*. 2013;72(7):1125-1135.

35. Watt FE, Gulati M. New drug treatments for osteoarthritis: what is on the horizon? *EMJ*. 2017;2(1):50-58.

36. Smolen JS, Aletaha D, McInnes IB. Rheumatoid arthritis. *Lancet*. 2016;388(10055):2023-2038. Erratum in: *Lancet*. 2016; 388(10055):1984.

37. Carmona L, Cross M, Williams B, Lassere M, March L. Rheumatoid arthritis. *Best Pract Res Clin Rheumatol*. 2010;24(6):733-745.

38. Potempa J, Mydel P, Koziel J. The case for periodontitis in the pathogenesis of rheumatoid arthritis. *Nat Rev Rheumatol*. 2017;13(10):606-620.

39. Mahdi H, Fisher BA, Kallberg H, et al. Specific interaction between genotype, smoking and autoimmunity to citrullinated alpha-enolase in the etiology of rheumatoid arthritis. *Nat Genet*. 2009;41(12):1319-1324.

40. Salliot C, Bombardier C, Saraux A, Combe B, Dougados M. Hormonal replacement therapy may reduce the risk for RA in women with early arthritis who carry HLA-DRB1 *01 and/or *04 alleles by protecting against the production of anti-CCP: results from the ESPOIR cohort. *Ann Rheum Dis*. 2010;69(9):1683-1686.

41. Williams RO, Feldmann M, Maini RN. Cartilage destruction and bone erosion in arthritis: the role of tumour necrosis factor alpha. *Ann Rheum Dis*. 2000;59(suppl 1):i75-i80.

42. Smolen JS, Aletaha D, Barton A, et al. Rheumatoid arthritis. *Nat Rev Dis Primers*. 2018;4:18001.

43. Wegner N, Lundberg K, Kinloch A, et al. Autoimmunity to specific citrullinated proteins gives the first clues to the etiology of rheumatoid arthritis. *Immunol Rev*. 2010;233(1):34-54.

44. Tan YK, Conaghan PG. Imaging in rheumatoid arthritis. *Best Pract Res Clin Rheumatol*. 2011;25(4):569-584.

45. Castañeda S, González-Juanatey C, González-Gay MA. Sex and cardiovascular involvement in inflammatory joint diseases [published online ahead of print August 29, 2017]. *Clin Rev Allergy Immunol*.

46. Monaco C, Nanchahal J, Taylor P, Feldmann M. Anti-TNF therapy: past, present and future. *Int Immunol*. 2015;27(1):55-62.

47. Walitt B, Pettinger M, Weinstein A, et al; Women's Health Investigators. Effects of postmenopausal hormone therapy on rheumatoid arthritis: the Women's Health Initiative randomized controlled trials. *Arthritis Rheum*. 2008;59(3):302-310.

48. Holroyd CR, Edwards CJ. The effects of hormone replacement therapy on autoimmune disease: rheumatoid arthritis and systemic lupus erythematosus. *Climacteric*. 2009;12(5):378-386.

49. Sieper J, Poddubnyy D. Axial spondyloarthritis. *Lancet*. 2017; 390(10089):73-84.

50. Strand V, Singh JA. Evaluation and management of the patient with suspected inflammatory spine disease. *Mayo Clin Proc*. 2017;92(4):555-564.

51. Mortezavi M, Thiele R, Ritchlin C. The joint in psoriatic arthritis. *Clin Exp Rheumatol*. 2015;33(5 suppl 93):S20-S25.

52. Dalbeth N, Merriman TR, Stamp LK. Gout. *Lancet*. 2016; 388(10055):2039-2052.

53. So AK, Martinon F. Inflammation in gout: mechanisms and therapeutic targets. *Nat Rev Rheumatol*. 2017;13(11):639-647.

54. Hamburger M, Baraf HS, Adamson TC 3rd, et al. 2011 recommendations for the diagnosis and management of gout and hyperuricemia. *Phys Sportsmed*. 2011;39(4):98-123.

55. Kydd AS, Seth R, Buchbinder R, Edwards CJ, Bombardier C. Uricosuric medications for chronic gout. *Cochrane Database Syst Rev*. 2014;(11): CD010457.

56. Molloy ES, McCarthy GM. Calcium crystal deposition diseases: update on pathogenesis and manifestations. *Rheum Dis Clin North Am*. 2006;32(2):383-400, vii.

57. Rubinow DR, Johnson SL, Schmidt PJ, Girdler S, Gaynes B. Efficacy of estradiol in perimenopausal depression: so much promise and so few answers. *Depress Anxiety*. 2015;32(8):539-549.

58. Lokuge S, Frey BN, Foster JA, Soares CN, Steiner M. Depression in women: windows of vulnerability and new insights into the link between estrogen and serotonin. *J Clin Psychiatry*. 2011;72(11): e1563-e1569.

59. Wittchen H-U, Becker E, Lieb R, Krause P. Prevalence, incidence and stability of premenstrual dysphoric disorder in the community. *Psychol Med.* 2002;32(1):119-132.

60. Bloch M, Rotenberg N, Koren D, Klein E. Risk factors for early postpartum depressive symptoms. *Gen Hosp Psychiatry.* 2006;28(1):3-8.

61. Yonkers KA, O'Brien PM, Eriksson E. Premenstrual syndrome. *Lancet.* 2008;371(9619):1200-1210.

62. Nelson HD. Menopause. *Lancet.* 2008;371(9614):760-770.

63. Joffe H, Massler A, Sharkey KM. Evaluation and management of sleep disturbance during the menopause transition. *Semin Reprod Med.* 2010;28(5):404-421.

64. Pérez-López FR, Pérez-Roncero G, Fernández-Iñarrea J, Fernández-Alonso AM, Chedraui P, Llaneza P; MARIA (MenopAuse RIsk Assessment) Research Group. Resilience, depressed mood, and menopausal symptoms in postmenopausal women. *Menopause.* 2014;21(2):159-164.

65. Bromberger JT, Harlow S, Avis N, Kravitz HM, Cordal A. Racial/ethnic differences in the prevalence of depressive symptoms among middle-aged women: The Study of Women's Health Across the Nation (SWAN). *Am J Public Health.* 2004;94(8):1378-1385.

66. Soares CN. Depression and menopause: current knowledge and clinical recommendations for a critical window. *Psychiatr Clin North Am.* 2017;40(2):239-254.

67. Schmidt PJ, Haq N, Rubinow DR. A longitudinal evaluation of the relationship between reproductive status and mood in perimenopausal women. *Am J Psychiatry.* 2004;161(12):2238-2244.

68. Bromberger JT, Kravitz HM, Chang YF, Cyranowski JM, Brown C, Matthews KA. Major depression during and after the menopausal transition: Study of Women's Health Across the Nation (SWAN). *Psychol Med.* 2011;41(9):1879-1888.

69. Freeman EW, Sammel MD, Boorman DW, Zhang R. Longitudinal pattern of depressive symptoms around natural menopause. *JAMA Psychiatry.* 2014;71(1):36-43.

70. Woods NF, Smith-DiJulio K, Percival DB, Tao EY, Mariella A, Mitchell S. Depressed mood during the menopausal transition and early postmenopause: observations from the Seattle Midlife Women's Health Study. *Menopause.* 2008;15(2):223-232.

71. Cohen LS, Soares CN, Vitonis AF, Otto MW, Harlow BL. Risk for new onset of depression during the menopausal transition: the Harvard study of moods and cycles. *Arch Gen Psychiatry.* 2006;63(4):385-390.

72. Bromberger JT, Kravitz HM, Matthews K, Youk A, Brown C, Feng W. Predictors of first lifetime episodes of major depression in midlife women. *Psychol Med.* 2009;39(1):55-64.

73. Kessler RC, McGonagle KA, Zhao S, et al. Lifetime and 12-month prevalence of DSM-III-R psychiatric disorders in the United States. Results from the National Comorbidity Survey. *Arch Gen Psychiatry.* 1994;51(1):8-19.

74. Joffe H, Chang Y, Dhaliwal S, et al. Lifetime history of depression and anxiety disorders as a predictor of quality of life in midlife women in the absence of current illness episodes. *Arch Gen Psychiatry.* 2012;69(5):484-492.

75. Calkins AW, Otto MW, Cohen LS, et al. Psychosocial predictors of the onset of anxiety disorders in women: results from a prospective 3-year longitudinal study. *J Anxiety Disord.* 2009;23(8):1165-1169.

76. Bromberger JT, Kravitz HM, Chang Y, et al. Does risk for anxiety increase during the menopausal transition? Study of Women's Health Across the Nation. *Menopause.* 2013;20(5):488-495.

77. Davison SN, Jhangri GS. The impact of chronic pain on depression, sleep, and the desire to withdraw from dialysis in hemodialysis patients. *J Pain Symptom Manage.* 2005;30(5):465-473.

78. McCall WV, Reboussin BA, Cohen W. Subjective measurement of insomnia and quality of life in depressed inpatients. *J Sleep Res.* 2000;9(1):43-48.

79. Joffe H, Soares CN, Thurston RC, White DP, Cohen LS, Hall JE. Depression is associated with worse objectively and subjectively measured sleep, but not more frequent awakenings, in women with vasomotor symptoms. *Menopause.* 2009;16(4):671-679.

80. Morrison JH, Brinton RD, Schmidt PJ, Gore AC. Estrogen, menopause, and the aging brain: how basic neuroscience can inform hormone therapy in women. *J Neurosci.* 2006;26(41):10332-10348.

81. Gundlah C, Lu NZ, Bethea CL. Ovarian steroid regulation of monoamine oxidase-A and -B mRNAs in the macaque dorsal raphe and hypothalamic nuclei. *Psychopharmacology (Berl).* 2002;160(3):271-282.

82. Bethea CL, Mirkes SJ, Su A, Michelson D. Effects of oral estrogen, raloxifene and arzoxifene on gene expression in serotonin neurons of macaques. *Psychoneuroendocrinology.* 2002;27(4):431-445.

83. Hiroi R, McDevitt RA, Neumaier JF. Estrogen selectively increases tryptophan hydroxylase-2 mRNA expression in distinct subregions of rat midbrain raphe nucleus: association between gene expression and anxiety behavior in the open field. *Biol Psychiatry.* 2006;60(3):288-295.

84. Srivastava DP, Woolfrey KM, Evans PD. Mechanisms underlying the interactions between rapid estrogenic and BDNF control of synaptic connectivity. *Neuroscience.* 2013;239:17-33.

85. Schmidt PJ, Ben Dor R, Martinez PE, et al. Effects of estradiol withdrawal on mood in women with past perimenopausal depression: a randomized clinical trial. *JAMA Psychiatry.* 2015;72(7):714-726.

86. Soares CN, Poitras JR, Prouty J, Alexander AB, Shifren JL, Cohen LS. Efficacy of citalopram as a monotherapy or as an adjunctive treatment to estrogen therapy for perimenopausal and postmenopausal women with depression and vasomotor symptoms. *J Clin Psychiatry.* 2003;64(4):473-479.

87. Soares CN, Arsenio H, Joffe H, et al. Escitalopram versus ethinyl estradiol and norethindrone acetate for symptomatic peri- and postmenopausal women: impact on depression, vasomotor symptoms, sleep, and quality of life. *Menopause.* 2006;13(5):780-786.

88. Joffe H, Soares CN, Petrillo LF, et al. Treatment of depression and menopause-related symptoms with the serotonin-norepinephrine reuptake inhibitor duloxetine. *J Clin Psychiatry.* 2007;68(6):943-950.

89. Joffe H, Groninger H, Soares CN, Nonacs R, Cohen LS. An open trial of mirtazapine in menopausal women with depression unresponsive to estrogen replacement therapy. *J Womens Health Gend Based Med.* 2001;10(10):999-1004.

90. Entsuah AR, Huang H, Thase ME. Response and remission rates in different subpopulations with major depressive disorder administered venlafaxine, selective serotonin reuptake inhibitors, or placebo. *J Clin Psychiatry.* 2001;62(11):869-877.

91. Soares CN, Thase ME, Clayton A, et al. Desvenlafaxine and escitalopram for the treatment of postmenopausal women with major depressive disorder. *Menopause.* 2010;17(4):700-711.

92. Soares CN, Kornstein SG, Thase ME, Jiang Q, Guico-Pabia CJ. Assessing the efficacy of desvenlafaxine for improving functioning and well-being outcome measures in patients with major depressive disorder: a pooled analysis of 9 double-blind, placebo-controlled, 8-week clinical trials. *J Clin Psychiatry* 2009;70(10):1365-1371.

93. Kornstein SG, Jiang Q, Reddy S, Musgnung JJ, Guico-Pabia CJ. Short-term efficacy and safety of desvenlafaxine in a randomized, placebo-controlled study of perimenopausal and postmenopausal women with major depressive disorder. *J Clin Psychiatry.* 2010;71(8):1088-1096.

94. Soares CN, Frey BN, Haber E, Steiner M. A pilot, 8-week, placebo lead-in trial of quetiapine extended release for depression in midlife women: impact on mood and menopause-related symptoms. *J Clin Psychopharmacol.* 2010;30(5):612-615.

95. Frey BN, Haber E, Mendes GC, Steiner M, Soares CN. Effects of quetiapine extended release on sleep and quality of life in midlife women with major depressive disorder. *Arch Womens Ment Health.* 2013;16(1):83-85.

96. Freeman MP, Cheng LJ, Moustafa D, et al. Vortioxetine for major depressive disorder, vasomotor, and cognitive symptoms associated with the menopausal transition. *Ann Clin Psychiatry.* 2017;29(4):249-257.

97. Soares CN, Almeida OP, Joffe H, Cohen LS. Efficacy of estradiol for the treatment of depressive disorders in perimenopausal women: a double-blind, placebo-controlled trial. *Arch Gen Psychiatry.* 2001;58(6):529-534.

98. Schmidt PJ, Nieman L, Danaceau MA, et al. Estrogen replacement in perimenopause-related depression: a preliminary report. *Am J Obstet Gynecol*. 2000;183(2):414-420.

99. Rasgon NL, Altshuler LL, Fairbanks L. Estrogen-replacement therapy for depression. *Am J Psychiatry*. 2001;158(10):1738.

100. Cohen LS, Soares CN, Poitras JR, Prouty J, Alexander AB, Shifren JL. Short-term use of estradiol for depression in perimenopausal and postmenopausal women: a preliminary report. *Am J Psychiatry*. 2003;160(8):1519-1522.

101. Schneider LS, Small GW, Clary CM. Estrogen replacement therapy and antidepressant response to sertraline in older depressed women. *Am J Geriatr Psychiatry*. 2001;9(4):393-399.

102. Morrison MF, Kallan MJ, Ten Have T, Katz I, Tweedy K, Battistini M. Lack of efficacy of estradiol for depression in postmenopausal women: a randomized, controlled trial. *Biol Psychiatry*. 2004;55(4):406-412.

103. Rudolph I, Palombo-Kinne E, Kirsch B, Mellinger U, Breitbarth H, Gräser T. Influence of a continuous combined HRT (2 mg estradiol valerate and 2 mg dienogest) on postmenopausal depression. *Climacteric*. 2004;7(3):301-311.

104. Joffe H, Petrillo LF, Koukopoulos A, et al. Increased estradiol and improved sleep, but not hot flashes, predict enhanced mood during the menopausal transition. *J Clin Endocrinol Metab*. 2011;96(7):E1044-E1054.

105. Santoro N, Teal S, Gavito C, Cano S, Chosich J, Sheeder J. Use of a levonorgestrel-containing intrauterine system with supplemental estrogen improves symptoms in perimenopausal women: a pilot study. *Menopause*. 2015;22(12):1301-1307.

106. Almeida OP, Lautenschlager NT, Vasikaran S, Leedman P, Gelavis A, Flicker L. A 20-week randomized controlled trial of estradiol replacement therapy for women aged 70 years and older: effect on mood, cognition and quality of life. *Neurobiol Aging*. 2006;27(1):141-149.

107. Soares CN. Mood disorders in midlife women: understanding the critical window and its clinical implications. *Menopause*. 2014;21(2):198-206.

108. Gordon JL, Rubinow DR, Eisenlohr-Moul TA, Xia K, Schmidt PJ, Girdler SS. Efficacy of transdermal estradiol and micronized progesterone in the prevention of depressive symptoms in the menopause transition: a randomized clinical trial. *JAMA Psychiatry*. 2018;75(2):149-157.

109. Saletu B, Brandstätter N, Metka M, et al. Double-blind, placebo-controlled, hormonal, syndromal and EEG mapping studies with transdermal oestradiol therapy in menopausal depression. *Psychopharmacology (Berl)*. 1995;122(4):321-329.

110. Dorsey CM, Lee KA, Scharf MB. Effect of zolpidem on sleep in women with perimenopausal and postmenopausal insomnia: a 4-week, randomized, multicenter, double-blind, placebo-controlled study. *Clin Ther*. 2004;26(10):1578-1586.

111. Boyle GJ, Murrihy R. A preliminary study of hormone replacement therapy and psychological mood states in perimenopausal women. *Psychol Rep*. 2001;88(1):160-170.

112. Gambacciani M, Ciaponi M, Cappagli B, et al. Effects of low-dose, continuous combined estradiol and noretisterone acetate on menopausal quality of life in early postmenopausal women. *Maturitas*. 2003;44(2):157-163.

113. Haines CJ, Yim SF, Chung TK, et al. A prospective, randomized, placebo-controlled study of the dose effect of oral oestradiol on menopausal symptoms, psychological well being, and quality of life in postmenopausal Chinese women. *Maturitas*. 2003;44(3):207-214.

114. Freeman MP, Hibbeln JR, Silver M, et al. Omega-3 fatty acids for major depressive disorder associated with the menopausal transition: a preliminary open trial. *Menopause*. 2011;18(3):279-284.

115. Masoumi SZ, Kazemi F, Tavakolian S, et al. Effect of citalopram in combination with omega-3 on depression in post-menopausal women: a triple blind randomized controlled trial. *J Clin Diagn Res*. 2016;10(10):QC01-QC05.

116. Sowers M, Luborsky J, Perdue C, Araujo KL, Goldman MB; SWAN. Thyroid stimulating hormone (TSH) concentrations and menopausal status in women at the mid-life: SWAN. *Clin Endocrinol (Oxf)*. 2003;58(3):340-347.

117. Hollowell JG, Staehling NW, Flanders WD, et al. Serum TSH, and thyroid antibodies in the United States population (1988 to 1994): National Health and Nutrition Examination Survey (NHANES III). *J Clin Endocrinol Metab*. 2002;87(2):489-499.

118. Garber JR, Cobin RH, Gharib H, et al; American Association of Clinical Endocrinologists and American Thyroid Association Taskforce on Hypothyroidism in Adults. Clinical practice guidelines for hypothyroidism in adults: cosponsored by the American Association of Clinical Endocrinologists and the American Thyroid Association. *Endocr Pract*. 2012;18(6):988-1028. Erratum in: *Endocr Pract*. 2013;19(1):175.

119. LeFevre ML; US Preventive Services Task Force. Screening for thyroid dysfunction: US Preventive Services Task Force recommendation statement. *Ann Intern Med*. 2015;162(9):641-650.

120. Biondi B, Wartofsky L. Treatment with thyroid hormone. *Endocr Rev*. 2014;35(3):433-512.

121. Chaker L, Bianco AC, Jonklaas J, Peeters RP. Hypothyroidism. *Lancet*. 2017;390(10101):1550-1562.

122. National Institute of Diabetes and Digestive and Kidney Diseases. *Hypothyroidism (Underactive Thyroid)*. National Institutes of Health. NIH Publication No. 13-6180. August 2016. www.niddk.nih.gov/health-information/endocrine-diseases/hypothyroidism. Accessed June 7, 2019.

123. Beck-Peccoz P, Rodari G, Giavoli C, Lania A. Central hypothyroidism—a neglected thyroid disorder. *Nat Rev Endocrinol*. 2017;13(10):588-598.

124. Persani L. Clinical review: central hypothyroidism: pathogenic, diagnostic, and therapeutic challenges. *J Clin Endocrinol Metab*. 2012;97(9):3068-3078.

125. Cooper DS, Biondi B. Subclinical thyroid disease. *Lancet*. 2012; 379(9821):1142-1154.

126. Aggarwal N, Razvi S. Thyroid and aging or the aging thyroid? An evidence-based analysis of the literature. *J Thyroid Res*. 2013;2013:481287.

127. Jonklaas J, Bianco AC, Bauer AJ, et al; Thyroid Association Task Force on Thyroid Hormone Replacement. Guidelines for the treatment of hypothyroidism: prepared by the American Thyroid Association Task Force on Thyroid Hormone Replacement. *Thyroid*. 2014;24(12):1670-1751.

128. Tahboub R, Arafah BM. Sex steroids and the thyroid. *Best Pract Res Clin Endocrinol Metab*. 2009;23(6):769-780.

129. Shifren J, Desindes S, McIlwain M, Doros G, Mazer NA. A randomized, open-label, crossover study comparing the effects of oral versus transdermal estrogen therapy on serum androgens, thyroid hormones, and adrenal hormones in naturally menopausal women. *Menopause*. 2007;14(6):985-994.

130. Peeters RP. Subclinical hypothyroidism. *N Engl J Med*. 2017; 376(26):2556-2565.

131. Taylor PN, Razvi S, Pearce SH, Dayan CM. Clinical review: a review of the clinical consequences of variation in thyroid function within the reference range. *J Clin Endocrinol Metab*. 2013;98(9):3562-3571.

132. Jabbar A, Pingitore A, Pearce SH, Zaman A, Lervasi G, Razvi S. Thyroid hormones and cardiovascular disease. *Nat Rev Cardiol*. 2017;14(1):39-55.

133. Hyland KA, Arnold AM, Lee JS, Cappola AR. Persistent subclinical hypothyroidism and cardiovascular risk in the elderly: the Cardiovascular Health Study. *J Clin Endocrinol Metab*. 2013;98(2):533-540.

134. Pasqualetti G, Tognini S, Polini A, Caraccio N, Monazni F. Is subclinical hypothyroidism a cardiovascular risk factor in the elderly? *J Clin Endocrinol Metab*. 2013;98(6):2256-2266.

135. LeGrys VA, Funk MJ, Lorenz CE, et al. Subclinical hypothyroidism and risk for incident myocardial infarction among postmenopausal women. *J Clin Endocrinol Metab*. 2013;98(6):2308-2317.

136. Rodondi N, den Elzen WP, Bauer DC, et al; Thyroid Studies Collaboration. Subclinical hypothyroidism and the risk of coronary heart disease and mortality. *JAMA*. 2010;304(12):1365-1374.

137. Rigge JB, Bougatsos C, Chou R. Screening and treatment of thyroid dysfunction: an evidence review for the US Preventive Services Task Force. *Ann Intern Med*. 2015;162(1):35-45.

138. Stott DJ, Rodondi N, Kearney PM, et al; TRUST Study Group. Thyroid hormone therapy for older adults with subclinical hypothyroidism. *N Engl J Med.* 2017;376(26):2534-2544.

139. Razvi S, Weaver JU, Butler TJ, Pearce SH. Levothyroxine treatment of subclinical hypothyroidism, fatal and nonfatal cardiovascular events, and mortality. *Arch Intern Med.* 2012;172(10):811-817.

140. Ross DS, Burch HB, Cooper DS, et al. 2016 American Thyroid Association Guidelines for diagnosis and management of hyperthyroidism and other causes of thyrotoxicosis. *Thyroid.* 2016;26(10):1343-1421.

141. Biondi B, Cooper DS. Subclinical hyperthyroidism. *N Engl J Med.* 2018;378(25):2411-2419.

142. Collet TH, Gussekloo J, Bauer DC, et al; Thyroid Studies Collaboration. Subclinical hyperthyroidism and the risk of coronary heart disease and mortality. *Arch Intern Med.* 2012;172(10):799-809.

143. Bauer DC, Ettinger B, Nevitt MC, Stone KL; Study of Osteoporotic Fractures Research Group. Risk for fracture in women with low serum levels of thyroid-stimulating hormone. *Ann Intern Med.* 2001;134(7):561-568.

144. Surks MI, Ortiz E, Daniels GH, et al. Subclinical thyroid disease: scientific review and guidelines for diagnosis and management. *JAMA.* 2004;291(2):228-238.

145. Blum MR, Bauer DC, Collet TH, et al; Thyroid Studies Collaboration. Subclinical thyroid dysfunction and fracture risk: a meta-analysis. *JAMA.* 2015;313(20):2055-2065.

146. Aubert CE, Floriani C, Bauer DC, et al; Thyroid Studies Collaboration. Thyroid function tests in the reference range and fracture: individual participant analysis of prospective cohorts. *J Clin Endocrinol Metab.* 2017;102(8):2719-2718.

147. Leader A, Ayzenfeld RH, Lishner M, Cohen E, Segev D, Hermoni D. Thyrotropin levels within the lower normal range are associated with an increased risk of hip fractures in euthyroid women, but not men, over the age of 65 years. *J Clin Endocrinol Metab.* 2014;99(8):2665-2673.

148. Greenspan SL, Greenspan FS. The effect of thyroid hormone on skeletal integrity. *Ann Intern Med.* 1999;130(9):750-758.

149. Haugen BR, Alexander EK, Bible KC, et al. 2015 American Thyroid Association Management Guidelines for Adult Patients with Thyroid Nodules and Differentiated Thyroid Cancer: The American Thyroid Association Guidelines Task Force on Thyroid Nodules and Differentiated Thyroid Cancer. *Thyroid.* 2016;26(1):1-133.

150. Gharib H, Papini E Garber JR, et al; AACE/ACE/AME Task Force on Thyroid Nodules. American Association of Clinical Endocrinologists, American College of Endocrinology, and Associazione Medici Endocrinologi Medical Guidelines for Clinical Practice for the Diagnosis and Management of Thyroid Nodules—2016 Update. *Endocr Pract.* 2016;22(5):622-639.

151. US Preventive Services Task Force, Bibbins-Domingo K, Grossman DC, Curry SJ, et al. Screening for thyroid cancer: US Preventive Services Task Force Recommendation Statement. *JAMA.* 2017;317(18):1882-1887.

152. Lin JS, Bowles EJA, Williams SB, Morrison CC. Screening for thyroid cancer: updated evidence report and systematic review for the US Preventive Services Task Force. *JAMA.* 2017;317(18):1888-1903.

153. Stinton LM, Shaffer EA. Epidemiology of gallbladder disease: cholelithiasis and cancer. *Gut Liver.* 2012;6(2):172-187.

154. Shaffer EA. Epidemiology and risk factors for gallstone disease: has the paradigm changed in the 21st century? *Curr Gastroenterol Rep.* 2005;7(2):132-140.

155. Everhart JE, Khare M, Hill M, Maurer KR. Prevalence and ethnic differences in gallbladder disease in the United States. *Gastroenterology.*1999;117(3):632-639.

156. Everhart JE. Gallstones and ethnicity in the Americas. *J Assoc Acad Minor Phys.* 2001;12(3):137-143.

157. O'Neill CJ, Gillies DM, Gani JS. Choledocholithiasis: overdiagnosed endoscopically and undertreated laparoscopically. *ANZ J Surg.* 2008;78(6):487-491.

158. Prat F, Meduri B, Ducot B, Chiche R, Salimbeni-Bartolini R, Pelletier G. Prediction of common bile duct stones by noninvasive tests. *Ann Surg.* 1999;229(3):362-368.

159. Collins C, Maguire D, Ireland A, Fitzgerald E, O'Sullivan GC. A prospective study of common bile duct calculi in patients undergoing laparoscopic cholecystectomy: natural history of choledocholithiasis revisited. *Ann Surg.* 2004;239(1):28-33.

160. Sieron D, Czerny B, Sieron-Stoltny K, et al. The effect of chronic estrogen application on bile and gallstone composition in women with cholelithiasis. *Minerva Endocrinol.* 2016;41(1):19-27.

161. Wang HH, Liu M, Clegg DJ, Portincasa P, Wang DQ. New insights into the molecular mechanisms underlying effects of estrogen on cholesterol gallstone formation. *Biochem Biophys Acta.* 2009;1791(11):1037-1047.

162. Everson GT, McKinley C, Kern F Jr. Mechanisms of gallstone formation in women. Effects of exogenous estrogen (Premarin) and dietary cholesterol on hepatic lipid metabolism. *J Clin Invest.* 1991;87(1):237-246.

163. Cirillo DJ, Wallace RB, Rodabough RJ, et al. Effect of estrogen therapy on gallbladder disease. *JAMA.* 2005;293(3):330-339.

164. Marjoribanks J, Farquhar C, Roberts H, Lethaby A. Long-term hormone therapy for perimenopausal and postmenopausal women. *Cochrane Database System Rev.* 2012;1:CD004143.

165. Simonsen MH, Erichsen R, Frøslev T, Rungby J, Sørensen HT. Postmenopausal estrogen therapy and risk of gallstone disease: a population-based case-control study. *Drug Saf.* 2013;36(12):1189-1197.

166. Talseth A, Ness-Jensen E, Edna TH, Hveem K. Risk factors for requiring cholecystectomy for gallbladder disease in a prospective population-based cohort study. *Br J Surg.* 2016;103(10):1350-1357.

167. Santen RJ, Allred DC, Ardoin SP, et al; Endocrine Society. Postmenopausal hormone therapy: an Endocrine Society scientific statement. *J Clin Endocrinol Metab.* 2010;95(7 suppl 1):S1-S66.

168. Manson JE, Chlebowski RT, Stefanick ML, et al. Menopausal hormone therapy and health outcomes during the intervention and extended poststopping phases of the Women's Health Initiative randomized trials. *JAMA.* 2013;310(13):1353-1368.

169. Liu B, Beral V, Balkwill A, Green J, Sweetland S, Reeves G; Million Women Study Collaborators. Gallbladder disease and use of transdermal versus oral hormone replacement therapy in postmenopausal women: prospective cohort study. *BMJ.* 2008;337:a386.

170. Uhler ML, Marks JW, Voigt BJ, Judd HL. Comparison of the impact of transdermal versus oral estrogens on biliary markers of gallstone formation in postmenopausal women. *J Clin Endocrinol Metab.*1998;83(2):410-414.

171. Racine A, Bijon A, Fournier A, et al. Menopausal hormone therapy and risk of cholecystectomy: a prospective study based on the French E3N cohort. *CMAJ.* 2013;185(7):555-561.

172. Brady CW. Liver disease in menopause. *World J Gastroenterol.* 2015;21(25):7613-7620.

173. Centers for Disease Control and Prevention. Division of STD Prevention. *Sexually Transmitted Disease Surveillance 2015.* Atlanta, Georgia: US Department of Health and Human Services; 2016.

174. Brooks JT, Buchacz K, Gobo KA, Mermin J. HIV infection and older Americans: the public health perspective. *Am J Public Health.* 2012;102(8):1516-1526.

175. Center for Disease Control and Prevention. *HIV Among People Aged 50 and Over.* Updated September 18, 2018. www.cdc.gov/hiv/group/age/olderamericans/. Accessed June 7, 2019.

176. Knight DA, Jarrett D. Preventive health care for women who have sex with women. *Am Fam Physician.* 2017;95(5):314-321.

177. Grimes DA, Schulz KF. Uses and abuses of screening tests. *Lancet.* 2002;359(9309):881-884.

178. California STD/HIV Prevention Training Center. California Department of Public Health-STD Control Branch. *California STD Screening Recommendations 2015.* November 18, 2015.

179. US Department of Health and Human Services. Centers for Disease Control and Prevention. *A Guide to Taking a Sexual History.* CDC publication 99-8445. Updated March 14, 2014. www.cdc.gov/std/treatment/sexualhistory.pdf. Accessed June 12, 2019.

180. Centers for Disease Control and Prevention. Recommendations for the laboratory-based detection of Chlamydia trachomatis and Neisseria gonorrhoeae—2014. *MMWR Recomm Rep*. 2014;63(RR-02):1-19.

181. Workowski KA, Bolan GA; Centers for Disease Control and Prevention. Sexually transmitted diseases treatment guidelines, 2015. *MMWR Recomm Rep*. 2015;64(RR-03):1-137. Erratum in: *MMWR Recomm Rep*. 2015;64(33):924.

182. LeFevre ML; US Preventive Services Task Force. Screening for Chlamydia and gonorrhea: US Preventive Services Task Force recommendation statement. *Ann Intern Med*. 2014;161(12):902-910.

183. Hogben M, Collins D, Hoots B, O'Connor K. Partner services in sexually transmitted disease prevention programs: a review. *Sex Transm Dis*. 2016;43(2 suppl 1):S53-S62.

184. Centers for Disease Control and Prevention. *Self-Study STD Modules for Clinicians: Genital Herpes Simplex Virus (HSV) Infection. Epidemiology*. Updated March 2014. https://www2a.cdc.gov/stdtraining/self-study/herpes/hsv_self_study_epidemiology.html. Accessed June 12, 2019.

185. Mark KE, Wald A, Magaret AS, et al. Rapidly cleared episodes of herpes simplex virus reactivation in immunocompetent adults. *J Infect Dis*. 2008;198(8):1141-1149.

186. US Preventive Services Task Force, Bibbins-Domingo K, Grossman DC, et al. Serologic screening for genital herpes infection: US Preventive Services Task Force recommendation statement. *JAMA*. 2016;316(23):2525-2253.

187. Centers for Disease Control and Prevention. *Self-Study STD Modules for Clinicians: Genital Herpes Simplex Virus (HSV) Infection. Clinical Manifestations and Sequelae*. Updated March 2014. https://www2a.cdc.gov/stdtraining/self-study/herpes/hsv_self_study_clinical.html. Accessed June 12, 2019.

188. Thurman AR, Doncel GF. Herpes simplex virus and HIV: genital infection synergy and novel approaches to dual prevention. *Int J STD AIDS*. 2012;23(9):613-619.

189. Schillie S, Harris A, Link-Gelles R, Romero J, ward J, Nelson N. Recommendations of the Advisory Committee on Immunization Practices for use of a hepatitis B vaccine with a novel adjuvant. *MMWR Morb Mortal Wkly Rep*. 2018;67(15):455-458.

190. Centers for Disease Control and Prevention. *Viral Hepatitis*. May 31, 2015. www.cdc.gov/hepatitis/hbv/. Accessed June 12, 2019.

191. LeFevre ML; US Preventive Services Task Force. Screening for hepatitis B virus infection in nonpregnant adolescents and adults: US Preventive Services Task Force recommendation statement. *Ann Intern Med*. 2014;161(1):58-66.

192. US Preventive Services Task Force. *Final Recommendation Statement: Hepatitis B Virus Infection: Screening, 2014*. June 2014. www.uspreventiveservicestaskforce.org/Page/Document/RecommendationStatementFinal/hepatitis-b-virus-infection-screening-2014. Accessed June 12, 2019.

193. Smith BD, Morgan RL, Beckett GA, et al; Centers for Disease Control and Prevention. Recommendations for the identification of chronic hepatitis C virus infection among persons born during 1945-1965. *MMWR Recomm Rep*. 2012;61(RR-4):1-32. Erratum in: *MMWR Recomm Rep*. 2012;61(43):886.

194. Moyer VA; US Preventive Services Task Force. Screening for HIV: US Preventive Services Task Force recommendation statement. *Ann Intern Med*. 2013;159(1):51-60.

195. Committee Opinion no 596: Committee on Gynecologic Practice: Routine human immunodeficiency virus screening. *Obstet Gynecol*. 2014;123(5):1137-1139.

196. Branson BM, Handsfield HH, Lampe MS, et al; Centers for Disease Control and Prevention (CDC). Revised recommendations for HIV testing of adults, adolescents, and pregnant women in health-care settings. *MMWR Recomm Rep*. 2006;55(RR-14):1-17.

197. Günthard HF, Saab MS, Benson CA, et al. Antiretroviral drugs for treatment and prevention of HIV infection in adults: 2016 recommendations of the International Antiviral Society-USA Panel. *JAMA*. 2016;316(2):191-210.

198. Practice Bulletin No. 167 summary: gynecologic care for women and adolescents with human immunodeficiency virus. *Obstet Gynecol*. 2016;128(4):920-922.

199. Lui-Filho JF, Valadares AL, Gomes Dde C, Amaral E, Pinto-Neto AM, Costa-Paiva L. Menopausal symptoms and associated factors in HIV-positive women. *Maturitas*. 2013;76(2):172-178.

200. Calvet GA, Grinsztejn BG, Quintana Mde S, et al. Predictors of early menopause in HIV-infected women: a prospective cohort study. *Am J Obstet Gynecol*. 2015;212(6):765.e1-765.e13.

201. Hartel D, Lo Y, Bauer C, et al. Attitudes toward menopause in HIV-infected and at-risk women. *Clin Interv Aging*. 2008;3(3):561-566.

202. Braaten KP, Laufer MR. Human papillomavirus (HPV), HPV-related disease, and the HPV vaccine. *Rev Obstet Gynecol*. 2008;1(1):2-10.

203. Petrosky E, Bocchini JA Jr, Hariri S, et al; Centers for Disease Control and Prevention (CDC). Use of 9-valent human papillomavirus (HPV) vaccine: updated HPV vaccination recommendations of the Advisory Committee on Immunization Practices. *MMWR Morb Mortal Wkly Rep*. 2015;64(11):300-304.

204. US Food and Drug Administration. FDA approves expanded use of Gardisil 9 to include individuals 27 through 45 years old [press release]. Last update October 9, 2018. www.fda.gov/newsevents/newsroom/pressannouncements/ucm622715.htm. Accessed June 12, 2019.

205. US Preventive Services Task Force (USPSTF), Bibbins-Domingo K, Grossman DC, et al. Screening for syphilis infection in nonpregnant adults and adolescents: US Preventive Services Task Force recommendation statement. *JAMA*. 2016;315(21):2321-2327.

206. Muzny CA, Schwebke JR. The clinical spectrum of Trichomonas vaginalis infection and challenges to management. *Sex Transm Infect*. 2013;89(6):423-425.

207. Sobel JD, Ferris D, Schwebke J, et al. Suppressive antibacterial therapy with 0.75% metronidazole vaginal gel to prevent recurrent bacterial vaginosis. *Am J Obstet Gynecol*. 2006;194(5):1283-1289.

7

Osteoporosis

Osteoporosis is a generalized skeletal disorder characterized by impaired bone strength that predisposes the patient to an increased risk of fractures, most importantly of the spine and hip. These and other serious osteoporosis-related fractures occur most commonly in older postmenopausal women and are often life-altering events; however, the bone loss that ultimately results in osteoporosis is most marked during the menopause transition and early menopause. Younger postmenopausal women with wrist fracture who have osteopenia or normal bone mineral density (BMD) are still at increased risk for future fracture, even if they do not have osteoporosis.

Women with osteoporosis and high risk of fracture can be readily identified, and both general and pharmacologic management strategies are available to slow or prevent bone loss and to reduce fracture risk. For these reasons, and because osteoporosis is such a common disorder, skeletal-health assessment should be a part of the routine evaluation of all postmenopausal women, and all providers caring for postmenopausal women should be competent and confident about undertaking that evaluation.

Pathophysiology

In adults, bone tissue undergoes constant change by a process called *bone remodeling*: old bone material is removed (resorbed) by osteoclasts and replaced with new healthy bone by osteoblasts. In young, healthy women, the resorption and formation components of remodeling are balanced; the amount of old bone resorbed is replaced with an almost equal amount of new bone. As a result, bone mass is usually quite stable in healthy premenopausal women. However, at the time of menopause,

in response to estrogen deficiency, bone resorption becomes more rapid, exceeding the ability of osteoblasts to form new bone, resulting in bone loss and a gradual but progressive deterioration of the microarchitecture of both trabecular and cortical bone. The imbalance in remodeling continues into advanced age, when an additional deficit in osteoblast function limits the rate of bone formation.

Rates of bone loss are highest at the time of menopause, with an average annual loss of about 2% beginning 1 to 3 years before menopause and lasting 5 to 10 years. Across the menopause transition, women experience an average loss of 10% to 12% (about one T-score) in the spine and hip.[1] Thereafter, rates of bone loss fall to about 0.5% per year. By the time a woman is aged 80 years, she has lost, on average, approximately 30% of her peak bone mass, and the average T-score in the hip at that age is about –2.5.

As bone loss occurs in the trabecular compartment of bone (mostly in the spine and ends of long bones), the once thick and numerous trabeculae become thinned and perforated and are often completely resorbed, resulting in empty spaces where bone tissue once existed. The thick outer shell of cortical bone is thinned from the inside and becomes porous because of the dominance of bone resorption over formation. The imbalance in bone remodeling can be accentuated by a very sedentary lifestyle, often resulting in an acceleration of bone loss in elderly, inactive women. In addition, many diseases and medications can amplify these effects by either increasing bone resorption or inhibiting bone formation.

There are other age-related changes in the quality of the bone tissue itself, including an increased number of microcracks and the accumulation of glycated end products. These combined changes in bone mass, structure, and quality result in impaired bone strength and the increased fracture risk that characterize postmenopausal osteoporosis.

Diagnosing osteoporosis

Although osteoporosis involves both low bone mass and altered bone structure and quality, the measurement of BMD by dual-energy X-ray absorptiometry (DXA) is the principal clinical tool used to assess skeletal health. Careful attention to the quality of both the acquisition and interpretation of DXA BMD tests is necessary.[2]

To standardize BMD values from different skeletal sites, results are reported as either a T-score or a Z-score, both expressed as standard deviation units.

The *T-score* is calculated by comparing a woman's BMD to the average BMD of normal, young adult white women. A T-score of +1 represents a value 1 standard deviation above the young normal mean, whereas a value of 2.5 standard deviations below the young normal mean would equate to a T-score of –2.5. The white young normal value serves as the reference for T-scores in women of all ethnicities. The normal range of BMD in healthy young women, defined as the mean +/–2 standard deviations, is expressed as a T-score –2 to +2. T-scores are used to make the diagnosis of osteoporosis in postmenopausal women.

The *Z-score* is the number of standard deviations above or below the average BMD for the average person of the same age, gender, and ethnicity. The Z-score allows comparison of a woman's BMD with her expected BMD. The normal range for the Z-score also is –2 to +2. The Z-score has limited value in postmenopausal women but is the preferred manner of expressing BMD results in premenopausal women.

The World Health Organization (WHO) defined osteoporosis in postmenopausal women as a BMD T-score value of –2.5 or lower.[3] In North America, the standard criterion for the diagnosis of osteoporosis in postmenopausal women is a T-score of –2.5 or lower at the lumbar spine (at least two vertebral levels measured in the posterior-anterior projection but not the lateral projection), femoral neck, or total hip by DXA testing.[4] Evidence supporting the use of T-scores in the forearm (radius) by DXA to diagnose osteoporosis is much weaker than that with hip and spine measurements. Postmenopausal women with T-score values between –1.0 and –2.49 are said to have low bone mass, or osteopenia, whereas T-score values greater than –1.0 are said to be normal. These criteria do not apply to premenopausal women;

the diagnosis of osteoporosis is made in premenopausal women who have low BMD (Z-score <–2.0) and a history of fragility fracture.

The diagnosis of *osteopenia* was described by WHO for epidemiologic purposes and has limited clinical use. Healthy postmenopausal women with T-score values in the low normal range (–1.0 to –2.0) will be diagnosed with osteopenia even though bone loss may not have occurred. Within the range of osteopenia are young postmenopausal women without other risk factors who are at low risk of fracture, as well as older women who, if they do have other risk factors, may be at very high risk of fracture.

Other methods of bone density assessment are available, including quantitative computed tomography (CT), densitometric measurements of the heel or fingers, and noninvasive ultrasound measurements at several skeletal sites. T-scores can be generated from these other methods, and measurements with some of the methods have been shown to predict fracture risk. However, the T-scores from these other measurements correlate only weakly with DXA T-scores and therefore cannot and should not be used to diagnose osteoporosis or low bone mass.

Historically, the diagnosis of osteoporosis was made in postmenopausal women who presented with nontraumatic fractures of their spine or hip. Recognizing that postmenopausal women with a history of a vertebral or hip fracture are at high risk of experiencing another fracture, these women are appropriately given the clinical diagnosis of osteoporosis, irrespective of their T-scores. There is less consensus about whether having other fragility fractures should be enough in the absence of low BMD or other risk factors to diagnosis osteoporosis.

In an effort to broaden insurance coverage of osteoporosis therapy in the United States, National Bone Health Alliance recommended that the clinical diagnosis of osteoporosis be made in postmenopausal women with a demonstrable elevated risk for future fractures, including a history of nontraumatic fractures of hip, vertebra, proximal humeral, pelvis, or in some cases, distal forearm or with an elevated estimated risk of fracture based on FRAX.[5] This expanded clinical definition of osteoporosis has not been endorsed by other organizations.

Prevalence

The prevalence of osteoporosis, as defined by low BMD, increases with age. Data from the Third National Health and Nutrition Examination Survey (NHANES) indicated that 15.4% of American women aged 50 years or older had osteoporosis, defined as a BMD T-score of −2.5 or lower at the femoral neck, and that another 51.4% had low bone mass.[6] The prevalence of osteoporosis rises from 6.8% in women aged 50 to 59 years to 34.9% in women aged 80 years and older. In 2010, there were an estimated 10.2 million adults in the United States with osteoporosis, and another 43 million had low bone density, most of whom were postmenopausal women. In the Canadian Multicentre Osteoporosis Study, 15.8% of Canadian women aged 50 years and older had osteoporosis by BMD criteria.[7]

More than 2 million fractures related to osteoporosis occur each year in the United States, including more than 700,000 clinical vertebral fractures and 300,000 hip fractures, resulting in more than 400,000 hospital admissions.[4,8] Most of these fractures occur in older postmenopausal women.

Between 40% and 50% of postmenopausal women experience a fracture related to osteoporosis during their lifetimes. In the United States, after adjusting for weight, BMD, and other covariates, whites and Hispanics had the highest risk for osteoporotic fracture, followed by American Indians, Asians, and blacks.[9] The incidence of vertebral fracture in Mexico and both vertebral and nonvertebral fractures in Canada also increase markedly with advancing age.[10,11] Age-adjusted rates of hip fracture in women in the United States and Canada appeared to be decreasing after 1997, soon after the availability of alendronate, but there is no clear evidence of a causal association. Data suggest that hip fracture rates have plateaued and may even be increasing again, perhaps related to the declining use of osteoporosis medications since 2008.[12] Even if the age-adjusted rate of fracture remains constant, the absolute number of women who have fractures will continue to increase, however, because of population growth.

Consequences of osteoporotic fractures

Hip fractures, which occur on average in women aged 82 years, elicit a particularly devastating clinical toll, resulting in higher cost, disability, and mortality than all other osteoporotic fracture types combined. Hip fractures are associated with a 5- to 8-fold increase in mortality in the first 3 months after the fracture and an excess mortality of more than 20% within 1 year of the fracture.[13] The increased mortality may persist for at least 10 years. Similarly, clinical or symptomatic vertebral fractures are associated with a 10% excess mortality in the year after the fracture.

Hip fracture is also associated with high morbidity, especially in older women. Up to 25% of women require long-term care after a hip fracture, and 50% will have some long-term loss of mobility. Vertebral fractures are associated with acute and chronic pain, height loss, and deformity and adversely affected ambulation, pulmonary function, and ability to perform routine chores.[14] Fractures of the humerus and distal forearm also are associated with substantial disability, lasting up to 6 months in many patients.[15]

Osteoporotic fractures take a psychological toll as well. Hip and vertebral fractures and the resultant pain, loss of mobility, changed body image, and loss of independence can have a strong negative effect on self-esteem and mood. Fear of falling after having had a fracture limits socialization and physical activity, contributing to the effect of fractures on the development of frailty.[16]

Risk factors

Osteoporosis or impaired bone strength is an important but not the only risk factor for fracture. It is necessary to distinguish between risk factors for osteoporosis and risk factors for fracture.

Risk factors for low bone mineral density

Advanced age
Bone loss decreases progressively with advancing age, and the prevalence of osteoporosis increases as women grow older.

Thinness
Bone mineral density in healthy women is strongly correlated with body weight. Thin women have lower BMD values than do heavier women.

Genetics
Family studies have demonstrated that 50% to 85% of the variance in BMD is genetically determined, and many genes have been weakly associated with low bone mass in humans.[17] In the United States, the rates of osteoporosis vary with ethnicity. In general, US Asian women have lower BMD than do white women, whereas BMD in black women is generally higher. Differences in body size explain the BMD difference in Asian women but do not entirely explain the BMD diffidence between blacks and whites.[9]

Smoking
Some but not all studies suggest that smokers have lower BMD than do nonsmokers. Possible explanations include

that women who smoke are generally thinner and have earlier menopause and lower serum estradiol levels than nonsmokers.

History of fracture
Because low BMD is a risk factor for fracture, it is not unexpected that women with a history of fragility fracture generally have lower BMD than those without a fracture history.

Diseases and drugs
Many if not most diseases adversely affect the skeleton. Particularly important secondary causes of bone loss (Table 1) include chronic inflammatory illnesses (rheumatoid arthritis), diseases causing malabsorption (celiac disease), and various endocrinopathies (hyperparathyroidism, Cushing syndrome).[18] Drugs can increase bone resorption causing bone loss (aromatase inhibitors [AIs]), impair vitamin D metabolism (phenytoin), or reduce bone formation (glucocorticoids).[19]

Notable risk factors *not* predictive of low BMD include low daily or lifetime intake of calcium or vitamin D, excessive alcohol intake, current or past physical activity, and reproductive history.

Risk factors for fracture
Based on large meta-analyses, independent risk factors for fracture in postmenopausal women have been identified.

Prior fragility fracture
Having or having had a fragility fracture is the most important and powerful risk factor for having another fracture.[20] The risk of refracture is especially high (4- to 8-fold increased risk) in women with recent fractures; 19% of women with osteoporosis who sustained a vertebral fracture had another vertebral fracture within 12 months.[21,22] The risk of another vertebral fracture also depends on the number and severity of previous vertebral fractures. The added risk after a fracture persists for at least 10 years, with the average risk over that time being 50% to 100% higher than expected for age and BMD. The high fracture risk after an incident fracture is the justification for secondary prevention programs such as Fracture Liaison Services, established in many health centers, to routinely assess fracture risk and to consider treatment for every patient who presents to a clinic, hospital, or health system with a fragility fracture.[23]

Low bone mineral density
Although low BMD at any site is correlated with fracture risk, the strongest correlation is with hip BMD.[24] Hip fracture risk increases by 2.6-fold for each age-adjusted standard deviation (one Z-score unit) decrease in femoral neck BMD and by 1.6-fold per standard deviation decrease in forearm BMD.

Age
For any BMD value, older women are at higher fracture risk than younger postmenopausal women.[25]

Smoking
Relative risk of fracture in postmenopausal women who smoke is increased about 30%, independent of BMD.[26] Some studies suggest that this added risk is lost on smoking cessation.[27]

Excessive alcohol intake
Consuming more than three servings of alcohol daily is associated with a 38% and 68% increase risk of osteoporotic and hip fracture, respectively.[28]

Parental history of hip fracture
The strongest component of a family history of osteoporosis or fracture predicting fracture risk is a parental history of hip fracture.

Diseases and drugs
In addition to diseases and drugs that cause bone loss, some diseases (type 2 diabetes mellitus and obesity) and some drugs (proton pump inhibitors) are associated with increased fracture risk not accounted for by changes in BMD.[29,30]

Falls
Most fractures, including many vertebral fractures, occur after a fall from a standing height or less. As a result, risk factors for falls, including a history of previous falls; weakness; impaired balance, coordination, vision, or hearing; obesity; and arthritis are also risk factors for fracture.

Assessing fracture risk
Dual-energy X-ray absorptiometry is a good predictor of relative fracture risk, with increases in risk of 1.6- to 2.6-fold per standard deviation decrease in age-adjusted BMD.[24] However, for estimation of absolute rather than relative risk of fracture, BMD must be combined with other important risk factors such as age and prior fracture history.

The FRAX tool, developed by a team at the University of Sheffield, combines eight risk factors based on meta-analyses of large observational cohorts.[31] The output of

Table 1. Secondary Causes of Bone Loss

Medications
- Aromatase inhibitors
- Cytotoxic agents
- Excessive thyroxine doses
- Gonadotropin-releasing hormone agonists or analogs
- Heparin
- Immunosuppressives (eg, cyclosporine)
- Intramuscular medroxyprogesterone
- Long-term use of certain anticonvulsants (eg, phenytoin)
- Oral or intramuscular use of glucocorticoids for >3 mo

Genetic disorders
- Hemochromatosis
- Hypophosphatasia
- Osteogenesis imperfecta
- Thalassemia

Disorders of calcium balance
- Hypercalciuria
- Vitamin D deficiency

Endocrinopathies
- Cortisol excess
- Cushing syndrome
- Gonadal insufficiency (primary and secondary)
- Hyperthyroidism
- Primary hyperparathyroidism
- Type 1 diabetes mellitus

Gastrointestinal diseases
- Billroth I gastroenterostomy
- Chronic liver disease (eg, primary biliary cirrhosis)
- Malabsorption syndromes (eg, celiac disease, Crohn disease)
- Total gastrectomy

Other disorders and conditions
- Ankylosing spondylitis
- Chronic renal disease
- Lymphoma and leukemia
- Multiple myeloma
- Nutritional disorders (eg, anorexia nervosa)
- Rheumatoid arthritis
- Systemic mastocytosis

Management of osteoporosis in postmenopausal women: 2010 position statement of The North American Menopause Society.[18]

FRAX is the 10-year probability of hip fracture or major osteoporotic fracture (hip, proximal humerus, distal radius, and symptomatic spine fractures). Bone mineral density input into FRAX is limited to femoral neck values because they were the only BMD values available in all the cohorts from which FRAX was developed. When BMD values are not available, FRAX can still be calculated using body mass index (BMI) as a surrogate for BMD. Because hip fracture rates differ so much among different populations, country-specific FRAX models are available for 63 countries, including the three North American countries. In the United States, four ethnic-specific FRAX databases (white, Hispanic, Asian, and black) are available. Many national societies have incorporated FRAX into their osteoporosis treatment guidelines. FRAX is appropriate for use in postmenopausal women aged 40 to 90 years.

In 2005, while awaiting the availability of FRAX, the Canadian Association of Radiologists and Osteoporosis Canada introduced a calculator to estimate a person's 10-year risk of fracture based on BMD (lowest T-score of hip and lumbar spine), age, gender, fracture history, and steroid use.[32] Bone mineral density input was subsequently limited to the femoral neck. The 10-year major osteoporosis fracture risk is categorized as low (<10%), moderate (10-20%), and high (>20%). The presence of either a fragility fracture or glucocorticoid use puts the woman at high fracture risk regardless of BMD result. The Canadian national guidelines state that either the Canadian Association of Radiologists and Osteoporosis Canada calculator or the Canadian version of the FRAX tool can be used for fracture risk assessment in Canada.[33]

Trabecular bone score is a special software available for DXA machines that analyzes the heterogeneity of density distribution on routine lumbar spine DXA images. Trabecular bone score measurements correlate with trabecular microarchitecture and, independent from BMD, predict fracture risk.[34] Trabecular bone score has been incorporated into the FRAX tool.[35] Adding the trabecular bone score value is most helpful in women whose fracture risk is near the treatment threshold.

Indications for bone mineral density testing

Guidance from the National Osteoporosis Foundation, The North American Menopause Society, American Association of Clinical Endocrinologists, Canadian Task Force on Preventive Health Care, and the Asociación Mexicana de Metabolismo Óseo y Mineral state that BMD testing by DXA should be performed in all postmenopausal women with risk factors for low BMD (Table 2).[4,18,33,36,37] This includes all women aged 65 years and older and also younger postmenopausal women with at least one other important risk factor for low BMD such as a personal or family history of fracture or low body weight (<127 lb). The US Preventive Services Task Force (USPSTF) had recommended BMD testing for women aged at least 65 years and for women aged 60 to 64 years with a FRAX estimate of major osteoporotic fracture risk equivalent to that of a 65-year-old women without other risk factors (9.3%).[38] The performance of this latter recommendation had been characterized as poor. Updated guidelines from the USPSTF again recommend BMD testing for all women aged 65 years and older and for women aged 60 to 64 years at risk for low BMD or fracture, based on FRAX or other screening tools such as the Osteoporosis Screening Tool or SCORE.[39]

Clinical evaluation of women with postmenopausal osteoporosis

Osteoporosis in healthy postmenopausal women because of a combination of low peak bone mass and bone loss related to estrogen deficiency and aging is called *primary osteoporosis*. When other diseases or medications adversely affect the skeleton, the diagnosis of *secondary osteoporosis* is made. Idiopathic osteoporosis is characterized by low bone density and fractures in young adults without known cause so a diagnosis is not commonly made in postmenopausal women.

A complete medical evaluation, including a detailed history of other diseases and medications, previous fractures and family history, a thorough physical examination and routine laboratory testing should be performed in all patients with osteoporosis before initiating therapy. The purpose of the evaluation is to assess the severity of osteoporosis, identify secondary causes of bone loss (especially the ones that can be corrected), and to identify contraindications to specific therapies.

The clinical history should ask about personal and family history of fractures, loss of weight or height, bone pain or muscle weakness and symptoms of other diseases. Risk factors for falls should also be evaluated. Physical examination should specifically include measurement of standing height with a stadiometer, evaluation for kyphosis, muscle strength, balance, bone tenderness (best elicited over the anterior tibia, rib cage or vertebrae), and joint laxity or blue sclerae (features of *osteogenesis imperfecta*).

Routine laboratory testing should include complete blood cell count and general serum chemistry, especially serum calcium, creatinine, alkaline phosphatase, albumin, and serum phosphate. Measurement of 24-hour urinary calcium excretion is useful to detect patients with poor calcium absorption (<100 mg/d) and those with hypercalciuria (>250 mg/d). In the presence of abnormal basic laboratory tests, clinical clues of other diseases, or unusual cases of osteoporosis special laboratory tests such as 24-hour urine free cortisol, 25-hydroxyvitamin D (25-OH D), serum and/or urine protein electrophoresis, thyroid-stimulating hormone, tissue transglutaminase antibody, and intact parathyroid hormone should be considered.

Management of osteoporosis

The objective of treating osteoporosis is to reduce the likelihood of fragility fractures. The available strategies are to decrease fall frequency or intensity and to strengthen the skeleton with general, nonpharmacologic measures and pharmacologic therapy. Comprehensive fall prevention programs, including home safety, exercises to promote strength and balance, correcting visual impairment, and appropriate use of walking aids may reduce fall frequency but have not been shown to reduce fracture risk.[40,41] A USPSTF report concluded that multifactorial and exercise interventions were associated with fall-related benefit, but evidence was most consistent across multiple fall-related outcomes for exercise.[42] Hip protectors may be considered in patients at high risk for falling, but evidence for their effectiveness exists only in supervised settings of long-term care facilities.[43]

General nonpharmacologic measures

General lifestyle measures (good nutrition, regular physical activity, avoiding harmful lifestyle habits) are usually recommended for all patients at risk for osteoporosis.[4,33,36] Much emphasis has been placed on providing adequate intakes of bone-healthy nutrients, especially calcium and vitamin D, so much so that a strong but incorrect perception exists that osteoporosis is the consequence of life-long calcium and/or vitamin D deficiency. Intakes of calcium and vitamin D are not different between women with or without osteoporosis and are not correlated with rates of bone loss or fracture risk.

The results of studies evaluating effects of calcium and vitamin D supplementation on fracture risk are inconsistent, perhaps because both these factors may be threshold nutrients (more is not better than enough) and because most of the studies, such as the Women's Health Initiative (WHI) in which the average daily calcium intake was 1,150 mg at baseline, have not evaluated outcomes specifically in patients deficient in calcium or vitamin D.[44] Any benefits of correcting deficiencies may be obscured by the absence of benefit when supplements

Table 2. Indications for BMD Testing by DXA in Postmenopausal Women

NAMS, NOF, AACE	Canadian Task Force on Preventive Health Care	USPSTF	AMMOM
All postmenopausal women with • Medical causes of bone loss • History of fragility fracture • Age ≥65 y Younger postmenopausal women with a risk factor: • Thinness (body weight <127 lb [57.7 kg] or BMI <21 kg/m²) • History of hip fracture in a parent • Current smoker • Rheumatoid arthritis • Alcohol intake >2 units/d (1 unit is 12 oz beer, 4 oz wine, or 1 oz liquor)	Postmenopausal women with one major and two minor clinical risk factors. **Major** • Age ≥65 y • Vertebral compression fracture • Fragility fracture after age 40 y • Family history of osteoporotic fracture (especially hip fracture in mother) • Systemic glucocorticoid therapy ≥3 mo • Malabsorption syndrome • Primary hyperparathyroidism • Propensity to falls • Appearance of osteopenia on radiograph • Hypogonadism and early menopause (<45 y) **Minor** • Rheumatoid arthritis • History of clinical hyperthyroidism • Long-term anticonvulsant therapy • Weight loss >10% of body weight at age 25 y • Weight <57 kg • Smoking • Excess alcohol intake • Excess caffeine intake • Low dietary calcium intake • Long-term heparin therapy	All women aged ≥65 y. Women aged 60-64 y with a FRAX estimate or risk equivalent to that of a 65-year-old women without other risk factors (10-y risk of major osteoporotic fracture, 9.3%)	All women aged ≥65 y. Younger postmenopausal women with risk factors for bone loss or fracture, including • History of fragility fracture after age 40 • Adults with some inflammatory disease (eg, rheumatoid arthritis) • Treatment with drugs associated with low bone mass or bone loss (eg, prednisone in daily doses ≥5 mg for ≥3 mo) • Osteopenia identified on radiograph

Abbreviations: AACE, American Association of Clinical Endocrinologists; AMMOM, Asociacion Mexicana de Metabolismo Oseo Y Mineral A.C.; BMD, bone mineral density; DXA, dual energy X-ray absorptiometry; NAMS, North American Menopause Society; NOF, National Osteoporosis Foundation; USPSTF, US Preventive Services Task Force.
Cosman F, et al[4]; Management of osteoporosis in postmenopausal women: 2010 position statement of The North American Menopause Society[18]; Papaioannou A, et al[33]; Camacho PM, et al[36]; Peña-Ríos DH, et al.[37]

are given to persons replete in calcium and vitamin D. Correcting clear deficiencies of these nutrients is appropriate. For calcium, this is achieved with a total daily intake of calcium of 800 mg to 1,200 mg (Table 3).[45] Excessive intake of calcium (>2,000 mg total daily)

should be avoided because this may be associated with an increased risk of renal stones, milk alkali syndrome and, less certainly, of cardiovascular (CV) events.[44,46]

Controversy exists about the optimal intake of vitamin D and appropriate target level for serum 25-OH D.

Table 3. Estimation of Daily Calcium Intake	
Dairy-free diet	300 mg
Servings of dairy products x 300 mg/serving	
___ servings =	___ mg
Calcium supplements	___ mg
Total Daily Intake	___ mg

Ross AC, et al.[45]

In otherwise healthy postmenopausal women, including those with osteoporosis the average serum 25-OH D level is about 20 ng/mL (the recommended daily intake is 600 international units (IU) for women aged 51 to 71 years and 800 IU for women aged older than 71 years).[45] There is very little evidence that having levels above that provides any clinical benefit. The studies demonstrating reductions in the risk of falls and hip fracture were performed in patients with marked vitamin D deficiency, and on-treatment 25-OH D levels were about 20 ng/mL.[47,48] Treatment with a very high dose of vitamin D once yearly was associated with higher rates of falls and fractures.[49] Meta-analyses have not supported a benefit of routine supplementation with vitamin D. The USPSTF concluded that evidence is insufficient to assess the balance of the benefits and harms of supplementation with daily doses greater than 400 IU of vitamin D and greater than 1,000 mg of calcium and recommends against daily supplementation with more than 400 IU of vitamin D and 1,000 mg of calcium for the primary prevention of fractures.[50] These USPSTF recommendations do not apply to adults with a preexisting diagnosis of osteoporosis who need adequate calcium and vitamin D.

In general, these nonpharmacologic measures can be recommended to all postmenopausal women. They may slow but do not prevent bone loss in either young or older postmenopausal women, do not restore BMD and are certainly not sufficient therapy for patients with osteoporosis at high risk of fracture.

Other supplements

Studies of relationships between protein intake and either bone mineral density or fracture risk have been inconsistent.[51] In fall-prone elderly patients who were losing weight, higher protein intake was associated with reduced fall frequency.[52]

Strontium is a heavier divalent cation than calcium and increases BMD by being deposited in the skeleton while having little to no effect on bone remodeling. Strontium ranelate, a proprietary strontium salt, was shown to reduce the risk of vertebral and nonvertebral fractures in postmenopausal women with osteoporosis.[53,54] This drug was approved as a treatment for osteoporosis in Europe but not in the United States or Canada, but its use is now severely restricted because of concerns about increased CV risk. Other strontium salts (citrate, chloride) are promoted in the United States for bone health, but there is no evidence of their effectiveness or safety.

Severe *magnesium* deficiency had adverse skeletal events in preclinical studies. Observational clinical studies have inconsistently demonstrated an association between magnesium intake and BMD. In the WHI, low dietary intake was associated with low BMD at some skeletal sites but was not related to fracture risk.[54] Low serum magnesium levels have been associated with fracture risk, but this was not related to magnesium intake.[55] Magnesium deficiency is uncommon in healthy adults with normal diets. Although providing magnesium supplements to patients with malabsorption may be warranted, routine magnesium supplementation cannot be recommended.

Vitamin K promotes carboxylation of osteocalcin, a protein that may have a role in bone mineralization. The use of various vitamin K preparations has been promoted to improve bone health. In a small (N=440) randomized trial in postmenopausal women, vitamin K1 had no effect on BMD, but fewer women in the vitamin K group had clinical fractures (9 vs 20; P=.04).[56] Adding vitamin K2 to risedronate had no effect on BMD or fractures.[57]

Phytoestrogens are plant-derived compounds with weak estrogenic activity. In this family are several soy isoflavones that have modest estrogen-like effects on the skeleton in animal models. Because studies evaluating the clinical effects isoflavones have inconsistently shown small effects on bone turnover or BMD, they cannot be recommended as effective strategies to prevent or treat postmenopausal osteoporosis.[58]

There also is no compelling evidence for beneficial effects of boron, zinc, black cohosh, berberine, or dehydroepiandrosterone (DHEA) on bone density or fracture risk in postmenopausal women.

Pharmacologic therapy

There is strong consensus among North American osteoporosis guidelines that pharmacologic therapy is appropriate for postmenopausal women at high risk of fracture and without contraindications to treatment. This includes postmenopausal women with a history of hip or vertebral fracture; BMD values in the lumbar spine or proximal femur (femoral neck or total hip regions) consistent with osteoporosis; low BMD (T-score values between −1 and −2.5) with 10-year fracture probability (by FRAX) of major osteoporosis fracture of 20% or more; or hip fracture risk of 3% or higher. Because of the lack of clinical trial data, some controversy exists among guidelines regarding optimal treatment of postmenopausal women and men who have low BMD plus elevated FRAX risk.[59]

Canadian guidelines recommend pharmacologic therapy in postmenopausal women with osteoporosis by DXA BMD testing or in women aged 65 years or older with T-score values of less than −2.0.[33]

Because no treatment "cures" osteoporosis, and the beneficial skeletal effects of most osteoporosis drugs wane quickly on stopping treatment, long-term management is required for this chronic disorder. Several drugs with differing mechanisms of action have been demonstrated to prevent bone loss in postmenopausal women and to reduce fracture risk in women with postmenopausal osteoporosis (Table 4).

The mechanisms of action of all osteoporosis drugs are to modulate (either to inhibit or to activate) bone remodeling. Antiremodeling agents, including estrogen-receptor (ER) agonists, bisphosphonates, and the RANK ligand inhibitor denosumab inhibit osteoclastic bone resorption and, secondarily and more slowly, inhibit bone formation. Remodeling spaces present at the beginning of treatment fill in and fewer new remodeling spaces are opened, resulting in modest increases in BMD and strengthening of the skeleton. However, these drugs do not improve or repair microarchitectural disruption of trabecular structure.

Potent antiremodeling agents such as denosumab improve cortical bone strength by increasing cortical thickness and reducing cortical porosity. Parathyroid hormone-receptor agonists teriparatide and abaloparatide, often referred to as anabolic agents, activate osteoblastic bone formation earlier and to a greater degree than resorption by osteoclasts, resulting in a positive remodeling balance, increased trabecular mass, and some improvement in trabecular microarchitecture. These agents also, at least transiently, increase cortical porosity but have been shown to improve bone strength in the hip as well as the spine. Clinicians can consider specialty consultation for patients in whom they are considering using anabolic agents.

Antiremodeling agents

Systemic estrogen therapy (ET), with or without a progestin, effectively prevents bone loss in postmenopausal women, and several oral and transdermal preparations of estrogen are approved for osteoporosis prevention in the United States. There are no clear differences in the BMD responses among different estrogen preparations or routes of administration. Conjugated estrogens, both as monotherapy and with medroxyprogesterone acetate (MPA), reduced the risk of vertebral and hip fractures by 34% in the low fracture risk population of the WHI.[60,61] However, estrogen is no longer approved as a treatment for established osteoporosis, in large part because estrogen has not specifically been shown to reduce fracture risk in women with known osteoporosis. Some guidelines recommend the use of estrogen to prevent bone loss in women when additional benefits of therapy, such as relief of menopause symptoms, are also accomplished and/or when alternate therapies are not appropriate in women at high risk of fracture.[33,36,62] Beginning estrogen in women more than 10 years beyond menopause is not recommended because of concerns about CV safety.[62]

The beneficial skeletal effects of estrogen abate within a few months after stopping therapy. Markers of bone turnover return to pretreatment values within a few months; relatively rapid bone loss occurs for 1 to 2 years, and protection from fracture partially or totally disappears within the first year of stopping therapy.[63-65] Switching from estrogen to alendronate (and probably other bisphosphonates or denosumab) prevents the rebound in remodeling and rapid bone loss.[66]

Tibolone. Tibolone is a synthetic hormone, derived from the Mexican yam, with weak estrogenic actions and with various metabolites that also have progestin and androgen effects in various tissues. Tibolone prevents bone loss In postmenopausal women.[67] Tibolone 2.5 mg daily is approved in Mexico for preventing osteoporosis. In women with postmenopausal osteoporosis treated for an average of 34 months, tibolone 1.25 mg daily significantly reduced the risks of vertebral and nonvertebral fracture and of both breast and colon cancer.[68] However, an increased risk of stroke was observed, resulting in the study being halted, and the drug was not submitted for regulatory approval in the United States or Canada.

Estrogen agonists/antagonists

These drugs, previously called selective estrogen receptor modulators, have weak estrogen agonist properties in bone while functioning as antiestrogens in female reproductive tissues.

Raloxifene. Raloxifene is a weak antiremodeling agent that induces small increases in BMD in postmenopausal

Table 4. Drugs Approved for Osteoporosis Management in North America

Drug		Route of administration	Dosing interval	Approved in United States		Approved in Canada	Approved in Mexico
				Treatment	Prevention		
Antiremodeling agents							
Estrogens	Estrogens	Oral, transdermal	Daily or continuous patch		✓	✓	✓
	Tibolone	Oral	Daily				✓
Bisphosphonates	Etidronate	Oral	Daily for 2 wk q 3rd mo			✓	
	Alendronate	Oral	Daily, weekly	✓	✓	✓	✓
	Risedronate	Oral	Daily, weekly, monthly	✓	✓	✓	✓ (monthly dose not available)
	Ibandronate	Oral, IV	Oral once monthly IV q 3rd mo	✓	✓		✓
	Zoledronic acid	IV	Once yearly	✓	✓	✓	✓
	Raloxifene	Oral	Daily	✓	✓	✓	✓
Estrogen agonists/ antagonists (SERMs)	BZA/CE	Oral	Daily		✓	✓	✓
RANK ligand inhibitor	Denosumab	Subcutaneous	Once q 6 mo	✓		✓	✓
Salmon calcitonin		Subcutaneous	Once daily	✓			
		Nasal	Once daily	✓			✓
Formation stimulators							
PTH-receptor agonists	Teriparatide	Subcutaneous	Once daily	✓		✓	✓
	Abaloparatide	Subcutaneous	Once daily	✓			

Abbreviations: BZA, bazedoxifene; CE, conjugated estrogens; SERM, selective estrogen-receptor modulator.

women.[69] In postmenopausal women with osteoporosis, raloxifene 60 mg daily for 3 years reduced the incidence of radiographic vertebral fractures by 30% (2.3% vs 4.5% with placebo) in those with no prior vertebral fracture and by 50% (14.7% vs 21.2%) in women with previous spine fractures.[70] However, no effects on nonvertebral or hip fracture were observed. Raloxifene may worsen hot flashes, was associated with an estrogen-like risk of venous thrombosis and, in elderly women at high risk of cardiovascular disease (CVD), an increased risk of death from stroke.[71] Therapy substantially reduced the risk of invasive breast cancer. The skeletal effects of raloxifene quickly abate when therapy is withdrawn.[72] Raloxifene is an appealing treatment option for younger postmenopausal women with osteoporosis at risk for vertebral but not hip fracture, without significant vasomotor symptoms (VMS), and who have no risk factors for venous thrombosis, especially if there is concern about breast cancer risk. As the patient ages and hip fracture becomes a greater clinical concern, switching to a drug known to reduce hip fracture risk would be appropriate.

Bazedoxifene. Bazedoxifene demonstrated similar fracture efficacy to raloxifene in a head-to-head comparison in women with postmenopausal osteoporosis.[73] Vertebral fracture risk was reduced by 42% over 3 years, with no difference in relative risk reduction between those with or without prior vertebral fracture. There was no overall effect on nonvertebral fracture risk. The safety profiles of bazedoxifene and raloxifene were similar, although no effect on breast cancer risk was observed in this study. Bazedoxifene has not been marketed as a treatment for osteoporosis. However, the combination of bazedoxifene 20 mg and 0.45 mg conjugated estrogen given daily improves VMS and prevents bone loss in young postmenopausal women.[74] This combination has been approved and is marketed in the United States and Mexico for the prevention of postmenopausal osteoporosis and for the management of moderate to severe VMS.

Bisphosphonates

Bisphosphonates are the most commonly used osteoporosis drugs. The four drugs in the class approved in the United States (alendronate, risedronate, ibandronate, and zoledronic acid) are aminobisphosphonates, which are more potent than the original bisphosphonates. These congeners of pyrophosphate bind to bone matrix at sites of active bone remodeling from where they are absorbed into osteoclasts. By interfering with important intracellular enzymes, osteoclast function is impaired; bone resorption is inhibited, and bone formation is reduced.[75] Alendronate, risedronate, and zoledronic acid effectively reduced the risk of vertebral, nonvertebral, and hip fracture in postmenopausal women with osteoporosis.[76] Ibandronate reduced spine fracture risk, but there was no overall effect on nonvertebral or hip fracture risk.[77]

Upper gastrointestinal symptoms appear to worsen with oral bisphosphonates, whereas flu-like symptoms occur in about one-third of patients with their first (but not subsequent) intravenous (IV) doses of zoledronic acid. Diffuse bone, muscle, or joint pain of unknown mechanism are described with both oral and IV bisphosphonates. These drugs, especially IV zoledronic acid, must be used with caution in patients with significantly impaired renal function or hypocalcemia. Osteonecrosis of the jaw (ONJ) occurs very infrequently in patients receiving osteoporotic doses of bisphosphonates. Invasive dental procedures and poor oral hygiene are risk factors for ONJ. Improving oral hygiene preoperatively and using topical antimicrobial therapy with dental extraction appear to reduce the risk of ONJ.[78] A duration-dependent risk of subtrochanteric or femoral shaft fractures with atypical radiologic features becomes evident after 2 to 3 years of therapy and in about 1/1,000 patients after 8 to 10 years

of therapy.[79] Most patients have pain in the thigh or groin several weeks to months before the atypical fracture occurs. For this reason, patients on bisphosphonate therapy for more than 3 years should be cautioned to report new thigh or groin pain so that radiographic evaluation can be undertaken. There is weak evidence that the risk of atypical fracture may decrease on discontinuation of oral bisphosphonates.[80]

Because these drugs bind to bone matrix with varying affinity, the effects of therapy on bone remodeling and protection from fracture wane slowly (over 1-5 y) when treatment is stopped. Markers of bone turnover return to baseline levels within 12 months of stopping risedronate, and inhibition of remodeling may persist for several years after withdrawal of alendronate or zoledronic acid.[81-83] Temporary withdrawal of therapy, a so-called "bisphosphonate holiday" may be considered if patients are at low risk of fracture after 3 to 5 years of therapy.[84] Reevaluation every 1 to 2 years is appropriate to determine when treatment should be restarted. If bone loss or fractures occur or if the patient meets the usual indications for therapy, restarting an osteoporosis drug should be considered. For patients who remain at high risk after 3 to 5 years of bisphosphonate therapy (including patients with a history of previous spine or hip fracture or multiple other fragility fractures, hip BMD values remaining in the osteoporosis range, or who have other important risk factors), continuing on an osteoporosis therapy is recommended. Bone mineral density in the hip region plateaus and then remains stable after about 5 years of bisphosphonate therapy. After 5 years of treatment in women at high risk, switching to denosumab should be considered because this results in additional gains in BMD.[81,83,85] Similarly, switching from a bisphosphonate to teriparatide results in additional gains in spine BMD and modest increases in BMD at the hip.[86]

Etidronate (not an aminobisphosphonate) was the first bisphosphonate evaluated as a treatment for osteoporosis. In a small study, cyclic etidronate, given daily for 2 weeks every third month, increased BMD and reduced vertebral fracture risk during the first 2 years of therapy.[87] By the end of the third year of the study, the effect on vertebral fractures was no longer evident. Etidronate is approved in Canada but not in the United States for treating postmenopausal osteoporosis.

Denosumab

This fully human monoclonal antibody binds to and inhibits RANK ligand, resulting in marked inhibition of bone remodeling. Administered by subcutaneous injection of 60 mg every 6 months, denosumab therapy for 3 years reduced the risk of vertebral fractures by 68% and hip fractures by 40% in postmenopausal women with osteoporosis.[88] These effects were evident within the first year of therapy. Bone mineral density increased progressively, and protection from fracture persisted or improved over 10 years of therapy.[89] Skin rash and infection occurred more frequently with denosumab than with placebo. The theoretical concern about possible immune dysfunction and increased risk of serious infection has not been observed in follow-up studies of up to 10 years. Very rare cases of atypical femoral fractures and ONJ were observed with long-term therapy, but the relationship between duration of denosumab therapy and these possible adverse events is unclear. There is no limit to the duration of denosumab therapy. On stopping treatment, indices of bone remodeling quickly rise above baseline levels before returning to pretreatment levels.[90] Rapid decreases in BMD and loss of vertebral fracture protection occur within a few months when treatment is stopped.[90,91] Case series of patients experiencing multiple vertebral fractures 3 to 18 months after stopping denosumab treatment have been reported.[92] These results emphasize the importance of having patients return for their injections at regular 6-month intervals. As with stopping estrogen, switching to another antiresorptive agent (eg, a bisphosphonate) should be considered if denosumab therapy is stopped.

Salmon calcitonin

Calcitonin is a hormone secreted primarily by the C-cells of the thyroid gland. In vitro, calcitonin is a potent inhibitor of bone resorption; however, the physiological role of calcitonin in humans is poorly understood. Clinical situations characterized by excess or deficiency of calcitonin are not associated with metabolic or skeletal abnormalities. Administration of pharmacologic doses of salmon calcitonin (much more potent than human calcitonin) results in very small decreases in markers of bone resorption and small increases in spine bone mineral density.

Salmon calcitonin by subcutaneous administration was originally approved for the treatment of osteoporosis in 1984 on the basis of total body calcium measurements. No studies have adequately evaluated the effects of subcutaneous calcitonin on fracture risk. Therapy was frequently limited by nausea. Nasal administration of salmon calcitonin had fewer AEs but even smaller effects on markers of bone remodeling and BMD. In a study in postmenopausal women with osteoporosis, one dose (200 µg/d) of three doses tested was associated with a small decrease in vertebral fracture risk.[93] Adverse events included nasal irritation and back pain. Nasal calcitonin was not effective in preventing bone loss in early postmenopausal women. This led to the approval of nasal calcitonin for the treatment of osteoporosis in postmenopausal women more than 5 years postmenopause. Because of limited evidence of efficacy and a possible association with increased cancer risk, nasal calcitonin was withdrawn from the Canadian market and a caution about the cancer risk was added to the American prescribing information. Where available, calcitonin should be used only when alternative treatments are not suitable.[36]

Parathyroid hormone receptor agonists

Two drugs, teriparatide and abaloparatide, activate bone remodeling through their interactions with the parathyroid hormone (PTH) receptor. They are the only available stimulators of bone formation; both are administered daily by subcutaneous injection.

Teriparatide is a recombinant 1-34 N-terminal fragment of PTH. When administered once daily, teriparatide stimulates osteoblastic bone formation but also increases bone resorption.[94] Trabecular architecture is improved; cortical thickness and porosity increase. Therapy for 18 to 24 months reduces the risk of vertebral and nonvertebral fracture by 65% and 35%, respectively.[95] In a head-to-head comparison study in women with previous vertebral fractures, teriparatide was significantly more effective in reducing fracture risk than was risedronate.[96] Adverse events have included hypercalciuria, mild and usually transient hypercalcemia, dizziness, and muscle pain. On discontinuing therapy, switching to a bisphosphonate or denosumab preserves or increases BMD.[97,98]

Abaloparatide is a synthetic analog of parathyroid hormone-related peptide (PTHrP) that has skeletal effects similar to that of teriparatide. Compared with placebo, new vertebral fractures were reduced by 86% and nonvertebral fractures by 43% over 18 months in postmenopausal women with osteoporosis.[99] Treating those patients with alendronate for an additional 6 months preserved the fracture-protecting effect of abaloparatide.[100] This drug was approved in the United States but is not yet available in Canada or Mexico.

Because of study results in rats, both teriparatide and abaloparatide carry a black box warning about a potential risk of osteosarcoma. Neither agent should be used in patients with hypercalcemia, at risk of osteosarcoma, or with known or possible skeletal metastases, and use of any PTH receptor agonist is limited to 24 months in a patient's lifetime.

Combining osteoporosis therapies

Unlike treating diabetes or hypertension, combining drugs to treat osteoporosis is not recommended by North American guidelines. There is no justification for using two antiremodeling agents simultaneously.[101] Combining bisphosphonates and teriparatide does not have meaningful benefit on BMD over monotherapy.[102,103] Beginning treatment with both teriparatide and denosumab results in faster and greater gains in BMD than with either therapy alone, but combined therapy is associated with a substantial decrease in markers of bone formation, perhaps reflecting mitigation of the anabolic effect of teriparatide.[104] Whether this combination results in greater protection from fracture is not known.

In contrast, using the drugs in sequence to accomplish long-term management is encouraged. Estrogen and raloxifene are appropriate in younger postmenopausal women, whereas teriparatide and abaloparatide have appeal in patients at high risk of vertebral fracture. Following each of these therapies with a bisphosphonate or denosumab should be considered in patents at high fracture risk to prevent bone loss and loss of fracture protection.

Monitoring therapy

The objectives of monitoring therapy are to enhance adherence with therapy and to identify those patients who continue to lose bone density in whom further evaluation or changing therapy would be considered. Follow-up contact by an office nurse may be the most effective means to enhance adherence to therapy.[105] Most guidelines recommend that BMD testing be repeated after 1 to 2 years, with careful attention to quality control of the repeat testing. For patients taking bisphosphonates, repeating BMD again at 5 years would be part of the determination of whether a "bisphosphonate holiday" would be considered.[84] In contrast, American College of Physician guidelines recommend that monitoring not be performed during 5 years of treatment, after which treatment should be discontinued.[59] The authors acknowledge that both the recommendation to limit therapy to 5 years and to not monitor treatment are based on weak evidence.

Biochemical markers reflecting bone resorption (serum C-terminal telopeptide of type 1 collagen) and bone formation (serum procollagen type 1 N-terminal propeptide) have been very useful in clinical research studies. Changes in these markers of bone remodeling

occur within a few weeks of beginning osteoporosis treatments, and specialists often use them to monitor adherence and effectiveness of therapy.[106]

Periodic evaluation of renal function in patients receiving bisphosphonates and of serum calcium in those receiving teriparatide or denosumab is appropriate.

Preventing bone loss and osteoporosis in postmenopausal women

The bone loss that occurs in aging postmenopausal women may be slowed but not stopped with general measures including adequate nutrition, regular physical activity and avoidance of harmful lifestyle habits such as smoking. That general measures do not prevent bone loss is especially true during the interval of relatively rapid bone loss that occurs in the first few years after menopause.[107] Many studies have documented that various oral and transdermal estrogen preparations can prevent bone loss in postmenopausal women of any age.[108-110] Several oral and transdermal estrogen preparations, the combination of bazedoxifene and conjugated estrogen, raloxifene, and four aminobisphosphonate drugs are approved for the prevention of osteoporosis on the basis of BMD endpoint studies in young postmenopausal women at low risk of fracture. A similar study demonstrated that denosumab 60 mg every 6 months effectively prevented bone loss in young postmenopausal women, but the prevention indication was not granted by FDA because the guidelines for osteoporosis treatment at the time of approval did not endorse the use of drugs for prevention.[111] Evidence for raloxifene being effective to prevent bone loss in early postmenopausal women is rather weak.[69] The doses of oral alendronate (5 mg/d; 35 mg/wk) and intravenous zoledronic acid (5 mg every 2 y) used for prevention are lower than the doses approved for treating osteoporosis.[112,113]

The studies leading to FDA approval for prevention have generally been only 2 years in duration. However, alendronate has been demonstrated to prevent bone loss in early postmenopausal women for at least 6 years and estrogen and tibolone for at least 10 years.[114-116] None of these studies was large enough to detect an effect of therapy on fracture rate, and none followed women long enough to evaluate the effect of preventing bone loss in early menopause on fracture risk in elderly women. The WHI did demonstrate that estrogen and estrogen plus progestin prevented both vertebral and hip fracture in women who were, on average, aged 63 years when the study began, most of whom did not have osteoporosis.[60,61] Despite these data, guidelines for treating osteoporosis since 2008, which place primary emphasis on prevention of fracture and on cost effectiveness, do not endorse the use of pharmacologic therapy, including estrogen, to treat women with the objective of preventing osteoporosis.

However, a strong clinical argument can be made for the use of estrogen, followed by a bisphosphonate, or by bisphosphonates if ET cannot be used, to prevent the rapid bone loss that occurs during the first 5 years of menopause in women who come to menopause with low bone mass.[117] On average, women lose about one T-score unit (10-12%) of bone mass across a normal menopause transition.[1,118] If a woman comes to menopause aged 50 years with a T-score of −1.5, it is very probable that she will have BMD values consistent with osteoporosis by age 60. With this rapid bone loss, significant and irreversible deterioration in trabecular microarchitecture occurs.[117] Despite the lack of hard clinical evidence that preventing bone loss in early menopause reduces fracture risk in later life, it seems obvious that preventing this rapid bone loss would be clinically useful if available therapies to prevent this loss have more benefit than risk for individual women.

Support for this reasoning is found in the treatment of women with nonmetastatic breast cancer who experience bone loss because of estrogen deficiency. Treatment of premenopausal women on a gonadotropin-releasing hormone agonist and an AI with bisphosphonates prevented bone loss and preserved trabecular microarchitecture.[119] Treatment of women on AIs with denosumab 60 mg every 6 months for a median time of 38 months (but some as long as 6 y) not only increased BMD but also reduced the incidence of vertebral fractures by 50% within the first year of treatment, including in women with normal BMD values at baseline.[120]

Emerging therapies

Odanacatib is a highly selective inhibitor of cathepsin K, the major proteolytic enzyme responsible for the degradation of bone collagen and other bone matrix proteins. This drug reduced bone resorption while having little or no effect on bone formation. Large, progressive increases in BMD were observed over 8 years of therapy.[121] In postmenopausal women with osteoporosis, odanacatib significantly reduced the risk of vertebral, nonvertebral, and hip fracture and was well tolerated as a once-weekly oral dose.[122] A modest, unexpected increase in the risk of stroke was observed, resulting in a halt to further clinical development or marketing of this drug.

Romosozumab, a humanized antibody that binds sclerostin, an osteocyte-derived inhibitor of bone formation, markedly but transiently activates bone formation while inhibiting bone resorption, resulting in large increases in BMD.[123] Results of two fracture end-point studies make it clear that beginning treatment with romosozumab therapy for 12 months, followed by either denosumab or alendronate, is superior to treatment with either denosumab or alendronate alone.[124,125] An increased risk of CV events with romosozumab was observed compared with alendronate but not compared with placebo.[125] Romosozumab received FDA approval in 2019 for the treatment of postmenopausal women at high risk for fracture. Romosozumab should not be initiated in patients who have had a myocardial infarction or stroke within the preceding year. Patients taking romosozumab should be monitored for symptoms of myocardial infarction or stroke, which are potential adverse events. Osteonecrosis of the jaw and atypical femoral fracture have been reported in patients treated with romosozumab in clinical trials.

To summarize

Bone loss, which almost always occurs in postmenopausal women, can lead to osteoporosis and, ultimately, to high fracture risk. Because all primary care providers who care for older women encounter many patients with or at risk for osteoporosis, they should be familiar with the evaluation and management of these women. For the smaller number of patients with unusual presentations of osteoporosis or who have complex medical stories, referral to an osteoporosis specialist could be considered.

Over the past 30 years, tools have been developed to diagnose osteoporosis and to identify women at high risk of fracture for whom pharmacologic therapy would be indicated. Practical guidelines for evaluating and treating osteoporosis are available. Multiple classes of drugs have proven effective in reducing fracture risk in women with postmenopausal osteoporosis. These benefits are clearly greater than the effects of good nutrition, dietary supplements, and regular exercise. In postmenopausal women with osteoporosis or with other important risk factors for fracture, the benefit-risk ratio for raloxifene, bisphosphonates, and denosumab is very favorable during the first several years of therapy. The skeletal benefits of all treatments, including bisphosphonates, wane, often quickly, when treatment is stopped. Although there are no studies evaluating the effects of treatment for more than 10 years, long-term management, by using different drugs in appropriate sequences, should be encouraged. For some women about to experience rapid bone loss (eg, during the menopause transition; discontinuing ET, discontinuing denosumab), short-term treatment with a long-acting bisphosphonate could be considered. There is not just one treatment formula. Decisions about treating each patient must be made individually.

REFERENCES

1. Greendale GA, Sowers M, Han W, et al. Bone mineral density loss in relation to the final menstrual period in a multiethnic cohort: results from the Study of Women's Health Across the Nation (SWAN). *J Bone Miner Res*. 2012;27(1):111-118.

2. Lewiecki EM, Binkley N, Morgan SL, et al; International Society for Clinical Densitometry. Best practices for dual-energy X-ray absorptiometry measurement and reporting: International Society for Clinical Densitometry guidance. *J Clin Densitom*. 2016;19(2):127-140.

3. Kanis JA, Melton LJ 3rd, Christiansen C, Johnston CC, Khaltaev N. The diagnosis of osteoporosis. *J Bone Miner Res*. 1994;9(8):1137-1141.

4. Cosman F, de Beur SJ, LeBoff MS, et al; National Osteoporosis Foundation. Clinician's guide to prevention and treatment of osteoporosis. *Osteoporos Int*. 2014;25:2359-2381.

5. Siris ES, Adler R, Bilezikian J, et al. The clinical diagnosis of osteoporosis: a position statement from the National Bone Health Alliance Working Group. *Osteoporos Int*. 2014;25(5):1439-1443.

6. Wright NC, Looker AC, Saag KG, et al. The recent prevalence of osteoporosis and low bone mass in the United States based on bone mineral density at the femoral neck or lumbar spine. *J Bone Miner Res*. 2014;29(11):2520-2526.

7. Tenenhouse A, Joseph L, Kreiger N, et al; CaMos Research Group. Canadian Multicentre Osteoporosis Study. Estimation of the prevalence of low bone density in Canadian women and men using a population-specific DXA reference standard: the Canadian Multicentre Osteoporosis Study (CaMos). *Osteoporos Int*. 2000;11(10):897-904.

8. Centers for Disease Control and Prevention. Hip fractures among older adults. www.cdc.gov/homeandrecreationalsafety/falls/adulthipfx.html. Last updated September 20, 2016. Accessed June 14, 2019.

9. Barrett-Connor E, Siris ES, Wehren LE, et al. Osteoporosis and fracture risk in women of different ethnic groups. *J Bone Miner Res*. 2005;20(2):185-194.

10. Clark P, Cons-Molina F, Deleze M, et al. The prevalence of radiographic vertebral fractures in Latin American countries: the Latin American Vertebral Osteoporosis Study (LAVOS). *Osteoporos Int*. 2009;20(2):275-282.

11. Papaioannou A, Joseph L, Ioannidis G, et al. Risk factors associated with incident clinical vertebral and nonvertebral fractures in postmenopausal women: the Canadian Multicentre Osteoporosis Study (CaMos). *Osteoporos Int*. 2005;16(5):568-578.

12. Michael Lewiecki E, Wright NC, Curtis JR, et al. Hip fracture trends in the United States, 2002 to 2015. *Osteoporos Int*. 2018;29(3):717-722.

13. Tran T, Bliuc D, Hansen L, et al. Persistence of excess mortality following individual nonhip fractures: a relative survival analysis. *J Clin Endocrinol Metab*. 2018;103(9):3205-3214.

14. Papaioannou A, Watts NB, Kendler DL, Yuen CK, Adachi JD, Ferko N. Diagnosis and management of vertebral fractures in elderly adults. *Am J Med*. 2002;113(3):220-228.

15. Fink HA, Ensrud KE, Nelson DB, et al. Disability after clinical fracture in postmenopausal women with low bone density: the fracture intervention trial (FIT). *Osteoporos Int*. 2003;14(1):69-76.

16. Guillemin F, Martinez L, Calvert M, et al. Fear of falling, fracture history, and comorbidities are associated with health-related quality of life among European and US women with osteoporosis in a large international study. *Osteoporos Int*. 2013;24(12):3001-3010.

17. Sigurdsson G, Halldorsson BV, Styrkarsdottir U, Kristjansson K, Stefansson K. Impact of genetics on low bone mass in adults. *J Bone Miner Res*. 2008;23(10):1584-1590.

18. Management of osteoporosis in postmenopausal women: 2010 position statement of The North American Menopause Society. *Menopause*. 2010;17(1):25-54.

19. Bours SP, van den Bergh JP, van Geel TA, Geusens PP. Secondary osteoporosis and metabolic bone disease in patients 50 years and older with osteoporosis or with a recent clinical fracture: a clinical perspective. *Curr Opin Rheumatol*. 2014;26(4):430-439.

20. Kanis JA, Johansson H, Odén A, et al. Characteristics of recurrent fractures. *Osteoporos Int*. 2018;29(8):1747-1757.

21. van Geel TA, Huntjens KM, van den Bergh JP, Dinant GJ, Geusens PP. Timing of subsequent fractures after an initial fracture. *Curr Osteoporos Rep*. 2010;8(3):118-122.

22. Lindsay R, Silverman SL, Cooper C, et al. Risk of new vertebral fracture in the year following a fracture. *JAMA*. 2001;285(3):320-323.

23. Osuna PM, Ruppe MD, Tabatabai LS. Fracture liaison services: multidisciplinary approaches to secondary fracture prevention. *Endocr Pract*. 2017;23(2):199-206.

24. Cummings SR, Black DM, Nevitt MC, et al. Bone density at various sites for prediction of hip fractures. The Study of Osteoporotic Fractures Research Group. *Lancet*. 1993;341(8837):72-75.

25. Kanis JA, Johnell O, Oden A, Dawson A, De Laet C, Jonsson B. Ten year probabilities of osteoporotic fractures according to BMD and diagnostic thresholds. *Osteoporos Int*. 2001;12(12):989-995.

26. Kanis JA, Johnell O, Oden A, et al. Smoking and fracture risk: a meta-analysis. *Osteoporos Int*. 2005;16(2):155-162.

27. Thorin MH, Wihlborg A, Åkesson K, Gerdhem P. Smoking, smoking cessation, and fracture risk in elderly women followed for 10 years. *Osteoporos Int*. 2016;27(1):249-255.

28. Kanis JA, Johansson H, Johnell O, et al. Alcohol intake as a risk factor for fracture. *Osteoporos Int*. 2005;16(7):737-742.

29. Vestergaard P. Discrepancies in bone mineral density and fracture risk in patients with type 1 and type 2 diabetes—a meta-analysis. *Osteoporos Int*. 2007;18(4):427-444.

30. Lau AN, Tomizza M, Wong-Pack M, Papaioannou A, Adachi JD. The relationship between long-term proton pump inhibitor therapy and skeletal frailty. *Endocrine*. 2015;49(3):606-610.

31. Kanis JA, McCloskey EV, Johansson H, Oden A, Ström O, Borgström F. Development and use of FRAX in osteoporosis. *Osteoporos Int*. 2010;21(suppl 2):S407-S413.

32. Leslie WD, Berger C, Langsetmo L, et al; Canadian Multicentre Osteoporosis Study Research Group. Construction and validation of a simplified fracture risk assessment tool for Canadian women and men: results from the CaMos and Manitoba cohorts. *Osteoporos Int*. 2011;22(6):1873-1883.

33. Papaioannou A, Morin S, Cheung AM, et al; Scientific Advisory Council of Osteoporosis Canada. 2010 Clinical practice guidelines for the diagnosis and management of osteoporosis in Canada: summary. *CMAJ*. 2010;182(17):1864-1873.

34. Nassar K, Paternotte S, Kolta S, Fechtenbaum J, Roux C, Briot K. Added value of trabecular bone score over bone mineral density for identification of vertebral fractures in patients with areal bone mineral density in the non-osteoporotic range. *Osteoporos Int*. 2014;25(1):243-249.

35. McCloskey EV, Odén A, Harvey NC, et al. Adjusting fracture probability by trabecular bone score. *Calcif Tissue Int*. 2015;96(6):500-509.

36. Camacho PM, Petak SM, Binkley N, et al. American Association of Clinical Endocrinologists and American College of Endocrinology clinical practice guidelines for the diagnosis and treatment of postmenopausal osteoporosis—2016. *Endocr Pract*. 2016;22(suppl 4):1-42.

37. Peña-Ríos DH, Cisneros-Dreinhofer FA, de la Peña-Rodriguez MP, et al. Consenso de diagnóstico y tratamiento de la osteoporosis en la mujer postmenopáusica Mexicana [article in Spanish]. *Med Int Méx*. 2015;31:596-610.

38. US Preventive Services Task Force. Screening for osteoporosis: US Preventive Services Task Force recommendation statement. *Ann Intern Med*. 2011;154(5):356-364.

CHAPTER 7

39. US Preventive Services Task Force, Curry SJ, Krist AH, et al. Screening for osteoporosis to prevent fractures: US Preventive Services Task Force recommendation statement. *JAMA.* 2018;319(24):2521-2531.

40. Gillespie LD, Robertson MC, Gillespie WJ, et al. Interventions for preventing falls in older people living in the community. *Cochrane Database Syst Rev.* 2012;(9):CD007146.

41. Tricco AC, Thomas SM, Veroniki AA, et al. Comparisons of interventions for preventing falls in older adults: a systematic review and meta-analysis. *JAMA.* 2017;318(17):1687-1699.

42. US Preventive Services Task Force, Grossman DC, Curry SJ, et al. Interventions to prevent falls in community-dwelling older adults: US Preventive Services Task Force recommendation statement. *JAMA.* 2018;319(16):1696-1704.

43. Santesso N, Carrasco-Labra A, Brignardello-Petersen R. Hip protectors for preventing hip fractures in older people. *Cochrane Database Syst Rev.* 2014;(3):CD001255.

44. Jackson RD, LaCroix AZ, Gass M, et al; Women's Health Initiative Investigators. Calcium plus vitamin D supplementation and the risk of fractures. *N Engl J Med.* 2006;354(7):669-683.

45. Ross AC, Manson JE, Abrams SA, et al The 2011 report on dietary reference intakes for calcium and vitamin D from the Institute of Medicine: what clinicians need to know. *J Clin Endocrinol Metab.* 2011;96(1):53-58.

46. Bolland MJ, Barber PA, Doughty RN, et al. Vascular events in healthy older women receiving calcium supplementation: randomised controlled trial. *BMJ.* 2008;336(7638):262-266.

47. Bischoff-Ferrari HA, Willett WC, Orav EJ, et al. A pooled analysis of vitamin D dose requirements for fracture prevention. *N Engl J Med.* 2012;367(1):40-49. Erratum in: *N Engl J Med.* 2012;367(5):481.

48. Chapuy MC, Arlot ME, Duboeuf F, et al. Vitamin D3 and calcium to prevent hip fractures in elderly women. *N Engl J Med.* 1992;327(23):1637-1642.

49. Sanders KM, Stuart AL, Williamson EJ, et al. Annual high-dose oral vitamin D and falls and fractures in older women: a randomized controlled trial. *JAMA.* 2010;303(18):1815-1822.

50. US Preventive Services Task Force, Grossman DC, Curry SJ, et al. Vitamin D, calcium, or combined supplementation for the primary prevention of fractures in community-dwelling adults: US Preventive Services Task Force recommendation statement. *JAMA.* 2018;319(15):1592-1599.

51. Shams-White MM, Chung M, Du M, et al. Dietary protein and bone health: a systematic review and meta-analysis from the National Osteoporosis Foundation. *Am J Clin Nutr.* 2017;105(6):1528-1543.

52. Zoltick ES, Sahni S, McLean RR, Quach L, Casey VA, Hannan MT. Dietary protein intake and subsequent falls in older men and women: the Framingham Study. *J Nutr Health Aging.* 2011;15(2):147-152.

53. Reginster JY, Seeman E, De Vernejoul MC, et al. Strontium ranelate reduces the risk of nonvertebral fractures in postmenopausal women with osteoporosis: Treatment of Peripheral Osteoporosis (TROPOS) study. *J Clin Endocrinol Metab.* 2005;90(5):2816-2822.

54. Orchard TS, Larson JC, Alghothani N, et al. Magnesium intake, bone mineral density, and fractures: results from the Women's Health Initiative Observational Study. *Am J Clin Nutr.* 2014;99(4):926-933.

55. Kunutsor SK, Whitehouse MR, Blom AW, Laukkanen JA. Low serum magnesium levels are associated with increased risk of fractures: a long-term prospective cohort study. *Eur J Epidemiol.* 2017;32(7):593-603.

56. Cheung AM, Tile L, Lee Y, et al. Vitamin K supplementation in postmenopausal women with osteopenia (ECKO trial): a randomized controlled trial. *PLoS Med.* 2008;5(10):e196. Erratum in: *PLoS Med.* 2008;5(12):e247.

57. Tanaka S, Miyazaki T, Uemura Y, et al. Comparison of concurrent treatment with vitamin K2 and risedronate compared with treatment with risedronate alone in patients with osteoporosis: Japanese Osteoporosis Intervention Trial-03. *J Bone Miner Metab.* 2017;35(4):385-395.

58. North American Menopause Society. The role of soy isoflavones in menopausal health: report of the North American Menopause Society/ Wulf H. Utian Translational Science Symposium in Chicago, IL (October 2010). *Menopause.* 2011;18(7):732-753.

59. Qaseem A, Forciea MA, McLean RM, Denberg TD; Clinical Guidelines Committee of the American College of Physicians. Treatment of low bone density or osteoporosis to prevent fractures in men and women: a clinical practice guideline update from the American College of Physicians. *Ann Intern Med.* 2017;166(11):818-839. Erratum in: *Ann Intern Med.* 2017;167(6)448.

60. Cauley JA, Robbins J, Chen Z, et al; Women's Health Initiative Investigators. Effects of estrogen plus progestin on risk of fracture and bone mineral density: the Women's Health Initiative randomized trial. *JAMA.* 2003;290(13):1729-1738.

61. Jackson RD, Wactawski-Wende J, LaCroix AZ, et al; Women's Health Initiative Investigators. Effects of conjugated equine estrogen on risk of fractures and BMD in postmenopausal women with hysterectomy: results from the Women's Health Initiative randomized trial. *J Bone Miner Res.* 2006;21(6):817-828.

62. The NAMS 2017 Hormone Therapy Position Statement Advisory Panel. The 2017 hormone therapy position statement of The North American Menopause Society. *Menopause.* 2017;24(7):728-753.

63. Wasnich RD, Bagger YZ, Hosking DJ, et al; Early Postmenopausal Intervention Cohort Study Group. Changes in bone density and turnover after alendronate or estrogen withdrawal. *Menopause.* 2004;11(6 pt 1):622-630.

64. Heiss G, Wallace R, Anderson GL, et al; WHI Investigators. Health risks and benefits 3 years after stopping randomized treatment with estrogen and progestin. *JAMA.* 2008;299(9):1036-1045.

65. Watts NB, Cauley JA, Jackson RD, et al; Women's Health Initiative Investigators. No increase in fractures after stopping hormone therapy: results From the Women's Health Initiative Investigators. *J Clin Endocrinol Metab.* 2017;102(1):302-308.

66. Ascott-Evans BH, Guanabens N, Kivinen S, et al. Alendronate prevents loss of bone density associated with discontinuation of hormone replacement therapy: a randomized controlled trial. *Arch Intern Med.* 2003;163(7):789-794.

67. Gallagher JC, Baylink DJ, Freeman R, McClung M. Prevention of bone loss with tibolone in postmenopausal women: results of two randomized, double-blind, placebo-controlled, dose-finding studies. *J Clin Endocrinol Metab.* 2001;86(10):4717-4726.

68. Cummings SR, Ettinger B, Delmas PD, et al; LIFT Trial Investigators. The effects of tibolone in older postmenopausal women. *N Engl J Med.* 2008;359(7):697-708.

69. Delmas PD, Bjarnason NH, Mitlak BH, et al. Effects of raloxifene on bone mineral density, serum cholesterol concentrations, and uterine endometrium in postmenopausal women. *N Engl J Med.* 1997;337(23):1641-1647.

70. Ettinger B, Black DM, Mitlak BH, et al. Reduction of vertebral fracture risk in postmenopausal women with osteoporosis treated with raloxifene: results from a 3-year randomized clinical trial. Multiple Outcomes of Raloxifene Evaluation (MORE) Investigators. *JAMA.* 1999;282(7):637-645.

71. Lewiecki EM, Miller PD, Harris ST, et al. Understanding and communicating the benefits and risks of denosumab, raloxifene, and teriparatide for the treatment of osteoporosis. *J Clin Densitom.* 2014;17(4):490-495.

72. Neele SJ, Evertz R, De Valk-De Roo G, Roos JC, Netelenbos JC. Effect of 1 year of discontinuation of raloxifene or estrogen therapy on bone mineral density after 5 years of treatment in healthy postmenopausal women. *Bone.* 2002;30(4):599-603.

73. Silverman SL, Christiansen C, Genant HK, et al. Efficacy of bazedoxifene in reducing new vertebral fracture risk in postmenopausal women with osteoporosis: results from a 3-year, randomized, placebo-, and active-controlled clinical trial. *J Bone Miner Res.* 2008;23(12):1923-1934.

74. Pinkerton JV, Pickar JH, Racketa J, Mirkin S. Bazedoxifene/conjugated estrogens for menopausal symptom treatment and osteoporosis prevention. *Climacteric.* 2012;15(5):411-418.

75. Russell RG, Rogers MJ. Bisphosphonates: from the laboratory to the clinic and back again. *Bone.* 1999;25(1):97-106.

76. McClung M, Harris ST, Miller PD, et al. Bisphosphonate therapy for osteoporosis: benefits, risks, and drug holiday. *Am J Med.* 2013;126(1):13-20.

77. Chesnut CH 3rd, Skag A, Christiansen C, et al; Oral Ibandronate Osteoporosis Vertebral Fracture Trial in North America and Europe (BONE). Effects of oral ibandronate administered daily or intermittently on fracture risk in postmenopausal osteoporosis. *J Bone Miner Res*. 2004;19(8):1241-1249.

78. Khan AA, Sándor GK, Dore E, et al; Canadian Taskforce on Osteonecrosis of the Jaw. Bisphosphonate associated osteonecrosis of the jaw. *J Rheumatol*. 2009;36(3):478-490.

79. Shane E, Burr D, Abrahamsen B, et al. Atypical subtrochanteric and diaphyseal femoral fractures: second report of a task force of the American Society for Bone and Mineral Research. *J Bone Miner Res*. 2014;29(1):1-23.

80. Schilcher J, Koeppen V, Aspenberg P, Michaëlsson K. Risk of atypical femoral fracture during and after bisphosphonate use. *N Engl J Med*. 2014;371(10):974-976.

81. Bone HG, Hosking D, Devogelaer JP, et al; Alendronate Phase III Osteoporosis Treatment Study Group. Ten years' experience with alendronate for osteoporosis in postmenopausal women. *N Engl J Med*. 2004;350(12):1189-1199.

82. Watts NB, Chines A, Olszynski WP, et al. Fracture risk remains reduced one year after discontinuation of risedronate. *Osteoporos Int*. 2008;19(3):365-372.

83. Black DM, Reid IR, Cauley JA, et al. The effect of 6 versus 9 years of zoledronic acid treatment in osteoporosis: a randomized second extension to the HORIZON-Pivotal Fracture Trial (PFT). *J Bone Miner Res*. 2015;30(5):934-944.

84. Adler RA, El-Hajj Fuleihan G, Bauer DC, et al. Managing osteoporosis in patients on long-term bisphosphonate treatment: report of a Task Force of the American Society for Bone and Mineral Research. *J Bone Miner Res*. 2016;31(1):16-35.

85. Kendler DL, Roux C, Benhamou CL, et al. Effects of denosumab on bone mineral density and bone turnover in postmenopausal women transitioning from alendronate therapy. *J Bone Miner Res*. 2010;25(1):72-81.

86. Obermayer-Pietsch BM, Marin F, McCloskey EV, et al; EUROFORS Investigators. Effects of two years of daily teriparatide treatment on BMD in postmenopausal women with severe osteoporosis with and without prior antiresorptive treatment. *J Bone Miner Res*. 2008;23(10):1591-1600.

87. Watts NB, Harris ST, Genant HK, et al. Intermittent cyclical etidronate treatment of postmenopausal osteoporosis. *N Engl J Med*. 1990;323(2):73-79.

88. Cummings SR, San Martin J, McClung MR, et al; FREEDOM Trial. Denosumab for prevention of fractures in postmenopausal women with osteoporosis. *N Engl J Med*. 2009;361(8):756-765.

89. Bone HG, Wagman RB, Brandi ML, et al. 10 years of denosumab treatment in postmenopausal women with osteoporosis: results from the phase 3 randomised FREEDOM trial and open-label extension. *Lancet Diabetes Endocrinol*. 2017;5(7):513-523.

90. Bone HG, Bolognese MA, Yuen CK, et al. Effects of denosumab treatment and discontinuation on bone mineral density and bone turnover markers in postmenopausal women with low bone mass. *J Clin Endocrinol Metab*. 2011;96(4):972-980.

91. Cummings SR, Ferrari S, Eastell R, et al. Vertebral fractures after discontinuation of denosumab: a post hoc analysis of the randomized placebo-controlled FREEDOM trial and its extension. *J Bone Miner Res*. 2018;33(2):190-198.

92. Anastasilakis AD, Polyzos SA, Makras P, Aubry-Rozier B, Kaouri S, Lamy O. Clinical features of 24 patients with rebound-associated vertebral fractures after denosumab discontinuation: systematic review and additional cases. *J Bone Miner Res*. 2017;32(6):1291-1296.

93. Chesnut CH 3rd, Silverman S, Andriano K, et al. A randomized trial of nasal spray salmon calcitonin in postmenopausal women with established osteoporosis: the Prevent Recurrence of Osteoporotic Fractures study. PROOF Study Group. *Am J Med*. 2000;109(4):267-276.

94. McClung MR, San Martin J, Miller PD, et al. Opposite bone remodeling effects of teriparatide and alendronate in increasing bone mass. *Arch Intern Med*. 2005;165(15):1762-1768. Erratum in: *Arch Intern Med*. 2005;165(18):2120.

95. Neer RM, Arnaud CD, Zanchetta JR, et al. Effect of parathyroid hormone (1-34) on fractures and bone mineral density in postmenopausal women with osteoporosis. *N Engl J Med*. 2001;344(19):1434-1441.

96. Kendler DL, Marin F, Zerbini CAF, et al. Effects of teriparatide and risedronate on new fractures in post-menopausal women with severe osteoporosis (VERO): a multicentre, double-blind, double-dummy, randomised controlled trial. *Lancet*. 2018;391(10117):230-240.

97. Leder BZ, Tsai JN, Uihlein AV, et al. Denosumab and teriparatide transitions in postmenopausal osteoporosis (the DATA-Switch study): extension of a randomised controlled trial. *Lancet*. 2015;386(9999):1147-1155.

98. Ebina K, Hashimoto J, Kashii M, et al. The effects of switching daily teriparatide to oral bisphosphonates or denosumab in patients with primary osteoporosis. *J Bone Miner Metab*. 2017;35(1):91-98.

99. Miller PD, Hattersley G, Riis BJ, et al; ACTIVE Study Investigators. Effect of abaloparatide vs placebo on new vertebral fractures in postmenopausal women with osteoporosis: a randomized clinical trial. *JAMA*. 2016;316(7):722-733.

100. Cosman F, Miller PD, Williams GC, et al. Eighteen months of treatment with subcutaneous abaloparatide followed by 6 months of treatment with alendronate in postmenopausal women with osteoporosis: results of the ACTIVExtend Trial. *Mayo Clin Proc*. 2017;92(2):200-210.

101. McClung MR. Using osteoporosis therapies in combination. *Curr Osteoporos Rep*. 2017;15(4):343-352.

102. Black DM, Greenspan SL, Ensrud KE, et al; PaTH Study Investigators. The effects of parathyroid hormone and alendronate alone or in combination in postmenopausal osteoporosis. *N Engl J Med*. 2003;349(13):1207-1215.

103. Cosman F, Eriksen EF, Recknor C, et al. Effects of intravenous zoledronic acid plus subcutaneous teriparatide [rhPTH(1-34)] in postmenopausal osteoporosis. *J Bone Miner Res*. 2011;26(3):503-511.

104. Leder BZ, Tsai JN, Uihlein AV, et al. Two years of Denosumab and teriparatide administration in postmenopausal women with osteoporosis (The DATA Extension Study): a randomized controlled trial. *J Clin Endocrinol Metab*. 2014;99(5):1694-1700.

105. Clowes JA, Peel NF, Eastell R. The impact of monitoring on adherence and persistence with antiresorptive treatment for postmenopausal osteoporosis: a randomized controlled trial. *J Clin Endocrinol Metab*. 2004;89(3):1117-1123.

106. Eastell R, Szulc P. Use of bone turnover markers in postmenopausal osteoporosis. *Lancet Diabetes Endocrinol*. 2017;5(11):908-923.

107. Hosking DJ, Russ PD, Thompson DE, et al. Evidence that increased calcium intake does not prevent early postmenopausal bone loss. *Clin Ther*. 1998;20(5):933-944.

108. Effects of hormone therapy on bone mineral density: results from the postmenopausal estrogen/progestin interventions (PEPI) trial. The Writing Group for the PEPI. *JAMA*. 1996;276(17):1389-1396.

109. Hosking D, Chilvers CE, Christiansen C, et al. Prevention of bone loss with alendronate in postmenopausal women under 60 years of age. Early Postmenopausal Intervention Cohort Study Group. *N Engl J Med*. 1998;338(8):485-492.

110. Adami S, Suppi R, Bertoldo F, et al. Transdermal estradiol in the treatment of postmenopausal bone loss. *Bone Miner*. 1989;7(1):79-86.

111. Bone HG, Bolognese MA, Yuen CK, et al. Effects of denosumab on bone mineral density and bone turnover in postmenopausal women. *J Clin Endocrinol Metab*. 2008;93(6):2149-2157

112. McClung M, Clemmesen B, Daifotis A, et al. Alendronate prevents postmenopausal bone loss in women without osteoporosis. A double-blind, randomized, controlled trial. Alendronate Osteoporosis Prevention Study Group. *Ann Intern Med*. 1998;128(4):253-261.

113. McClung M, Miller P, Recknor C, Mesenbrink P, Bucci-Rechtweg C, Benhamou CL. Zoledronic acid for the prevention of bone loss in postmenopausal women with low bone mass: a randomized controlled trial. *Obstet Gynecol*. 2009;114(5):999-1007.

114. McClung MR, Wasnich RD, Hosking DJ, et al; Early Postmenopausal Intervention Cohort Study. Prevention of postmenopausal bone loss: six-year results from the Early Postmenopausal Intervention Cohort Study. *J Clin Endocrinol Metab*. 2004;89(10):4879-4885.

115. Moore M, Bracker M, Sartoris D, Saltman P, Strause L. Long-term estrogen replacement therapy in postmenopausal women sustains vertebral bone mineral density. *J Bone Miner Res*. 1990;5(6):659-664.

116. Rymer J, Robinson J, Fogelman I. Ten years of treatment with tibolone 2.5 mg daily: effects on bone loss in postmenopausal women. *Climacteric*. 2002;5(4):390-398.

117. McClung MR. Osteopenia: to treat or not to treat? *Ann Intern Med*. 2005;142(9):796-797.

118. Recker R, Lappe J, Davies K, Heaney R. Characterization of perimenopausal bone loss: a prospective study. *J Bone Miner Res*. 2000;15(10):1965-1973.

119. Gnant M, Mlineritsch B, Schippinger W, et al; ABCSG-12 Trial Investigators. Endocrine therapy plus zoledronic acid in premenopausal breast cancer. *N Engl J Med*. 2009;360(7):679-691. Erratum in: *N Engl J Med*. 2009;360(22):2379.

120. Gnant M, Pfeiler G, Dubsky PC, et al; Austrian Breast and Colorectal Cancer Study Group. Adjuvant denosumab in breast cancer (ABCSG-18): a multicentre, randomised, double-blind, placebo-controlled trial. *Lancet*. 2015;386(9992):433-443.

121. Rizzoli R, Benhamou CL, Halse J, et al. Continuous treatment with odanacatib for up to 8 years in postmenopausal women with low bone mineral density: a phase 2 study. *Osteoporos Int*. 2016;27(6):2099-2107.

122. Bone HG, Dempster DW, Eisman JA, et al. Odanacatib for the treatment of postmenopausal osteoporosis: development history and design and participant characteristics of LOFT, the Long-Term Odanacatib Fracture Trial. *Osteoporos Int*. 2015;26(2):699-712. Erratum in: *Osteoporos Int*. 2015;26(11):2721.

123. McClung MR, Grauer A, Boonen S, et al. Romosozumab in postmenopausal women with low bone mineral density. *N Engl J Med*. 2014;370(5):412-420.

124. Cosman F, Crittenden DB, Adachi JD, et al. Romosozumab treatment in postmenopausal women with osteoporosis. *N Engl J Med*. 2016;375(16):1532-1543.

125. Saag KG, Petersen J, Brandi ML, et al. Romosozumab or alendronate for fracture prevention in women with osteoporosis. *N Engl J Med*. 2017;377(15):1417-1427.

8

Cardiometabolic Disorders in Midlife Women

Cardiovascular Health

Cardiovascular disease (CVD) is an inclusive term used to describe many conditions (Table 1) and is the leading killer of women worldwide. More women die from CVD than from all cancers, tuberculosis, HIV/AIDS, and malaria combined.[1] In 2014, 399,028 US women died from heart disease, accounting for almost half of all deaths in women. Although rates of CVD in the United States are declining because of significant advancements in prevention, diagnosis, and treatment, one in three women will die of heart disease regardless of ethnicity.[2] Mortality rates from CVD in women have exceeded mortality rates in men every year from 1984 to 2013, with deceleration in the decline in mortality in both sexes and all race and ethnic groups since 2011.[3]

Heart disease awareness in women is increasing, yet only 52% of women identify heart disease as the leading cause of death in women. Awareness is particularly low in black and Hispanic women, with only 30% of those aged 25 to 34 years aware.[4]

Etiology

Proper function of the myocardium depends on a positive balance of oxygen and nutrient supply and demand. Angina is most often associated with the narrowing or dysfunction of coronary arteries, caused by the formation of atherosclerotic plaques in the epicardial coronary arteries or abnormal vasomotor function of microvasculature in the heart. Chronic narrowing of the lumen of the coronary artery is most commonly associated with a continuous process of plaque formation, disruption, reorganization, and reformation that begins early in life and may lead to stable angina or even sudden death. Genetic, metabolic, behavioral, and environmental factors can all contribute to the process.

Myocardial infarction (MI) usually occurs when a previously narrowed artery suddenly becomes completely occluded with a thromboembolism (often associated with atherosclerotic plaque erosion or rupture) and less commonly because of microvascular dysfunction or coronary dissection, which are relatively more prevalent in women.[5]

Diseased peripheral blood vessels can lead to conditions such as stroke, transient ischemic attack, and hypertension (HTN). In addition, peripheral vascular disease can result in difficulty walking and, if severe, amputation of the affected limb.

Menopause and risk of cardiovascular disease

Most CVD in women occurs during the postmenopause period or after age 55 years. Premature or early onset of natural or surgical menopause is an established risk factor for CVD. This has contributed to the idea that menopause

---

Table 1. Cardiovascular Diseases

- Arrhythmias
- Atherosclerosis
- Congenital cardiovascular defect
- Heart failure
- Coronary heart disease and ischemic heart disease
  - Myocardial infarction
  - Angina pectoris
  - Microvascular coronary dysfunction
- Hypertension
- Stroke and transient ischemic attack
- Valvular heart disease
- Peripheral arterial disease
- Aortic disease
- Arterial and venous thrombosis and pulmonary embolism

results in an increased risk for CVD. However, the relationship between menopause itself and the risk of CVD remains controversial, and the Atherosclerosis Risk in Communities surveillance study (1985-2016) from the National Heart, Lung, and Blood Institute shows no acceleration of absolute CVD rates after menopause in most women. Further, menopause does not modulate the relation between blood pressure (BP) and CVD, independent of age.[6] In fact, increasing systolic blood pressure (SBP) confers a higher CVD risk in premenopausal women compared with the same increase in SBP in postmenopausal women. Menopause does, however, appear to result in an accelerated increase in low-density lipoprotein cholesterol (LDL-C) and total cholesterol (TC) during the year immediately after the final menstrual period, whereas other risk factors (glycated hemoglobin A_{1c} [HbA_{1c}] and BP) appear to maintain their usual trajectories during this transition period.[6,7] Progression of carotid atherosclerosis has been shown to accelerate during the late perimenopause, controlling for age.[8] Metabolic syndrome (MetS) is more prevalent during these years as well.[9]

Menopause-related hormone changes also may have direct vascular effects. Estrogen and progesterone receptors are present in vascular tissues, including coronary arteries.[10] Coagulation balance also may play a role in the hormone-vascular interaction during menopause changes. Certain fibrinolytic factors (eg, antithrombin III and plasminogen) increase, along with some procoagulation factors (eg, factor VII and fibrinogen). After menopause, blood flow in all vascular beds decreases, prostacyclin decreases, endothelin levels increase, and vasoconstriction occurs in response to acetylcholine challenges. Circulating plasma levels of nitric oxide increase, and levels of angiotensin-converting enzyme (ACE) decrease.

Palpitations

During menopause-related vasomotor episodes, the heart rate can increase seven to fifteen beats per minute. Some women may interpret the perceived increase as palpitation. Although most are benign, the differential diagnosis for palpitations can be extensive and includes cardiac disorders, anemia, medication or caffeine use, and thyroid and anxiety disorders. Although it is unlikely that palpitations associated with vasomotor symptoms (VMS) in perimenopausal and postmenopausal women are related to serious cardiac abnormalities, caution should be exercised if syncope or presyncope is reported. A stress test should be conducted if symptoms are accompanied by exercise intolerance, shortness of breath, or chest pain. Women with a high risk of coronary heart disease (CHD) or with a strong family history of early cardiac death (ie, first-degree male relatives aged <50 y or female relatives aged <60 y) also should be assessed. The American College of Cardiology (ACC)/American Heart Association (AHA) global risk scores (or other risk score instruments such as Framingham Risk, Reynolds Risk, or Multi-ethnic Study of Atherosclerosis Risk) should be used for risk stratification. Although each of these tools can overestimate risk, especially in women, they remain widely used.

Sex-specific initiatives and intervention

Early menopause is related to an increased incidence of CVD morbidity and mortality. Menopause before age 35 years has been associated with a 2- to 3-fold increased risk of MI. The Nurses' Health Study found an overall significant association between younger age at menopause and higher risk of CVD in women who experienced natural menopause and never used hormone therapy (HT).[11] An increased risk was observed in current smokers and not in participants who never smoked.[12] Conversely, other data suggest that processes that increase the risk for CVD may be a determinant of early menopause rather than the presumed reverse scenario[13] or that the relationship is bidirectional.[14] One study reported that for each 1% increase in the premenopausal Framingham Risk Score, there was an associated 1.8-year decrease in age at menopause.

Lipid changes

Low-density lipoprotein cholesterol and very-low-density lipoprotein cholesterol increase in women at menopause, and there is enhanced oxidation of LDL-C postmenopause. There also is an increase in non-high-density lipoprotein cholesterol (TC minus high-density lipoprotein cholesterol [HDL-C]), a variable that includes apolipoprotein B (apoB) atherogenic triglyceride (TG) metabolized particles and very-low-density lipoprotein cholesterol. Non-high-density lipoprotein cholesterol is an excellent marker for increased risk when it is elevated. In a cross-sectional analysis of 9,309 women who had never used HT, the increases in TC, LDL-C, and TG from premenopause to postmenopause were 3% to 4% after adjusting for covariates such as smoking and age.[15] Adverse LDL-C changes and changes in apoB levels occur independently of age during the menopause transition.[7]

The Women's Healthy Lifestyle Project, however, found that the menopause-related rise in LDL-C can be reduced through a lifestyle intervention program that focuses on two factors: decreasing saturated fat and cholesterol intake and preventing excess weight gain through increased physical activity and exercise and reduced calorie and fat intake.[16]

Women who are healthy and not obese experience a decrease in carbohydrate tolerance as insulin resistance increases in postmenopause, which is aggravated in women who are obese.[17] Stress reactivity is exaggerated in postmenopausal women compared with younger women[18]; however, the role of diminished estrogen in these effects is not yet clear.

Risk factors

Major modifiable risk factors associated with CVD in women include increasing traditional and emerging risk factors (Figure 1).[19] Whether obesity and MetS are independent CVD risk factors or simply represent a clustering of risk is unclear.[20-23] It remains controversial whether a decline in estrogen levels is an independent risk factor through either direct or indirect mechanisms.

The 2011 AHA guidelines on CVD prevention in women defines how risk is stratified (Table 2).[24] The greater the risk, the more aggressive the prevention strategy should be; AHA guidelines note that a Framingham

Risk Score of more than 10% could be used to identify a woman at high risk, but less than 10% is not sufficient to assure low risk.[24,25] The guidelines focus on the lifetime risk for CVD and emphasize that at age 50 years, even one single risk factor increases lifetime risk for women.[26]

The AHA guidelines also highlight the CV and metabolic changes that occur during pregnancy, such as preeclampsia and gestational diabetes, as CVD risk factors.[27] This unique time of increased cardiac output and circulating blood volume provides a natural stress test for CV health. In a meta-analysis of eight studies, women with preeclampsia were found to have a 1.65- to 3.61-fold increased risk in ischemic heart disease (IHD) later in life.

Screening

Developing a standardized procedure for evaluating and managing women at risk for CVD is important.

The 2013 ACC/AHA guidelines on the assessment of CV risk includes a gender- and ethnicity-based prediction risk assessment for heart attack and stroke.[26] The risk assessment tool is a formula based on age, sex, race, cholesterol, BP, diabetes mellitus (DM), and smoking status and will provide a short-term (10 y) as well as a

Figure 1. Traditional and Nontraditional Atherosclerotic Cardiovascular Disease (ASCVD) Risk Factors in Women

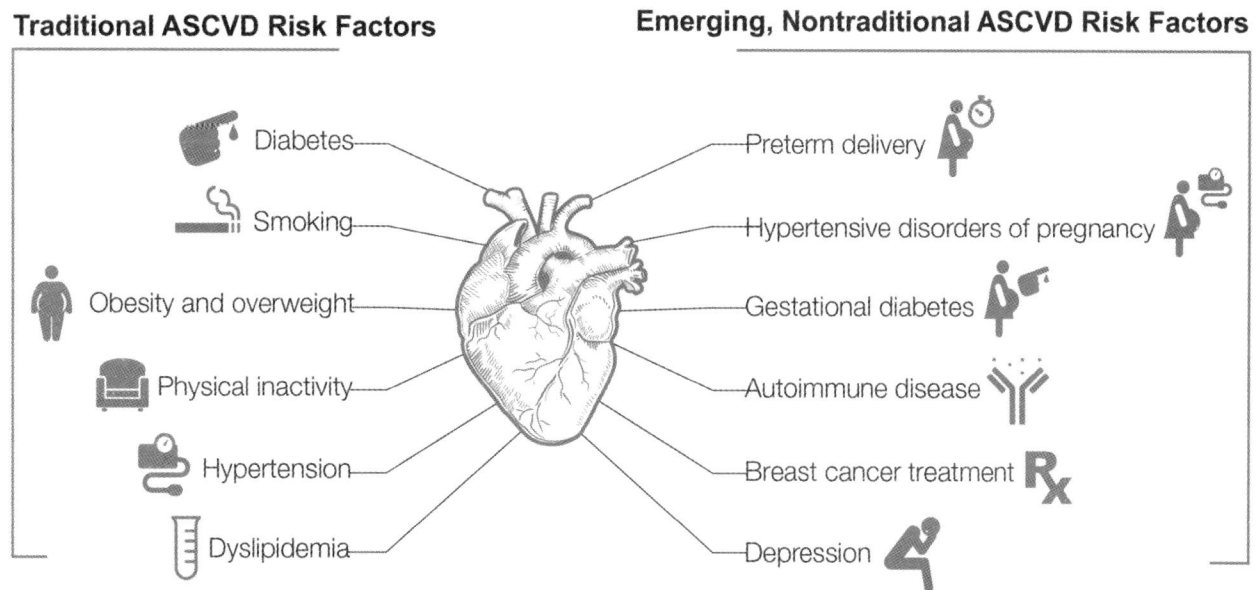

Traditional ASCVD Risk Factors
- Diabetes
- Smoking
- Obesity and overweight
- Physical inactivity
- Hypertension
- Dyslipidemia

Emerging, Nontraditional ASCVD Risk Factors
- Preterm delivery
- Hypertensive disorders of pregnancy
- Gestational diabetes
- Autoimmune disease
- Breast cancer treatment
- Depression

Increasing in women and more affective traditional ASCVD risk factors include diabetes mellitus, hypertension, dyslipidemia, smoking, obesity, and physical inactivity. Emerging, nontraditional ASCVD risk factors include preterm delivery, hypertensive pregnancy disorders, gestational diabetes mellitus, breast cancer treatments, autoimmune diseases, and depression.
Garcia J, et al.[19] Reproduced with permission from Wolters Kluwer Health, Inc. © 2016.

Table 2. 2011 AHA Guidelines CVD Risk Stratification

Risk level	Definition
High risk (one or more)	• Established CHD • Cerebrovascular disease • PAD • Abdominal aortic aneurysm • End-stage or CKD • DM • 10-year predicted CVD ≥10%
At risk (one or more)	• Cigarette smoking • SBP ≥120 mm Hg; DBP ≥80 mm Hg; or treated HTN • TG ≥200 mg/dL • HDL-C >50 mg/dL or treated dyslipidemia • Obesity, particularly central adiposity • Poor diet • Physical inactivity • Family history of premature CVD in first-degree relatives (men <55 y or women <65 y) • MetS • Evidence of advanced subclinical atherosclerosis (eg, coronary calcification, carotid plaque, or intimal medial thickness) • Poor exercise capacity on treadmill test or abnormal heart rate recovery after stopping exercise • Systemic autoimmune collagen-vascular disease (eg, lupus or rheumatoid arthritis) • History of preeclampsia, gestational diabetes, or pregnancy-induced HTN
Ideal CV health (all of these)	• TC <200 mg/dL (untreated) • BP <120/80 mm Hg (untreated) • Fasting blood glucose <100 mg/dL (untreated) • BMI <25 kg/m2 • No smoking • Moderate-intensity physical activity ≥150 min/wk or vigorous intensity ≥75 min/wk or a combination • Healthy diet

Abbreviations: AHA, American Heart Association; BMI, body mass index; BP, blood pressure; CHD, coronary heart disease; CKD, chronic kidney disease; CV, cardiovascular; CVD, cardiovascular disease; DBP, diastolic blood pressure; DM, diabetes mellitus; HDL-C, high-density lipoprotein cholesterol; HTN, hypertension; MetS, metabolic syndrome; PAD, peripheral artery disease; TC, total cholesterol; TG, triglycerides. Mosca L, et al.[24]

lifetime risk of developing heart disease and stroke for persons aged 40 to 79 years. Risk factors include age, TC, HDL-C, SBP, ongoing treatment for HTN, black ethnicity, and active cigarette smoking. The pooled risk equation estimates are more robust for atherosclerotic CVD (ASCVD) prediction because of the inclusion of black populations and stroke. Low-density lipoprotein cholesterol remains the primary target of therapy.

The Framingham Risk Score has been validated in Canada and also is recommended by the Canadian Cardiovascular Society.[28] The Reynolds Risk Score was developed to better estimate risk in patients in the intermediate-risk category.[29] High-sensitivity C-reactive protein (hsCRP) is used as a screening and monitoring tool.[30,31] Oral estrogen is associated with elevated hsCRP, which can limit the use of this blood test as a predictor of increased CVD risk in women using oral estrogen.[32]

Lifestyle modification

Women with modifiable CVD risk factors should be urged to initiate lifestyle changes to decrease overall risk.[24] American Heart Association guidelines for the prevention of CVD in women define lifestyle interventions as tobacco cessation counseling, physical activity, dietary intake, weight maintenance and reduction, cardiac rehabilitation after a recent acute coronary event, and omega-3 fatty acids to lower TG. The 2013 ACC/AHA guidelines on lifestyle management to reduce cardiovascular (CV) risk were published with the intent of evaluating diet, nutritional intake, and physical activity.[33] The key recommendations include eating a diet consistent with the Mediterranean or Dietary Approaches to Stop Hypertension (DASH) diets, which is based on fruits, vegetables, and lean meats and restricting saturated and *trans* fats, sugar, and sodium. These lifestyle interventions are important, not only because of their potential to reduce clinical CVD but also because heart-healthy lifestyles may prevent the development of major risk factors. Such prevention may minimize the need for more intensive future interventions and revascularization.[34,35]

Cigarette smoking

Use of tobacco is the single most important preventable risk factor for CVD in women. A woman who smokes is two to six times more likely to have a heart attack than a woman who does not smoke. The effect of smoking on risk of fatal CVD is dose related (ie, heavier smokers have a greater relative risk). One meta-analysis confirms that even smoking a single cigarette a day portends a significant risk of developing CVD, just half that for people who smoke 20 cigarettes a day.[36] The AHA guidelines for smoking cessation include counseling at each encounter, nicotine replacement, and other pharmacotherapy as indicated, in conjunction with a behavior program or formal smoking-cessation program.[24]

Women also should avoid environmental (ie, secondhand) smoke. Although oral contraceptive use does not appreciably increase CVD risk in nonsmokers, use of oral contraceptives synergistically increases CVD risk, especially MI, in women who do smoke.[19,37] Studies have shown an increased risk of MI with the number of cigarettes smoked per day. Oral contraceptives are therefore not recommended for women who smoke, especially those aged 35 years or older.[38]

Physical activity

Middle-aged women who exercise regularly have lower weight, BP, and plasma glucose levels, as well as more favorable lipid profiles, than sedentary women. Regular physical activity, particularly aerobic exercise, promotes CV health. Adoption of a regular aerobic exercise program reduces the risk of coronary events in women. The AHA recommends that women accumulate at least 150 minutes per week of moderate-intensity exercise (eg, brisk walking), 75 minutes per week of vigorous exercise, or a combination equal to both aerobic activities.[24] The guidelines also recommend that the aerobic activity be performed in at least 10-minute sessions, spread throughout the week. Resistance training for 20 minutes, two to three times a week on nonconsecutive days, also helps to build muscle mass, reduce insulin resistance, and facilitate weight loss.[39]

Nutrition

The AHA guidelines suggest a heart-healthy nutrition strategy that includes intake of a variety of fruits and vegetables (≥4.5 cups/d) and whole-grain and high-fiber foods.[24] A modified Mediterranean or DASH diet, tested in randomized trial settings, is the most practical way to implement a heart-healthy diet to reduce cardiometabolic risk and should include oily fish at least twice a week. Intake of saturated fat (<7% of total energy) and cholesterol (<150 mg/d) should be limited, avoiding *trans* fatty acids. Sodium intake should be limited to less than 1.5 g per day (approximately one-third teaspoon salt), although some other guidelines, including the Institute of Medicine, allow up to 2.4 g per day. As an adjunct to diet, omega-3 fatty acid supplementation may be considered in women with severe hypertriglyceridemia. Several nonpharmacologic, nutritional strategies are available to reduce dyslipidemia.[40]

Antioxidants. Epidemiologic studies have shown a lower incidence of heart disease in those who eat more fruits and vegetables high in antioxidants and whole grains. To date, however, no large randomized, controlled trials (RCTs) have established any CV benefit of taking antioxidant vitamin supplements such as vitamin C, vitamin E, beta-carotene, or lycopene. Some studies suggest that supplements may cause harm. The AHA guidelines indicate that antioxidant vitamin supplements should not be used for primary or secondary prevention of CVD.[24]

B vitamins. Supplements of the B vitamins folic acid, B_6, and B_{12} will lower homocysteine levels, although multiple studies have failed to demonstrate benefit of folic acid with or without other B vitamins for CVD prevention. Although important during pregnancy to prevent neural tube and other birth defects, folic acid supplementation should not be used for the primary or secondary prevention of CVD.[24,41]

Vitamin D. A growing number of studies suggest that there may be an association between low vitamin D and heart health. In several meta-analyses, vitamin D deficiency has been associated with increased BP, higher risk of heart attacks, and early death.[42,43] The Multi-ethnic Study of Atherosclerosis, however, found that such association varies by race and ethnicity and was not associated with greater risk in black or Hispanics.[44] These findings suggest that there are likely biologic variations in the metabolism of vitamin D. Also, the correlations seen in observational studies may not reflect cause-and-effect relationships. Randomized trials including the Vitamin D Assessment Study in New Zealand[45] and the Vitamin D and Omega-3 Trial[46] have not shown benefits of moderate to high dose supplementation with vitamin D for CVD prevention. There are no formal recommendations for vitamin D supplementation and heart disease. While awaiting results of additional RCTs, clinicians should be cautious to avoid overtreatment with high-dose vitamin D supplementation, as well as undertreatment, until the true risks and benefits are known.[47]

Plant sterols and stanols. Naturally occurring plant sterols and stanols may help to reduce the risk of CVD by lowering blood cholesterol levels.[48] These compounds chemically resemble cholesterol and inhibit cholesterol absorption in the small intestine and have been incorporated into low-fat foods including bread, cereals, dressings, low-fat milk and yogurt, and fruit juice.[49] Food products, such as spreads containing stanols and sterols, are available, as well as soft gel dietary supplements. The AHA, in its diet and lifestyle recommendations, advocates consumption of plant sterols and stanols from a variety of foods and beverages similar to cholesterol-lowering medication to maintain LDL-C reductions.[50] The AHA also noted that maximal effects are achieved at intakes of about 2 g per day. This is consistent with the Third Report of the National Cholesterol Education Program Expert Panel on Detection, Evaluation, and Treatment of High Blood Cholesterol in Adults Treatment Panel evidence statement that daily intakes of 2 g to 3 g per day will reduce LDL-C by 6% to 15%.[20,51]

Patients on statin therapy may achieve further reductions in their blood cholesterol levels when consuming a diet rich in plant sterols and stanols. These compounds seem to be somewhat more effective than doubling the statin dose, which usually produces an additional lowering of LDL-C levels by only 8% to 9%.[52] One review suggested that long-term use of plant sterols or stanols resulted in a 20% reduction in the incidence of CHD.[53] Incorporating plant sterols or stanols into a healthy diet in older adults can help prevent aging-associated diseases.[54]

Soy isoflavones. Although not mentioned specifically in the AHA diet and lifestyle recommendations, an AHA science advisory panel reviewed the use of soy and isoflavones and their effects on CV health in 22 RCTs.[55] Isolated soy protein supplementation with isoflavones led to minimal LDL-C reductions, in the range of 3%. No significant effects on HDL-C, TG, lipoprotein(a), or BP were evident. Further review of 19 studies of soy isoflavones showed no effect on LDL-C or other lipid risk factors. Use of isoflavone supplements in food or pills was not recommended. The review does note, however, that soy products may be beneficial to health as a replacement for animal protein because of their high content of polyunsaturated fats, fiber, vitamins, and minerals and their low content of saturated fat.

Other dietary considerations. A large RCT demonstrated the efficacy of Mediterranean-style nutrition that included supplemented daily tree nuts or virgin olive oil and demonstrated reduction in CVD events in women and men with risk factors.[56] Flavonoids in foods such as soy, as well as fruits and nuts, may be beneficial, but the effect of over-the-counter supplements on disease prevention requires further study.[57]

Alcohol consumption. The ACC/AHA guidelines encourage limiting alcohol consumption to no more than one drink per day (a drink being equal to a 12-oz bottle of beer, a 5-oz glass of wine, or 1.5 oz of 80-proof spirit).[24] Some evidence suggests that light to moderate use of alcohol lowers CVD mortality in women aged older than 50 years who are at greater risk for CHD; however, higher levels (>7 drinks/wk) may increase risk of HTN, stroke, and IHD.[58] Furthermore, even moderate alcohol intake may increase the risk of breast cancer.[59]

Body weight

Maintaining an ideal body weight is important for optimal CV health. Central obesity (ie, apple shape) is more dangerous than subcutaneous obesity for heart health.[60] The AHA recommends weight maintenance or reduction through an appropriate balance of physical activity, caloric intake, and formal behavior programs, when indicated, to maintain or achieve a body mass index (BMI) between 18.5 kg/m^2 and 24.9 kg/m^2 and a waist circumference of less than 35 inches (88 cm) or 31.5 in (80 cm] for women of South Asian descent.[61]

For women who need to lose weight or sustain prior weight loss, the AHA guidelines recommend a minimum of 60 to 90 minutes of moderate-intensity exercise on most and preferably all days of the week. A combined approach of exercise and diet is superior to diet only. Three 10-minute exercise sessions have been shown to be as least as effective as one 30-minute session. A reasonable goal is losing 10% of body weight over a 6-month period. (See also "Body Weight" in Chapter 2.)

Psychosocial factors

Although RCTs have failed to demonstrate CVD reduction, postmenopausal women should be evaluated for depression and treated appropriately for quality-of-life and mental health considerations. (See also "Depression" in Chapter 6.)

Aspirin

The benefit of aspirin use in secondary prevention for women and men with established CVD remains unchallenged, and the use of daily low-dose aspirin (81 mg) to prevent recurrence of MI, stroke, and TIA has become common practice. Dozens of studies have shown that aspirin impairs platelet function and reduces vascular inflammation.[62]

However, randomized trials of aspirin in primary prevention, including ARRIVE,[63] ASCEND,[64] and ASPREE,[65] have led to diminished enthusiasm for the use of aspirin in patients without CVD unless they are at markedly elevated risk. Guidelines from the ACC[66] and the AHA[67] generally advise against the use of aspirin for primary prevention on the basis of these trials, and a meta-analysis of trials suggests that the increased risk of bleeding may offset any CVD benefits. The guidelines advise that aspirin should not be initiated for primary prevention in patients aged 70 years or older or in those at high bleeding risk but may be considered in patients aged 40 to 69 years at high risk for ASCVD and low risk for bleeding.

An earlier large-scale trial of aspirin for primary prevention in women had shown more favorable results.[68] Aspirin 100 mg every other day for primary prevention in women was evaluated in the Women's Health Study, which demonstrated reductions in stroke of 17%, including a 24% reduction in the risk of ischemic stroke, with a nonsignificant increase in the risk of hemorrhagic stroke and reduction in MI in those aged 65 years and older. There was a significant 40% increase in gastrointestinal (GI) bleeding.

The decision to initiate low-dose aspirin use for the primary prevention of CVD in women aged 40 to 69 years still needs to be an individualized one that involves shared decision making with the patient. Women who are not at increased risk for bleeding, are at higher risk of CVD, have a life expectancy of at least 10 years, and are willing to take low-dose aspirin daily for at least 10 years are more likely to benefit.[69]

Aspirin use has been shown to significantly increase the rate of upper GI bleeding and is contraindicated in those who have an allergy to aspirin, a tendency for bleeding, recent GI bleeding, or clinically active hepatic disease. Even enteric-coated or buffered aspirin may damage the intestinal lining. However, studies have shown that patients who regularly take aspirin (and other anti-inflammatory drugs) have unusually low rates of digestive tract cancers. Data are not clear regarding an adverse association with cancers of the pancreas, prostate, and breast.

Hormone therapy

Initiation of HT in women aged 50 to 59 years or in those within 10 years of menopause to treat typical menopause symptoms (eg, VMS, vaginal symptoms) does not seem to increase the risk of CV events.[70,71] Observational data and reanalysis of older studies by age or time since menopause, including the Women's Health Initiative (WHI), suggest that for healthy, recently menopausal women with bothersome menopause symptoms, the benefits of HT are likely to outweigh its risks, including fewer coronary events in younger versus older women.[72]

Three primary CV outcomes have been studied in relation to HT: CHD, stroke, and venous thromboembolism (VTE). Hormone therapy is not recommended for CV protection in women of any age.

Hormone therapy and coronary heart disease

Although most observational and preclinical studies support the potential benefits of systemic HT in reducing the risk of CHD, most RCTs do not. However, the characteristics of women participating in observational studies are different from those of women enrolled in RCTs, which may influence baseline CV risk and the HT effects.[73]

The results of the WHI RCTs demonstrate that in postmenopausal women (mean age, 63 y), HT is not cardioprotective for CHD and that estrogen therapy (ET) and estrogen-progestin therapy (EPT) may even increase the population risk for thrombosis and stroke. Subsequent WHI analyses stratified by age at HT initiation demonstrate that the risk of CHD is not increased in women closer to the onset of menopause but increases with time since menopause.[71]

The Kronos Early Estrogen Prevention Study was a double-blind, placebo-controlled trial that addressed the question of whether HT slows atherosclerosis progression when given soon after menopause rather than later.[74] Over 4 years, 727 women within 3 years of menopause were randomized to oral or transdermal estrogen with cyclic progesterone to assess the progression of atherosclerosis. Results showed a similar rate of progression for all treatment groups over the study period as measured by carotid intimal medial thickness and coronary calcium score. Although the study demonstrated no harm in progression of atherosclerosis, there was no evidence of a cardioprotective benefit.

Data indicate that the disparity in findings between observational studies and RCTs may be related in part to the timing of initiation of HT in relation to age and proximity to menopause.[75] Most women studied in observational studies of CHD risk were aged younger than 55 years at the time HT was initiated and within 2 to 3 years of menopause, whereas the women enrolled in the CV RCTs were aged, on average, older than 63 years and were more than 10 years beyond menopause onset.[73,76] A secondary analysis of the WHI data found a significant reduction in the composite endpoint of MI, coronary artery revascularization, and coronary death in women who were randomized to ET when aged 50 to 59 years.[76]

Some observational studies of coronary artery calcifications suggested a benefit of HT in early postmenopausal women, but other RCTs have provided inconsistent results.[74-76]

A 2015 Cochrane review of RCT data found that HT initiated fewer than 10 years after menopause onset lowered CHD in postmenopausal women (relative risk [RR], 0.52; 95% confidence interval [CI], 0.29-0.96).[77] It also found a reduction in all-cause mortality (RR, 0.70; 95% CI, 0.52-0.95) and no increased risk of stroke but an increased risk of VTE (RR, 1.74; 95% CI, 1.11-2.73), similar to the findings of an earlier meta-analysis of studies in women who initiated HT within 10 years of menopause onset or in women aged younger than 60 years.[78]

Hormone therapy and stroke

The WHI reported an approximate 40% increase in the risk of stroke with both HT regimens, but absolute risks of stroke were low in younger women.[71] A meta-analysis of studies found no increased risk of stroke in women aged younger than 60 years or who were fewer than 10 years from menopause onset.[77] Based only on observational studies, lower doses of either oral[79] or transdermal[80] estrogen may have less risk of stroke; no clear association with age has been found. No head-to-head trials comparing oral to transdermal estrogen have been large enough to assess clinical stroke outcomes.

Stroke risk was not significantly increased in the Heart and Estrogen/Progestin Replacement Study.[81] The Women's International Study of Long Duration Oestrogen After Menopause found no excess of stroke in EPT users compared with women on placebo in 1 year.[82] Postmenopause HT has not been shown to be effective for reducing the risk of a recurrent stroke in women with established CVD or for prevention of a first stroke, and it may increase the rate of first strokes, particularly in women initiating HT at an age older than 60 years.

Hormone therapy and venous thromboembolism

Data from observational studies and from RCTs demonstrate an increased risk of VTE with oral HT. In the WHI, there were eight additional cases of VTE per 10,000 women per year of EPT and seven additional cases of VTE per 10,000 women per year of ET when the entire cohort was analyzed.[83,84] Risk for VTE in RCTs emerges soon after HT is initiated (ie, during the first 1-2 y), but the magnitude of the excess risk seems to decrease somewhat over time. In the WHI, the absolute excess VTE risk associated with either EPT or ET was lower in women who started HT at an age younger than 60 years than in women who initiated HT aged 60 years or older.[85,86] In

women aged 50 to 59 years at randomization, there were seven additional cases of VTE per 10,000 woman-years of EPT therapy and four additional cases of VTE per 10,000 woman-years of ET.

In a meta-analysis of trials in women who began HT fewer than 10 years after menopause onset or who were aged younger than 60 years, strong evidence of increased risk of VTE was found in HT groups compared with placebo (RR, 1.74; 95% CI, 1.11-2.73).[77] Lower doses of oral ET may confer less risk of VTE than higher doses,[87] but comparative RCT data are lacking. Micronized progesterone may be less thrombogenic than other progestins.[88] Limited observational data suggest less risk with transdermal HT than with oral.[80,85,88] No excess risk has been seen with vaginal ET.

The baseline risk of VTE also increases relative to BMI. For women who are obese (BMI >30 kg/m²), the baseline risk was 3-fold greater than a woman who was not obese. At any BMI, the risk of VTE doubled with HT and returned to baseline soon after discontinuation.[89] Growing evidence suggests that women with a prior history of VTE or women who possess factor V Leiden are at increased risk with HT use.[90]

Hormone therapy is not recommended by The North American Menopause Society, the AHA, or other US or Canadian organizations for the primary or secondary prevention of CVD. For women with or at increased risk of CVD, it would be prudent to emphasize CV risk reduction with established evidence-based treatments.

Hypertension, hyperlipidemia, and diabetes mellitus

Primary prevention of CVD in postmenopausal woman should include treatment of all identified risk factors to goal. Hypertension, hyperlipidemia, and DM are three such risk factors that must be evaluated and treated.

Treatment for established cardiovascular disease

Postmenopausal women with established CVD have a high risk for recurrent IHD events, congestive heart failure, and CV mortality. Therapies that result in even a small reduction in CVD risk can have a major effect on public health. In postmenopausal women with preexisting CVD, dietary and pharmacologic management of HTN, dyslipidemia, and DM should be initiated when appropriate, according to established guidelines from leading US and Canadian organizations, including the AHA, the ACC, the National Lipid Association, and the International Atherosclerosis Association. Aspirin, statins, beta-blockers,

ACE inhibitors/angiotensin II receptor blockers (ARBs), aldosterone blockade, and other therapies are important to consider, often in consultation with the patient's cardiologist. (See also "Hypertension," "Hyperlipidemia," and "Metabolic Syndrome, Prediabetes, and Diabetes" in this Chapter.)

Hypertension

Hypertension (HTN) is one of the greatest risk factors for CVD in men and women and is a leading cause of morbidity and mortality worldwide.[91] In 2015, according to the Global Burden of Diseases, Injuries, and Risk Factors Study, HTN was associated with the highest burden of morbidity and mortality among all risk factors—causing an even greater disease burden than smoking and obesity.[92] The overall prevalence of HTN in the US adult population (surveyed 2011-2014) was 30.0% for men and 28.1% for women (Figure 2).[93]

The prevalence of HTN strongly correlates with age, with a steady rise in SBP with increasing age. Men have a higher prevalence of HTN than women until approximately age 60 years. After age 60 years, women have a higher prevalence than men.[93] More than 75%

of US women aged older than 60 years and at least 41% of postmenopausal women have HTN.[94] In fact, the steady increase in BP that happens over time has a step up, or a "bump," around the time of menopause (Figure 3).[95] Observational studies have shown that there is an approximately 4 mm to 5 mm Hg increase in SBP after menopause.[96] Menopause-related increase in BP may be because of estrogen withdrawal; weight gain; neurohumoral influences (ie, endogenous vasoconstrictors such as angiotensin or increased sympathetic activity); salt sensitivity; decreased endothelial nitric oxide production; upregulation of the angiotensin II subtype 1 receptor; or other undefined influences.[97,98] It is estimated that both men and women aged older than 55 years have a 90% lifetime risk of developing HTN.[99]

The consequences of untreated HTN in older women are myriad. It is one of the leading causes of CHD,[100] HF,[101] atrial fibrillation,[102] dementia,[103] and stroke.[104]

Management of hypertension in postmenopausal women

In 2014, the Report of the Eighth Joint National Committee HTN guidelines were released.[105] One of the most controversial features of those guidelines was the

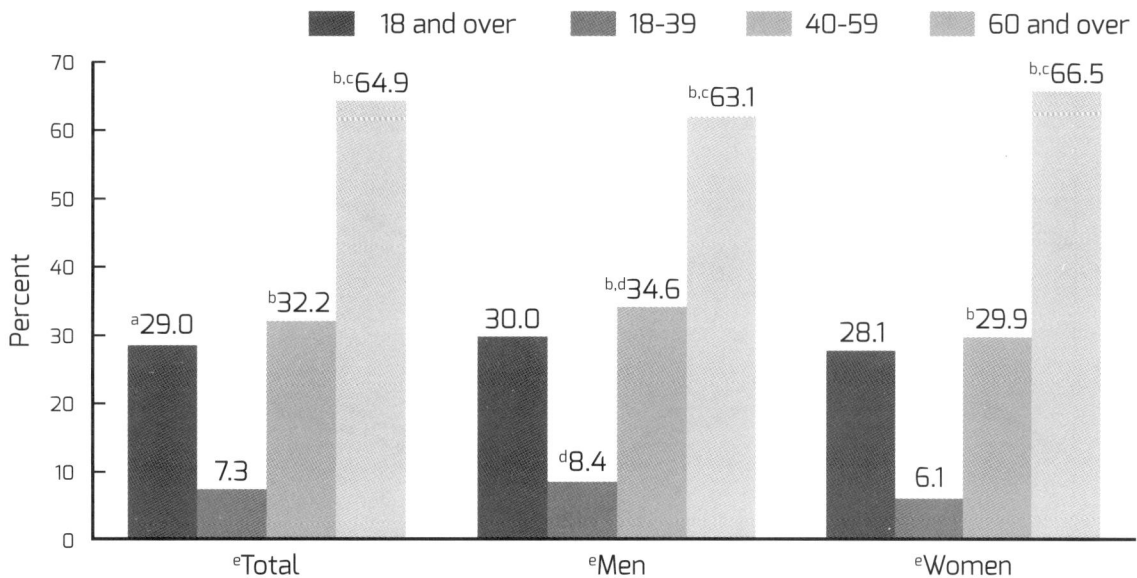

Figure 2. Prevalence of Hypertension in US Adults Aged 18 Years and Older by Sex and Age: 2011-2014

Estimates for the 18 year-old and older category were age adjusted by the direct method to the 2000 US census population.
[a]Crude estimates are 31.3% for total, 31.0% for men, and 31.5% for women.
[b]Significant difference from age group 18-39 years.
[c]Significant difference from age group 40-59 years.
[d]Significant difference from women for same age group.
[e]Significant linear trend.
Yoon SS, et al.[93]

recommendation to increase the threshold for treatment of BP in patients aged older than 60 years to greater than 150/90 mm Hg. This recommendation was substantially different from the Seventh Report of the Joint National Committee on Prevention, Detection, Evaluation, and Treatment of High Blood Pressure guidelines (JNC7) (Table 3)[106,107] and was opposed by many HTN specialists. It was even opposed by several members of the guideline-writing committee, who published a dissenting opinion because they believed that the recommendation to raise the threshold for treatment of persons aged older than 60 years lacked support from the available data and would possibly result in increased risk of CV events.[108]

Shortly after those recommendations were published, results of a large, open-label RCT funded by the National Institutes of Health comparing an SBP goal of less than 120 mm Hg to a goal of less than 140 mm Hg were published.[109] The Systolic Blood Pressure Intervention Trial randomized participants with HTN to intensive (<120 mm Hg) versus standard (<140 mm Hg) BP control. The trial included 9,361 participants without DM or stroke but who were at elevated CV risk.

At 1 year, BP in the intensive arm averaged 121/68 mm Hg versus 136/76 mm Hg in the standard arm. The number of antihypertensive medications averaged 2.8 and 1.8, respectively. Median follow-up was 3.26 years out of the planned 5 years, and the trial was stopped prematurely because of the benefit of the intensive BP goal in reducing the primary outcome (first occurrence of MI, acute coronary syndrome, stroke, HF, or CV mortality) and reduction in total mortality. Rates of the primary outcome were 5.2% in the intensive arm versus 6.8% in the standard arm (hazard ratio [HR], 0.75; 95% CI, 0.64-0.89; $P<.001$; number needed to treat [NNT], 61). Rates of all-cause mortality were 3.3% in the intensive arm versus 4.5% in the standard arm (HR, 0.73; 95% CI, 0.60-0.90; $P=.003$; NNT, 90).

In a prespecified subgroup analysis, participants aged older than 75 years had the same benefit as seen in the overall cohort. There was no heterogeneity by sex. Although significant benefits were noted in the intensive arm, there were also some harms. The rates of serious adverse events (AEs) possibly or definitely associated with the intervention were 4.7% in the intensive arm versus 2.5% in the standard arm (HR, 1.88; $P<.001$; number needed to harm [NNH], 45). Also seen more frequently in the intensive arm were hypotension: 2.4% versus 1.4% (HR, 1.67; $P=.001$; NNH, 100); syncope: 2.3% versus 1.7% (HR, 1.33; $P=.05$; NNH, 167);

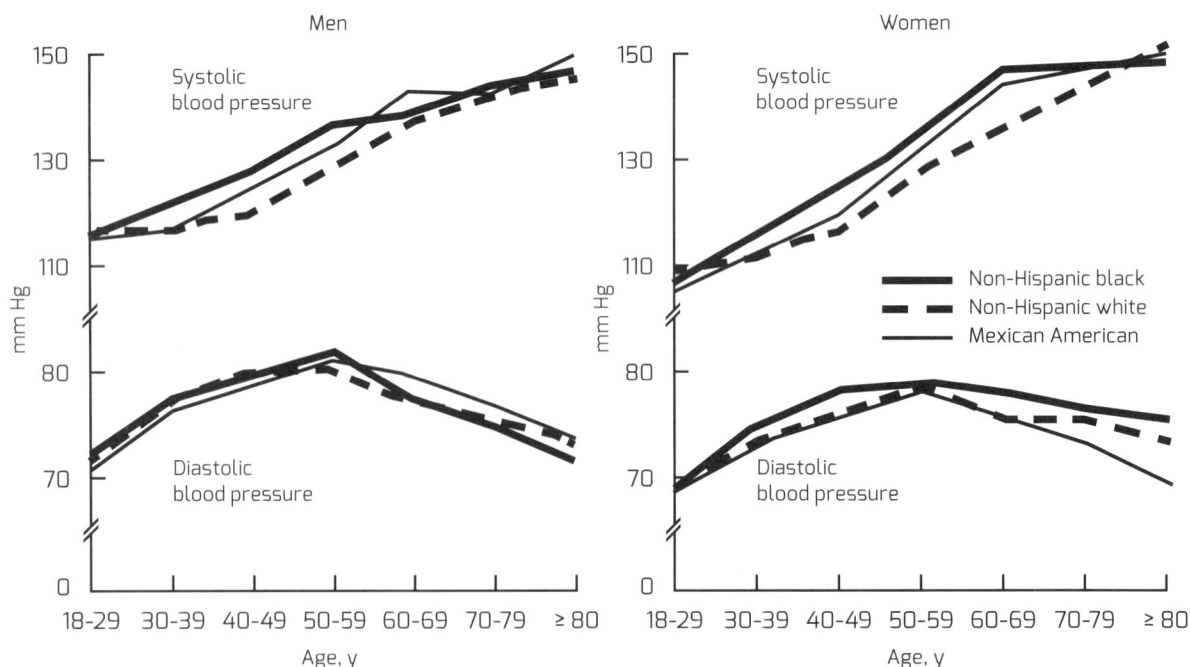

Figure 3. Mean Systolic and Diastolic Blood Pressures by Age and Race/Ethnicity for US Men and Women Aged 18 Years and Older

Table 3. BP Classification by JNC7 and 2017 ACC/AHA HTN Guidelines

Systolic/Diastolic, mm HG	JNC7	2017 ACC/AHA
<120/<80	Normal BP	Normal BP
120-129/<80	Prehypertension	Elevated BP
130-139 or 80-89	Prehypertension	Stage 1 HTN
140-159 or 90-99	Stage 1 HTN	Stage 2 HTN
≥160 or ≥100	Stage 2 HTN	N/A

Abbreviations: ACC, American College of Cardiology; AHA, American Heart Association; BP, blood pressure; HTN, hypertension; JNC7, Seventh Report of the Joint National Committee on Prevention, Detection, Evaluation, and Treatment of High Blood Pressure.
Chobanian AV, et al[106]; Whelton PK, et al.[107]

bradycardia: 1.9% versus 1.6% (HR, 1.19; P=.28); acute kidney injury/acute renal failure: 4.1% versus 2.5% (HR, 1.66; P<.001; NNH, 63); and electrolyte abnormality: 3.1% versus 2.3% (HR, 1.35; P=.02; NNH, 125).

In November 2017, new HTN guidelines were released by the ACC and the AHA. The recommendations were largely informed by results of the Systolic Blood Pressure Intervention Trial. The 2017 ACC/AHA/AAPA/ABC/ACPM/AGS/APhA/ASH/ASPC/NMA/PCNA Guideline for the Prevention, Detection, Evaluation, and Management of High Blood Pressure in Adults incorporated several changes.[107] Perhaps the two most transformative changes were a new risk-based approach to decision-making for treating HTN and lower targets for BP during the management of HTN. The guidelines are not sex-specific. The new guidelines classify HTN differently than the earlier JNC7 guidelines (Table 3).[106,107]

The new guidelines also introduced a risk-based treatment algorithm with recommendations for therapy varying by level of risk (Table 4; Table 5).[107] Although recommendations are similar in women and men, women may tend to have higher risk of AEs from drugs. Drug therapy is recommended for all patients with BP greater than 140/90 mm Hg and select patients with lower BP levels.

Four drug classes are recommended as options for initial choice of antihypertensive drug therapy (thiazide diuretics, calcium channel blockers, ACE inhibitors, and ARBs) in adults who do not have a compelling need for a specific BP-lowering medication from another class to manage other illness (Table 6).[107] There are also nonpharmacologic management recommendations (Table 7).[107]

In black patients, thiazides and calcium antagonists are recommended as monotherapy because of their greater relative BP-lowering efficacy. Chlorthalidone is the preferred thiazide diuretic because of its prolonged duration of action and proven CVD risk reduction.

Not all medical societies agree with these guideline recommendations. The American College of Physicians

Table 4. HTN Management Recommendations in 2017 ACC/AHA Guidelines

<120 and <80	• Healthy lifestyle choices • Yearly check-ups
120-129 and <80	• Healthy lifestyle changes • Reassess in 3-6 mo

130-139 or 80-89	• 10-year heart disease and stroke risk assessment >10% risk
	  — Lifestyle changes
	  — Reassess in 3-6 mo
	• 10-year heart disease and stroke risk assessment ≥10% risk
	  — Lifestyle changes
	  — Medication
	  — Monthly follow-up until BP is under control

>140/90	• Lifestyle changes • Consider initiation of therapy with two different classes of medications • Monthly follow-up until BP is under control • If BP ≥160/100 mm Hg, treat promptly, monitor carefully, and adjust medication dose upward as necessary to achieve control

Abbreviations: ACC, American College of Cardiology; AHA, American Heart Association; BP, blood pressure; HTN, hypertension.
Whelton PK, et al.[107]

Table 5. 2017 ACC/AHA HTN Guidelines for Treatment and Treatment Targets

Clinical condition(s)	Threshold for treatment, mm HG	BP goal, mm HG
General		
Clinical CVD or 10-year ASCVD risk ≥10%	≥130/80	<130/80
No clinical CVD and 10-year ASCVD risk <10%	≥140/90	<130/80
Older persons (≥65 y; noninstitutionalized, ambulatory, community living)	≥130 (SBP)	<130 (SBP)
Specific comorbidities		
DM	≥130/80	<130/80
CKD	≥130/80	<130/80
CKD after renal transplantation	≥130/80	<130/80
Heart failure	≥130/80	<130/80
Stable IHD	≥130/80	<130/80
Secondary stroke prevention	≥140/90	<130/80
Secondary stroke prevention (lacunar)	≥130/80	<130/80
PAD	≥130/80	<130/80

Abbreviations: ACC, American College of Cardiology; AHA, American Heart Association; ASCVD, atherosclerotic cardiovascular disease; BP, blood pressure; CKD, chronic kidney disease; CVD, cardiovascular disease; DM, diabetes mellitus; HTN, hypertension; IHD, ischemic heart disease; PAD, peripheral artery disease; SBP, systolic blood pressure. Whelton PK, et al.[107]

(ACP) and American Academy of Family Physicians (AAFP) released their own guidelines for treatment of HTN in persons aged older than 60 years, which continue to recommend a goal BP of less than 150/90 mm Hg.[110]

Hypertension is very prevalent in postmenopausal women, and in light of the aging population, in which women tend to live longer than men, significant attention must be paid to this group. Blood pressure levels are typically lower in premenopausal women than age-matched men. After menopause, however, BP levels rise in women, meet, then exceed those of men. Unfortunately many national surveys continue to show low rates of HTN awareness, treatment, and control in women.[111] Appropriate management of BP can significantly reduce morbidity and mortality, thus attention to this risk factor is paramount.

Hyperlipidemia

The TG and cholesterol-rich apoB-containing lipoproteins, as measured by LDL-C and non-HDL-C, are important risk factors for ASCVD in both men and women. Low-density lipoprotein-cholesterol and other apoB lipoproteins increase within 1 year of menopause, but levels are not clearly distingushable from aging-related changes in the later stages of menopause.[7,112]

Risk factors

Major risk factors for ASCVD (advancing age, smoking, elevated BP, and DM) are also similar in men and women around the world.[113-115] Cardiovascular disease risk factors are largely driven by unhealthy lifestyle habits over the life course.

Risk assessment

Women with clinical CVD or an LDL-C level of 190 mg/dL and above are at high risk of an ASCVD event (nonfatal and fatal MI and stroke), and no further risk assessment is recommended before initiating statin therapy.[116,117] In women without clinical CVD and an LDL-C level less than 190 mg/dL, the 2013 ACC/AHA risk-assessment guideline recommends estimating the 10-year and lifetime risk of ASCVD starting at age 20 years and again every 4 to 6 years up to age 79 years.[118] The presence of risk factors and the disease-risk estimates can then be used to counsel patients on the need for lifestyle modification or preventive medications.

Age, race (white or black), current smoking, HTN, SBP level, DM, TC, and HDL-C can be entered into the ACC

Table 6. 2017 ACC/AHA Guidelines (Oral Agents) HTN Pharmacologic Management

Class	Agents	Notes
Thiazide (type) diuretics	• Chlorthalidone • Hydrochlorothiazide • Indapamid • Metolazone	• Chlorthalidone preferred • Monitor electrolytes • Caution if history of gout
ACE inhibitors	• Benazapril • Captopril • Enalapril • Fosinopril • Lisinopril • Moexipril	• Do not use in combination with ARBs • Caution in use with K+ supplements or K+ sparing diuretics • May cause acute renal failure if bilateral renal artery stenosis is present • Potential for angioedema • Avoid in pregnancy
ARBs	• Azilsartan • Candesartan • Eprosartan • Irbesartan • Losartan • Olmesartan • Telmisartan • Valsartan	• Do not use in combination with ACE inhibitors • Caution in use with K+ supplements or K+-sparing diuretics • May cause acute renal failure if bilateral renal artery stenosis is present • Potential for angioedema • Avoid in pregnancy
CCBs Dihydropyridines	• Amlodipine • Felodipine • Isradipine • Nicardipine SR • Nifedipine LA • Nisoldipine	• Avoid in patients with HFrEF • May cause dose-related pedal edema, (women>men)
Nondihydropyridines	• Diltiazem SR • Diltiazem ER • Verapamil IR • Verapamil SR • Verapamil ER	• Avoid use with beta blockers • Do not use in patients with HFrEF • Potential for drug interactions of diltiazem and verapamil with CYP 3A4

Abbreviations: ACC, American College of Cardiology; ACE, angiotensin-converting enzyme; AHA, American Heart Association; ARBs, angiotensin receptor blockers, CCBs, calcium channel blockers; CYP 3A4, cytochrome P450 3A4; ER, extended release; HFrEF, heart failure with reduced ejection fraction; IR, immediate release; K+, potassium; LA, long acting; SR, sustained release.
Whelton PK, et al.[107]

disease-risk calculator (http://tools.acc.org/ASCVD-Risk-Estimator-Plus/#!/calculate/estimate/ or as a downloadable app for mobile devices; Figure 4). The disease-risk calculator estimates lifetime risk in persons aged 20 to 59 years and 10-year disease risk in persons aged 40 to 79 years. The pooled cohort equations used by the disease-risk calculator to predict MI and stroke risk perform quite well in the broad population of white and black US women.[119,120]

Estimates of 10-year disease risk provided by the ASCVD risk calculator may be adjusted on the basis of several considerations.[118] Nonwhite race/ethnicity may increase the 10-year ASCVD risk estimate for

Table 7. 2017 ACC/AHA Guidelines Nonpharmacologic Management of HTN

Strategy	Goal
Weight loss	• Optimum goal is ideal body weight but can expect 1 mm Hg for every 1 kg reduction

Diet	• DASH diet: Fruits and vegetables, whole grains, low-fat dairy products, reduced saturated and total fat
	• Other diets with supportive evidence
	  — Low in calories from carbohydrates
	  — High-protein diets
	  — Vegetarian diets
	  — Mediterranean dietary pattern
	• Sodium: Goal, <1,500 mg/d but aim for at least a 1,000-mg/d reduction
	• Potassium: Goal, 3,500-5,000 mg/d, preferably through diet

Exercise	• Aerobic: 90-150 min/wk; 65-75% heart rate reserve • Dynamic resistance exercise (eg, weight lifting 90-150 min/wk) • Isometric resistance (eg, hand grip 4 × 2 min; 3 sessions/wk)
Alcohol	• Women: ≤1 drink/d • Men: ≤2 drinks/d

Abbreviations: ACC, American College of Cardiology; AHA, American Heart Association; DASH, Dietary Approaches to Stop Hypertension; HTN, hypertension. Whelton PK, et al.[107]

some groups (eg, American Indian, Pacific Islander, and South Asian ancestry and some Hispanics, such as those with Puerto Rican ancestry) or decrease the 10-year risk estimate in other groups (eg, East Asian ancestry and some Hispanics, such as Mexicans). Women with higher levels of education or socioeconomic status may also be at lower-than-predicted risk.[121,122] Other characteristics also may influence ASCVD risk estimates, such as an LDL-C between 160 mg/dL and 189 mg/dL; premature family history of ASCVD, with onset younger than 55 years in a first-degree male relative or younger than 65 years in a first-degree female relative; elevated coronary artery calcium (≥300 Agatston units or ≥75th percentile for age); hsCRP 2 mg/L and above; ankle-brachial index less than 0.9; or elevated lifetime risk.[116,118]

The 2013 ACC/AHA risk assessment did not formally assess reproductive factors for ASCVD risk prediction in women. A history of polycystic ovary syndrome (POS), preeclampsia, gestational HTN or diabetes, pregnancy loss, delivery of a preterm or small-for-gestational age infant, and lack of breastfeeding are associated with increased CV risk later in life.[19,123,124]

Lipid measurement

Fasting is not mandatory for lipid measurement, although knowing a patient's fasting status is helpful for interpretation of the results, especially for TG levels, which can be acutely elevated after a meal.[20] Total cholesterol and HDL-C are not sensitive to fasting, so even if the patient did not fast, the non-HDL-C level can be used. If TG levels are greater than 400 mg/dL, the test should be repeated after fasting for at least 8 hours. Non-HDL-C is measured by subtracting HDL-C from the TC and is generally about 30 mg/dL higher than the LDL-C level when TG are lower than 500 mg/dL.

Cholesterol

Cholesterol is a well-established risk factor for ASCVD and is primarily transported in the blood by the apoB-containing atherogenic lipoproteins: low-density lipoprotein, very-low-density lipoprotein, and intermediate-density lipoprotein.

About 1 in 250 women will have a monogenetic cause for familial hypercholesterolemia and a 20-fold higher lifetime risk of ASCVD, with the highest risk in those with other CV risk factors.[125,126] All women should have their LDL-C levels checked by age 21 because heterozygous familial hypercholesterolemia is essentially curable with existing LDL-C-lowering therapies.[126] However, many women with elevated LDL-C levels have a polygenic predisposition to hypercholesterolemia, which is exacerbated by lifestyle habits. Nonetheless, they still have a 5-fold higher lifetime risk of CVD. The family members of all women with LDL-C levels of 190 mg/dL and above should be screened for familial hypercholesterolemia.

Treatment of blood lipids

The 2013 ACC/AHA cholesterol guidelines recommend that lifestyle modification is the foundation for CV risk-reduction efforts and for lowering LDL-C (Table 8).[33,127]

Low-density lipoprotein cholesterol-lowering drugs such as statins, ezetimbe, and proprotein convertase subtilisin/kexin type 9 (PCSK9) inhibitors have been shown to reduce ASCVD events in proportion to the magnitude of LDL-C reduction.[128] Statins reduce the risk of CHD events and stroke by 25% to 45% and reduce risk similarly in women and in men and in

Figure 4. American College of Cardiology ASCVD Risk Estimator Plus

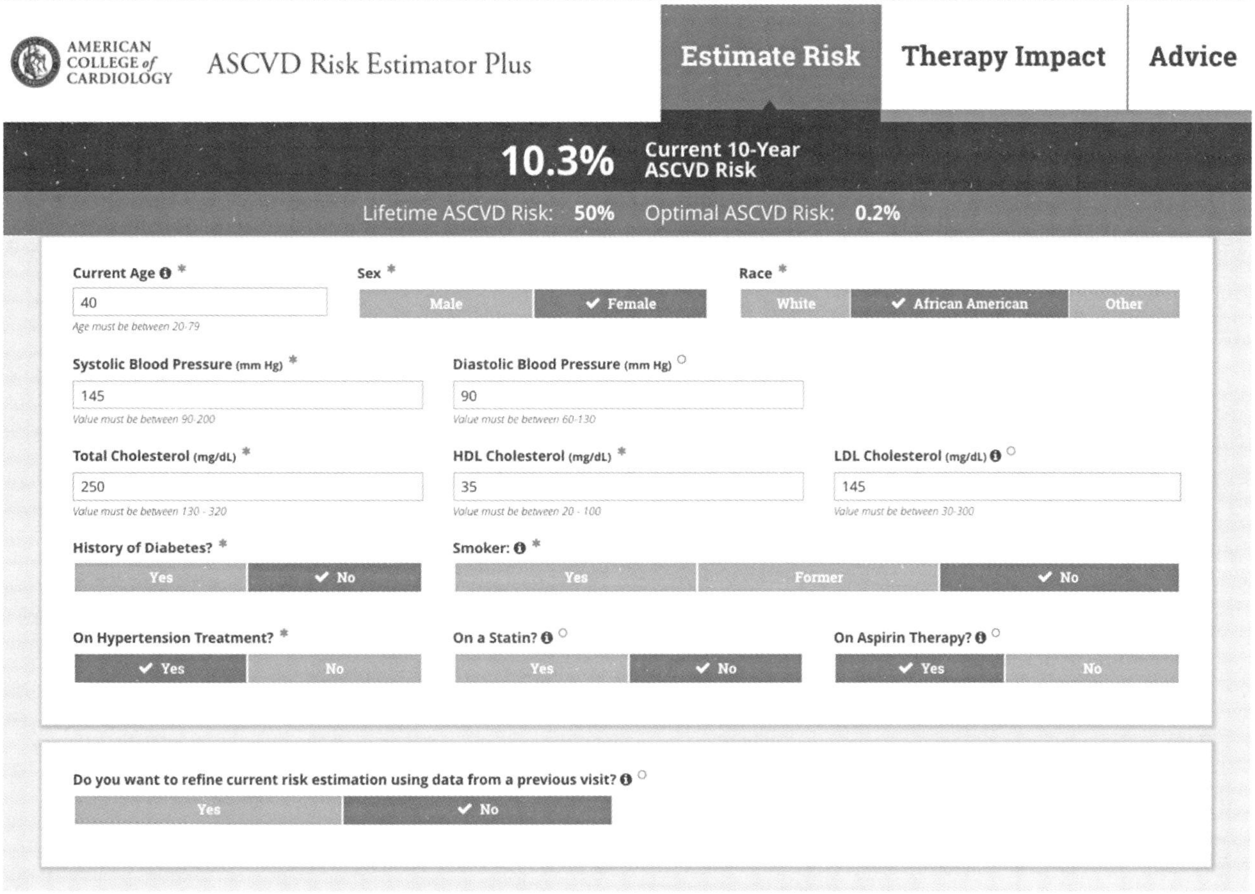

Reproduced with permission from the American College of Cardiology. © 2019 American College of Cardiology Foundation.

primary and secondary prevention.[129-131] Ezetimibe and PCSK9 inhibitors may be indicated in select women at high CVD risk whose LDL-C levels remain elevated despite maximal statin therapy.[132,133]

On the basis of a systematic review of RCT evidence, the guideline has moved away from targeting specific lipid levels and instead focuses on identifying persons most likely to benefit from statin therapy.[116] Although the guideline was initially met with some skepticism, subsequent evaluations have found this new treatment paradigm to be a superior approach for preventing CV events compared with other guideline approaches.[134,135]

The 2013 ACC/AHA cholesterol guidelines recommend moderate- or high-intensity statin therapy for four patient groups most likely to benefit (Table 9).[33,127] Statin therapy can be considered for other patients, but there is less clinical-trial evidence to determine the potential for net benefit. High-intensity statin therapy (which on average lowers LDL-C by 50% or more)

Table 8. 2013 ACC/AHA Cholesterol Guidelines Lifestyle Modifications Recommendations to Lower LDL-C

- A dietary pattern emphasizing intake of vegetables, fruits, and whole grains and includes low-fat dairy products, poultry, fish, legumes, nontropical vegetable oils, and nuts. Limits intake of sweets, sugar-sweetened beverages, and red meats. This pattern can be achieved by following diet plans such as the DASH dietary pattern, the USDA Food Pattern, or the AHA diet.

- Limiting daily calories to just 5% to 6% from saturated fats.

- Avoiding *trans* fats.

- Engaging in regular physical activity at least 3-4 times/wk, lasting on average 40 min per session and involving moderate to vigorous physical activity.

- Weight reduction in persons who are overweight and obese.

Abbreviations: AHA, American Heart Association; DASH, Dietary Approaches to Stop Hypertension; LDL-C, low-density lipoprotein cholesterol; USDA, US Food and Drug Administration.
Eckel RH, et al[33]; Jensen MD, et al.[127]

reduces CV risk more than moderate-intensity statin therapy (which, on average, lowers LDL-C between 30% and 50%; Table 10).[116]

Women with clinical evidence of CVD are at the highest risk of an ASCVD event in the next 10 years and have the highest priority for preventive therapies. High-intensity statin therapy is recommended for women aged up to 75 years with clinical CVD, as well as for women with genetic hypercholesterolemia as evidenced by an LDL-C of 190 mg/dL and above, unless there are safety concerns. Additional research on the benefits and risks of statin use in women is needed.

Statin safety

Statins are contraindicated during pregnancy and lactation. A woman with reproductive potential who requires statin therapy, and her partner if appropriate, should be counseled on the need to avoid statins unless effective contraception is used.

Many patients will have muscle symptoms, including muscle pain, tenderness, stiffness, cramping, weakness, and/or fatigue, during statin therapy, but established statin intolerance is uncommon. Rates of muscle AEs in statin trials were the same as in the control groups.[136] Statins modestly increase the risk of DM in patients with risk factors for DM; however, onset is only about 2 to 4 months earlier in statin-treated patients compared with controls.[137] Statins do not increase liver function abnormalities, and there is no need for routine monitoring.[116]

Monitoring response to therapy

After initiating statin therapy or altering treatment regimens, women should return for a fasting lipid panel after 4 to 12 weeks to assess response.[116] If the reduction in LDL-C is less than expected (30-50% for moderate-intensity statins and ≥50% for high-intensity statins) or further LDL-C reduction is needed, lifestyle adherence should be reinforced, and an increase in statin dose or intensity may be considered. Patients should continue to be reassessed regularly until desired levels of lifestyle, adherence, and LDL-C levels are achieved.

Symptoms during statin therapy

Muscle and other symptoms are common during statin therapy. However, in clinical trials, more than 75% of

---

Table 9. Patient Groups Most Likely to Benefit From Moderate- or High-Intensity Statin Therapy

- Those with CVD
- Those with LDL-C ≤190 mg/dL
- Those with DM (type 1 or 2) aged 40 to 75 years and LDL-C between 70 mg/dL and 189 mg/dL
- Those with a 10-year risk of ≤7.5% (using the ASCVD risk calculator) aged 40 to 75 years with LDL-C between 70 mg/dL and 189 mg/dL

Abbreviations: AHA, American Heart Association; ASCVD, atherosclerotic cardiovascular disease; CVD, cardiovascular disease; DM, diabetes mellitus; LDL-C, low-density lipoprotein cholesterol.
Eckel RH, et al[33]; Jensen MD, et al.[127]

Table 10. Intensity of Statin Therapy

High intensity	Moderate intensity	Low intensity
Daily dose lowers LDL-C, on average, by ≥50%	Daily dose lowers LDL-C, on average, by 30% to <50%	Daily dose lowers LCL-C, on average, by <30%
• Atorvastatin (40)[a]-80 mg	• Atorvastatin 10 (20)[a] mg	• Simvastatin 10 mg
• Rosuvastatin 20 (40)[a] mg	• Rosuvastatin (5)[a] 10 mg	• Pravastatin 10-20 mg
	• Simvastatin 20-40 mg[b]	• Lovastatin 20 mg
	• Pravastatin 40 (80)[a] mg	• Fluvastatin 20-40 mg
	• Lovastatin 40 mg	• Pitavastatin 1 mg
	• Fluvastatin XL 80 mg	
	• Fluvastatin 40 mg bid	
	• Pitavastatin 2-4 mg	

Individual responses to statin therapy varied in RCTs and should be expected to vary in clinical practice. There might be a biologic basis for a less-than-average response.
Abbreviations: LDL-C, low-density lipoprotein cholesterol; RCT, randomized, controlled trial.
[a]Parenthesis indicate evidence from one RCT only: down-titration if unable to tolerate atorvastatin 80 mg or efficacy from manufacturer's prescribing information
[b]Although simvastatin 80 mg was evaluated in RCTs, initiation of simvastatin 80 mg or titration to 80 mg is not recommended by FDA because of the increased risk of myopathy, including rhabdomyolysis.
Stone NJ, et al.[116]

patients who report intolerance to two or more statins were able to tolerate a moderate-intensity statin, atorvastatin 20 mg, when taken in a blinded fashion[138]; therefore, it is important to work with patients to find a dose of statin that they can take because greater CV risk reduction occurs from greater reductions in LDL-C. For example, rosuvastatin 10 mg weekly can lower LDL-C by about 25%.[139] Most patients with symptoms during statin therapy can be successfully rechallenged with statin therapy (Table 11).[116]

Nonstatin therapy

Once a patient is taking the maximally tolerated intensity of statin therapy, nonstatin therapy is an option in selected high-risk patients who might benefit from additional LDL-C lowering.[132,133] Ezetimibe and PCSK9 inhibitors have both been shown to reduce CV events when added to background statin therapy.[140,141]

High-density lipoprotein-cholesterol

High-density lipoprotein-cholesterol has historically been considered atheroprotective because HDL-C levels are inversely associated with CV risk in observational epidemiologic studies. However, drugs to raise HDL-C have not been shown to reduce CV events and in some cases have been harmful.[116] Therefore, HDL-C remains only a risk marker but is not a target of therapy.

Triglycerides

Triglycerides are transported in the blood on apoB-containing atherogenic lipoproteins, along with cholesterol, and in chylomicrons, which transport TG from the intestine to the liver.[142] Blood TG levels per se are not clearly related to CV risk, but elevated levels of TG-rich atherogenic apoB lipoproteins are associated with increased CV risk, especially in women.[143,144] Thus, reduction of CV risk in a patient with elevated TG should be focused on lifestyle modification and LDL-C-lowering drugs that have been shown to reduce CV risk. Blood TG 500 mg/dL and above are considered severely elevated, often because of secondary causes including exogenous oral estrogen, poorly controlled DM, obesity, or a high-fat diet.[116] These patients should be referred for additional evaluation if TG levels remain at 500 mg/dL or above after a trial of a low-fat diet, regular physical activity, and modest weight loss. Triglyceride levels greater than about 1,000 mg/dL are often because of monogenetic disorders and may be associated with an increased risk of pancreatitis.[145,146] Triglyceride-lowering drug therapies, including fenofibrate, gemfibrozil (contraindicated with statins),

and high-dose omega-3 marine fatty acids are often used in these patients.

Metabolic Syndrome, Prediabetes, and Diabetes

Postmenopausal women have an increased risk for four related, but not identical, issues regarding glucose metabolism and insulin resistance. First, women are at risk for features of MetS (HTN, dyslipidemia, central obesity, or increased fasting glucose level), which is thought to be primarily caused by a state of insulin resistance and increases the risk for CVD.

Second, women can have specific abnormalities of glucose metabolism—prediabetes, type 1 DM, and type 2 DM. Prediabetes and type 2 DM are a spectrum of elevation in blood glucose levels, with cut points defined by glucose levels. The risk for these two conditions increases with ethnicity, age, and obesity. Type 1 DM is an autoimmune disease, which can be diagnosed in women of any age, although half have had the disease since childhood.

Women with prediabetes and type 1 or type 2 DM may or may not have MetS.[147] MetS confers an additional risk for CVD and must be considered when individualizing treatment for postmenopausal women.[148] Conversely, not all people with MetS have prediabetes or DM. Although these overlaps can seem confusing, key to treatment is lifestyle, weight reduction (if overweight or obese), and management of glycemia, lipid disorders, and HTN.

Metabolic syndrome

Metabolic syndrome is common in postmenopausal women—50% to 85% will have at least one feature, and rates vary on the basis of ethnicity and socioeconomic status.[149] Historically, there have been multiple definitions for MetS, although a 2009 consensus statement is the most widely used and accepted definition.[150]

Although visceral adiposity is directly related to the risk of CVD, it is difficult to measure it in a standard way in clinical practice, and it varies on the basis of ethnicity. Additionally, it is not independent of BMI, and most people with MetS have a BMI of 30 kg/m^2 or more.[151] Routine measurement of specific markers of insulin resistance or inflammation such as hsCRP or C-peptide/insulin levels is not recommended in clinical practice, although these are often used as research tools.[152] Metabolic syndrome is also associated with nonalcoholic steatohepatitis, chronic kidney disease, and POS.

Table 11. Management of Symptoms During Statin Therapy

Choice of statin and dose

To maximize the safety of statins, selection of the appropriate statin and dose in men and nonpregnant or nonnursing women should be based on patient characteristics, level of CVD risk, and potential for AEs. Moderate-intensity statin therapy should be used in persons in whom high-intensity statin therapy would otherwise be recommended when characteristics predisposing them to statin-associated AEs are present. Characteristics predisposing persons to statin AEs include but are not limited to

- Multiple or serious comorbidities, including impaired renal or hepatic function
- History of previous statin intolerance or muscle disorders
- Unexplained ALT elevations ≥3 times ULN
- Patient characteristics or concomitant use of drugs affecting statin metabolism
- Age >75 y

Additional characteristics that could modify the decision to use higher statin intensities might include but are not limited to

- History of hemorrhagic stroke
- Asian ancestry

Symptom management

Most patients with symptoms during statin therapy can be successfully rechallenged with statin therapy. It is reasonable to evaluate and treat muscle symptoms, including pain, tenderness, stiffness, cramping, weakness, or fatigue, in statin-treated patients according to this management algorithm:

- To avoid unnecessary discontinuation of statins, obtain a history of prior or current muscle symptoms to establish a baseline before initiation of statin therapy.
- If unexplained severe muscle symptoms or fatigue develop during statin therapy, promptly discontinue the statin and address the possibility of rhabdomyolysis by evaluating CK and creatinine and performing urinalysis for myoglobinuria.
- If mild to moderate muscle symptoms develop during statin therapy
  - Discontinue the statin until the symptoms can be evaluated.
  - Evaluate the patient for other conditions that might increase the risk for muscle symptoms (eg, hypothyroidism, reduced renal or hepatic function, rheumatologic disorders such as polymyalgia rheumatica, steroid myopathy, vitamin D deficiency, or primary muscle diseases).
  - If muscle symptoms resolve and if no contraindication exists, give the patient the original or a lower dose of the same statin to establish a causal relationship between the muscle symptoms and statin therapy.
  - If a causal relationship exists, discontinue the original statin. Once muscle symptoms resolve, use a low dose of a different statin.
  - Once a low dose of a statin is tolerated, gradually increase the dose as tolerated.
  - If, after 2 mo without statin treatment, muscle symptoms or elevated CK levels do not resolve completely, consider other causes of muscle symptoms.
  - If persistent muscle symptoms are determined to arise from a condition unrelated to statin therapy or if the predisposing condition has been treated, resume statin therapy at the original dose.

Monitoring

- CK: Do not routinely measure CK levels (although baseline levels may be helpful in patients with a history of statin intolerance or if muscle symptoms develop).
- Hepatic transaminases: Do not routinely measure hepatic transaminases (unless baseline ALT is elevated or symptoms of hepatoxicity develop).
- Glucose and HBA$_{1c}$: Do not routinely monitor glycemic parameters. Patients should be monitored as recommended by expert guidelines.

Abbreviations: AEs, adverse events; ALT, alanine aminotransferase; CK, creatine kinases; CVD, cardiovascular disease; HBA$_{1c}$, hemoglobin A1c; ULN, upper limits of normal. Stone NJ, et al.[116]

The Metabolic Syndrome

The metabolic syndrome includes a cluster of signs and is closely associated with a generalized metabolic disorder of central obesity, HTN, and insulin resistance. Criteria for diagnosing the metabolic syndrome are not universally accepted. Many healthcare clinicians, particularly in North America, use criteria proposed in the Third Report of the National Cholesterol Education Program Expert Panel on Detection, Evaluation, and Treatment of High Blood Cholesterol in Adults (NCEP).

The NCEP defines the metabolic syndrome as the presence of three or more of these factors:
- Central obesity (≥35-in or 88-cm waist measurement; 31.5 in women of South Asian descent)
- Elevated serum TG ≥150 mg/dL (1.70 mmol/L)
- Low serum HDL-C <50 mg/dL (1.3 mmol/L)
- Elevated BP (≥130/85 mm Hg)
- Fasting plasma glucose level ≥110 mg/dL (6.105 mmol/L)

The NCEP did not find conclusive evidence to recommend routine measurement of insulin resistance, prothrombotic state, or proinflammatory state. However, universal waist measurements using the National Health and Nutrition Examination Survey method are recommended.

Underlying causes of this syndrome are overweight/obesity, physical inactivity, and genetic factors. Women with the metabolic syndrome are at increased risk of CVD, stroke, peripheral vascular disease, type 2 DM, and subclinical atherosclerosis.

If a woman has features of MetS, it increases her risk for the development of prediabetes and type 2 DM (if a woman does not yet have increased glucose levels), as well as CVD.[150,153] The treatment is to reduce overall CVD risk through lifestyle modification and treatment of HTN and abnormal lipids, as they exist. Use of aspirin may also be recommended.

Type 1 diabetes

Type 1 DM is an autoimmune disease in which beta cells are destroyed by circulating antibodies. Although it used to be considered a pediatric disease, approximately 83% of persons with type 1 DM are adults.[154] Type 1 DM can occur at any age—half of all new-onset cases are now diagnosed at age 20 years and older.[155] This is often called *latent autoimmune diabetes of the adult* and can be diagnosed by measuring antibodies, most commonly the anti-glutamic acid decarboxylase antibody and zinc transporter-8.[156]

Stages of type 1 DM have been delineated (Table 12).[157] If a woman has positive antibodies, she would fit into one of several classifications.[158]

Type 1 DM is, at least in part, genetic and associated with other forms of autoimmunity such as Hashimoto thyroiditis and celiac disease.[159] Because of advances in disease treatment, women are living longer, and there are now many older women with type 1 DM, which poses particular challenges because rates of severe hypoglycemia are

higher in older persons.[160] Issues associated with frailty, such as osteoporosis, dementia, and CVD, are increased in these women.[161] It is important to note that women can have MetS plus type 1 DM—so-called "double diabetes"—which means that they have an increased risk for CVD in addition to the risk conferred by their type 1 DM.[162]

Prediabetes and type 2 diabetes

Prediabetes is a risk for the progression along the glucose spectrum from normal glucose tolerance to DM.[163] Most often the diagnosis is made based on a fasting blood glucose level or an HbA$_{1C}$ test (a test that shows the average

Table 12. Stages of Type 1 Diabetes

	1	2	3
Characteristics	Autoimmunity	Autoimmunity	New-onset hyperglycemia
	Presymptomatic	Presymptomatic	Often symptomatic
Diagnostic criteria	Multiple autoantibodies	Multiple autoantibodies	Multiple autoantibodies
Glucose levels	Normal	Prediabetes	Diabetes

Insel RA, et al.[157]

level of glucose in the blood for the past 3 months) result (Table 13).[158] Oral glucose tolerance tests (GTT) are rarely required, except in pregnancy.

Prediabetes and type 2 DM occur in people with a genetic susceptibility to developing type 2 DM as well as in those with environmental factors such as weight gain and physical inactivity. The two fundamental defects that lead to hyperglycemia are some form of beta-cell dysfunction or failure that renders the beta cells unable to increase insulin production in the face of insulin resistance, as well as the development of insulin resistance.[147] What comes first is much debated, although insulin resistance alone does not cause DM (there are many women who are obese with extreme insulin resistance who do not develop DM because their beta cells can keep up with the demand). Therefore, an inability of the beta cells to respond to the demand is required for the development of type 2 DM. Regardless of the pathophysiology of type 2 DM, reducing insulin resistance through weight loss and exercise can have a profound effect on blood glucose levels and is generally the cornerstone of therapy for prediabetes and type 2 DM.[164]

Epidemiology

Type 1 diabetes

The incidence of type 1 DM is increasing in children but not in adults.[154,165] However, because of the longer time span of adulthood (defined as age 20-64 y), there are a greater number of new cases in adults compared with youth.[154] Type 1 DM is diagnosed somewhat more often in males than in females, with a male-to-female incidence rate ratio of 1.32 (95% CI, 1.30-1.35). The male predominance is seen by age 10 and persists throughout adulthood. Latent autoimmune diabetes of the adult can often be misdiagnosed as type 2 DM initially, but a failure to respond to noninsulin medications, along with positive autoantibodies, suggests the diagnosis.

Prediabetes

The percentage of US women with prediabetes is 31% compared with 37% of men. Only 14% of women were aware they had prediabetes.[166]

Type 2 diabetes

In 2015, 11.7% of US women of all ages had DM (diagnosed and undiagnosed).[166] This is roughly the same as the percentage of men who have DM (12.7%). The percentage increases overall to 25% in those aged 65 years and older. Based on ethnicity, the highest rate (15.3%) is in American Indian/Alaska Native women. In non-Hispanic black women, it is 13.2%, in Hispanic women it is 11.7%, in Asian women it is 7.3%, and the lowest rate is in non-Hispanic white women at 6.8%. Rates of obesity and type 2 DM have increased over the past decade in women.

Screening for prediabetes and type 2 diabetes

Screening (and diagnosing) prediabetes and type 2 DM is usually done through a fasting glucose test or an HbA$_{1C}$ test. A 2-hour value on a 75 g oral GTT can be used but is not generally measured in clinical practice (Table 13).[158] To diagnosis prediabetes, a screening test needs to be done only once, whereas to diagnose DM, the test must be repeated to confirm the diagnosis.

Screening should be considered for all women beginning at age 45 years and repeated every 3 years. It should be done sooner in women with a BMI of 25 kg/m² or higher (≥23 kg/m² in women of Asian descent) and with one or more additional risk factors (Table 14).[158] Women with prediabetes should be tested yearly. Women who have had a diagnosis of gestational diabetes should be tested at least every 3 years after the birth of the baby.

If test results are normal, testing should be done at least every 3 years, but more frequent testing may be needed if initial results are abnormal or risk is considered to be high.

Diabetes prevention

The Diabetes Prevention Program (DPP) suggests that a lifestyle intervention consisting of moderate weight loss

Table 13. Diagnostic Criteria for Prediabetes and Diabetes

	Prediabetes		
	FPG	**HbA$_{1C}$**	**2-h PG during 75 g OGTT**
Diagnosis if any one of these are present	100-125 mg/dL	5.7-6.4%	140-199 mg/dL
	Diabetes (for asymptomatic persons)		
	FPG	**HbA$_{1C}$**	**2-h PG during 75 g OGTT**
Diagnosis requires repeat confirmatory test	≥126 mg/dL	≥6.5%	≥200 mg/dL

In a woman with classic symptoms of hyperglycemia or hyperglycemic crisis, a random plasma glucose of ≥200 mg/dL is diagnostic.
Abbreviations: FPG, fasting plasma glucose; HbA$_{1c}$, glycated hemoglobin A$_{1c}$; OGTT, oral glucose tolerance test; PG, plasma glucose.
American Diabetes Association.[158]

Table 14. Risk Factors for DM

- BMI ≥25 kg/m² (≥23 kg/m² in women of Asian descent)
- First-degree relative with DM
- High-risk ethnicity (eg, black, Latino, American Indian, Asian, Pacific Islander)
- History of CVD
- HTN (≥140/90 mm Hg or on therapy for HTN)
- HDL-C <35 mg/dL or TG >250 mg/dL
- Women with POS
- Physical inactivity
- Other clinical conditions associated with insulin resistance

Abbreviations: BMI, body mass index; CVD, cardiovascular disease; DM, diabetes mellitus; HDL-C, high-density lipoprotein cholesterol; HTN, hypertension; POS, polycystic ovary syndrome; TG, triglycerides.
American Diabetes Association.[158]

and physical activity significantly reduced the progression to DM in high-risk men and women.[167] This benefit was seen to persist for at least 10 years in women with a history of gestational diabetes.[168] Additionally, particularly in younger, heavier persons, metformin reduced progression to DM. It was not helpful in older persons and thus would be less useful for DM prevention in postmenopausal women.[167] Use of pioglitazone was shown to prevent progression to DM in Hispanic women with prediabetes after gestational diabetes.[169] It has been shown to prevent progression to DM in both younger and older women,[170] but because of a variety of AEs, including weight gain and edema, it is not commonly used in clinical practice for DM prevention.

Programs such as the DPP are a covered benefit through Medicare. Postmenopausal women with prediabetes and Medicare should be encouraged to seek out and register for these programs.

Complications of diabetes

There are both microvascular and macrovascular complications caused by DM.[171] There is no sex difference in terms of the risk for complications. Retinopathy, nephropathy, and neuropathy are the major microvascular complications and are directly related to the level of glycemia over time. Other factors, such as BP, appear to play a role. The macrovascular complications—coronary artery disease, stroke, PAD—are caused by a multitude of factors, glucose being one of them, but HTN and dyslipidemia play a significant role. The American Diabetes Association (ADA) recommends screening for complications (Table 15),[153] and postmenopausal women with DM should add screening for complications to their list of

healthy preventive care measures, with particular attention to the increased risk for macrovascular complications.

Menopause risk factors

In postmenopausal women, as in men, the same risk factors, such as weight gain and physical inactivity, increase the risk for developing DM. So does advancing age, which increases insulin resistance and reduces insulin secretion. Hormone changes associated with menopause can increase central fat accumulation, which can increase insulin resistance and contribute to the development of the metabolic syndrome. It is difficult to prove, however, that menopause is an independent risk factor for the development of worsening glucose metabolism, given that it coexists with so many additional risk factors for diabetes.[172]

Hormone therapy may help attenuate the abdominal fat accumulation and weight gain seen with menopause.[72] Hormone therapy also may reduce the risk for developing DM. In the WHI, women receiving HT had a 14% to 19% reduction in the incidence of type 2 DM.[71] A US Preventive Services Task Force systematic review showed a similar reduction in the development of DM in postmenopausal woman treated with HT.[173]

In general, recommendations for the use of HT should be individualized on the basis of age and CVD risk and should follow the general guidelines for HT use.[72,173] These recommendations state that in women aged 60 years and older, the benefit-risk ratio appears less favorable because of the greater absolute risks of CHD, stroke, VTE, and dementia. It is not recommended to use HT to reduce the risk for MetS or to slow the progression to DM.

Diabetes treatment: lifestyle

Lifestyle management is the foundation for DM treatment for both type 1 and type 2 DM in the postmenopausal woman. Many advocate that treatment of obesity should be the starting point in the management of DM in the person who is overweight or obese.[174] However, management of hyperglycemia should not be delayed while weight loss is attempted but rather done concurrently. More recently released antihyperglycemic agents, such as glucagon-like peptide-1 receptor agonists and sodium-glucose cotransporter 2 inhibitors, provide glucose lowering as well as weight loss and should be considered in women for whom both outcomes are desired (Figure 5).

Ideally, women should not start on a diet per se but should strive to make lifelong changes in dietary habits. In the DPP[167] and Look AHEAD (Action for Health in Diabetes) program,[175] in which weight-loss interventions were employed in prediabetes and DM, respectively, older women responded at least as well as younger women. Thus, dietary interventions are useful in the postmenopausal age group. A variety of dietary patterns, such as the DASH and the Mediterranean diets, may reduce BP, improve lipids, reduce inflammation, and reduce risk for CVD, as well as improve blood sugar levels.[176-178]

Physical activity reduces insulin resistance and can aid in efforts to prevent and treat DM. Postmenopausal women may need to modify exercise based on their functional status, but simply walking 30 minutes daily can improve health.[179] It is important for each person to start slowly and increase gradually in order to avoid injury.

A lifestyle program should be individualized depending on a woman's preferences, health, and life circumstances. Many resources exist, including referral to a dietitian and/or nutrition classes, as well as local facilities where classes and supervision are provided.

Alcohol is not necessarily harmful to women with prediabetes and DM but should be consumed in moderation (no more than one drink/d).[164] Alcohol can cause a reduction of hepatic glucose production and can cause hypoglycemia in a woman on an agent (such as a sulfonylurea agent or insulin) that can cause hypoglycemia.

Smoking cessation is vital and should be addressed at every visit if a woman is actively smoking.

Pharmacotherapy: type 1 diabetes

Women are living longer with type 1 DM. Additionally, older women also can be diagnosed with type 1 DM. The biggest issue with the use of insulin for treating type 1 DM is that rates of hypoglycemia increase with advancing age.[160] This can be particularly frightening for women who live alone and is worse if they have developed early dementia. Additionally, women with longstanding type 1 DM are more likely to have CVD and other DM complications, adding to the difficulty in their management.[180] It is very important to adjust HbA1c targets upward in older women with type 1 DM, especially those having frequent episodes of hypoglycemia. However, a higher target doesn't necessarily reduce the risk. It may be more important to reduce the variance, or time in range, to lower the risk for hypoglycemia.

Degludec, a long-acting insulin analog, reduces rates of both mild and severe hypoglycemia in persons with type 1 DM.[181] It may reduce the variability of blood glucose levels.[182] Some women prefer insulin pump therapy, and this should be continued for as long as possible. In general, pump or multiple daily insulin therapy is similar

Table 15. Routine Screening Tests for Women With Diabetes

	Measure	Initial/Annual	3-6 mo follow-up
Physical examination	Height (measure initially		
	Weight/BMI	X	X
	BP	X	X
	Infusion/Injection sites	X	X
	Foot examination	Comprehensive examination	Visual inspection
Lab tests	HbA1c	X	X
	Lipids	X	
	Liver function	X	
	Spot A/C ratio	X	
	Serum creatinine/eGFR	X	
	TSH (type 1 DM)	X	
	Vitamin B12 (on metformin)	X	
	Serum potassium (if on ACE-I, ARB, or diuretic)	X	
Other	Dilated retinal exam	Every 1-2 y	
	EKG (screening of asymptomatic women for heart is not recommended unless EKG is abnormal)	X	

Abbreviations: A/C, albumin to creatinine; ACE-I, angiotensin-converting enzyme inhibitor; ARB, angiotensin II receptor blocker; BMI, body mass index; BP, blood pressure; DM, diabetes mellitus; eGFR, estimated glomerular filtration rate; EKG, electrocardiogram; HbA1c, glycated hemoglobin A1c; TSH, thyroid-stimulating hormone. American Diabetes Association.[153]

Figure 5. Treatment for Type 2 Diabetes Mellitus

Step 1.

Assess A_{1C}, symptoms, clinical characteristics. Treat obesity concurrently if present.

Likely T2DM, no or minimal symptoms—start lifestyle, DMSE, metformin. ($A_{1C} > 9\%$, consider dual combination therapy.)

Higher A_{1C} (>10%), +/− moderate/severe symptoms, leaner: start lifestyle, DMSE, metformin + injectable (GLP-1 RA, or insulin).

Set A_{1C} target and determine whether history of CVD.

Step 2. Known CVD

If patient not at target,[a] add second-line therapy. If patient with CVD already on dual therapy without one of these agents, consider switching.

eGFR >45 , add SGLT-2 I with FDA-approved CVD benefit (empagliflozin) or GLP-1 RA with CVD benefit (liraglutide).

eGFR <45, add GLP-1 RA with FDA-approved CVD benefit (liraglutide).

If not at target, add the other agent with CVD benefit.

If not at target but close and not at risk for CHF, add DPP-4 I or low-dose TZD; otherwise add basal insulin with lowest risk for hypoglycemia.

Step 2. No Known CVD

If patient not at target, add second-line therapy (or third-line therapy if already on dual combination therapy).

If cost and/or formulary is biggest consideration, add SU. Remember risk for hypoglycemia/weight gain when dosing.

Assess patient characteristics, goals (such as weight loss), contraindications. Add SGLT-2 I, low-dose TZD, DPP-4 I, or GLP-1 RA.

If not at target, add additional agents (SGLT-2 I, GLP-1 RA, TZD, or basal insulin as dictated by prescribing constraints).

If not at target with dual combination therapy, add third agent. If not already started, this will often be a GLP-1 RA, especially if desired reduction in $A_{1C} \geq 1\%$. Stop DPP-4 I when adding GLP-1 RA.

Step 3. With and Without CVD

If patient not at target on prior combinations, continue metformin, SGLT-2 I, and GLP-1 RA (if on one—try GLP-1 RA before insulin if possible). If on SU, reduce dose by 50%. Stop TZD, DPP-4 I.

Add basal insulin. Adjust to fasting target.

If not at target, add prandial insulin, starting with largest meal. Consider insulin pump therapy. Continue metformin when on prandial insulin. Continue SGLT-2 I and/or GLP-1 RA if known CVD.

[a]If at target with metformin, consider switching to monotherapy with CVD risk-reducing agent or lowering target.
Abbreviations: A$_{1c}$, glycated hemoglobin A$_{1c}$; CHF, coronary heart failure; CVD, cardiovascular disease; DPP-4 I, dipeptidyl peptidase-4 inhibitor; DMSE, diabetes mellitus self-management education; eGFR, estimated glomerular filtration rate; GLP-1 RA; glucagon-like peptide-1 receptor agonist; SGLT-2 I, sodium/glucose cotransporter-2 inhibitor; SU, sulfonylurea; T2DM, type 2 diabetes mellitus; TZD, thiazolidinedione.

with regards to HbA_{1C} reduction,[183] but women often have preferences for one therapy over another.

Continuous glucose monitoring is a tool that has been shown to lower HbA_{1C} levels and reduce episodes of hypoglycemia in persons with type 1 DM.[183] These systems measure glucose levels every few minutes and allow users to check their glucose levels as frequently as needed without finger sticks. The devices provide trend arrows so that the user can see whether blood glucose levels are rising, falling, or staying flat, which means that insulin and food can be adjusted based on the direction glucose levels are trending.[184] The data can also be downloaded for retrospective review. Some of the devices offer the advantage of real-time transmission to another's smart phone (a feature unfortunately not covered by Medicare) so that a family member or caregiver can remotely monitor a patient's glucose levels. For women living alone, this can be a comfort as well as an important safety measure.

Newer systems, often described as an "artificial pancreas" but are really a hybrid closed-loop system, use an algorithm to take sensor data and use it to automatically adjust the basal rate throughout the day. Persons still have to enter their carbohydrate intake, but these systems are evolving rapidly and may soon be fully automated. When these systems are more widely available and user friendly, they may greatly simplify the management of type 1 DM.

Pharmacotherapy: type 2 diabetes

In every study powered to show a difference, tighter blood glucose control reduced the risk of microvascular complications—retinopathy, nephropathy, and neuropathy. These complications can be very distressing to the quality of a woman's life, and because of the longer life expectancy (and thus potentially longer life expectancy of a woman with DM), it is important to control glucose levels. However, it is important to reduce any harm from medications that lower blood glucose, in particular agents that cause hypoglycemia. Medications, both old (metformin) and new (glucagon-like peptide-1 receptor agonists, dipeptidyl peptidase-4 inhibitors, sodium-glucose cotransporter-2 inhibitors) that do not cause hypoglycemia or excessive weight gain may be better tolerated with less risk of hypoglycemia (Figure 5).

Large CV outcomes trials have demonstrated much about the CVD safety and even benefits associated with newer agents (Table 16).[185-194] Two agents, empagliflozin[193] and liraglutide,[191] are labeled by FDA for prevention of CHD events in persons with type 2 DM who have known CVD. Thus, these agents are both glucose and CVD risk reducing and are incorporated into guidelines to use as second-line therapy in women with preexisting CVD.

The use of antihyperglycemic medications is outlined in the ADA Standards of Care[195] and the American Association of Clinical Endocrinologists (AACE) guidelines.[196] There are no known gender differences with regards to the use of these drugs. For each woman, the choice of agent(s) should be made individually on the basis of efficacy, AEs, cost, hypoglycemia risk, and weight change. Most women will end up on more than one agent, and cost of medications can become prohibitive for women living on a fixed income. Ideally, agents would be used that do not cause hypoglycemia because of the dangers associated with it[197] and lack of desire for weight gain. The ADA and most other professional societies continue to recommend metformin as the first-line pharmacologic therapy, unless contraindicated, because of its efficacy, safety profile, weight neutrality, and reasonable cost.

The recommendation for the choice of the second-line therapy has changed.[195] After metformin and lifestyle, a woman with known CVD should be treated with an agent shown to reduce CV events and CV mortality (liraglutide and empagliflozin). Canagliflozin also reduces CV events and may be considered. For women without known CVD, any agent can be used on the basis of the woman's clinical circumstances. The commonly used options include sulfonlyurea agents, dipeptidyl peptidase-4 inhibitors, thiazolidinediones, meglinitidines, sodium-glucose cotransporter-2 inhibitors, glucagon-like peptide-1 receptor agonists, and/or insulin. In a woman with a higher initial HBA_{1C} level and/or catabolic symptoms, use of dual agents or insulin may be required (Figure 5).

Although sulfonylurea agents are often less preferred because of their risk for hypoglycemia, cost may drive their use.[198] Thus, when using sulfonylurea agents, the lowest effective dose should be used. Insulin can also cause hypoglycemia, so the dose should be adjusted to avoid causing this AE. Women on agents that can cause hypoglycemia should be educated regarding the signs and symptoms of hypoglycemia, as well as how to prevent and treat it. Family members and caregivers should be trained on the use of glucagon for women with either type 1 or type 2 DM who are on intensive insulin therapy and/or who have episodes of severe hypoglycemia.

Treatment goals

It is extremely important to set appropriate targets for each postmenopausal woman when starting DM treatment.[199,200] Each woman should be assessed for her predicted remaining life expectancy and the risks-benefits of treatment. Lowering HbA$_{1C}$ levels has been unequivocally shown to reduce the risk of microvascular complications—retinopathy, nephropathy, neuropathy.[171] If tight control is started early in the disease, persons followed over time show a reduction in macrovascular complications, as well as in people with both type 1 and type 2 DM.[201,202] However, in the Action to Control Cardiovascular Risk in Diabetes (ACCORD) trial, which targeted an HbA$_{1C}$ of less than 6.0%, there was an increase in overall mortality in persons with CVD who were treated aggressively with insulin and other therapies that can cause hypoglycemia.[203] It is known from ACCORD and other studies that if a woman has an episode of severe hypoglycemia, her mortality risk is increased over the next year or more.[197] However, documented severe hypoglycemia was not the reason for the mortality excess in ACCORD.

The ADA recommends adjusting the HbA$_{1C}$ target upward, especially in persons on medications that can cause hypoglycemia as well as in those with a limited life expectancy (Table 17).[204] A healthy woman aged in her early 60s has a reasonable predicted life expectancy and may choose to have a HbA$_{1C}$ target of less than 7% because she could live long enough to develop microvascular complications. However, women aged in their 80s and 90s are unlikely to have much benefit from tight glycemic control, and a target of less than 8% is reasonable.

Macrovascular risk

Postmenopausal women should be treated for their CV risks per current guidelines.[205,206] There are no differences in terms of the recommendations for men or women, and by the time a woman reaches menopause, it is likely that she is old enough to require statin therapy (statin therapy is recommended for all with DM who are aged older than 40 years), aspirin (should be considered in women with DM aged 50 years and older who have one additional risk factor), and appropriate antihypertensive therapy.[205] Comprehensive assessment and treatment of CVD risk factors is of vital importance in all women with the metabolic syndrome, prediabetes, or type 1 or type 2 DM.

Reducing cardiovascular risk

Historically we have used "diabetes medications" to lower blood sugar levels and statins, ARBs/ACE inhibitors, and aspirin to lower CV risk. However, from the large CV outcomes trials mandated by FDA, there are data to suggest that certain antihyperglycemic medications such as empagliflozin,[193] canagliflozin,[194] liraglutide,[191] and semaglutide[190] further reduce CVD risk in persons with known CVD. Although the Cardiovascular Outcome Trials were conducted mainly in men, their large sample sizes included enough women to show no gender differences.

Table 16. Cardiovascular Outcomes Trials

	Trial	Drug	N	Reported	Outcome	Other
DPP-4 I	Savor	Saxagliptin	16,492	2013	Neutral	Increased CHF
	Examine	Alogliptin	5,380	2013	Neutral	Increased CHF
	Sitagliptin	Sitagliptin	14,735	2015	Neutral	None
GLP-1 RA	ELIXA	Lixisenatide	6,068	2015	Neutral	None
	FREEDOM-CVO	Exenatide	4,000	2016	Neutral	None
	LEADER	Liraglutide	9,340	2016	Benefit	Renal benefit
	SUSTAIN 6	Semaglutide	3,297	2016	Benefit	Worsening of retinopathy
	EXSCEL	Exenatide	14,752	2017	Neutral	None
SGLT-2 I	EMPA-Reg	Empagliflozin	7,028	2015	Benefit	Reduction in CHF, hospitalization, and progression of renal insufficiency
	CANVAS	Canagliflozin	10,142	2017	Benefit	Increased risk of lower extremity amputation and fracture

Abbreviations: CANVAS, Canagliflozin Cardiovascular Assessment Study; CHF, congestive heart failure; CVO, cardiovascular outcomes; DPP-4 I, dipeptidyl peptidase-4 inhibitor; ELIXA, Evaluation of Lixisenatide in Acute Coronary Syndrome; EMPA-Reg, Empagliflozin, Cardiovascular Outcomes, and Mortality in Type 2 Diabetes; EXSCEL, Exenatide Study of Cardiovascular Event Lowering; GLP-1 RA, glucagon-like peptide-1 receptor agonist; LEADER, Liraglutide Effect and Action in Diabetes: Evaluation of Cardiovascular Outcome Results; SGLT-2 I, sodium-glucose cotransporter 2 inhibitor; SUSTAIN, Semaglutide in Subjects With Type 2 Diabetes trial.
Scirica BM, et al[185]; White WB, et al[186]; Green JB, et al[187]; Pfeffer MA, et al[188]; Gerstein HC, et al[189]; Marso SP, et al[190]; Marso SP, et al[191]; Holman RR, et al[192]; Zinman B, et al[193]; Neal B, et al.[194]

Table 17. Glycemic Recommendations for Nonpregnant Women With Diabetes

HbA$_{1C}$	<7.0%[a]
Preprandial capillary plasma glucose	80-130 mg/dL[a]
Peak postprandial capillary plasma glucose[b]	<180 mg/dL[a]

[a]More or less stringent glycemic goals may be appropriate for individual patients. Goals should be individualized based on duration of diabetes, age/life expectancy, comorbid conditions, known cardiovascular disease or advanced microvascular complications, hypoglycemia unawareness, and individual patient considerations.
[b]Postprandial glucose may be targeted if HbA$_{1C}$ goals are not met despite reaching preprandial glucose goals. Postprandial glucose measurements should be made 1-2 h after the beginning of the meal, generally peak levels in patients with diabetes.
Abbreviation: HbA$_{1c}$, glycated hemoglobin A$_{1c}$.
American Diabetes Association.[204]

Therefore, DM medications can have an independent role in CVD risk reduction and are preferred in women who have type 2 DM and known CVD.[195,196,205]

REFERENCES

1. World Health Organization. *World Health Statistics 2017: Monitoring Health for the SDGs, Sustainable Development Goals*. Geneva: World Health Organization; 2017.

2. Benjamin EJ, Virani SS, Callaway CW, et al; American Heart Association Council on Epidemiology and Prevention Statistics Committee and Stroke Statistics Subcommittee. Heart disease and stroke statistics—2018 update: a report from the American Heart Association. *Circulation*. 2018;137(12): e67-e492.

3. Sidney S, Quesenberry CP, Jaffe MG, et al. Recent trends in cardiovascular mortality in the United States and public health goals. *JAMA Cardiol*. 2016;1(5):594-599.

4. Mosca L, Hammond G, Mochari-Greenberger H, Towfighi A, Albert MA; American Heart Association Cardiovascular Disease and Stroke in Women and Special Populations Committee of the Council on Clinical Cardiology; Council on Epidemiology and Prevention, Council on Epidemiology and Prevention; Council on Cardiovascular Nursing; Council on High Blood Pressure Research; Council on Nutrition, Physical Activity, and Metabolism. Fifteen-year trends in awareness of heart disease in women: results of a 2012 American Heart Association national survey. *Circulation*. 2013;127(11):1254-1263, e1-e29.

5. Shaw LJ, Bugiardini R, Merz CN. Women and ischemic heart disease: evolving knowledge. *J Am Coll Cardiol*. 2009;54(17):1561-1575.

6. Gierach GL, Johnson BD, BaireyMerz CN, et al; WISE Study Group. Hypertension, menopause, and coronary artery disease in the Women's Ischemia Syndrome Evaluation (WISE) Study. *J Am Coll Cardiol*. 2006;47(3 suppl):S50-S58.

7. Matthews KA, Crawford SL, Chae CU, et al. Are changes in cardiovascular disease risk factors in midlife women due to chronological aging or to the menopausal transition? *J Am Coll Cardiol*. 2009;54(25):2366-2373.

8. El Khoudary SR, Wildman RP, Matthews K, Thurston RC, Bromberger JT, Sutton-Tyrrell K. Progression rates of carotic intima-media thickness and adventitial diamter during the menopausal transition. *Menopause*. 2013;20(1):8-14.

9. Thurston RC, Karvonen-Gutierrez CA, Derby CA, El Khoudary SR, Kravitz HM, Manson JE. Menopause versus chronologic aging: their roles in women's health. *Menopause*. 2018;25(8):849-854.

10. Mendelsohn ME, Karas RH. Molecular and cellular basis of cardiovascular gender differences. *Science*. 2005; 308(5728): 1583-1587.

11. Hu FB, Grodstein F, Hennekens CH, et al. Age at natural menopause and risk of cardiovascular disease. *Arch Intern Med*. 1999;159(10):1061-1066.

12. Murabito JM, Yang Q, Fox C, Wilson PW, Cupples LA. Heritability of age at natural menopause in the Framingham Heart Study. *J Clin Endocrinol Metab*. 2005;90(6):3427-3430.

13. Kok HS, van Asselt KM, van der Schouw YT, et al. Heart disease risk determines menopausal age rather than the reverse. *J Am Coll Cardiol*. 2006;47(10):1976-1983.

14. Manson JE, Woodruff TK. Reproductive health as a marker of subsequent cardiovascular disease: the role of estrogen. *JAMA Cardiol*. 2016;1(7):776-777.

15. de Aloysio D, Gambacciani M, Meschia M, et al. The effect of menopause on blood lipid and lipoprotein levels. The Icarus Study Group. *Atherosclerosis*. 1999;147(1):147-153.

16. Kuller LH, Simkin-Silverman LR, Wing RR, Meilahn EN, Ives DG. Women's Healthy Lifestyle Project: a randomized clinical trial: results at 54 months. *Circulation*. 2001;103(1):32-37.

17. Feng Y, Hong X, Wilker E, et al. Effects of age of menarche, reproductive years, and menopause on metabolic risk factors for cardiovascular diseases. *Atherosclerosis*. 2008;196(2):590-597.

18. Lobo R. Menopause and aging. In: *Yen & Jaffe's Reproductive Endocrinology: Physiology, Pathophysiology, and Clinical Management*. 7th ed. Strauss JF, Barbieri RL, eds. Philadelphia, Pennsylvania: Elsevier Saunders; 2014:308.e8-339.e8.

19. Garcia M, Mulvagh SL, Merz CN, Buring JE, Manson JE. Cardiovascular disease in women: clinical perspectives. *Circ Res*. 2016;118(8):1273-1293.

20. National Cholesterol Education Program (NCEP) Expert Panel on Detection, Evaluation, and Treatment of High Blood Cholesterol in Adults (Adult Treatment Panel III). Third Report of the National Cholesterol Education Program (NCEP) Expert Panel on Detection, Evaluation, and Treatment of High Blood Cholesterol in Adults (Adult Treatment Plan III) final report. *Circulation*. 2002;106(25):3143-3421.

21. US Department of Health and Human Services. National Heart, Lung, and Blood Institute. *Assessing Cardiovascular Risk: Systematic Evidence Review From the Risk Assessment Work Group, 2013*. www.nhlbi.nih.gov/sites/default/files/media/docs/risk-assessment.pdf. Accessed June 24, 2019.

22. Genest J, Frohlich J, Fodor G, McPherson R; Working Group on Hypercholesterolemia and Other Dyslipidemias. Recommendations for the management of dyslipidemia and prevention of cardiovascular disease: 2003 update. *CMAJ*. 2003;168(9):921-924.

23. Kramer H, Cao G, Dugas L, Luke A, Cooper R, Durazo-Arvizu R. Increasing BMI and waist circumference and prevalence of obesity among adults with type 2 diabetes: the National Health and Nutrition Examination Surveys. *J Diabetes Complications*. 2010;24(6):368-374.

24. Mosca L, Benjamin EJ, Berra K, et al; American Heart Association. Effectiveness-based guidelines for the prevention of cardiovascular disease in women—2011 update: a guideline from the American Heart Association. *J Am Coll Cardiol*. 2011;57(12):1404-1423.

25. Grundy SM, Cleeman JI, Merz CN, et al; National Heart, Lung, and Blood Institute; American College of Cardiology Foundation; American Heart Association. Implications of recent clinical trials for the National Cholesterol Education Program Adult Treatment Panel III guidelines. *Circulation*. 2004;110(2):227-239.

26. Goff DC Jr, Lloyd-Jones DM, Bennett G, et al; American Cardiology/American Heart Assocaition Task Force on Practice Guidelines. 2013 ACC/AHA guideline on the assessment of cardiovascular risk: a report of the American College of Cardiology/American Heart Association Task Force on Practice Guidelines. *Circulation*. 2014;129(25 suppl 2):S49-S73.

27. Bellamy L, Casas JP, Hingorani AD, Williams DJ. Pre-eclampsia and risk of cardiovascular disease and cancer in later life: systematic review and meta-analysis. *BMJ*. 2007;335(7627):974.

28. Anderson TJ, Grégoire J, Pearson GJ, et al. 2016 Canadian Cardiovascular Society guidelines for the management of dyslipidemia for the prevention of cardiovascular disease in the adult. *Can J Cardiol*. 2016;32(11):1263-1282.

29. Ridker PM, Buring JE, Rifai N, Cook NR. Development and validation of improved algorithms for the assessment of global cardiovascular risk in women: the Reynolds Risk Score. *JAMA*. 2007;297(13):611-619.

30. Ridker PM, Wilson PW, Grundy SM. Should C-reactive protein be added to metabolic syndrome and to assessment of global cardiovascular risk? *Circulation*. 2004;109(23):2818-2825.

31. Ridker PM, Rifai N, Cook NR, Bradwin G, Buring JE. Non-HDL cholesterol, apolipoproteins A-1 and B100, standard lipid measures, lipid ratios, and CRP as risk factors for cardiovascular disease in women. *JAMA*. 2005;294(3):326-333.

32. Walsh BW, Paul S, Wild RA, et al. The effects of hormone replacement therapy and raloxifene on C-reactive protein and homocysteine in healthy postmenopausal women: a randomized, controlled trial. *J Clin Endocrinol Metab*. 2000;85(1):214-218.

33. Eckel RH, Jakicic JM, Ard JD, et al; American College of Cardiology/American Heart Association Task Force on Practice Guidelines. 2013 AHA/ACC guideline on lifestyle management to reduce cardiovascular risk: a report of the American College of Cardiology/American Heart Association Task Force on Practice Guidelines. *J Am Coll Cardiol*. 2014;63(25 pt B):2960-2984.

34. Mosca L, Linfante AH, Benjamin EJ, et al. National study of physician awareness and adherence to cardiovascular disease and prevention guidelines. *Circulation*. 2005;111(4):499-510.

35. Mosca L, Merz NB, Blumenthal RS, et al. Opportunity for intervention to achieve American Heart Association guidelines for optimal lipid levels in high-risk women in a managed care setting. *Circulation*. 2005;111(4):488-493.

36. Hackshaw A, Morris JK, Boniface S, Tang J, Milenković. Low cigarette consumption and risk of coronary heart disease and stroke: meta-analysis of 141 cohort studies in 55 study reports. *BMJ*. 2018;360:J5855.

37. Chasan-Taber L, Stampfer MJ. Epidemiology of oral contraceptives and cardiovascular disease. *Ann Intern Med*. 1998;128(6):467-477.

38. Centers for Disease Control and Prevention. US medical eligibility criteria for contraceptive use, 2010. *MMWR Recomm Rep*. 2010;59(RR-4):1-86.

39. Fukushima Y, Kurose S, Shinno H, et al. Importance of lean muscle maintenance to improve insulin resistance by body weight reduction in female patients with obesity. *Diabetes Metab J*. 2016;40(2):147-153.

40. Houston MC, Faxio S, Chilton FH, et al. Nonpharmacologic treatment of dyslipidemia. *Prog Cardiovasc Dis*. 2009;52(2):61-94.

41. Dazzano LA, Reynolds K, Holder KN, He J. Effect of folic acid supplementation on risk of cardiovascular disease: a meta-analysis of randomized controlled trials. *JAMA*. 2006;296(22):2720-2726.

42. Brøndum-Jacobsen P, Benn M, Jensen GB, Nordestgaard BG. 25-hydroxyvitamin D levels and risk of ischemic heart disease, myocardial infarction, and early death: population-based study and meta-analysis of 18 and 17 studies. *Arterioscler Thromb Vasc Biol*. 2012;32(11):2794-2802.

43. Wang L, Song Y, Manson JE, et al. Circulating 25-hydrosy-vitamin D and risk of cardiovascular disease: a meta-analysis of prospective studies. *Circ Cardiovasc Qual Outcomes*. 2012;5(6):819-829.

44. Robinson-Cohen C, Hoofnagle AN, Ix JH, et al. Racial differences in the association of serum 25-hydroxyvitamin D concentrations with coronary heart disease events. *JAMA*. 2013;310(2):179-188.

45. Scragg R, Stewart AW, Waayer D, et al. Effect of monthly high-dose vitamin D supplementation on cardiovascular disease in the Vitamin D Assessment Study: a randomized clinical trial. *JAMA Cardiol*. 2017;2(6):608-616.

46. Manson JE, Cook NR, Lee IM, et al; VITAL Research Group. Vitamin D supplements and prevention of cancer and cardiovascular disease. *N Engl J Med*. 2018;380(1):33-44.

47. Schnatz PF, Manson JE. Vitamin D and cardiovascular disease: an appraisal of the evidence. *Clin Chem*. 2014;60(4):600-609.

48. Katan MB, Grundy SM, Jones P, Law M, Miettinen T, Paoletti R; Stresa Workshop Participants. Efficacy and safety of plant stanols and sterols in the management of blood cholesterol levels. *Mayo Clin Proc*. 2003;78(8):965-978.

49. Devaraj S, Jialal I, Vega-López S. Plant sterol-fortified orange juice effectively lowers cholesterol levels in mildly hypercholesterolemic healthy individuals. *Arterioscler Thromb Vasc Biol*. 2004;24(3):e25-e28.

50. American Heart Association Nutrition Committee, Lichtenstein AJ, Appel LJ, et al. Diet and lifestyle recommendations revision 2006: a scientific statement from the American Heart Association Nutrition Committee. *Circulation*. 2006;114(1):82-96. Erratum in: *Circulation*. 2006;114(23):e629; *Circulation*. 2006;114(1):e27.

51. Marangoine F, Poli A. Phytosterols and cardiovascular health. *Pharmacol Res*. 2010;61(3):193-199.

52. Han S, Jiao J, Xu J, Zimmerman D, et al. Effects of plant stanol or sterol-enriched diets on lipid profiles in patients treated with statins: systematic review and meta-analysis. *Sci Rep*. 2016;6:31337.

53. Gylling H, Miettinen TA. Plant stanol consumption for cardiovascular health: what do we know about efficacy and safety? *Clin Lipidol*. 2010;5(6):827-833.

54. Rudkowska I. Plant sterols and stanols for healthy ageing. *Maturitas*. 2010;66(2):158-162.

55. Sacks FM, Lichtenstein A, Van Horn L, Harris W, Kris-Etherton P, Winston M; American Heart Association Nutrition Committee. Soy protein, isoflavones, and cardiovascular health: an American Heart Association Science Advisory for professionals from the Nutrition Committee. *Circulation*. 2006;113(7):1034-1044.

56. Estruch R, Ros E, Salas-Salvadó J, et al; PREDIMED Study Investigators. Primary prevention of cardiovascular disease with a Mediterranean diet. *N Engl J Med*. 2013;368(14):1279-1290. Erratum in: *N Engl J Med*. 2014;370(9):886.

57. Prasain JK, Carlson SH, Wyss JM. Flavonoids and age-related disease: risk, benefits and critical windows. *Maturitas*. 2010;66(2):163-171.

58. Bell S, Daskalopoulou M, Rapsomaniki E, et al. Association between clinically recorded alcohol consumption and initial presentation of 12 cardiovascular diseases: population based cohort study using linked health records. *BMJ*. 2017;356:j909

59. Willet WC, Stampfer MJ, Colditz GA, Rosner BA, Hennekens CH, Speizer FE. Moderate alcohol consumption and the risk of breast cancer. *N Engl J Med*. 1987;316(19):1174-1180.

60. Tankó LB, Bagger YZ, Qin G, Alexandersen P, Larsen PJ, Christiansen C. Enlarged waist combined with elevated triglycerides is a strong predictor of accelerated atherogenesis and related cardiovascular mortality in postmenopausal women. *Circulation*. 2005;111(15):1883-1890.

61. Jensen MD, Ryan DH, Apovian CM, et al; American College of Cardiology/American Heart Association Task force on Practice Guidelines; Obesity Society. 2013 AHA/ACC/TOS guideline for the management of overweight and obesity in adults: a report of the American College of Cardiology/American Heart Association Task Force on Practice Guidelines and the Obesity Society. *Circulation*. 2014;129(25 suppl 2):S102-S138.

62. Smith SC Jr, Benjamin EJ, Bonow RO, et al. AHA/ACCF secondary prevention and risk reduction therapy for patients with coronary and other atherosclerotic vascular disease: 2011 update: a guideline from the American Heart Association and American College of Cardiology Foundation endorsed by the World Heart Federation and the Preventive Cardiovascular Nurses Association. *J Am Coll Cardiol*. 2011;58(23):2432-2446.

63. Gaziano JM, Brotons C, Coppolecchia R, et al; ARRIVE Executive Committee. Use of aspirin to reduce risk of initial vascular events in patients at moderate risk of cardiovascular disease (ARRIVE): a randomised, double-blind, placebo-controlled trial. *Lancet*. 2018;391(10152):1036-1046.

64. ASCEND Study Collaborative Group, Bowman L, Mafham M, et al. Effects of aspirin for primary prevention in persons with diabetes mellitus. *N Engl J Med*. 2018;379(16):1529-1539.

65. McNeil JJ, Wolfe R. Woods RL, et al; ASPREE Investigator Group. Effect of aspirin on cardiovascular events and bleeding in the healthy elderly. *N Engl J Med*. 2018;379(16):1509-1518.

66. Arnett DK, Blumenthal RS, Albert MA, et al. 2019 ACC/AHA guideline on the primary prevention of cardiovascular disease: a report of the American College of Cardiology/American Heart Association Task Force on clinical Practice Guidelines. [published online ahead of print March 17, 2019]. *J Am Coll Cardiol*.

67. Arnett DK, Blumenthal RS, Albert MA, et al. 2019 ACC/AHA guideline on the primary prevention of cardiovascular disease [published online ahead of print March 17, 2019]. *Circulation*.

68. Ridker PM, Cook NR, Lee IM, et al. A randomized trial of low-dose aspirin in the primary prevention of cardiovascular disease in women. *N Engl J Med*. 2005;352(13):1293-1304.

69. Bibbins-Domingo K; US Preventive Services Task Force. Aspirin use for the primary prevention of cardiovascular disease and colorectal cancer: recommendation statement. *Ann Intern Med*. 2016;164(12):836-845.

70. Rossouw JE, Prentice RL, Manson JE, et al. Postmenopausal hormone therapy and risk of cardiovascular disease by age and years since menopause. *JAMA*. 2007;297(13):1465-1477.

71. Manson JE, Chlebowski RT, Stefanick ML, et al. Menopausal hormone therapy and health outcomes during the intervention and extended poststopping phases of the Women's Health Initiative randomized trials. *JAMA*. 2013;310(13):1353-1368.

72. The NAMS 2017 Hormone Therapy Position Statement Advisory Panel. The 2017 hormone therapy position statement of the North American Menopause Society. *Menopause*. 2017;24(7):728-753.

73. Prentice RL, Langer RD, Stefanick ML, et al; Women's Health Initiative Investigators. Combined analysis of Women's Health Initiative observational and clinical trial data on postmenopausal hormone treatment and cardiovascular disease. *Am J Epidemiol*. 2006;63(7):589-599.

74. Harman SM, Black DM, Naftolin F, et al. Arterial imaging outcomes and cardiovascular risk factors in recently menopausal women: a randomized trial. *Ann Intern Med*. 2014;161(4):249-260.

75. Hodis HN, Mack WJ, Henderson VW, et al; ELITE Research Group. Vascular effects of early versus late postmenopausal treatment with estradiol. *N Engl J Med*. 2016;374(13):1221-1231.

76. Manson JE, Bassuk SS. Invited commentary: hormone therapy and risk of coronary heart disease why renew the focus on the early years of menopause? *Am J Epidemiol*. 2007;166(5):511-517.

77. Boardman HM, Hartley L, Eisinga A, et al. Hormone therapy for preventing cardiovascular disease in post-menopausal women. *Cochrane Database Syst Rev*. 2015;(3):CD002229.

78. Salpeter SR, Cheng J, Thabane L, Buckley NS, Salpeter EE. Bayesian meta-analysis of hormone therapy and mortality in younger postmenopausal women. *Am J Med*. 2009;122(11):1016-1022.

79. Canonico M, Carcaillon L, Plu-Bureau G, et al. Postmenopausal hormone therapy and risk of stroke: impact of the route of estrogen administration and type of progestogen. *Stroke*. 2016;47(7):1734-1741.

80. Renoux C, Dell×aniello S, Garbe E, Suissa S. Transdermal and oral hormone replacement therapy and the risk of stroke: a nested case-control study. *BMJ*. 2010;340:c2519.

81. Grady D, Herrington D, Bittner V, et al; HERS Research Group. Cardiovascular disease outcomes during 6.8 years of hormone therapy: Heart and Estrogen/Progestin Replacement Study follow-up (HERS II). *JAMA*. 2002;288(1):49-57. Erratum: *JAMA*. 2002;288(9):1064.

82. Vickers MR, MacLennan AH, Lawton B, et al; WISDOM group. Main morbidities recorded in the women's international study of long duration oestrogen after menopause (WISDOM): a randomised controlled trial of hormone replacement therapy in postmenopausal women. *BMJ*. 2007;335(7613):239.

83. Rossouw JE, Anderson GL, Prentice RL, et al; Writing Group for the Women's Health Initiative Investigators. Risks and benefits of estrogen plus progestin in healthy postmenopausal women: principle results from the Women's Health Initiative randomized controlled trial. *JAMA*. 2002;288(3):321-333.

84. Anderson GL, Limacher M, Assaf AR, et al; Women's Health Initiative Steering Committee. Effects of conjugated equine estrogen in postmenopausal women with hysterectomy: the Women's Health Initiative randomized controlled trial. *JAMA*. 2004;291(14):1701-1712.

85. Canonico M, Oger E, Plu-Bureau G, et al; Estrogen and Thromboembolism Risk (ESTHER) Study Group. *Circulation*. 2007;115(7):840-845.

86. Canonico M, Plu-Bureau G, Lowe GD, Scarabin PY. Hormone replacement therapy and risk of venous thromboembolism in postmenopausal women. *BMJ*. 2008;336(7655):1227-1231.

87. Speroff L. Transdermal hormone therapy and the risk of stroke and venous thrombosis. *Climacteric*. 2010;13(5):429-432.

88. Canonico M, Alhenc-Gelas M, Plu-Bureau G, Olié V, Scarabin PY. Activated protein C resistance among postmenopausal women using transdermal estrogens: importance of progestogen. *Menopause*. 2010;17(6):1122-1127.

89. Eisenberger A, Westhoff C. Hormone replacement therapy and venous thromboembolism. *J Steroid Biochem Mol Biol*. 2014;142:76-82.

90. Cushman M, Kuller LH, Prentice R, et al; Women's Health Initiative Investigators. Estrogen plus progestin and risk of venous thrombosis. *JAMA*. 2004;292(13):1573-1580.

91. Lim SS, Vos T, Flaxman AD, et al. A comparative risk assessment of burden of disease and injury attributable to 67 risk factors and risk factor clusters in 21 regions, 1990-2010: a systematic analysis for the Global Burden of Disease Study 2010. *Lancet*. 2013;380(9859):2224-2260.

92. GBD 2015 Risk Factors Collaborators. Global, regional, and national comparative risk assessment of 79 behavioural, environmental and occupational, and metabolic risks or clusters of risks, 1990-2015: a systematic analysis for the Global Burden of Disease Study 2015. *Lancet*. 2016;388(10053):1659-1724.

93. Yoon SS, Fryar CD, Carroll MD. *Hypertension Prevalence and Control Among Adults: United States, 2011-2014*. NCHS data brief, no 220. Hyattsville, MD: National Center for Health Statistics; 2015.

94. National Center for Health and Statistics. *Health, United States, 2010: With Special Feature on Death and Dying*. Hyattsville MD: US Department of Health and Human Services; 2011.

95. Burt VL, Whelton P, Roccella EJ, et al. Prevalence of hypertension in the US adult population. Results from the Third National Health and Nutrition Examination Survey, 1988-1991. *Hypertension*. 1995;25(3):305-313.

96. Hage FG, Mansur SJ, Xing D, Oparil S. Hypertension in women. *Kidney Int Suppl (2011)*. 2013;3(4):352-356.

97. Igho Pemu P, Ofili E. Hypertension in women: part I. *J Clin Hypertens (Greenwich)*. 2008;10(5):406-410.

98. Lima R, Wofford M, Reckelhoff JF. Hypertension in postmenopausal women. *Curr Hypertens Rep*. 2012;14(3):254-260.

99. Vasan RS, Beiser A, Seshadri S, et al. Residual lifetime risk for developing hypertension in middle-aged women and men: The Framingham Heart Study. *JAMA*. 2002;287(8):1003-1010.

100. Escobar E. Hypertension and coronary heart disease. *J Hum Hypertens*. 2002;16(suppl 1):S61-S63.

101. Eaton CB, Pettinger M, Rossouw J, et al. Risk factors for incident hospitalized heart failure with preserved versus reduced ejection fraction in a multiracial cohort of postmenopausal women. *Circ Heart Fail*. 2016;9(10):e002883.

102. Rodriguez F, Stefanick ML, Greenland P, et al. Racial and ethnic differences in atrial fibrillation risk factors and predictors in women: findings from the Women's Health Initiative. *Am Heart J*. 2016;176:70-77.

103. Haring B, Leng X, Robinson J, et al. Cardiovascular disease and cognitive decline in postmenopausal women: results from the Women's Health Initiative Memory Study. *J Am Heart Assoc*. 2013;2(6):e000369.

104. Howe MD, McCullough LD. Prevention and management of stroke in women. *Expert Rev Cardiovasc Ther*. 2015;13(4):403-415.

105. James PA, Oparil S, Carter BL, et al. 2014 evidence-based guideline for the management of high blood pressure in adults: report from the panel members appointed to the Eighth Joint National Committee (JNC 8). *JAMA*. 2014;311(5):507-520. Erratum in: *JAMA*. 2014;311(17):1809.

106. Chobanian AV, Bakris GL, Black HR, et al; National Heart, Lung, and Blood Institute Joint National Committee on Prevention, Detection, Evaluation, and Treatment of High Blood Pressure; National High Blood Pressure Education Program Coordinating Committee. The Seventh Report of the Joint National committee on Prevention, Detection, Evaluation, and Treatment of High Blood Pressure: the JNC 7 report. *JAMA*. 2003;289(19):2560-2572. Erratum in: *JAMA*. 2003;290(2):197.

107. Whelton PK, Carey RM, Aronow WS, et al. 2017 ACC/AHA/AAPA/ABC/ ACPM/AGS/APhA/ASH/ASPC/NMA/PCNA guideline for the prevention, detection, evaluation, and management of high blood pressure in adults a report of the American College of Cardiology/American Heart Association Task Force on Clinical Practice Guidelines. *J Am Coll Cardiol.* 2018;71(19):e127-e248. Erratum in: *J Am Coll Cardiol.* 2018;71(19):2275-2279.

108. Wright JT Jr, Fine LJ, Lackland DT, Ogedegbe G, Dennison-Himmelfarb CR. Evidence supporting a systolic blood pressure goal of less than 150 mm Hg in patients aged 60 years or older: the minority view. *Ann Intern Med.* 2014;160(7):499-503.

109. SPRINT Research Group. Wright JT Jr, Williamson JD, et al. A randomized trial of intensive versus standard blood-pressure control. *N Engl J Med.* 2015;373(22):2103-2116.

110. Qaseem A, Wilt TJ, Rich R, Humphrey LL, Frost J, Forciea MA; Clinical Guidelines Committee of the American College of Physicians and the Commission on Health of the Public and Science of the American Academy of Family Physicians. Pharmacologic treatment of hypertension in adults aged 60 years or older to higher versus lower blood pressure targets: a clinical practice guideline from the American College of Physicians and the American Academy of Family Physicians. *Ann Intern Med.* 2017;166(6):430-437.

111. Ong KL, Cheung BM, Man YB, Lau CP, Lam KS. Prevalence, awareness, treatment, and control of hypertension among United States adults 1999-2004. *Hypertension.* 2007;49(1):69-75.

112. Derby CA, Crawford SL, Pasternak RC, Sowers M, Sternfeld B , Matthews KA. Lipid changes during the menopause transition in relation to age and weight: the Study of Women's Health Across the Nation. *Am J Epidemiol.* 2009;169(11):1352-1361.

113. Yusuf S, Rangarajan S, Teo K, et al; PURE Investigators. Cardiovascular risk and events in 17 low, middle-, and high-income countries. *N Engl J Med.* 2014;371(9):818-827.

114. Pencina MJ, D'Agostino RB Sr, Larson MG, Massaro JM, Vasan RS. Predicting the 30-year risk of cardiovascular disease: the Framingham Heart Study. *Circulation.* 2009;119(24):3078-3084.

115. Mozaffarian D, Benjamin EJ, Go AS, et al; American Heart Association Statistics Committee and Strok Statistics Subcommittee. Heart disease and stroke statistics—2015 update: a report from the American Heart Association. *Circulation.* 2015;131(4): e29-e322.

116. Stone NJ, Robinson JG, Lichtenstein AH, et al; American College of Cardiology/American Heart Association Task Force on Practice Guidelines. 2013 ACC/AHA guideline on the treatment of blood cholesterol to reduce atherosclerotic cardiovascular risk in adults: a report of the American College of Cardiology/American Heart Association Task Force on Practice Guidelines. *J Am Coll Cardiol.* 2014;63(25 pt B):2889-2934.

117. Gidding SS, Champagne MA, de Farranti SD, et al; American Heart Association Atherosclerosis, Hypertenseion, and Obesity in Young Committee of Council on Cardiovascular Disease in Young, Council on Cardiovascular and Stroke Nursing, Council on Functional Genomics and Translational Biology, and Council on Lifestyle and Cardiometabolic Health. The Agenda for Familial Hypercholesterolemia: a scientific statement from the American Heart Association. *Circulation.* 2015;132(22):2167-2192. Erratum in: *Circulation.* 2015.

118. Goff DC Jr, Lloyd-Jones DM, Bennett G, et al; American College of Cardiology/American Heart Association Task Force on Practice Guidelines. 2013 ACC/AHA guideline on the assessment of cardiovascular risk: a report of the American College of Cardiology/ American Heart Association Task Force on Practice Guidelines. *J Am Coll Cardiol.* 2014;63(25 pt B):2935-2959. Erratum in: *J Am Coll Cardiol.* 2014;63(25 pt B):3026.

119. Muntner P, Colantonio LD, Cushman M, et al. Validation of the atherosclerotic cardiovascular disease pooled cohort risk equations. *JAMA.* 2014;311(14):1406-1415.

120. Karmali KN, Goff DC Jr, Ning H, Lloyd-Jones DM. A systematic examination of the 2013 ACC/AHA pooled cohort risk assessment tool for atherosclerotic cardiovascular disease. *J Am Coll Cardiol.* 2014;64(10):959-968.

121. Rana JS, Tabada GH, Solomon MD, et al. Accuracy of the atherosclerotic cardiovascular risk equation in a large contemporary, multiethnic population. *J Am Coll Cardiol.* 2016;67(18):2118-2130.

122. Cook NR, Ridker PM. Calibration of the pooled cohort equations for atherosclerotic cardiovascular disease: an update. *Ann Intern Med.* 2016:165(11):786-794.

123. Sanghavi M, Parikh NI. Harnessing the power of pregnancy and pregnancy-related events to predict cardiovascular disease in women. *Circulation.* 2017;135(6):590-592.

124. Parikh NI, Jeppson RP, Berger JS, et al. Reproductive risk factors and coronary heart disease in the Women's Health Initiative Observational Study. *Circulation.* 2016;133(22):2149-2158.

125. Wiegman A, Gidding SS, Watts GF, et al; European Atherosclerosis Society Consensus Panel. Familial hypercholesterolaemia in children and adolescents: gaining decades of life by optimizing detection and treatment. *EurHeart J.* 2015;36(36):2425-2437.

126. Perak AM, Ning H, de Ferranti SD, Gooding HC, Wilkins JT, Lloyd-Jones DM. Long-term risk of atherosclerotic cardiovascular disease in US adults with the familial hypercholesterolemia phenotype. *Circulation.* 2016;134(1):9-19.

127. Jensen MD, Ryan DH, Apovian CM, et al; American College of Cardiology/American Heart Association Task Force on Practice Guidelines; Obesity Society. 2013 AHA/ACC/TOS guideline for the management of overweight and obesity in adults: a report of the American College of Cardiology/American Heart Association Task Force on Practice Guidelines and the Obesity Society. *J Am Coll Cardiol.* 2014;63(25 pt B):2985-3023. Erratum in: *J Am Coll Cardiol.* 2014;63(25 pt B):3029-3030.

128. Silverman MG, Ference BA, Im K, et al. Association between lowering LDL-C and cardiovascular risk reduction among different therapeutic interventions: a systematic review and meta-analysis. *JAMA.* 2016;316(12):1289-1297.

129. Cholesterol Treatment Trialists' (CTT) Collaboration, Baigent C, Blackwell L, et al. Efficacy and safety of more intensive lowering of LDL cholesterol: a meta-analysis of data from 170,000 participants in 26 randomised trials. *Lancet.* 2010;376(9753):1670-1681.

130. Cholesterol Treatment Trialists' (CTT) Collaborators, Mihaylova B, Emberson J, et al. The effects of lowering LDL cholesterol with statin therapy in people at low risk of vascular disease: meta-analysis of individual data from 27 randomised trials. *Lancet.* 2012;380(9841):581-590.

131. Cholesterol Treatment Trialists' (CCT) Collaborators, Fulcher J, O'Connell R, et al. Efficacy and safety of LDL-lowering therapy among men and women: meta-analysis of individual data from 174,000 participants in 27 randomized trials. *Lancet.* 2015;385(9976):1397-1405.

132. Writing Committee, Lloyd-Jones DM, Morris PB, et al. 2016 ACC expert consensus decision pathway on the role of non-statin therapies for LDL-cholesterol lowering in the management of atherosclerotic cardiovascular disease risk: a report of the American College of Cardiology Task Force on Clinical Expert Consensus Documents. *J Am Coll Cardiol.* 2016;68(1):92-125.

133. Robinson JG, Huijgen R, Ray K, Persons J, Kastelein JJ, Pencina MJ. Determining when to add nonstatin therapy: a quantitative approach. *J Am Coll Cardiol.* 2016;68(22):2412-2421.

134. Hofer TP, Sussman JB, Hayward RA. New studies do not challenge the American College of Cardiology/American Heart Association lipid guidelines. *Ann Intern Med.* 2016;164(10):683-684.

135. Shah R, Spahillari A, Mwasongwe S, et al. Subclinical atherosclerosis, statin eligibility, and outcomes in African American individuals: the Jackson Heart Study. *JAMA Cardiology.* 2017;2(6):644-652.

136. Collins R, Reith C, Emberson J, et al. Interpretation of the evidence for the efficacy and safety of statin therapy. *Lancet.* 2016;388(10059):2532-2561.

137. Robinson JG. Statins and diabetes risk: how real is it and what are the mechanisms? *Curr Opin Lipidol.* 2015;26(3):228-235.

138. Moriarty PM, Thompson PD, Cannon CP, et al; ODYSSEY ALTERNATIVE Investigators. Efficacy and safety of alirocumab vs ezetimibe in statin-intolerant patients, with a statin rechallenge arm: The ODYSSEY ALTERNATIVE randomized trial. *J Clin Lipidol.* 2015;9(6):758-769.

139. Backes JM, Ruisinger JF, Gibson CA, Moriarty PM. Statin-associated muscle symptoms—managing the highly intolerant. *J Clin Lipidol.* 2017;11(1):24-33.

140. Cannon C, Blazing MA, Giugliano RP, et al; IMPROVE-IT Investigators. Ezetimibe added to statin therapy after acute coronary syndromes. *N Engl J Med.* 2015;372(25):2387-2397.

141. Sabatine MS, Giugliano RP, Keech AC, et al; FOURIER Steering Committee and Investigators. Evolocumab and clinical outcomes in patients with cardiovascular disease. *N Engl J Med.* 2017;376(18):1713-1722.

142. Miller M, Stone NJ, Ballantyne C, et al; American Heart Association Clinical Lipidology, thrombosis, and Prevention Committee of the Council on Nutrition, Physical Activity, and Metabolism; Council on Arteriosclerosis, Thrombosis and Vascular Biology; Council on Cardiovascular Nursing; council on the Kidney in Cardiovascular Disease. Triglycerides and cardiovascular disease: a scientific statement from the American Heart Association. *Circulation.* 2011;123(20):2292-2333.

143. Nordestgaard BG, Benn M, Schnor P, Tybjaerg-Hansen A. Nonfasting triglycerides and risk of myocardial infarction, ischemic heart disease, and death in men and women. *JAMA.* 2007;298(3):299-308.

144. Rosenson RS, Davidson MH, Hirsch BJ, KathiresanS, Gaudet D. Genetics and causality of triglyceride-rich lipoproteins in atherosclerotic cardiovascular disease. *J Am Coll Cardiol.* 2014;64(23):2525-2540.

145. Hegele RA, Ginsberg HN, Chapman MJ, et al; European Atherosclerosis Society Consensus Panel. The polygenic nature of hypertriglcyeridaemia: implications for definition, diagnosis, and management. *Lancet Diab Endocrinol.* 2014;2(8):655-666.

146. Brunzell JD. Clinical practice. Hypertriglyceridemia. *N Engl J Med.* 2007;357(10):1009-1017.

147. Skyler JS, Bakris GL, Bonifacio E, et al. Differentiation of diabetes by pathophysiology, natural history, and prognosis. *Diabetes.* 2017;66(2):241-255.

148. Chae CU, Derby CA. The menopausal transition and cardiovascular risk. *Obstet Gynecol Clin North Am.* 2011;38(3):477-488.

149. Kazlauskaite R, Avery-Mamer EF, Li H, et al. Race/Ethnic comparisons of waist-to-height ratio for cardiometabolic screening: the study of Women's Health Across the Nation. *Am J Hum Biol.* 2017;29(1):doi: 10.1002/ajhb.22909.

150. Alberti KG, Eckel RH, Grundy SM, et al; International Diabetes Federation Task Force on Epidemiology and Prevention; National Heart, Lung, and Blood Institute; American Heart Association; World Heart Federation; International Atherosclerosis Society; International Association for the Study of Obesity. Harmonizing the metabolic syndrome: a joint interim statement of the International Diabetes Federation Task Force on Epidemiology and Prevention; National Heart, Lung, and Blood Institute; American Heart Association; World Heart Federation; International Atherosclerosis Society; and International Association for the Study of Obesity. *Circulation.* 2009;120(16):1640-1645.

151. Grundy SM. Metabolic syndrome update. *Trends Cardiovasc Med.* 2016;26(4):364-373.

152. Sperling LS, Mechanick JI, Neeland IJ, et al. The CardioMetabolic Health Alliance: working toward a new care model for the metabolic syndrome. *J Am Coll Cardiol.* 2015;66(9):1050-1067.

153. American Diabetes Association. 3. Comprehensive medical evaluation and assessment of comorbidities: standards of medical care in diabetes—2018. *Diabetes Care.* 2018;41(suppl 1):S28-S37.

154. Rogers MAM, Kim C, Banerjee T, Lee JM. Fluctuations in the incidence of type 1 diabetes in the United States from 2001 to 2015: a longitudinal study. *BMC Med.* 2017;15(1):199.

155. Thomas NJ, Jones SE, Weedon MN, Shields BM, Oram RA, Hattersley AT. Frequency and phenotype of type 1 diabetes in the first six decades of life: a cross-sectional, genetically stratified survival analysis from UK Biobank. *Lancet Diabetes Endocrinol.* 2018;6(2):122-129.

156. Sosenko JM, Skyler JS, Palmer JP, et al; Type 1 Diabetes TrialNet Study Group; Diabetes Prevention Trial-Type 1 Study Group. The prediction of type 1 diabetes by multiple autoantibody levels and their incorporation into an autoantibody risk score in relatives of type 1 diabetic patients. *Diabetes Care.* 2013;36(9):2615-2620.

157. Insel RA, Dunne JL, Atkinson MA, et al. Staging presymptomatic type 1 diabetes: a scientific statement of JDRF, the Endocrine Society, and the American Diabetes Association. *Diabetes Care.* 2015;38(10):1964-1974.

158. American Diabetes Association. 2. Classification and diagnosis of diabetes: standards of medical care in diabetes—2018. *Diabetes Care.* 2018;41(suppl 1):S13-S27.

159. Hughes JW, Riddlesworth TD, DiMeglio LA, Miller KM, Rickels MR, McGill JB; T1D Exchange Clinic Network. Autoimmune diseases in children and adults with type 1 diabetes from the T1D Exchange clinic registry. *J Clin Endocrinol Metab.* 2016;101(12):4931-4937.

160. Weinstock RS, Xing D, Maahs DM, et al; T1D Exchange Clinic Network. Severe hypoglycemia and diabetic ketoacidosis in adults with type 1 diabetes: results from the T1D Exchange clinic registry. *J Clin Endocrinol Metab.* 2013;98(8):3411-3419.

161. Kalyani RR, Tian J, Xue Q-L, et al. Hyperglycemia and incidence of frailty and lower extremity mobility limitations in older women. *J Am Geriatr Soc.* 2012;60(9):1701-1707.

162. Kilpatrick ES, Rigby AS, Atkin SL. Insulin resistance, the metabolic syndrome, and complication risk in type 1 diabetes: "double diabetes" in the Diabetes Control and Complications Trial *Diabetes Care.* 2007;30(3):707-712.

163. Genuth S, Alberti KG, Bennett P, et al; Expert Committee on the Diagnosis and Classification of Diabetes Mellitus. Follow-up report on the diagnosis of diabetes mellitus. *Diabetes Care.* 2003;26(11):3160-3167.

164. American Diabetes Association. 4. Lifestyle management: standards of medical care in diabetes—2018. *Diabetes Care.* 2018;41 (suppl 1):S38-S50.

165. Mayer-Davis EJ, Lawrence JM, Dabelea D, et al. SEARCH for Diabetes in Youth Study. Incidence trends of type 1 and type 2 diabetes among youths, 2002-2012. *N Engl J Med.* 2017;376(15):1419-1429.

166. Centers for Disease Control and Prevention. National Center for Chronic Disease Prevention and Health Promotion. Division of Diabetes Translation. *National Diabetes Statistics Report, 2017: Estimates of Diabetes and Its Burden in the United States.* www.cdc.gov/diabetes/pdfs/data/statistics/national-diabetes-statistics-report.pdf. Accessed June 24, 2019.

167. Knowler WC, Barrett-Connor E, Fowler SE, et al; Diabetes Prevention Program Research Group. Reduction in the incidence of type 2 diabetes with lifestyle intervention or metformin. *N Engl J Med.* 2002;346(6):393-403.

168. Aroda VR, Christophi CA, Edelstein SL, et al; Diabetes Prevention Program Research Group. The effect of lifestyle intervention and metformin on preventing or delaying diabetes among women with and without gestational diabetes: the Diabetes Prevention Program outcomes study 10-year follow-up. *J Clin Endocrinol Metab.* 2015;100(4):1646-1653.

169. Xiang AH, Peters RK, Kjos SL, et al. Effect of pioglitazone on pancreatic beta-cell function and diabetes risk in Hispanic women with prior gestational diabetes. *Diabetes.* 2006;55(2):517-522.

170. Espinoza SE, Wang CP, Tripathy D, et al. Pioglitazone is equally effective for diabetes prevention in older versus younger adults with impaired glucose tolerance. *Age (Dordr).* 2016;38(5-6):485-493.

171. Nathan DM. Diabetes: advances in diagnosis and treatment. *JAMA.* 2015;314(10):1052-1062.

172. Soriguer F, Morcillo S, Hernando V, et al. Type 2 diabetes mellitus and other cardiovascular risk factors are no more common during menopause: longitudinal study. *Menopause.* 2009;16(4):817-821.

173. Gartlehner G, Patel SV, Feltner C, et al. Hormone therapy for the primary prevention of chronic conditions in postmenopausal women: evidence report and systematic review for the US Preventive Services Task Force. *JAMA.* 2017;318(22):2234-2249.

174. Mechanick JI, Hurley DL, Garvey WT. Adiposity-based chronic disease as a new diagnostic term: the American Association of Clinical Endocrinologists and American College of Endocrinology position statement. *Endocr Pract.* 2017;23(3):372-378.

175. Rejeski WJ, Ip EH, Bertoni AG, et al; LookAHEAD Research Group. Lifestyle change and mobility in obese adults with type 2 diabetes. *N Engl J Med.* 2012;366(13):1209-1217.

176. Eckel RH, Jakicic JM, Ard JD, et al; American College of Cardiology/American Heart Association Task Force on Practice Guidelines. 2013 AHA/ACC guideline on lifestyle management to reduce cardiovascular risk: a report of the American College of Cardiology/American Heart Association Task Force on Practice Guidelines. *Circulation*. 2014;129(25 suppl 2):S76-S99.

177. MacLeod J, Franz MJ, Handu D, et al. Academy of Nutrition and Dietetics Nutrition practice guideline for type 1 and type 2 diabetes in adults: nutrition intervention evidence reviews and recommendations. *J Acad Nutr Diet*. 2017;117(10):1637-1658.

178. Howard BV, Aragaki AK, Tinker LA, et al. A low-fat dietary pattern and diabetes: a secondary analysis from the Women's Health Initiative Dietary Modification trial. *Diabetes Care*. 2018;41(4):680-687.

179. Manson JE, Greenland P, LaCroix AZ, et al. Walking compared with vigorous exercise for the prevention of cardiovascular events in women. *N Engl J Med*. 2002;347(10):716-725.

180. Agiostratidou G, Anhalt H, Ball D, et al. Standardizing clinically meaningful outcome measures beyond HbA1C for type 1 diabetes: a consensus report of the American Association of Clinical Endocrinologists, the American Association of Diabetes Educators, the American Diabetes Association, the Endocrine Society, JDRF International, the Leona M. and Harry B. Helmsley Charitable Trust, the Pediatric Endocrine Society, and the T1D Exchange. *Diabetes Care*. 2017;40(12):1622-1630.

181. Lane W, Bailey TS, Gerety G, et al; Group Information; Switch 1. Effect of insulin degludec vs insulin glargine U100 on hypoglycemia in patients with type 1 diabetes: the SWITCH 1 randomized clinical trial. *JAMA*. 2017;318(1):33-44.

182. Marso SP, McGuire DK, Zinman B, et al; DEVOTE Study Group. Efficacy and safety of degludec versus glargine in type 2 diabetes. *N Engl J Med*. 2017;377(8):723-732.

183. Peters AL, Ahmann AJ, Battelino T, et al. Diabetes technology-continuous subcutaneous insulin infusion therapy and continuous glucose monitoring in adults: an Endocrine Society clinical practice guideline. *J Clin Endocrinol Metab*. 2016;101(11):3922-3937.

184. Aleppo G, Laffel LM, Ahmann AJ, et al. Continuous glucose monitoring trend arrows in the management of adults with diabetes: a practical approach to using the Dexcom G5 CGM system. *J Endocr Soc*. 2017;12:1445-1460.

185. Scirica BM, Bhatt DL, Braunwald E, et al; SAVOR-TIMI 53 Steering Committee and Investigators. Saxagliptin and cardiovascular outcomes in patients with type 2 diabetes mellitus. *N Engl J Med*. 2013;369(14):1317-1326.

186. White WB, Cannon CP, Heller SR, et al; EXAMINE Investigators. Alogliptin after acute coronary syndrome in patients with type 2 diabetes. *N Engl J Med*. 2013;369(14):1327-1335.

187. Green JB, Bethel MA, Armstrong PW, et al; TECOS Study Group. Effect of sitagliptin on cardiovascular outcomes in type 2 diabetes. *N Engl J Med*. 2015;373(3):232-242.

188. Pfeffer MA, Claggett B, Diaz R, et al; ELIXA Investigators. Lixisenatide in patients with type 2 diabetes and acute coronary syndrome. *N Engl J Med*. 2015;373(23):2247-2257.

189. Gerstein HC, Colhoun HM, Dagenais GR, et al; REWIND Trial Investigators. Design and baseline characteristics of participants in the Researching cardiovascular Events with a Weekly INcretin in Diabetes (REWIND) trial on the cardiovascular effects of dulaglutide. *Diabetes Obes Metab*. 2018;20(1):42-49.

190. Marso SP, Bain SC, Consoli A, et al; SUSTAIN-6 Investigators. Semaglutide and cardiovascular outcomes in patients with type 2 diabetes. *N Engl J Med*. 2016;375(19):1834-1844.

191. Marso SP, Daniels GH, Brown-Frandsen K, et al; LEADER Steering Committee; LEADER Trial Investigators. Liraglutide and cardiovascular outcomes in type 2 diabetes. *N Eng J Med*. 2016;375(4):311-322.

192. Holman RR, Bethel MA, Mentz RJ, et al; EXSCEL Study Group. Effects of once-weekly exenatide on cardiovascular outcomes in type 2 diabetes. *N Engl J Med* 2017;377(13):1228-1239.

193. Zinman B, Wanner C, Lachin JM, et al; EMPA-REG OUTCOME Investigators. Empagliflozin, cardiovascular outcomes, and mortality in type 2 diabetes. *N Engl J Med*. 2015;373(22):2117-2128.

194. Neal B, Perkovic V, Mahaffey KW et al; CANVAS Program Collaborative Group. Canagliflozin and cardiovascular and renal events in type 2 diabetes. *N Engl J Med*. 2017;377(7):644-657.

195. American Diabetes Association. 8. Pharmacologic approaches to glycemic treatment: standards of medical care in diabetes—2018. *Diabetes Care*. 2018;41(suppl 1):S73-S85.

196. Garber AJ, Abrahamson MJ, Barzilay JI, et al. Consensus Statement by the American Association of Clinical Endocrinologists and American College of Endocrinology on the comprehensive type 2 diabetes management algorithm—2018 Executive Summary. *Endocr Pract*. 2018;23(2):207-238.

197. Lee AK, Warren B, Lee CJ, et al. The association of severe hypoglycemia with incident cardiovascular events and mortality in adults with type 2 diabetes. *Diabetes Care*. 2018;41(1):104-111.

198. Yu O, Azouly L, Yin H, Filion KB, Suissa S. Sulfonylureas as initial treatment for type 2 diabetes and the risk of severe hypoglycemia. *Am J Med*. 2018;131(3):317.e11-317.e22.

199. Kirkman MS, Briscoe VJ, Clark N, et al. Diabetes in older adults. *Diabetes Care*. 2012;35(12):2650-2664.

200. Sussman JB, Kerr EA, Saini SD, et al. Rates of deintensification of blood pressure and glycemic medication treatment based on levels of control and life expectancy in older patients with diabetes mellitus. *JAMA Intern Med*. 2015;175(12):1942-1949.

201. Nathan DM, Cleary PA, Backlund JY, et al; Diabetes Control and Complications Trial/Epidemiology of Diabetes Interventions and Complications (DCCT/EDIC) Study Research Group. Intensive diabetes treatment and cardiovascular disease in patients with type 1 diabetes. *N Engl J Med*. 2005;353(25):2643-2653.

202. Holman RR, Paul SK, Bethel MA, Matthews DR, Neil HA. 10-year follow-up of intensive glucose control in type 2 diabetes. *N Engl J Med*. 2008;359(15):1577-1589.

203. The Action to Control Cardiovascular Risk in Diabetes Study Group, Gerstein HC, Miller ME, et al. Effects of intensive glucose lowering in type 2 diabetes. *N Engl J Med*. 2008;358(24):2545-2559.

204. American Diabetes Association. 6. Glycemic targets: standards of medical care in diabetes—2018. *Diabetes Care*. 2018;41(suppl 1):S55-S64.

205. American Diabetes Association. 9. Cardiovascular disease and risk management: standards of medical care in diabetes—2018. *Diabetes Care*. 2018;41(suppl 1):S86-S104.

206. de Ferranti SD, de Boer IH, Fonseca V, et al. Type 1 diabetes mellitus and cardiovascular disease: a scientific statement from the American Heart Association and American Diabetes Association. *Circulation*. 2014;130(13):1110-1130.

9

Cancers Common in Midlife Women

Women have a one-in-three chance of developing cancer in their lifetimes.[1] Some cancers are unique to women—cervical, uterine, and ovarian—and other cancers have a unique natural history when diagnosed in women. In reality, squamous and basal cell skin cancers are the most commonly diagnosed cancers. However, because these cancers are not included in tumor registries, breast, lung, colorectal, and uterine cancers are listed as the most common cancers in women.

A woman's lifetime risk for developing cancer continues to increase primarily because of two factors: aging and obesity. Generally, cancer is a disease of the elderly. As the population continues to age, the incidence and prevalence of cancer increase.[2]

Obesity is a recognized risk for developing cancer, and 2015-2016 National Health and Nutrition Examination Survey data found that 39.8% of adult Americans are obese.[3] The highest incidence of obesity is in non-Hispanic black and Hispanic women, 54.8% and 50.6%, respectively. The incidence is only slightly lower in non-Hispanic white women at 38%.

Obesity plays a significant role in the increased risk for breast, uterine, ovarian, and colorectal cancers. Initially, it was thought that breast and uterine cancers were more common in women who are obese or overweight because of higher estrogen levels produced by fat. The mechanism is more complex and is likely to be attributed to metabolic changes such as metabolic syndrome and alterations in fatty acid metabolism.[4-6]

Because of an increased awareness of cancer symptoms and routine screening, many women are diagnosed with early stage cancers. This and improved therapies have resulted in improved cancer-specific outcomes and many more survivors of cancer.[7,8] Survivorship care often falls on the shoulders of primary care providers (PCPs) to ensure that lipid profiles have been checked, that bone health has been addressed, and that screening for other cancers is performed. A discussion and education about healthy lifestyle behaviors such as exercise, healthy diet, weight loss, and smoking cessation have the potential to decrease the incidence of cancers in women and improve the outcomes of those who have been diagnosed.

Breast Cancer

Breast cancer is the most common cancer in women in the United States and worldwide. After the Women's Health Initiative (WHI) reported an increased incidence of breast cancer in postmenopausal women treated with combined estrogen and progestin therapy (EPT),[9] use of hormone therapy (HT) declined, and the incidence of breast cancer also declined. In recent years, the incidence of breast cancer in the United States has increased slightly; however, over the past few decades, the risk of dying from breast cancer has steadily decreased.[10] It is likely that the improvement in survival is because of early detection and improved treatment. The increase in survivors makes it imperative that PCPs understand the unique health issues facing the more than 3.5 million survivors of breast cancer.

Risk factors

The risk for developing breast cancer may be categorized as nonmodifiable, modifiable, and treatment-associated (Table 1).[1,11-24] Nonmodifiable factors such as sex, age, menstrual life, and genetics are those that cannot be changed. Modifiable factors such as obesity and alcohol intake are those that can be changed. Treatment-related factors

Table 1. Risk Factors for Developing Breast Cancer

Nonmodifiable	
Sex	99.5% of breast cancers are diagnosed in women.
Age	The median age for breast cancer is 61 years. The increased incidence of breast cancer is largely attributed to the aging population.
Prolonged menstrual life	Early menarche (before age 11 years); late menopause (≥55 years).
Genetic predisposition	5-10% of breast cancers are diagnosed in women who have a genetic mutation that is associated with an increased risk for breast cancer. *BRCA 1/2* mutations are most common. Mutations in eight additional genes have also been associated with an increased risk for breast cancer: *PALB2, CHEK2, CDH1, PTEN, STK11, ATM, NMB, NF1.* Women with a strong family history should be referred for genetic counseling.
High breast density	The amount of glandular tissue relative to fatty tissue measured on a mammogram.
Modifiable	
Obesity	Obesity and weight gain increase the risk of breast cancer, and cancers that occur in women who are obese tend to have a more aggressive natural history.
Alcohol	The use of alcohol has been associated with increased risk.
Treatment-Associated	
Hormone therapy	The use of estrogen and progestin as hormone therapy is associated with an increased risk for breast cancer. Estrogen alone did not increase breast cancer incidence in the Women's Health Initiative. However, women on estrogen alone had undergone hysterectomy, and many had bilateral salpingo-oophorectomy, which may reduce breast cancer risk.
X-ray therapy to the thoracic region	Women who have received thoracic radiation therapy as treatment for lymphoma, especially before the age of 30 years, are at extremely high risk (55-fold increase) for development of breast cancer.

American Cancer Society[1]; Antoniou A, et al[11]; Antoniou AC, et al[12]; Antoniou AC, et al[13]; Chlebowski RT, et al[14]; Chlebowski RT, et al[15]; Dignam JJ, et al[16]; Eliassen A, et al[17]; Ewertz M, et al[18]; Hancock SL, et al[19]; Hill DA, et al[20]; Pharoah PD, et al[21]; White AJ, et al[22]; Yang XR, et al[23]; Zhang SM, et al.[24]

include HT and thoracic radiation therapy as treatment for lymphoma, especially before the age of 30 years.

Screening mammography

Screening mammography guidelines have been modified over the past decade, and different societies and organizations differ slightly in their recommendations (Table 2).[25-27] Women who are at high risk for breast cancer but choose not to undergo a risk-reduction strategy should be considered for additional imaging. In women with a known *BRCA1* or *BRCA2* mutation, the addition of annual magnetic resonance imaging (MRI) to mammography has been shown to identify small primary cancers, with no interval cancers (cancers that develop in between mammographic screenings).[28-30]

Presentation and workup

Despite the success of screening programs, most women diagnosed with breast cancer still present because a breast lump has been identified, either through self-examination or by a PCP. Most breast cancers (95%) are diagnosed with stage I to stage III disease, and the remaining 5% present with de novo metastatic disease. The initial workup includes a thorough physical examination, bilateral diagnostic mammography, and biopsy of suspicious lesions. In women who have dense or heterogeneous breast tissue, breast ultrasound or MTI also may be indicated. With a diagnosis of breast cancer, the woman should be referred for interdisciplinary care, starting with the breast surgeon.

Therapy

For women eligible for breast-conserving therapy, lumpectomy followed by radiation has been found to have an equivalent survival rate as mastectomy.[31,32] Postoperative systemic (adjuvant) therapy is administered according to tumor characteristics and risk of recurrence. In women with estrogen and/or progesterone receptor-positive, human epidermal growth factor receptor (HER)2-negative disease, and three or fewer positive lymph nodes, the need for chemotherapy is based on the tumor's Onco*type* Recurrence Score—a 21-gene assay that is prognostic and predictive of chemotherapy benefit.[33,34] Those with low recurrence scores (<25) derive no benefit from chemotherapy, whereas those with a score of 25 or greater clearly will benefit from chemotherapy.[34] The importance of tumor biology in determining prognosis and need for chemotherapy led the American Joint Committee on Cancer to include molecular assessment of hormone receptor(HR)-positive breast cancers by Onco*type*

Table 2. Breast Cancer Mammography Screening Guidelines

	ACS	NCCN	USPSTF
Age at first screen	45 y (average risk)	≥40 y (average risk)	Before age 50 y (based on individual risk)
Frequency	Age 45-54 y, annual Age >55 y, biannual	Annual	Age 50-74 y, biannual
Upper age	Life expectancy ≥10 y	Insufficient data	

Abbreviations: ACS, American Cancer Society; NCCN, National Comprehensive Cancer Network; USPSTF, US Preventive Services Task Force.
Oeffinger KC, et al[25]; NCCN Clinical Practice Guidelines in Oncology[26]; Siu AL, et al.[27]

Recurrence Score, Mammaprint, Prosigna, EndoPredict, or Breast Risk Index as a component in the new staging of postmenopause HR-positive breast cancers starting in January 2018.[35]

Women who have localized triple negative disease (estrogen receptor[ER]-negative, progesterone receptor [PR]-negative, and HER2-negative) and women with positive lymph nodes should receive anthracycline and taxane chemotherapy unless contraindicated.[36] The addition of HER2-directed therapy has altered the natural history of an aggressive subtype of breast cancer, HER2-positive. For women with HER2-positive cancers that are 2 cm or smaller with negative lymph nodes, weekly taxol for 12 weeks combined with trastuzumab for 1 year is associated with a 4-year overall survival of 95%.[37] For women with larger HER2-positive cancers and cancers with nodal metastases, chemotherapy with 1 year of trastuzumab (and possibly also pertuzumab) has been shown to increase overall survival compared with chemotherapy alone.[38,39]

For women presenting with larger tumors who desire breast conservation, and in women with locally advanced disease, initial treatment (neoadjuvant) with chemotherapy or endocrine therapy may downstage the tumor.[40-42] In HER2-positive cancers, trastuzumab and pertuzumab are administered in combination with chemotherapy.[43,44] The addition of 14 cycles of trastuzumab emtansine postoperatively has been shown to increase survival, especially in women with residual disease at surgery.[45] The order of systemic therapy (preoperative vs postoperative) has no effect on overall survival. As a result of tumor shrinkage from neoadjuvant chemotherapy, less breast tissue may be removed, and more

women become eligible for breast-conserving surgery. Neoadjuvant therapy also is associated with fewer surgical complications.[46]

All women with HR-positive disease should receive adjuvant endocrine therapy with tamoxifen for 10 years for women diagnosed when premenopausal and 5 years of an aromatase inhibitor (AI) for those diagnosed after menopause.[47,48] Ten years of adjuvant tamoxifen has been demonstrated to be superior to 5 years, although there is no proven advantage for more than 5 years of an AI.[49,50]

Survivorship care

Most breast cancers are diagnosed in women after menopause, but a significant number of premenopausal women who receive adjuvant chemotherapy will become permanently amenorrheic.[51,52] The management of symptoms and silent signs of menopause are critical to the quality and quantity of life and may be especially important in the follow-up care of younger women. The diagnosis and treatment of breast cancer becomes the central focus of healthcare in newly diagnosed women and in women who become nonadherent, with medications needed for other medical problems.[53] Women treated for early stage breast cancer are more likely to die of cardiovascular disease (CVD), and healthcare providers need to focus on health maintenance and prevention.[54]

Vasomotor symptoms

Hot flashes and night sweats are the most common symptoms experienced by survivors of breast cancer. These symptoms may be because of menopause or endocrine therapies such as tamoxifen and AIs.[55,56] For many women, the administration of gabapentin (escalating from 300 mg to 900 mg at night) is associated with improvement in sleep and vasomotor symptoms (VMS). Tamoxifen is a prodrug, which is bioactivated via cytochrome P450 2D6 (CYP2D6) to its active component, endoxifen. Selective serotonin reuptake inhibitors are often effective in minimizing VMS and improving sleep. For women on tamoxifen, it is preferred to use drugs that have minimal or no effect on CYP2D6, such as sertraline or the selective serotonin norepinephrine reuptake inhibitor, venlafaxine.[57]

Musculoskeletal pain

Muscle and joint pain may occur after menopause. However, a unique musculoskeletal syndrome has been reported in as many as half of women treated with an AI and is the cause of noncompliance in 20% because of the pain.[57-59] Women generally complain of joint pain in the hands and knees within 8 to 12 weeks of initiating an AI. The mechanism for this is unclear because acute-phase reactants are not elevated, anti-inflammatory medications are ineffective, and damage to the joints has not been documented. Magnetic resonance images of the hands have demonstrated tenosynovial fluid, which may explain why some women describe stiffness in the hands that is worse in the morning and dissipates with activity as the day progresses.[60] Although one trial suggested that vitamin D therapy improves symptoms, there is no consensus on how to best manage an adverse event (AE) that occurs in 30% to 50% of women on an AI. Carpal tunnel syndrome and trigger fingers also are increased with these agents.[61] When musculoskeletal pain is severe enough to compromise quality of life and risks noncompliance with medication, discontinuation of the AI and switching to tamoxifen is prudent.

Bone health

Empiric bone-directed therapy has been recommended as adjuvant treatment for women with postmenopause ER-positive and/or PR-positive breast cancer.[62] Attention to bone health and assessment of bone mineral density with dual-energy X-ray absorptiometry should be included in the follow-up of women with HR-negative breast cancer, especially those who are rendered postmenopausal as a result of adjuvant chemotherapy. With the new treatment guidelines, 4 mg intravenous zoledronic acid every month for 6 months or 1,600 mg clodronate per day for 2 to 3 years should be added to the adjuvant therapy of all postmenopausal women and premenopausal women who become postmenopausal as a result of chemotherapy.

Bone-directed therapy as adjuvant treatment

Studies have demonstrated that women who have T-scores less than −1.5 at initiation of an AI are at increased risk for developing osteoporosis over the subsequent 5 years and that the administration of a bisphosphonate (most often zoledronic acid 4 mg every 6 mo for 6 doses) is associated with an improvement in T-score.[63] A decrease in breast cancer recurrence has been seen in meta-analyses of adjuvant bone-directed therapies.[64] As a result, breast cancer treatment guidelines have recently been amended to include the use of bone-directed therapy in postmenopausal women with ER-positive and/or PR-positive breast cancers.[62]

Cardiovascular issues

Women with breast cancer are more likely to die of CVD than of breast cancer.[65] Early menopause secondary to chemotherapy and possible increases in cholesterol associated with the AIs require that patients have a lipid-profile assessment on an annual basis.[65,66]

Gynecologic follow-up

The estrogen agonist effects of tamoxifen are observed as endometrial thickening in excess of the 5 mm threshold used to determine the need for endometrial biopsy. Studies have looked at empiric follow-up with annual vaginal ultrasounds and/or endometrial biopsy, and neither of these strategies identified early uterine cancer.[67] The 2014 guidelines from the American College of Obstetrics and Gynecology recommend that a pretamoxifen ultrasound be considered and that follow-up care in low-risk women should be the same as women not taking tamoxifen.

Sexual functioning

Decreased libido and dyspareunia are common sequelae of natural aging and chemotherapy-induced menopause. Both tamoxifen and AIs adversely affect receptive intercourse.[68] Topical agents such as moisturizers, lubricants, or aqueous lidocaine may be helpful in treating dyspareunia.[69,70] Nonrandomized studies have failed to show an increased risk for breast cancer recurrence in women treated with oral or vaginal estrogens.[71,72] Nonetheless, the American College of Obstetricians and Gynecologists recommends that the decision to use vaginal estrogen be made jointly with a woman's oncologist and should be reserved for women with severe urogenital symptoms who have not responded to other measures.[73]

Weight management and exercise

Survivors of breast cancer who are obese and those who gain weight after treatment are more likely to develop disease recurrence, and stage-for-stage, women who are overweight have a worse prognosis compared with women of normal weight.[74] Adjuvant chemotherapy has been shown to cause weight gain as well as the metabolic syndrome.[75,76] Women should be counseled on the importance of healthy eating, maintaining a normal weight, and exercising at least 30 to 60 minutes, three to five times per week.

Further cancer screening

In the absence of disease recurrence, diagnostic mammography should be performed annually for 5 years after diagnosis of breast cancer. Thereafter, an annual screening mammogram may be considered adequate.

Women who are breast cancer survivors may be at increased risk of other primary cancers, including lung and colorectal cancer. Smokers have an increased risk of complications associated with breast irradiation, may have a higher risk of breast cancer recurrence, and are at increased risk for lung cancer. To screen for lung cancer, the US Preventive Services Task Force (USPSTF) recommends annual low-dose computerized tomography in persons aged 55 to 80 years with at least a 30-pack per-year history of smoking or who have quit smoking within the prior 15 years.[77]

The US preventive Services Task Force recommendations for colon cancer screening include a colonoscopy beginning at age 50 years and every 5 to 10 years until age 75 years.[78] For those women with a hereditary predisposition for cancer, an earlier age and more frequent colonoscopy may be appropriate.

Risk-reduction strategies

Genetic predisposition, family history, and lifetime risk for developing breast cancer based on models should be considered for risk-reduction interventions, and women at high risk for developing breast cancer should be considered for risk-reduction strategies.[26] Women with deleterious mutations of *BRCA1*, *BRCA2*, *PTEN*, and *p53* are at high risk. In the absence of a known mutation, high risk may be defined by a family history in which a single family member has two or more breast cancer primaries; two or more primaries on the same side of the family, one of whom is aged 50 years or younger; a family history of male breast cancer; a first- or second-degree relative aged 45 years or younger with breast cancer; a family history of ovarian, fallopian tube, or peritoneal cancers; and families with multiple primary cancers. Women who have received thoracic radiation and those who have been diagnosed with atypical ductal hyperplasia or lobular carcinoma in situ are at high risk for breast cancer.

The Gail model is a risk-prediction model that is of value in women with an "average risk" of breast cancer.[79] The model focuses on a person's risk for breast cancer, estimating both the 5-year and lifetime risk. For inclusion in chemoprevention trials, a 1.7% risk of developing breast cancer is used. The Gail model has been updated to include a more accurate risk assessment in African American women.[80]

Surgical risk-reduction strategies

Data from randomized, clinical trials (RCTs) are lacking, and support for prophylactic mastectomy is derived from retrospective studies. Women with deleterious mutations of *BRCA1* or *BRCA2* have a lifetime risk for developing breast cancer, as high as 72%, and bilateral risk-reducing breast surgery is associated with a significant decreased

incidence of breast cancer.[80] Women who are *BRCA1* or *BRCA2* mutation carriers are at risk for ovarian cancer. Bilateral salpingo-oophorectomy (BSO) has been shown to decrease the incidence of ovarian, fallopian tube, and peritoneal cancers by 80%, as well as a 50% reduction in breast cancer.[82-84]

Chemoprevention

Tamoxifen

Tamoxifen was the first agent proven to be an effective chemoprevention agent. In premenopausal and postmenopausal women aged 35 years and older with a Gail model risk of at least 1.7% of developing breast cancer in the next 5 years or a biopsy confirmation of lobular carcinoma in situ, 5 years of tamoxifen decreased the incidence of breast cancer by 48% compared with those receiving a placebo. For women with a history of atypical ductal hyperplasia, a 50% decrease was seen at 5 years, and a 65% decrease at 10 years.[85,86] (The modified Gail model no longer includes atypical ductal hyperplasia.) Although generally well tolerated, tamoxifen is associated with an increased risk for venous thromboembolism and uterine cancer in women aged 50 years and older. A retrospective assessment of a small subset of women with *BRCA1* or *BRCA2* mutations suggests a possible benefit.[87]

Raloxifene

Raloxifene, also a selective estrogen receptor modifier, has been tested as chemoprevention only in postmenopausal women with a Gail model risk of 1.7% over 5 years or a history of lobular carcinoma in situ.[88] Risk reduction with tamoxifen was superior to raloxifene, but the toxicity profile favored raloxifene. Whereas the incidence of VMS and thromboembolism is comparable for the two drugs, raloxifene has no deleterious effects on the uterus.

Aromatase inhibitors

The AIs anastrozole and exemestane have been studied only in postmenopausal women. Exemestane in women with a Gail model risk of 1.7% over 5 years or a history of lobular carcinoma in situ reduced the risk of breast cancer by 65%.[89] In high-risk women aged 40 to 70 years, anastrozole reduced the relative risk of breast cancer by 53%.[90]

Risks and benefits

The greatest benefit from chemoprevention is seen in younger women and should be reserved for women with a life expectancy of at least 10 years. The data for using chemoprevention is based on trials that enrolled predominantly white women, with risk defined by the Gail model and with no genetic predisposition. The benefits should not be extrapolated to all populations. Ultimately, the selection of a chemopreventive agent is based on menopause status, age, and comorbidities, balancing the potential benefits and possible long-term toxicities.

Endometrial Cancer

Endometrial cancer is the fourth most common cancer in women after breast, lung, and colorectal cancer and the most common cancer of the female reproductive organs. The American Cancer Society (ACS) estimates that 63,230 new cases of cancer of the body of the uterus (uterine body or corpus) will be diagnosed in 2018, and about 11,350 women will die from cancers of the uterine body.[91] Although endometrial cancer is the fourth leading cancer in women, it accounts only for 4% of cancer deaths.[92]

Endometrial cancer is uncommon in women aged younger than 45 years. Although endometrial cancer occurs more frequently in white women, mortality rates are higher in black women, 3.9 per 100,000 versus 7.1 per 100,000, respectively.[93] The etiology of the ethnic disparities is multifactorial and may relate to access to care.[94] The differences in outcomes in different ethnicities are still present in the 5-year disease-specific survival of endometrial cancer in white, Asian, and Hispanic women (85.9%, 87.2%, and 85.5%, respectively) compared with black women at 66.9%.[95] A recent simulation provides evidence that by improving early diagnosis and surgical rates, the outcome differences between white women and black women with endometrial cancer can be narrowed.[96]

Most uterine cancers arise from the endometrial glands, but 8% of uterine cancers are sarcomas.[97] Endometrial cancers are classified into type 1 and type 2 on the basis of their etiology, HR, and histologic grade (Table 3).[98-105]

Type 1 tumors consist of endometrioid tumors that are low grade and HR-positive.[106] They are common, comprising approximately 80% of endometrial cancers. The precursor of type 1 endometrial cancer is endometrial hyperplasia—15% to 50% of endometrial biopsy specimens interpreted as atypical endometrial hyperplasia are associated with an invasive endometrial cancer at the time of hysterectomy.[107] It is classified according to the severity of glandular crowding and the presence of nuclear atypia.[108] The World Health Organization categorizes hyperplasia as simple hyperplasia, complex

Table 3. Endometrial Cancer Types

Characteristic	Type 1	Type 2
Percentage of cases	80	20
Main histologic features	Endometrioid	Papillary serous or clear cell
Common tissue background	Endometrial hyperplasia	Atrophic endometrium
Usual precursor	Atypical complex hyperplasia	Endometrial intraepithelial carcinoma
Hyperestrogenism	+	–
Menopause status	Early	Late
Grade (at diagnosis)	Usually low	Usually high
Confined to uterus	>70% of cases	<40% of cases
Extramural spread	<25% of cases	>60% of cases
5-year survival rate	>85%	<50%

Bokhman JV[98]; Creasman WT, et al[99]; Levine RL, et al[100]; Emons G, et al[101]; Clement PB, et al[102]; Amant F, et al[103]; Hamilton CA, et al[104]; Leslie WD, et al.[105]

hyperplasia, simple atypical hyperplasia, or complex atypical hyperplasia.[109] A study in women with non-atypical hyperplasia showed only moderate increase in risk of endometrial cancer, from 1.2% to 4.6% over 19 years. In contrast, in women with atypical endometrial hyperplasia, the risk of endometrial cancer increased from 8.2% to 27.5% over 19 years.

Type 2 cancers are nonendometriod, HR-negative, aggressive malignancies that arise in atrophic endometrium and spread intraperitoneally, similar to ovarian epithelial tumors (Table 4).[110] Women with type 2 cancers are more likely to be older at diagnosis, of non-white ethnicity, and have a history of additional primary tumors. They are less likely to be obese and have a significantly worse prognosis compared with type 1.[111]

Risk factors and pathophysiology

Epidemiologic and experimental studies have identified factors associated with endometrial cancer (Table 5).[112] These factors can prospectively identify some women at risk of developing type 1 endometrial cancer. Type 2 endometrial cancer often develops in normoestrogenic women who are not obese and who may have a family history of endometrial cancer. Although some risk factors for type 1 and type 2 endometrial cancer may overlap, this

Table 4. Routes of Type 2 Endometrial Cancer Metastases

- Contiguous extension (associated with grade 3 disease and lymphovascular invasion)
- Hematogenous dissemination (associated with myometrial invasion)
- Lymphatic embolization (associated with cervical and lymph node invasion)
- Exfoliation with intraperitoneal spread (observed in advanced stages of the disease)

Mariani A, et al.[110]

classification is helpful in understanding the pathogenesis of the disease[113] but does not contribute to the staging or treatment of endometrial cancer. Increasingly mutational profiles are being used to distinguish more aggressive cancers and to aide in identifying women who may have a genetic predisposition for uterine cancer, such as in Lynch syndrome. The goal is to identify reproducible molecular profiles that will further characterize tumor aggression and will be used to individualize treatment.[106]

Hyperestrogenic endometrial milieu

Type 1 endometrial cancer is associated with exposure to estrogen. Mitogenic stimuli in the endometrium are associated with ER-α.[114] Estrogen stimulates endometrial cell proliferation, inhibits apoptosis, and promotes angiogenesis.[115] Endometrial hyperestrogenic milieu and excessive activation of the ER-α pathway have been associated with a number of origins and conditions (Table 6).[116-126]

Type 2 endometrial cancers are not affected by the ER pathways and are unrelated to hyperestrogenism.

Estrogen-like effects

Estrogen-like effects bypass the ER mechanism. The effect of hyperinsulinemia and type 2 diabetes mellitus (DM), for example, is mediated in part by obesity; the mechanism involves activation of signaling cascades downstream of the ER (eg, the insulin-like growth factor).[127] Another example is aberrant activity of intracellular pathways (eg, tumor protein 53, human epidermal growth factor receptor 2, and others).[128-130]

Defective control of estrogen endometrial effects

The endometrial effects of estrogen are physiologically controlled by progesterone and by the action of proapoptotic pathways. Attenuated control of estrogen endometrial effects can be associated with endometrial cancer by a history of low progestinic activity (nulliparity, anovulatory cycles, polycystic ovary syndrome, infertility)[131] and defective activity of proapoptotic pathways such as the $P2X_7$ mechanism and mitochondrial DNA polymorphism.[132,133]

Obesity

In the United States and other developed countries, obesity has become an epidemic that can pose an increasing endometrial cancer risk for women. Obesity increases the risk of endometrial cancer by a number of mechanisms. In premenopausal women, obesity causes insulin resistance, ovarian androgen excess, anovulation, and chronic progesterone deficiency.[103] Obesity is associated with excess white adipose tissue, which can metabolize and store steroid hormones.[134] White adipose tissue is involved in the elaboration of vascular endothelial cell growth factor, interlukin-6, and tumor necrosis factor-α, all of which have been implicated in "crosstalking" with

Table 5. Endometrial Cancer Risk Factors

- Age (>50 y)
- Hyperestrogenic endometrial milieu
  - History of hyperestrogenism (early menarche, nulliparity, unovulatory cycles, infertility, late menopause)
  - Unopposed estrogen use
  - Long-term SERM use
  - Defective estrogen metabolization
- Polymorphic variations in the estrogen receptor-α-1 gene
- Estrogen-like effect
  - Hyperinsulinemia and activation of insulin-growth-factor-1 pathways
  - Aberrant activation of intracellular pathways
- Defective control of estrogen endometrial effects
  - History of hypoprogesteronism (nulliparity, unovulatory cycles, PCOS)
  - Defective activity of proapoptotic pathways
- Obesity and high caloric intake
- Physical inactivity and sedentary lifestyle
- Diabetes mellitus
- Genetic factors and familial traits
  - Hereditary nonpolyposis colorectal cancer syndrome (Lynch II)
  - Familial predisposition for endometrial cancer
  - Familial breast cancer or endometrial cancer

Abbreviations: PCOS, polycystic ovary syndrome; SERM, selective estrogen receptor modulator.
Morice P, et al.[112]

Table 6. Conditions Leading to Endometrial Hyperestrogenic Milieu and Excessive Activation of the Estrogen Receptor-α Pathway

- A history of hyperestrogenism before menopause (early menarche, nulliparity, anovulation, infertility, late menopause).

- Unopposed exogenous estrogen use after menopause, regardless of the route of administration, which can result in endometrial hyperplasia, atypical hyperplasia, or eventually type 1 endometrial cancer. The effect is dose and duration dependent. When used for 5 or more years, the risk of endometrial cancer is increased by more than 6-fold, and the increased risk can persist for several years after discontinuing estrogen. The risk of endometrial cancer is lower in women in whom estrogen treatment is opposed by the concurrent use of a progestin and in women with decreased estrogen levels.

- Use of estrogen agonists/antagonists. In the uterus, raloxifene and tamoxifen impart estrogenic effects that involve stimulation of estrogen receptor-α. Tamoxifen is associated with the development of endometrial polyps, endometrial hyperplasia, and endometrial cancer. Raloxifene has only mild uterine proestrogenic effects, and in postmenopausal women, its use is associated with a lower risk of type 1 endometrial cancer compared with tamoxifen or estrogen users.

- In situ production of estrogen.

- Polymorphic variations in the estrogen receptor-α-1 gene, which are associated with endometrial cancer risk.

Mishra GD, et al[116]; Setiawan VW, et al[117]; Pocobelli G, et al[118]; Phipps AI, et al[119]; Wiederpass E, et al[120]; Hill DA, et al[121]; Shang Y, et al[122]; Polin SA, et al[123]; DeMichele A, et al[124]; Bulun SE, et al[125]; Wedrén S, et al.[126]

endometrial cancer and other gynecologic cancers. Adipose tissue is a primary source of extragonadal estrogens via aromatase-induced conversion of androgens. In postmenopausal women, peripheral conversion of androgens to estrogens is enhanced in peripheral fat stores, leading to increased blood concentrations of estrogens and an increased risk of endometrial cancer.[135]

A body mass index (BMI) greater than 25 kg/m^2 doubles a woman's risk of endometrial cancer; a BMI above 30 kg/m^2 triples the risk.[136,137] Two studies, one a review of the Swedish obesity database and the other a systematic review, indicate that bariatric surgery reduces the incidence of endometrial cancer.[138,139]

Diabetes mellitus

Diabetes mellitus (DM) increases the risk of endometrial cancer via factors related to hyperinsulinemia and obesity.[140,141] Mechanisms related to hyperinsulinemia involve, in part, an increase in free estrogen levels via decreased sex hormone-binding globulin, effects on the insulin-growth factor system, and increased levels of insulin-growth factor-1 and of insulin-growth factor-binding protein-1.[120,141,142]

Physical inactivity and sedentary lifestyle

A sedentary lifestyle has been correlated with increased endometrial cancer risk.[143] In contrast, studies have found an inverse, independent association between physical activity and the risk for endometrial cancer after adjusting for BMI and other risk factors.[144]

Genetic factors and familial traits

As reported in a population-based study, a history of endometrial cancer in a first-degree relative increases its risk by 2-fold after adjusting for age, obesity, and number of relatives.[145] Several genetic mutations have been found to be associated with endometrial cancer, and approximately 10% of cases of endometrial cancer have a familial-hereditary basis, including Lynch syndrome and Cowden syndrome.[146]

Hereditary nonpolyposis colorectal cancer, also known as Lynch syndrome, is an inherited disorder characterized by a defect in mismatch repair genes. It has a high penetrance (80-85%) and an early age of onset for a number of neoplasms (colorectal, endometrial, gastric, ureteral, ovarian, skin cancers).[147] Four genes are associated with Lynch syndrome: *MLH1*, *MSH2*, *MSH6*, and *PMS2*. Although generally considered a risk for colorectal cancer, women with *hMLH1* and *hMSH2* mutations have a 40% to 60% risk for endometrial cancer.[148,149] Loss of function of the *PTEN* gene in Cowden syndrome confers a lifetime risk of endometrial cancer as high as 28%.[150] Prophylactic hysterectomy may be considered for these women after childbearing.[145]

Alcohol consumption

A prospective-questionnaire, multiethnic cohort study on the effect of alcohol intake on endometrial cancer risk in postmenopausal women showed that alcohol consumption of two drinks per day was associated with a relative risk of 2.01, but there was no increased risk associated with fewer drinks per day than that.[151]

Cigarette smoking

The risks for endometrial hyperplasia with atypia and of endometrial cancer appear to be lower in cigarette smokers, possibly through the antiestrogenic effects of nicotine on estrogen production and metabolism.[152]

Antioxidants

No association was found in the Nurses' Health Study between endometrial cancer risk (or reduced risk) and the intake of vitamins A, C, or E or carotenoids from foods or supplements.[153]

Diagnosis and staging

Diagnosis usually results from evaluation of a woman's report of abnormal uterine bleeding (AUB). Although 90% of women diagnosed with uterine cancer present with AUB, postmenopausal women who present with AUB are diagnosed with endometrial cancer in only 5%.[154] Other causes of endometrial bleeding include endometrial hyperplasia, endometrial polyps, or other pathology of the endometrium in 20% of these women. However, in about 50% to 70% of these women, no organic cause of bleeding is found, and the postmenopausal AUB is often attributed to endometrial or vaginal atrophy. Nevertheless, any postmenopausal bleeding warrants an initial evaluation for endometrial cancer. (See also "Abnormal Uterine Bleeding" in Chapter 5.)

Although dilation and curettage of the uterus was standard evaluation in the past, less-invasive methods (eg, blind endometrial biopsy) can be used initially in an office setup without anesthesia. This is only a stopping point if it is positive for cancer or atypical hyperplasia. When pathology occupies less than 50% of the uterine surface and blind biopsy is not sensitive enough, even in cases of known carcinoma, alternative approaches to evaluate AUB, such as office hysteroscopy or transvaginal sonography and saline infusion sonohysterography, are indicated.

In 2009, the Féderation Internationale de Gynécologie et d'Obstétrique (FIGO) published a revised staging system for endometrial cancer based on surgical findings that better predicts a women's stage-dependent prognosis (Table 7).[155] Exclusive endometrial glandular involvement is considered stage I regardless of tumor grade because there were no significant differences in 5-year survival rates in these cases. Pelvic and para-aortic lymph node involvement has been separated because the involvement of para-aortic lymph nodes carries a worse prognosis. Positive cytology has been excluded as a factor for defining the new FIGO surgical staging, but it should be noted separately.

A key point of the revised FIGO staging system is that every woman with endometrial cancer should undergo surgery as part of management staging and planning.

Table 7. 2009 FIGO Staging System for Endometrial Cancer

IA	Tumor confined to the uterus; <50% myometrial invasion
IB	Tumor confined to the uterus; ≥50% myometrial invasion
II	Cervical stromal invasion but not beyond uterus
IIIA	Tumor invades serosa or adnexa
IIIB	Vaginal and/or parametrial involvement
IIIC1	Tumor invades serosa or adnexa
IIIC2	Para-aortic involvement
IVA	Tumor invasion bladder and/or bowel mucosa
IVB	Distant metastases including abdominal metastases and/or inguinal lymph nodes

Abbreviation: FIGO, Féderation Internationale de Gynécologie et d'Obstétrique. Creasman W, et al.[155]

Treatment of precursor lesions

The use of office-based diagnostic techniques results in earlier diagnosis of endometrial hyperplasia. Hyperplasia without atypia, either simple or complex, has a low likelihood (<5%) of progressing to carcinoma; however, women with increased risk factors for developing endometrial cancer should be treated with a progestin (eg, medroxyprogesterone acetate [MPA] or megestrol acetate), administered either in a cyclic or in a continuous fashion.[156,157]

Treatment with a progestin-releasing intrauterine device has a higher regression rate and a lower relapse rate than oral progestogen therapy.[158] Fertility-sparing treatments using progestin with or without a progestin-releasing intrauterine device have similar outcomes. The progestin-releasing intrauterine device alone was associated with a poorer obstetric outcome in the women who became pregnant compared with women using both progestin plus a progestin-releasing intrauterine device.[159]

Perimenopausal women with oligo-ovulatory or anovulatory cycles can be prescribed oral contraceptives (OCs) if there is no contraindication. In women at high risk for developing endometrial cancer, follow-up endometrial evaluation is recommended every 3 to 6 months until regression to normal endometrium occurs.[160] If abnormal vaginal bleeding resumes, endometrial evaluation should be performed more often. Postmenopausal women at risk for developing endometrial cancer who have hyperplasia without atypia may be considered for hysterectomy.

Hysterectomy and bilateral adnexal removal is the recommended treatment for women with atypical hyperplasia because atypical hyperplasia is the immediate precursor to endometrial cancer. Women with atypical hyperplasia have an estimated 30% risk of developing invasive carcinoma, and about one-third of women with a histologic finding of atypical hyperplasia in their dilation and curettage specimen already have invasive carcinoma in their hysterectomy specimen.[109,161]

Conservative treatment with high-dosed progestin therapy (PT) may be implemented in compliant younger women seeking to preserve fertility or in poor surgical candidates, but it requires a meticulous follow-up. Conservative treatment in such cases carries a 30% chance of recurrence, and those women should be carefully followed and advised to undergo surgical treatment after their last pregnancy.[162] Atypical hyperplasia can regress after treatment with progestogens in 60% to 95% of women, but close follow-up is indicated.[156,163] On the basis of a meta-analysis of 28 studies, a 71% complete response of atypical hyperplasia and stage I endometrial cancer has been found.[159] Pregnancy rates after the levonorgestrel-releasing intrauterine device (IUD), PT, and levonorgestrel-releasing IUD plus progestin were 18%, 34%, and 40%, respectively, with an approximately 50% take-home baby rate.

Treatment of invasive endometrial cancer

Standard therapy for endometrial cancer is surgery, including hysterectomy and removal of adnexal structures, as well as surgical staging, including pelvic and para-aortic lymph node sampling in women considered at risk for extrauterine disease.[103] The surgical findings will provide disease staging and prognosis and serve as the guide for further lymph node dissection and adjuvant therapy. Most endometrial cancers are diagnosed at an early stage (I-II) and have an excellent 5-year survival with surgery.

Routine pelvic and para-aortic lymphadenectomy as part of the surgical treatment of endometrial cancer remains controversial. Proponents suggest that pelvic and para-aortic lymph node dissection could be used as a diagnostic tool to determine the need for and extent of postoperative treatment, as a staging tool to define the extent of disease spread, and as a therapeutic modality.[164-167] Data tend to support use of lymphadenectomy

to prolong survival in advanced-stage endometrial carcinoma and in poorly differentiated stage I carcinoma.[168,169]

Postoperative adjuvant treatment options depend on surgical staging and pelvic and para-aortic lymph node assessment. Recurrences usually occur in women with high-grade tumors or with deep myometrial invasion and usually involve the vaginal apex.[170] Vaginal brachytherapy and/or external pelvic radiotherapy may be used postoperatively in such women.[103] External pelvic radiotherapy improves local control of the disease, but it does not substantially increase survival.[171] The Post Operative Radiation Therapy in Endometrial Carcinoma-2A RCT of adjuvant external teletherapy versus vaginal brachytherapy showed no significant differences with respect to vaginal recurrence rates, the occurrence of distant metastases, disease-free survival, or overall survival.[172] However, women who had received only vaginal brachytherapy had significantly fewer AEs and reported a better quality of life.[173]

In the adjuvant setting of stage III disease, adjuvant chemotherapy may improve cancer-specific survival. In women with recurrent or metastatic disease, chemotherapy is used for palliation. The most active chemotherapy agents include platinum agents, taxanes, and anthracyclines, which produce response rates of 20% to 35%. In select patients, HT with progestins can produce 20% response rates.[174]

Endometrial cancer and hormone therapy

Bilateral salpingo-oophorectomy in young women results in early menopause and its associated long-term health problems such as bone fractures from osteoporosis and cardiovascular complications. Estrogen therapy (ET) has generally been avoided because of concern of cancer recurrence. Although one study reported a low risk of cancer recurrence with ET, confirmatory data from an RCT are lacking.[175,176]

Prescribing either ET or EPT for women after endometrial cancer remains controversial. In the absence of data from well-designed studies, the decision to recommend HT for women after endometrial cancer should be based on prognostic indicators, including depth of invasion, degree of differentiation, and cell type. Moreover, careful counseling regarding perceived benefits and risks should be conducted to assist each woman in making an informed decision. The need for adding a progestin is undetermined, although progestogen supplementation has not been found to affect the recurrence rate.[177] One review indicates that data are currently lacking on use of hormones for menopause symptoms in women with hormone-dependent cancers.[178] Early stage disease without evidence of hormone dependency appears to be relatively safe for use of HT.

Preventive measures

The data do not support screening for uterine cancer in the absence of symptoms. Women should undergo a gynecologic exam according to current screening guidelines. Lifestyle modifications (eg, diet control, structured physical exercise) have been shown to reduce the risks of a number of medical conditions, including endometrial cancer, DM, and hypertension, which may prolong life.

Preventive considerations

Perimenopause can be a time of relative progesterone deficiency. Anovulatory cycles and intermittently high estrogen levels may lead to an estrogen-dominant hormone milieu. Use of a menstrual calendar may facilitate identification of this imbalance, so that measures can be taken to restore a balance of progestogen, continuous progestogen, low-dose hormonal contraception, or a progestogen-containing intrauterine system, depending on the needs and preferences of the woman.

After menopause, use of ET alone should be reserved for women who have undergone hysterectomy. If ET is used by a woman with a uterus despite this recommendation, women should undergo an endometrial evaluation at baseline and periodically thereafter. Endometrial evaluation should be performed after any episode of AUB; reevaluation is necessary when AUB is persistent.

Women with a uterus using EPT after menopause should undergo endometrial evaluation if AUB persists for more than 6 months after beginning therapy or sooner if there are other risk factors such as obesity, DM, or family history of endometrial cancer. The use of progestin reduces the risks of endometrial hyperplasia and endometrial cancer induced by estrogen therapy to the level found in women not taking hormones. In the WHI, postmenopausal women taking oral conjugated estrogens (CE) 0.625 mg per day plus MPA 2.5 mg per day did not experience a significant increase in endometrial cancer, and no appreciable differences were found in the distribution of tumor histology, stage, or grade compared with women assigned to placebo.[179] However, women taking EPT required significantly more endometrial biopsies for AUB than women taking placebo.

When an oral progestogen used in a cyclic regimen combined with a standard estrogen dose (eg, CE 0.625 mg,

1 mg oral estradiol, or 0.05 mg patch), the minimum effective dose for endometrial protection is 5 mg per day (or equivalent) for 12 to 14 days each month. With oral micronized progesterone, the dose is 200 mg per day for 12 to 14 days each month. Progestin-containing intrauterine devices or vaginal gels offer another possibility for endometrial protection, but long-term efficacy data are lacking regarding their protection against endometrial cancer, and they are not FDA approved for this purpose. Continuous-combined EPT dose schedules, in which a smaller amount of progestin is taken daily along with estrogen, usually result in amenorrhea over time. However, some women (particularly those who are recently postmenopausal) may have uterine spotting and bleeding during the first year or so of this regimen. With continuous-combined EPT, the minimum effective dose of oral progestogen for endometrial protection against standard doses of estrogen is 2.5 mg per day of MPA (or equivalent) or 100 mg per day of oral micronized progesterone. The continuous-combined regimen is the most popular regimen in the United States.

A way to reduce HT-induced uterine bleeding includes dosing progestogen less frequently, but these dosing regimens are not recommended and may require uterine evaluation periodically to monitor for endometrial proliferation changes. Women using these regimens should be encouraged to report any AUB.

Cervical Cancer

Cervical cancer is diagnosed in more than 13,000 US women per year and results in more than 4,000 deaths.[1] Relatively uncommon in developed nations, cervical cancer represents a major global health threat as the fourth most common cancer in women worldwide, with 528,000 new cases and 266,000 deaths annually.[180] Of these, more than 84% are diagnosed in developing nations.

Squamous cell carcinoma is the predominant subtype (80% of cases); adenocarcinoma makes up less than 20%, with histologic subtypes such as clear cell and small cell carcinoma, lymphoma, or sarcoma encountered rarely.[181-183] Incidence of adenocarcinoma has increased somewhat, possibly because cervical cytology screening is less effective than in squamous cell carcinoma.

Causes

Invasive cervical cancer develops in the setting of persistent human papillomavirus (HPV) infection of the genital mucosa after contracting the virus through sexual activity.

Human papillomavirus infection is highly prevalent in sexually active women, and although most HPV infections go away by themselves within 1 to 2 years, about 10% persist and can lead to invasive cervical cancer.[184] Four steps are required for the development of invasive cervical cancer: oncogenic HPV infection of cervical epithelium at the transition zone; persistent HPV infection; clonal progression of precancerous cells to high-grade dysplasia; and development of frank carcinoma with invasion of the epithelial basement membrane.[185] The HPV infection alone is insufficient for the development of invasive cancer.

The latency between HPV infection and development of invasive cancer is about 15 years.[186] Duration of active HPV infection is associated with progression of cervical dysplasia, with one report demonstrating high-grade dysplasia developing a median of 26 months from first diagnosis of cervical HPV infection.[187]

Additional risk factors supporting the development of cervical cancer include smoking, likely through accelerated progression of dysplasia to invasive squamous cell carcinoma; use of OCs; longer duration of OC use; early age at first sexual intercourse; larger number of sexual partners; high-risk sexual partners; and a history of sexually transmitted infections.[188] Women exposed in utero to diethylstilbestrol are at lifelong increased risk for both cervical and vaginal clear cell carcinoma.[189] Although not well defined to date, genetic factors influence risk for invasive cervical cancer, and there is an increased risk of cervical cancer within families.[190] Inherited gene polymorphisms regulate immunity, susceptibility of HPV infection, cytokine production, angiogenesis, and tumor-suppressor pathways.[191] Women with chronic immune suppression, such as those with HIV, solid-organ transplant recipients, or those requiring immunosuppressive therapy for chronic disease, have decreased capacity of viral clearance and accelerated progression from precancerous lesions to invasive cancer.[192,193] Women who are chronically immunocompromised have a higher risk of cervical cancer, likely because of enhanced susceptibility to sexual transmission of viruses and accelerated transition from dysplasia to invasive carcinoma.[194]

Screening

The Papanicolaou (Pap) test was developed in the 1960s to detect the cervical cytologic abnormalities associated with preinvasive findings such as dysplasia as well as frank cervical cancer. Removal of preinvasive lesions prevents their progression to more invasive pathology and predicts those at future risk. A diagnosis of moderate to severe cervical dysplasia, cervical intraepithelial neoplasia (CIN) 2

or 3, or adenocarcinoma in situ requires complete excision of affected cervical mucosa to optimally reduce recurrence.[195] The Pap test is likely responsible for declining mortality because of cervical cancer in developed nations such as the United States, but sadly, Pap screening is not widely available in developing nations.

Consensus guidelines recommend that women aged 21 to 29 years deemed at standard risk for cervical cancer undergo cervical cytology screening every 3 years, with reflex HPV testing of residual liquid if cytologic abnormalities, such as atypical cells of undetermined significance or dysplasia, are detected.[196] Women aged 30 to 65 years are recommended to undergo cotesting with cervical cytology and high-risk HPV screening every 5 years, or if cotesting is unavailable, cervical cytology every 3 years. Women aged older than 65 years are advised to discontinue testing if they had negative screening on three consecutive tests or two negative cotesting results in the prior 10 years.[197] Women at high risk, such as those with HIV infection, history of diethylstilbestrol exposure, prior history of cervical dysplasia or cancer, or chronic immunosuppression, should undergo annual cervical cytology with reflex HPV screening or cotesting every 3 years.

Presentation and diagnosis

Early symptoms of cervical cancer may include a watery vaginal discharge, intermittent vaginal spotting, or postcoital bleeding. However, early cervical cancer is frequently asymptomatic.

Cervical cytology or Pap tests and cervical biopsies are the primary means for diagnosis and secondary prevention of invasive cervical cancer by identifying cervical dysplasia that may be treated before progression to invasive cervical cancer. Cervical cytology may be less accurate in diagnosing adenocarcinoma because this affects the regions of the cervix that are less superficial and harder to sample, such as the endocervical canal. Cervical cone biopsy is undertaken if cervical biopsy is insufficient to exclude invasion and requires the en bloc removal of the ectocervix and the endocervical canal with cold knife or loop electrosurgical excision procedure.

Staging

Staging of cervical cancer is primarily clinical and requires assessment of primary tumor size and involvement of paracervical tissues. The FIGO clinical staging system continues in wide use because it ensures an unbiased comparison of outcomes between surgical and nonsurgical treatment approaches.[198] However, additional clinical variables, specifically lymph node involvement and lymphovascular space invasion, affect prognosis and treatment decisions.

Cervical cancer spreads by direct extension to the uterine corpus, vagina, parametria, bladder, or rectum. Lymphatic spread to obturator, pelvic, sidewall, and para-aortic lymph nodes increases with increasing depth of invasion of the primary tumor. Hematogenous spread is most common to lungs, liver, and bone. However, additional clinical variables, specifically lymph node involvement and lymphovascular space invasion, affect prognosis and treatment decisions.

Treatment

Because cervical cancer is almost universally associated with HPV infection (99.7% of cancers),[199] vaccination against HPV in presexual females is anticipated to dramatically decrease the incidence of invasive cervical cancer as well as cervical cancer mortality when there is worldwide implementation of vaccines. Treatment aims to control local disease and generally involves a combination of surgery, radiation therapy, and chemotherapy.[200] After a cervical cancer diagnosis, the progression-free survival is highly correlative with overall survival, consistent with a low rate of salvage in the event of recurrent or metastatic disease.

Women with early stage disease (<2 cm primary tumor) may be eligible for fertility-sparing resection.[201] Radical trachelectomy resects the cervix and vaginal margins with lymph node dissection while the main body of the uterus remains intact. Studies have shown successful pregnancy in more than 50% of women after this procedure; however, miscarriage and preterm labor is common.

The preferred curative surgical approach for women with early stage disease (stage IA_2-IIA_1) is the radical hysterectomy, which includes wide paracervical margins and bilateral pelvic lymph node dissection.[202] Surgical cure in early stage disease exceeds 80%.[203] Evolving technical expertise has made laparoscopic and robotic surgical approaches feasible, and studies have shown comparable outcomes to open abdominal procedures.[204,205] Women with high-risk features after resection, including at least two of these: lymphovascular space invasion, tumor 4 cm or more, or invasion of more than one-third of the cervical stroma, benefit from the addition of external-beam radiotherapy.[206] The addition of external-beam radiotherapy improves disease-free survival compared with no adjuvant therapy, and adjuvant chemoradiotherapy is associated with improved overall survival.[207] The combination of radical surgery

and radiation therapy is associated with a high rate of toxic effects, so clinical assessment of risk at time of diagnosis is essential to inform treatment.

In the United States, definitive chemoradiation is preferred for women with bulky, local disease (≥IB_2 stage tumors), on the basis of the results of 19 RCTs of more than 4,500 patients.[208] These trials showed that cisplatin-based chemotherapy concurrent with external-beam radiotherapy to the whole pelvis leads to a 30% to 50% decreased risk of death compared with radiation therapy alone. The best-studied chemotherapy regimens are weekly cisplatin 40 mg/m^2 or cisplatin and fluorouracil by continuous infusion (4 g/m^2 over 96 h) on days 1 and 29 of radiation therapy, although weekly cisplatin combined with 6 weeks of external-beam radiotherapy is the standard approach in the United States.[209]

Brachytherapy, or the placement of radioactivity close to the tumor in the vagina, an adjuvant radiation, follows the external-beam radiotherapy and permits maximal dosing of radiation to tumor tissue.[210,211] The radiation therapy course must be completed within 7 to 8 weeks in order to optimize outcomes.

For recurrent or persistent cancers involving the central pelvis without distant metastasis, a percentage of women may be cured through surgical pelvic exenteration (removal of the urinary bladder, urethra, rectum, and anus).[212] However, in general, metastatic cervical cancer or distant spread beyond periaortic lymph nodes or to solid organs is incurable, and treatment aims at prolonging life and palliating symptoms. Standard therapy in this setting includes cisplatin chemotherapy and is associated with a 20% to 30% response rate. For women naive to cisplatin, there is improved disease-free and overall survival with doublet therapy, generally the combination of cisplatin and paclitaxel.[213,214] Newer, targeted agents offer promise for additional benefits and include bevacizumab[213] and immune checkpoint inhibitors.[215]

Vaccination

There are approximately 40 HPV serotypes capable of infecting genital mucosa, and of these, 15 are known to be oncogenic. Of these, subtypes 16 and 18 are found in more than 70% of all cervical cancers.[216,217] Immunization against HPV by the FDA-approved quadrivalent vaccine Gardasil prevents infection by HPV associated with invasive cancer through antibody-mediated immunity.[218] This immunity is anticipated to prevent HPV-associated cancers, including squamous and adenocarcinoma of the cervix. Encouraging reports correlate increased vaccination rates with decreased incidence of high-grade cervical dysplasia.[219]

The Advisory Committee on Immunization Practices recommends vaccinating all children at 11 or 12 years old, as well as young women through age 26, with the nonavalent HPV vaccine.[220] This strategy is predicted to reduce cervical cancer incidence by 73% and mortality by 49%.[221]

Vaccination demonstrates a reduced risk of CIN; however, the larger questions regarding the effectiveness of vaccination in reducing the risk of invasive cervical cancer and its attendant mortality, the duration of immunity after vaccination, and the worldwide applicability of the vaccination approach remain unanswered. Certainly poised to dramatically improve cervical cancer incidence and survival in the United States, if vaccination were universally applied, the worldwide benefit in lives saved would be remarkable.

Ovarian Cancer

Epithelial ovarian cancer (EOC) is the leading cause of death from gynecologic cancer in the United States and the fifth most common cause of cancer mortality in women. In 2018, it is estimated that 22,240 new diagnoses and 14,070 deaths from this neoplasm will occur in the United States.[222] Less than 25% of cases are diagnosed in the early stages. The 5-year survival rate for all stages is 47% but drops to less than 30% for patients with distant metastases.[223] The median age at the time of diagnosis is 63 years, and more than 70% of patients present with advanced disease.

Classification

The traditional classification of EOC was based on the histopathologic appearance of tumors. However, the gene-expression profiling of EOC identified molecular subtypes, which demonstrated that pathologic variances were linked to different epidemiologic and genetic risk factors, precursor lesions, response to chemotherapy, and prognosis.

The classification of EOC was revised in 2014 to integrate the scientific knowledge accumulated in recent years.[224] The new classification recognizes serous, mucinous, seromucinous endometrioid, clear cell, and Brenner tumors EOC subtypes that account for more than 95% of cases. Each subtype includes benign, borderline, and malignant tumors.

High-grade serous subtype

The high-grade serous subtype comprises most of all EOCs and demonstrates the most aggressive disease course. The high-grade serous subtype may be associated with *BRCA1* and *BRCA2* mutations, and many of these tumors likely develop from tubal precancerous lesions.[225] The improved understanding of the pathogenesis of serous carcinomas had surgical implications leading to the consideration of bilateral salpingectomy with preservation of the ovaries followed by postmenopause oophorectomy as prophylactic surgery in high-risk populations.[226] This would avoid the detrimental AEs of oophorectomy in premenopausal women.

Mucinous subtype

Primary mucinous ovarian tumors are rare, and metastases of an extragenital malignancy need to be excluded before classifying them as tumors originating from the ovarian epithelium.

Seromucinous and endometrioid subtype

Seromucinous and endometrioid ovarian cancer may be associated with atypical glandular epithelial changes and endometriosis as precursor lesions. *ARID1A* mutations can be seen in both histologic types.[224] In addition, endometrioid epithelial ovarian cancer may harbor *PIK3CA* and *PTEN* mutations similar to endometrial carcinoma.[227]

Clear cell subtype

Clear cell carcinoma is a rare histologic type of EOC diagnosed with higher frequency in women with atypical endometriosis and Lynch syndrome compared with the low incidence in the general population.[228] It is the most common ovarian cancer associated with paraneoplastic symptoms (thromboembolism or hypercalcemia).[229,230]

Brenner tumor subtype

Brenner tumors are replacing the previous category of *transitional cell tumors*. Most of them are benign, although borderline or malignant transformation can be seen in up to 5% of these tumors.[231]

Risk factors

Most ovarian cancers are sporadic, but up to 15% of cases are associated with hereditary susceptibility.[228] Within this group, germline mutations in *BRCA1* or *BRCA2* genes account for most cases. In the general population, the average lifetime risk of developing EOC is 1% to 2%.[222] A woman with a *BRCA* mutation has up to a 46% lifetime risk of ovarian cancer and up to an 85% lifetime risk of breast cancer.[232]

The next most common genetic syndrome associated with EOC is Lynch syndrome, also known as hereditary nonpolyposis colorectal cancer. This condition increases a woman's risk of ovarian and uterine cancer. It is caused by mutations in several different genes, called mismatch repair genes. Women with Lynch syndrome or hereditary nonpolyposis colorectal cancer syndrome have a 40% to 60% lifetime risk of both endometrial and colorectal cancer, as well as a 9% to 12% lifetime risk of EOC.[232] Other genetic conditions that cause EOC include Li-Fraumeni syndrome, ataxia-telangiectasia, Peutz-Jeghers syndrome, and nevoid basal cell carcinoma syndrome.

Reproductive history correlates with EOC risk.[233] Factors associated with increased ovarian activity are more important than the duration of estrogen and progesterone exposure. Therefore, factors associated with increased ovarian activity such as nulliparity or infertility are more important than the age of menarche and menopause. Factors that reduce ovulation such as OC use, pregnancy, and breastfeeding are associated with lower ovarian cancer risk.

Oral contraception for 5 years can decrease EOC risk by 50% compared with women who have never used this method of contraception.[233,234] Studies suggest that use of HT, especially long-term use, can increase the risk of EOC.[233] However, it remains unclear whether the use of fertility drugs affects EOC risk.[235]

Aging is another recognized risk factor for EOC, and women aged 60 years or more are more likely to develop this malignancy.[222]

Endometriosis is a risk factor for specific subtypes of EOC, such as clear cell, low-grade serous, and endometrioid invasive EOC.[236] A retrospective analysis of 13 EOC case-control studies, part of the Ovarian Cancer Association Consortium, found no association between endometriosis and risk of mucinous or high-grade serous invasive EOC.

Similarly, data from 15 case-control studies participating in the Ovarian Cancer Association Consortium were analyzed to evaluate the link between BMI and EOC risk.[237] This association was further analyzed by histologic subtype, menopause status, and postmenopause hormone use. High BMI was associated with increased risk of the less common histologic subtypes of EOC: borderline serous (odds ratio [OR], 1.24; 95% confidence interval [CI], 1.18-1.30), low-grade serous invasive tumors (OR, 1.13; 95% CI, 1.03-1.25), invasive endometrioid (OR, 1.17; 95% CI, 1.11-1.23), and invasive mucinous (OR, 1.19; 95% CI, 1.06-1.32), but there was no association with high-grade serous invasive cancer (OR, 0.98; 95% CI, 0.94-1.02), which is the most common histologic subtype.

Therefore, reducing BMI is unlikely to directly influence most deaths from EOC.

Symptoms

Most women with EOC present with symptoms of an advanced stage, such as ascites, bowel obstruction, pleural effusions, and malnutrition. Early symptoms are nonspecific and include bloating or change in bowel or bladder habits. These atypical symptoms many times prompt the initiation of a workup for gastrointestinal or urinary problems, causing delays in the diagnosis of EOC. Lack of awareness regarding the signs and symptoms of EOC among patients and health professionals appears to be one of the main reason for time delays in the diagnosis of EOC.[238] Educational programs and public awareness on early diagnosis may be useful tools for detection of early stage disease.

Diagnosis

A physical examination is unremarkable for women with early stage EOC but can confirm the clinical diagnosis of small bowel obstruction or ascites in patients with advanced disease. A pelvic examination is frequently unrevealing.

Many women undergo intravaginal ultrasound as an initial test for identification of ovarian masses. Computed tomography (CT), MRI, and positron emission tomography–computed tomography can provide additional details on the extent of EOC and can help plan the surgical approach.

The glycoprotein CA125 has been used as a standard tumor biomarker to detect ovarian malignancy. The normal value is less than 35 IU/mL. A high CA125 can be seen in other cancers or nonmalignant situations such as inflammatory or benign gynecologic conditions.[239] Histologic confirmation of EOC may occur before surgery (by peritoneal cytology or image guided biopsy of an amenable lesion), during surgery, or postoperatively.

Prevention

There is no acceptable method of screening for EOC, although measurement of CA125 levels and transvaginal ultrasound have been used. The Society of Gynecologic Oncology has developed guidelines to assist physicians and other health professionals in identifying patients who may benefit from EOC prevention strategies, which include 1) OC use, 2) tubal sterilization, 3) risk-reducing salpingo-oophorectomy for the prevention of *BRCA*-associated breast and ovarian cancer, 4) genetic counseling and testing for women with EOC, and 5) salpingectomy, after childbearing is complete (at the time of elective pelvic surgeries and as an alternative to tubal ligation).[240]

Treatment

The primary treatment for EOC consists of aggressive surgical staging followed by platinum/taxane-based chemotherapy in virtually all patients.[241] At least 60% to 80% of newly diagnosed women with EOC are expected to respond to platinum-based chemotherapy.[242,243]

Despite effective adjuvant chemotherapy, most women with EOC will eventually relapse. Patients who relapse 6 months or more after initial platinum-based chemotherapy are considered "platinum sensitive" and are treated with platinum-based combination chemotherapy.[244-246] In this setting, the expected response to platinum chemotherapy varies between 25% to 60%, based on the platinum-free interval.[247]

Disease recurring within 6 months of platinum-based chemotherapy is classified as platinum resistant. Patients with relapsed platinum-resistant disease may be treated with a variety of agents that all have an approximately 20% chance of objective response.[248,249] They are not considered to benefit from additional platinum-based therapy.

Patients with platinum-resistant EOC have a poor prognosis. It is increasingly important to identify new agents with increased efficacy and to develop better selection of patients for a particular treatment.

Several nonchemotherapy treatment options are available in the recurrent setting. Estrogen and progesterone receptors are widely expressed in normal and cancerous ovarian tissues.[250] For this reason, tamoxifen and AIs have been used in patients with recurrent EOC who have progressed after platinum-based chemotherapy.[251] These agents are administered to patients with isolated biochemical relapse or evidence of tumor progression.[252,253] However, ER or PR expression does not always correlate with the response to HT.[254]

Poly(ADP-ribose) polymerase inhibitors have emerged as an effective new class of agents for EOC, especially for high-grade ovarian carcinoma with a *BRCA* mutation. Poly(ADP-ribose) polymerase inhibition leads to double-strand DNA breaks during replication and persistent DNA lesions normally repaired by homologous recombinational repair, causing apoptosis of the *BRCA*-deficient cells.

Three poly(ADP-ribose) polymerase inhibitors are now FDA approved, and their efficacy depends on the *BRCA* status (and other molecular "signatures"), platinum sensitivity, and prior lines of therapy.[255-257] These agents can be used as maintenance therapy in patients with recurrent platinum-sensitive EOC or can be used for progressive disease after failure to prior lines of chemotherapy in women with *BRCA*-mutated EOC.

New treatments such as immunotherapy are being actively pursued. These agents are reprogramming the immune system to fight cancer, with the potential for long-term tumor immunity. This approach remains investigational in EOC.

Despite recent progress in EOC treatment, new treatment strategies are warranted for women with EOC to optimize early detection and improve the cure rate.

Lung Cancer

Each year, more people die of lung cancer than of colon, breast, and prostate cancers combined. It is estimated that there will be 234,030 new cases and 155,870 deaths in 2018 in the United States, and an estimated 105,510 and 71,280 women will be diagnosed and die from this disease, respectively.[92] Since 1998, the incidence of lung cancer has steadily declined in both sexes and across all racial and ethnic groups. This decline has been steeper in men than women. For persons born in the 1960s, lung cancer rates are higher in white and Hispanic women than in men. This difference is not explained by higher rates of smoking. Although hypothetical, it has been suggested by epidemiologists that women are more susceptible to the carcinogenic effects of tobacco than men. As many as 15% of the lung cancers develop in nonsmoking women. Most are adenocarcinomas, yet there is no clear explanation for this.[258,259] It has been 50 years since the first report of the US Surgeon General linking cigarette smoking to lung cancer, and smoking prevalence has been decreasing because of anti-smoking campaigns and taxation on cigarettes, yet smoking still accounts for 80% of lung cancer deaths.[258] The implication here is that lung cancer is a largely preventable disease, which provides on opportunity for PCPs to discuss smoking cessation.

Lung cancers are divided into two major subtypes, small cell and non-small cell lung cancer. Non-small cell is more common, accounting for approximately 85% of all cases, and includes the histologic subtypes, with adenocarcinoma (40%), squamous cell (25-30%), and large cell (15%). Small cell accounts for 10% to 15% of all lung cancers.[260]

Risk factors

Most lung cancers develop in persons with a history of smoking. Yet most smokers never develop lung cancer, and lung cancers develop in nonsmokers. Other accepted risks for developing lung cancer include genetics, environmental factors, pollution, and prior therapy (Table 8).[261-271]

Cooking fumes are a major risk factor in developing countries and have been shown as a contributor to a significant increased risk in development of lung cancer.[267] Bituminous coal, which is associated with more smoke while cooking, carries an increased risk opposed to cleaner-cooking anthracite coal. Wood burning has been shown to carry a similar associated increased risk.[268]

Treatment-associated cancers

Chronic obstructive pulmonary disease (COPD) has been shown to be associated with increased risk of lung cancer.[272] Aside from smoking, it is the most common independent risk factor for lung cancer. Though this remains in debate, discerning between increased risk caused by COPD compared with smoking is difficult because COPD is primarily caused by smoking.

It has not been shown that diets high in fruits and vegetables can alter risk for lung cancer. Beta-carotene was previously shown in observational studies to possibly lower lung cancer risk, but randomized data show that not only does it not decrease risk of lung cancer, there was an increase in incidence in lung cancer in smokers who took beta-carotene supplements.[273]

Screening

The National Lung Screening Trial, which involved 53,454 high-risk patients aged 55 to 74 years randomized to 3 years of annual screening with either CT or chest X-ray,

---

Table 8. Risk Factors for Developing Lung Cancer

Nonmodifiable	
Age	Most lung cancer is diagnosed in patients aged older than 65 years.
Genetic predisposition	It is estimated that 8% of lung cancers are associated with a genetic predisposition. A number of candidate genes are under investigation.
Modifiable	
Smoking	Direct and indirect exposure to tobacco smoke is the predominant risk factor. Eighty percent of lung cancer in the United States can be attributed to tobacco smoking. Smoking cessation decreases the risk of lung cancer up to 90% in some cases.
Environmental	
Pollution	Polycystic aromatic hydrocarbons from incomplete combustion, fuels, exhaust, and vehicle emissions are associated with an increased risk for lung cancer.
Asbestos	The type of fiber and nature of exposure predict risk. Occupational exposure, such as working in a factory with asbestos, carries a much higher and more defined risk than nonoccupational environmental exposure. In those patients with a smoking history and associated with asbestos exposure, there appears to be a significant increased risk of lung cancer.
Radon	Increased radon concentrations are associated with a small significant increase in risk of lung cancer. Radon exposure is varied in incidence by geography. Higher concentrations are identified in rural areas because radon is present in soil, rock, and groundwater.
Cooking fumes	Cooking fumes are a major risk factor in developing countries and have been shown as a contributor to a significant increased risk in development of lung cancer. Bituminous coal, which is associated with more smoke while cooking, carries an increased risk as opposed to cleaner-cooking anthracite coal. Wood burning has been shown to carry a similar associated increased risk.
Treatment-Associated	
Radiation therapy to the thoracic region	Patients who have received radiation therapy for breast cancer and lymphomas have an increased risk for developing lung cancer and that risk is magnified if they are also smokers.
	Data remain limited regarding risks of developing a second primary malignancy in patients previously diagnosed with a primary cancer. In patients diagnosed with lung cancer, those who had a previous diagnosis of cancer were more likely to be women, with the most common previous cancers being colorectal (22.0%), breast (18.4%), and gastric (14.4%).

Torre LA, et al[261]; Kanwal M, et al[262]; Peto R, et al[263]; Reid A, et al[264]; Hessel PA, et al[265]; Darby S, et al[266]; Barone-Adesi F, et al[267]; Barcenas CH, et al[268]; Neugat AI, et al[269]; Schoenfeld JD, et al[270]; Shan S, et al.[271]

demonstrated a 20% reduction in lung cancer mortality in the CT arm.[274] This and other studies led the USPSTF to recommend annual low-dose CT as screening in high-risk persons, defined as asymptomatic persons aged 55 to 80 years with a 30-pack-year smoking history who currently smoke or quit within in the past 15 years.[77]

Hormone therapy

Preclinical data in animal models suggest that non-small cell lung cancers can have ERs and respond to estradiol, with increased gene transcription and growth.[275] In humans, ERs and aromatase, the enzyme that synthesizes 17β-estradiol, also have been identified in non-small cell lung cancers.[276] In women with lung cancer, higher estrogen levels have been correlated with higher cancer mortality. Observational studies of EPT and lung cancer incidence and outcome have provided mixed results.[277] In the WHI, postmenopausal women who took EPT had a nonsignificant increase in lung cancer incidence (219 in the hormone-intervention group vs 184 in the placebo group) and deaths from lung cancer (153 vs 132).[278] However, although women who were on the intervention had significantly more lung cancer deaths observed with HT, this difference resolved with discontinuation of the hormone.

Data for the use of HT and its association with lung cancer incidence and survival are limited, with conflicting results. Additional research is needed to evaluate the significance of long-term use of HT on outcomes in lung cancer, including characterization of tumors for ERs and PRs. Research is focusing on differences in female physiology, including bronchial responsiveness, airway size, cytochrome P450, and differences in DNA repair.[279-281] Early limited studies have suggested that antiestrogen agents may improve lung cancer outcomes, which could have substantial implications for clinical practice.[282]

Treatment

Non-small cell lung cancer that is localized should still be treated with surgical resection with or without adjuvant chemotherapy. Localized or unresectable cancer may be treated with a combination of chemotherapy or immunotherapy with radiation. Patients with advanced-stage disease are candidates for systemic therapy with chemotherapy, immunotherapy, and/or targeted agents according to the unique natural history and molecular features of the disease (Table 9).[283-291] Small cell lung cancers rarely present as solitary lesions that are curable with surgical resection. Locally advanced cancers are treated with chemotherapy and radiation therapy. Metastatic disease is treated with chemotherapy.

Colorectal Cancer

Colorectal cancer is the third most commonly diagnosed cancer in the United States, with an estimated 71,420 and 64,010 new cases in men and women, respectively, in 2017.292 In US women, colorectal cancer remains the third leading cause of cancer death, with an estimated 23,110 deaths in 2017 after deaths caused by lung (71,280) and breast cancer (40,610).[92] From 2006 to 2015, incidence rates declined by an average of 2.6% per year, and death rates declined by an average of 2.4% per year. The 2011-2015 incidence ranged from 28.6 per 100,000 per year in Hispanic women to 41.9 per 100,000 per year in black women. The age-adjusted mortality rate for women is 12.2 per 100,000 per year.[223] Approximately 4.2% of Americans are expected to develop the disease in their lifetimes, and the estimated 5-year survival is 64.5%.

In men and women combined, the death rate from colorectal cancer has dropped 51% from its peak of 28.6 per 100,000 in 1976 to 14.1 per 100,000 in 2014.[292] Reductions in colorectal cancer mortality through 2000 have been attributed to better therapies (12%), changing patterns in risk factors for colorectal cancer (35%), and implementation of screening practices (53%).[293] The most important reason for the decline in colorectal cancer is thought to be the removal of polyps at the first screening colonoscopy. The lifetime risk of colorectal cancer is 4.2%, or 1 in 24. The median age at diagnosis is 67 years.[223] Most (82.5%) cases of colorectal cancer are diagnosed in men and women aged between 45 and 84 years. The incidence of colorectal cancer is highest in black women and lowest in Asian women. Expected survival rates depend on the stage of the cancer at diagnosis. From 2008 to 2014, the overall 5-year survival rate was 89.8% for localized disease and 13.8% for distant disease.

Risk factors

Various nonmodifiable and modifiable risk factors for colorectal cancer have been identified (Table 10).[294-300] One inherited form of colorectal cancer is known as *hereditary nonpolyposis colorectal cancer*, or Lynch syndrome.[301] It is caused by germline mutations in mismatch repair genes. It is characterized by an increased risk of colon cancer as well as cancers of the urinary tract, brain, skin, endometrium, ovary, stomach, small intestine, and hepatobiliary

Table 9. Clinical Characteristics and Treatment According to Molecular Subtype of Non-Small Cell Lung Cancer

	Molecular Target			
	EGFR	**ALK**	**ROS1**	**PD-L1**
Molecular findings	Deletion or exon 2 substitution or mutation	Gene rearrangement	Translocation	Overexpression
Clinical characteristics	Nonsmokers or low-burden smokers, East Asians, adenocarcinomas	Tend to be younger, light smokers, adenocarcinomas	Mostly women, tend to be younger, adenocarcinomas	No clear association with smoking or sex. Tend to be high-grade histology.
Treatments	Erlotinib, gefitinib, afatinib, osimertinib	Crizotinib, ceritinib, alectinib	Crizotinib	Pembrolizumab or nivolumab in conjunction with platinum chemotherapy
Adverse events	Diarrhea, rash, cough, dyspnea, dry skin, decreased appetite, stomatitis	Nausea, vomiting, diarrhea, increased ALT	Nausea, vomiting, diarrhea, increased ALT, visual disturbances, constipation	Autoimmune disease, diarrhea, fatigue, pyrexia

Abbreviations: ALK, anaplastic lymphoma kinase; ALT, alanine aminotransferase; EGFR, epidermal growth factor receptor; PD-L1, programmed cell death ligand-1; ROS1, proto-oncogene 1, receptor tyrosine kinase.
Chia PL, et al[283]; Dugay F, et al[284]; Kang JK, et al[285]; Kim HR, et al[286]; Kim H, et al[287]; Prabhakar CN[288]; Reck M, et al[289]; Shigematsu H, et al[290]; Wang A, et al.[291]

tract.[302] Patients with Lynch syndrome have a 52% to 82% lifetime risk for colorectal cancer (mean age at diagnosis, 44-61 y).[303] The risk for other Lynch syndrome-related cancers is lower, although substantially increased over general population rates.[304]

Another inherited condition is *familial adenomatous polyposis*, in which people develop hundreds to thousands of adenomatous polyps in the colon and rectum.[305] There is nearly a 100% risk of developing cancer by age 40 years, with some patients developing cancer by age 20 years. This condition accounts for less than 1% of all colorectal cancers.

Of the modifiable risk factors, the influence of the Western diet is increasingly becoming recognized as a contributor of risk for colorectal cancer. The intake of red and processed meat, a part of the Western diet, has been associated with increased risk for colorectal cancer.[306] Furthermore, obesity and physical inactivity are known risk factors for colorectal cancer, with comparable risks in men and women,[307,308] as well as for the development of DM.[309]

Dietary intake of vitamin D alone has not been shown to predict risk for colorectal cancer. However, persons with serum 25-hydroxyvitamin D [25(OH)D], or vitamin D_3, levels of 30 ng/mL had a 33% lower risk of colorectal cancer than those with levels of 5 ng/mL.[310] In a meta-analysis evaluating blood levels of vitamin D, persons with the lowest quintile of 25-hydroxyvitamin D were compared with those with levels in the highest quintile; the latter had a 30% lower risk of developing colorectal adenomas (precursors to colorectal cancers) than those in the lowest quintile.[311] Lower levels of 25-hydroxyvitamin D have also been associated with increased risk of incident colon, prostate, and breast cancer, along with higher mortality from these cancers, according to prospective and retrospective epidemiologic studies.[312] An RCT of vitamin D_3 1,000 IU daily, calcium 1,200 mg daily, or both did not significantly reduce the risk of recurrent colorectal adenomas over 3 to 5 years.[313] Although investigations are ongoing, levels of vitamin D_3 appear associated with colorectal cancer risk, but a clear cause-and-effect relationship has yet to be established. Its role as a definitive risk factor for colorectal cancer therefore remains unclear.

Screening

The goals of screening are prevention and early detection of colorectal cancer. The primary screening tests for detecting colorectal cancer are fecal occult blood testing (FOBT), flexible sigmoidoscopy, colonoscopy, barium enema, and CT colonoscopy, with colonoscopy being the gold standard. Women at average risk of colorectal cancer should be screened with a colonoscopy every 10 years, beginning at age 50 years, as recommended by most major societies and groups (Table 11).[78,294,314,315] The ACS

Table 10. Risk Factors for Colorectal Cancer

Nonmodifiable

- Ethnicity
- Age (risk increases markedly after age 50 y)
- Family history of colorectal cancer
- Inherited syndromes such as familial adenomatous polyposis coli
- Personal history of inflammatory bowel disease
- Prior colon cancer
- Prior polyps

Modifiable

- Type 2 diabetes mellitus
- Diet high in red meats and processed meats
- Physical inactivity
- Obesity
- Smoking
- Heavy alcohol use

American Cancer Society[294]; Bardou M, et al[295]; Cho EL, et al[296]; Doubeni CA, et al[297]; Mills KT, et al[298]; Nimptsch K, et al[299]; Zgaga L, et al.[300]

recently updated their guidelines to recommend screening for colorectal cancer starting at the age of 45 years instead of 50 years for persons of average risk.[294] However, several groups have argued for caution in implementing the ACS guidelines given that they were derived from complex modeling studies of the natural history of colonic neoplasia and screening performance rather than a large, prospective clinical study.[316] Other societies, including the USPSTF, continue to recommend screening to begin at age 50 years for average-risk persons.[78] Furthermore, the ACS recognizes that the Affordable Care Act requires private insurers and Medicare to cover costs of colorectal cancer screening tests as recommended by the USPSTF; at this time, insurers are not required to and may not cover the cost of screening before age 50 years.[294]

Stool blood testing

The purpose of the FOBT is to detect the presence of blood in the gastrointestinal tract that is not visible to the naked eye.[317] The guiaic-based method, which is still in use, was among the earliest approaches to colorectal cancer screening and remains among the least expensive test available for this purpose. It results in a change in dye color when hemoglobin is present. Although the guiaic-based test has good clinical specificity, it has low analytical and clinical sensitivity. Follow-up of a false-positive test can result in discomfort, cost, and occasional complications from unnecessary tests.

A more advanced type of the FOBT is achieved by using an immunochemical method. This method uses an antibody to the hemoglobin protein in order to detect the presence of blood in the stool. At a relatively low cost, the fecal immunochemical test (FIT) has fair one-time sensitivity (79%) and appears to have better sensitivity for colorectal cancer and precursor lesions, as well greater participation rates, compared with the guiaic-based test. This test is about five times more expensive than the guiaic-based test.[314,317] The FIT is considered a cancer-detecting test and is recommended annually.[314] A stool DNA test combining a FIT with testing of several markers for colon cancer was approved by FDA in 2014 after showing the ability to detect more colorectal cancers than the FIT alone (92% vs 74% sensitivity) but had a higher number of false positives and likelihood of follow-up colonoscopy and associated AEs.[318] Although originally not recommended for colorectal cancer screening in average-risk adults by the USPSTF in 2008, this test is now recognized by the ACS and the 2016 USPSTF.[78,294]

Sigmoidoscopy

Sigmoidoscopy uses a flexible sigmoidoscope to examine the colon from the anus to the proximal descending colon.[315] Its primary use is to detect left-sided cancers. Randomized clinical trials have shown a 29% to 76% reduction in distal and rectosigmoid colon cancer incidence and/or mortality with flexible sigmoidoscopy.[314] Flexible sigmoidoscopy has a lower cost and risk, requires no sedation, and requires more limited bowel preparation compared with colonoscopy. However, flexible sigmoidoscopy is inferior to colonoscopy in detecting right-sided colon cancer.

Colonoscopy

Colonoscopy is the examination of the large intestine with a flexible fiber-optic colonoscope. Air introduced through the colonoscope distends the intestinal walls to enhance visualization. Colonoscopy evaluates polypoid lesions that are beyond the reach of a sigmoidoscope. During colonoscopy, polyps are removed for histologic evaluation, and photographs of visualized lesions are taken. Colonoscopy is repeated at more frequent intervals when women have a prior history of polyps, colon cancer, or high-risk factors such as family history or genetic predisposition.

Colonoscopy is widely considered the gold standard for screening because of its ability to visualize, sample, and remove lesions from the entire colon. Data from a large study revealed an expected perforation rate of

0.082%, which is lower than previously thought.[319] Risk factors for perforation include increasing age, significant comorbidity, female sex, hospital setting, and invasive interventions during the procedure. There is a higher perforation rate when nongastroenterologists perform the procedure, perhaps because of the lower volume and differences in training.[320]

Obstruction is a contraindication for colonoscopy. Colonoscopy combined with polypectomy has been shown to decrease morbidity and mortality from colorectal cancer. Updated data from the National Polyp Study calculated an expected mortality reduction from colorectal cancer to be 53%.[321] The observed decrease is thought to reflect the effect of the initial colonoscopy with polyp removal.

Barium enema

Barium enema with air contrast increases the quality of X-rays of the rectum. The sensitivity of this procedure, however, is only 48% for polyps 1 cm and larger.[322] Barium enema has effectively been replaced by CT colonography, given efficacy and tolerability considerations.[314]

Computed tomography colonography

Computed tomography colonography can be used to examine the colon and reconstruct the images in a 3-dimensional format, so-called *virtual colonoscopy*.[323] It can be used as a follow-up examination when traditional colonoscopy could not be completed for technical reasons or when colonoscopy is contraindicated because of a medical reason such as anticoagulation or an inherited coagulation defect. Bowel preparation is still required. Radiologists may not identify lesions smaller than 5 mm. There is a perforation rate associated with this procedure, estimated to be 0.02%, secondary to insufflation with air for visualization of the mucosal wall.[324]

Alternative testing to colonoscopy

There are some alternative screening methods to colonoscopy that have been recognized by the ACS (Table 11).[78,294,314,315] The ColoGuard assay, a stool DNA test, offers a noninvasive and relatively sensitive alternative to colonoscopy, although abnormal findings will require a follow-up colonoscopy, with potential AEs from additional procedures. Flexible sigmoidoscopy every 10 years in combination with an annual FIT is an alternative option for persons who want endoscopic screening but wish to avoid colonoscopy.[78] Computed tomography colonography can be offered every 5 years, and a bowel preparation is

Table 11. Screening Tests and Guidelines for Colorectal Cancer in Average-Risk Women, Beginning at Age 45-50 Years

Tests that detect adenomatous polyps and cancer
- Colonoscopy every 10 y
- Flexible sigmoidoscopy every 5 y[a]
- Computed tomography colonography or virtual colonoscopy every 5 y[a]

Tests that mainly detect colorectal cancer
- Guaiac-based FOBT every y[a,b]
- FIT every y[a,b]
- Stool DNA every 3 y[a]

The American Cancer Society has updated their guidelines to recommend screening for colorectal cancer starting at the age of 45 instead of 50 for persons at average risk. Other societies, including the US Preventive Services Task Force, continue to recommend that screening begin at age 50 for average-risk persons.
[a]Follow-up with colonoscopy if positive.
[b]A take-home multiple sample method should be used with highly sensitive versions of these tests. An FOBT or FIT done from a digital rectal exam at the physician's office is not sufficient for screening.
Abbreviations: FOBT, fecal occult blood test; FIT, fecal immunochemical test.
US Preventive Services Task Force[78]; American Cancer Society[294]; Rex DK, et al[314]; Levin B, et al.[315]

necessary as for routine colonoscopy. Furthermore, CT colonography is performer dependent and not widely adopted. Abnormal findings will lead to another procedure (colonoscopy), with potential AEs related to additional testing. Screening barium enema can be offered every 5 years and may require follow-up colonoscopy if one or more polyps 6 mm or larger is detected; a complete bowel prep also is required.[315]

Risk-specific testing

More intensive screening for colorectal cancer should be done when a patient's family history is positive for colorectal cancer. When a patient has a single first-degree relative diagnosed with colorectal cancer or adenomatous polyp when aged younger than 60 years or has two first-degree relatives with colorectal cancer or adenomatous polyps at any age, the recommended screening is every 5 years with colonoscopy starting at age 40 years or 10 years younger than the age at diagnosis of the youngest affected relative.[315] In persons with a single first-degree relative aged older than 60 years diagnosed with colorectal cancer or adenomatous polyps or in two or more second-degree relatives at any age, recommendations include screening with the same test options and frequency as those with average-risk but starting at the age of 40 years. Recommendations for screening and surveillance colonoscopy during the perioperative period and postoperative period in patients diagnosed with resectable colorectal cancer should be made in a multidisciplinary setting with a medical oncologist, surgeon, and/or gastroenterologist.

Familial adenomatous polyposis

Genetic counseling is recommended for women at risk of familial adenomatous polyposis, based on family history. Given a 100% risk of colorectal cancer by age 40 years, an annual flexible sigmoidoscopy or colonoscopy is recommended starting at age 10 to 12 years until colectomy is deemed appropriate.[315] Additional screening is recommended for noncolorectal tumors associated with this syndrome.[325]

Hereditary nonpolyposis colorectal cancer

Patients who meet the Bethesda criteria should have genetic testing for Lynch syndrome.[326] The American Society of Clinical Oncology now recommends universal testing for mismatch repair deficiency or microsatellite instability in all patients with colorectal cancer.[325] Those with microsatellite instability colorectal cancer should undergo genetic germline testing for Lynch syndrome. Microsatellite instability, when present and not caused by MLH1 promoter methylation or its surrogate *BRAF* mutation, is a strong predictor of Lynch syndrome, whereas the presence of either MLH1 promoter methylation or *BRAF* mutation in the setting of microsatellite instability indicates a sporadic case of colorectal cancer.[304] Therefore, genetic testing should be performed in patients with microsatellite instability colorectal cancer without somatic *BRAFV600E* mutation or without MLH1 promoter hypermethylation. Those with positive testing or at increased risk for Lynch syndrome should undergo colonoscopy every 1 to 2 years beginning at age 20 to 25 years or 10 years before the youngest case in the immediate family.[315] Additional screening is recommended for noncolorectal tumors associated with Lynch syndrome.[325]

Inflammatory bowel disease

In persons with chronic ulcerative colitis or Crohn disease, referral to an experienced center for surveillance and management of inflammatory bowel disease is recommended.[315,327] Here, colonoscopy with biopsies every 1 to 2 years are important to assess for cancer because significant risk begins 8 years after the start of pancolitis or 12 to 15 years after the start of left-sided colitis.[294,315] Additionally, several other societies have put forth their recommendations for colorectal cancer surveillance with

noted differences in the frequency of colonoscopies that may depend on the institution and intensity of colitis.[327]

Lifestyle modification

Colorectal cancer risk may be lowered by exercise and lower fat intake. Populations with a fat intake significantly lower than the US population have one-third the risk of colorectal cancer. However, the WHI Dietary Modification Trial (a randomized trial involving 48,835 postmenopausal women) demonstrated that reducing fat ingestion and increasing intake of fruits, vegetables, and grains did not reduce the incidence of colorectal cancer.[328] In that trial, intervention-group participants reduced fat as a percentage of energy intake by 10.7% more than the control group at 1 year, and most maintained this difference (8.1%) at 6 years. There was no evidence that this intervention reduced colorectal cancer incidence in subsequent years. However, many women in the study were taking aspirin, HT, and calcium and vitamin D supplementation, which may have influenced the findings.

These findings were consistent with those of the Polyp Prevention Trial, which showed no reduction in polyp formation in 2,079 participants followed for 4 years.[329] The results were also consistent with a pooled analysis of prospective cohort studies evaluating dietary fiber intake and the risk of colorectal cancer.[330] Despite conflicting evidence, a growing number of healthcare providers and researchers agree that diet and lifestyle modifications should complement colorectal cancer screening and potentially reduce risk in addition to benefits in preventing other comorbidities such as CVD.[331]

Postpolypectomy guidelines

In 1990, a different type of precancerous polyp, called a *serrated polyp*, was described.[332] This is a type of hyperplastic polyp that tends to be found in the right side of the colon, is more common in women, and has a shorter progression to cancer than the traditional tubular adenoma. The traditional tubular adenoma is more likely to be found in the left side of the colon, is more common in men, and has at least a 10-year interval progression to colon cancer. There are different mutations involved. The serrated polyps can be difficult to detect because they are usually flatter. Postpolypectomy guidelines now reflect this classification so that practitioners will see different recommendations after polyp removal than in the past.[333]

For patients with one or two small tubular adenomas (≤1 cm) with low-grade dysplasia, colonoscopy is recommended 5 to 10 years after the initial polypectomy.[294,315]

For those with three to 10 adenomas, any adenomas with high-grade dysplasia or villous features, or a large (≥1 cm) adenoma, colonoscopy is recommended 3 years after polyp removal. In patients with more than 10 adenomas on a single exam, genetic testing should be considered, and a colonoscopy is recommended within 3 years of removal of polyps. In patients with sessile adenomas that are removed in pieces, a repeat colonoscopy is recommended 2 to 6 months after removal. Women with small rectal hyperplastic polyps can be followed with the same test options and frequency as for average-risk women.

Chemoprevention

There is evidence that use of aspirin and nonsteroidal anti-inflammatory drugs (NSAIDs) are associated with reduced risk of colorectal cancer.[331,334] For primary prevention, regular aspirin use has been shown to be effective in reducing colorectal polyps and colorectal cancer.[335,336] Aspirin 100 mg per day also prevents the development of colorectal cancer in patients with familial adenomatous polyposis syndrome.[337] The NSAIDs celocoxib (400 mg twice/d) and sulindac (150 mg twice/d) also have been shown to significantly reduce the number of colorectal polyps in familial adenomatous polyposis syndrome.[338,339] The USPSTF recommends low-dose daily aspirin for at least 10 years for the primary prevention of CVD and colorectal cancer in persons aged 50 to 59 years with 10% or greater 10-year CVD, a life expectancy of at least 10 years, and no increased risk for bleeding.[340]

There is also some evidence that a daily folate supplement may be chemopreventive in a subset of patients with colon cancer[341]; however, there is no generally accepted recommendation for any of these supplements because there is no single strategy that is applicable to all of the different types of colon cancer.

Randomized, controlled trials, including the WHI, have shown that EPT is associated with decreased risk of colorectal cancer, with six fewer cases per 10,000 women over 1 year.[342] In this trial, 16,608 postmenopausal women were randomized to receive EPT as a single tablet or identical-appearing placebo. After an average follow-up of 5.6 years, 43 invasive colorectal cancers were discovered in the hormone group compared with 72 in the placebo group (hazard ratio, 0.56; 95% CI, 0.38-0.81; P=.003). Overall, this translated to a 44% decrease in the risk for colorectal cancer in the EPT group. However, the colorectal tumors diagnosed in EPT users tended to have more lymph node involvement, although there were no statistically significant

differences in tumor grades, stage, and deaths compared with placebo. One of the noted differences between the groups was that the women in the EPT group had more vaginal bleeding than did women in the placebo group, which may have delayed their evaluation for colorectal cancer.[343] Data are insufficient to support a global recommendation for use of EPT to reduce the risk of colorectal cancer in postmenopausal women.

Investigations are ongoing regarding the secondary prevention of colorectal cancer with various chemopreventive strategies. In resected colorectal cancer, regular aspirin use has been associated with significantly reduced rates of recurrence in colorectal polyps and colorectal cancer.[344,345] A prospective study showed that tree-nut consumption (≥2 servings/wk) in those with stage III colorectal cancer had significantly reduced cancer recurrence.[346]

Halting screening

The age at which to stop screening should be individualized on the basis of risk factors and symptoms. Asymptomatic women aged between 50 and 75 years should be screened regularly.[78] Routine screening of asymptomatic persons aged between 76 and 85 years should be done on an individual basis. Screening is not recommended in asymptomatic persons aged older than 85 years who have previously been adequately screened.

Treatment

The treatment of colorectal cancer is multidisciplinary and dependent on stage.[347,349] Stage I colon and rectal cancers are curative and treated with surgery alone. Stage II and III rectal cancers are considered locally advanced, and neoadjuvant chemoradiation followed by surgery and postoperative chemotherapy to complete a total of 6 months of perioperative chemotherapy is currently the standard of care.[348] Stage III colon cancers are treated with surgery followed by fluoropyrimidine-based adjuvant or postoperative chemotherapy of 3 to 6 months based on risk features.[347] Stage II colon cancers are similarly treated with surgery, but decisions on adjuvant chemotherapy are based on risk features, with the option to forgo adjuvant chemotherapy in specific populations. Most patients with stage IV colorectal cancer have incurable disease except for those with isolated metastases that are potentially curable with surgery. The current standard therapy for stage IV colorectal cancer involves combination chemotherapy with cytotoxics, including 5-fluorouracil, oxaliplatin, and/or irinotecan and biologic agents, some of which are dependent on the molecular features of the tumor.[349] In microsatellite instability metastatic colorectal cancer, immunotherapy in the form of checkpoint inhibitors is now available for patients who are refractory to standard therapies.[347]

Skin Cancer

Skin cancers include a diverse spectrum of cutaneous malignancies and include basal cell carcinoma, squamous cell carcinoma, and melanoma. The nonmelanoma skin cancers, basal cell and squamous cell carcinoma, are the most commonly diagnosed cancers, and 2012 estimates exceeded 5.4 million cases worldwide.[350] In contrast, an estimated 87,110 new cases of melanoma will be diagnosed in the United States in 2017.[92] Despite accounting for the vast minority of skin cancers, melanoma is responsible for most of skin cancer deaths.

Ultraviolet light exposure is an important risk factor for all of the most common skin cancers, making past blistering sunburns and use of tanning beds important elements of a patient's history.[351] Patients with a history of skin cancer have a significantly increased risk of developing new skin cancers, and elderly patients have high rates of posttreatment complications. These factors highlight the importance of preventive measures such as annual full body skin checks and sun protection and avoidance.

Malignant lesions

Actinic keratosis

Actinic keratoses are among the most common of dermatologic findings and are the result of cumulative sun damage to the skin, thus they arise on sun-exposed areas.[352] Actinic keratoses generally appear as scaly outgrowths with an erythematous base and may cause tenderness or burning. Because of their sandpaper-like texture, they are often diagnosed by gentle palpation rather than visual inspection. These lesions represent a premalignant proliferation of keratinocytes, with potential to progress to squamous cell carcinoma. Cryotherapy (via liquid nitrogen) or topical treatments such as topic 5-fluorouracil or imiquimod can be used to prevent the development of squamous cell carcinoma.[351]

Squamous cell carcinoma

Squamous cell carcinoma is commonly characterized by persistent crusting and ulceration with induration and ill-defined edges.[353] It will appear on sun-exposed areas of the skin and may be heralded by a precursor lesion, such as an actinic keratosis. Compared with other skin cancers, it is most closely related to chronic sun exposure. Other risk factors include age, fair skin, and immunosuppression, with as much as a 250-fold increase in risk in white organ transplant recipients. Women have a decreased risk of nearly 3-fold compared with men.[354] Squamous cell carcinoma is the second most common malignancy of the skin, behind only basal cell carcinoma.[353]

Basal cell carcinoma

The lifetime risk of developing basal cell carcinoma in the United States is 28% to 33%.[354] The average age of diagnosis for women is in the sixth decade of life. It may present as a persistent nonhealing sore or a shiny nodule with telangiectasia on sun-exposed areas of the skin. Another common presentation includes a chronic erythematous patch with rolled borders, a presentation that is more likely to be found on the trunk. Patients may also complain of tenderness or pruritus. For both squamous and basal cell carcinoma, biopsy is performed to confirm diagnosis, and treatment is excisional (eg, Mohs surgery). Cure rates can reach 96% to 99%.[353,354]

Melanoma

Melanoma arises because of a malignant proliferation of melanocytes and is the most deadly form of skin cancer. Risk factors include fair skin with an inability to tan, ultraviolet (UV) light exposure (especially at a young age), advancing age (median age at diagnosis, 64 y), positive family history, and the presence of atypical nevi/moles.[223,355] Naevi and solar keratoses are usually mutually exclusive as risk factors for melanoma, and this highlights the fact that different skin phenotypes can lead to melanoma. Additionally, the more nevi a patient has, the greater the risk.[355,356] Progression of a nevus into melanoma may occur but is not always the case. It has been shown that a low vitamin D level is associated with a worse prognosis. This finding presents an interesting paradox in the primary prevention of melanoma because sun exposure is a source of vitamin D but is a major risk factor for the development of melanoma.[356]

Characteristic lesions are usually pigmented and possess one or more features of the "ABDCE" rule (Table 12).[357-359] Other clues toward diagnosis include a nevus that appears different from the patient's other nevi ("ugly duckling sign")[359,360] and an existing nevus that has become pruritic or burns.[361] Diagnosis is confirmed with a biopsy

Table 12.	Lesion Characteristics of Melanoma: "ABCDE" Criteria
A	Asymmetry
B	Irregular border
C	Color is variable
D	Diameter >6 mm
E	Evolving or changing

Friedman RJ, et al[357]; Abbasi NR, et al[358]; Ilyas M, et al.[359]

and histopathologic evaluation. Tumor staging, which may include sentinel lymph node biopsy, will determine whether systemic therapy is necessary in addition to surgical excision.[362]

Merkel cell carcinoma

Merkel cell carcinoma is a rare but aggressive neuroendocrine tumor, with a mortality rate greater than that of melanoma, lending to this malignancy's propensity for misdiagnosis and metastasis.[363] The primary lesion will most commonly appear as a subepidermal red or pink cyst-like growth on sun-exposed areas of the skin. Clinical characteristics can be summarized using the "AEIOU" mnemonic (Table 13).[364] Merkel cell polyomavirus has been implicated in the pathogenesis of this deadly skin cancer.[363] Biopsy is necessary for diagnosis, as well as sentinel lymph node biopsy for staging, followed with excision and adjuvant radiotherapy for treatment.

Dermatofibrosarcoma protuberans

Dermatofibrosarcoma protuberans is a rare (4.2/million persons), soft-tissue neoplasm arising from the dermis, carries low risk for metastasis, and has a good prognosis (99.2% 5-y survival).[365,366] However, this tumor is associated with significant morbidity because of local infiltration and a high rate of postsurgical recurrence. It appears as a red-blue plaque on the trunk that may rapidly progress into one or more nodules. Incidence is highest in blacks, with some studies indicating a higher incidence in women.[366] Diagnosis is established via biopsy, and treatment involves wide local excision.

Dermatofibrosarcoma protuberans is typically caused by a translocation between chromosomes 17 and 22, leading to overexpression of platelet-derived growth factor.[365] The drug imatinib targets this pathway and is FDA approved for the treatment of select cases, including cases of local recurrence. Current recommendations

suggest follow-up with a dermatologist or surgical oncologist at 6- to 12-month intervals.

Benign lesions

Seborrheic keratosis

Seborrheic keratoses are benign proliferations of keratinocytes that are often sharply demarcated, pigmented, round, and elevated. They usually appear oily and possess a "stuck-on" appearance. Seborrheic keratoses have roughly equal prevalence in men and women, with a clear correlation with increasing age, beginning at age 30 years.[367] Indications for therapy include mechanical irritation or uncertain diagnosis because this lesion can mimic the appearance of malignant lesions such as melanoma.[368] Treatment options include cryotherapy, electrocautery, shave excision (preferred if biopsy is necessary), laser therapy, and topical vitamin D.[367,368]

Nevi/Solar lentigo

Acquired melanocytic nevi and solar lentigines are benign pigmented lesions caused by proliferation of melanocytes.[367,369] Acquired melanocytic nevi (moles) have a wide range of appearances, but they will most often have a well-circumscribed, rounded shape with even pigmentation. They are associated with sun exposure, and high mole counts confer an increased risk of melanoma. Nevi peak in number in young adulthood and spontaneously regress thereafter, with most disappearing by age 60 years.[367]

Solar lentigines (actinic lentigines, aging spots, liver spots) are a form of freckling that present as flat brown spots that are caused by chronic sun exposure.[369] They are most common on the face or dorsum of the hands in persons aged older than 50 years with darker skin. In contrast, freckles in young people (ephelides) are seen

Table 13.	Clinical Characteristics of Merkel Cell Carcinoma: "AEIOU" Mnemonic	
A	Asymptomatic
E	Expanding rapidly (≤3 mo)
I	Immunosupression
O	Older than 50 years
U	UV-exposed areas

Abbreviation: UV, ultraviolet.
Heath M, et al.[364]

in persons with light skin and/or red hair and become more apparent after sun exposure.

Cherry angioma

Cherry angiomas are small, red, dome-shaped, blanching, vascular lesions that most commonly appear on the trunk.[367] They are very common and increase in number with age beginning in the third decade of life. Treatment is elective and options include electrocautery, laser coagulation, and shave excision.

Lipoma

Lipomas are slow-growing adipose tumors that present as nontender, rounded, mobile subcutaneous masses with a characteristic doughy feel.[370] They usually appear between ages 40 and 60 years and are more common in women. Treatment is based on the aesthetic concerns of the patient, and options include surgery, liposuction, and lipolysis (eg, phosphatidylcholine injections).[371]

Dermatofibroma

Dermatofibromas present as firm, well-defined oval nodules with overlying pigmentation, most commonly arising on the distal lower extremities. These benign lesions are 25 times more common in women and can form secondary to local trauma.[372,373] They follow a gradual course, taking months to develop.[367] Excision or cryotherapy is usually not necessary for reasons other than cosmesis.

Warts

Cutaneous viral warts are caused by HPV and come in a variety of shapes and sizes.[374] Plantar warts, for example, present on the sole of the foot as a rough, white plaque with black dots, which represent thrombosed capillaries. Warts are more common in children and young adults, but states of immunosuppression can lead to wart development in older adults. Spontaneous resolution generally occurs in months to years in immunocompetent patients, but treatment options include duct tape, salicylic acid, imiquimod cream, and cryotherapy.

Sun protection

A broad-spectrum sunscreen that blocks both UVA and UVB radiation with a sun protection factor greater than 30 should be applied daily to sun-exposed skin. Sunscreen needs to be reapplied every 60 to 90 minutes, even with water-resistant brands. A wide-brimmed (≥3 in) hat and sun-protective clothing (UV protection factor 50) are often easier for patient compliance than applying and reapplying sunscreens. Spray sunscreens can be effective, but they need to be rubbed in after spraying to make sure the product is physically in contact with the skin. Ultraviolet radiation exposure peaks between 10 AM and 2 PM, so patients should seek shade during these hours. Sunburns can occur even on cloudy days. Reflectance off of water, sand, and snow can increase the amount UV exposure, so advise patients to be especially careful in these situations. An annual skin examination is recommended for patients with a personal or family history of skin cancer. Suspicious lesions should be evaluated and biopsied in a timely fashion, because early detection will have the best outcomes for skin cancers.

Skin care after menopause

The barrier function of the skin diminishes with aging, frequently causing dryness. Dry, brittle skin predisposes to many types of rash, including xerotic eczema and allergic contact dermatitis. Dry skin care involves a number of different strategies that will help to maintain and preserve the barrier function of the skin. Use of a good emollient moisturizer on a daily or twice daily basis will help maintain and support the skin's barrier function. Most dermatologists recommend plain 100% petrolatum ointment because it has no fragrance or preservative. If the greasy feel of petrolatum is not tolerated, then any thick cream that is fragrance and dye free can be used. Lotions in pumps generally contain too much water and are not as effective. Soap use should be minimized because even the gentlest cleanser will cause some drying of the skin. Prolonged, hot showers should be avoided, because this habit can also cause excessive drying. Although less satisfying, brief, lukewarm showers are best for itchy, dry skin. Finally, switching to fragrance- and dye-free personal care products is highly recommended, especially for patients with sensitive skin. Patients with persistent rash or pruritus should be evaluated by a dermatologist, and patch testing may be required. Additional patient-oriented information on skin-related topics can be found on the American Academy of Dermatology website (www.aad.org). (See also "Skin Changes" in Chapter 2.)

REFERENCES

1. American Cancer Society. *Cancer Facts & Figures 2018*. Atlanta, Ga: American Cancer Society; 2018.

2. Edwards BK, Howe HL, Ries LA, et al. Annual report to the nation on the status of cancer, 1973-1999, featuring implications of age and aging on the US cancer burden. *Cancer*. 2002;94(10):2766-2792.

3. National Center for Health Statistics. National Health and Nutrition Examination Survey. *NCHS Fact Sheet*. December 2017. www.cdc.gov/nchs/data/factsheets/factsheet_nhanes.pdf. Accessed July 3, 2019.

4. Bianchini F, Kaaks R, Vainio H. Overweight, obesity, and cancer risks. *Lancet Oncol.* 2002;3(9):565-574.

5. Bultman SJ. A reversible epigenetic link between obesity and cancer risk. *Trends Endocrinol Metab.* 2018:29(8):529-531.

6. Lohmann AD, Goodwin PJ, Chlebowski RT, Pan K, Stambolic V, Dowlin RJ. Association of obesity-related metabolic disruptions with cancer risk and outcome. *J Clin Oncol.* 2016;34(35):4249-4255.

7. Coleman MP, Forman D, Bryant H, et al; ICBP Module 1 working Group. Cancer survival in Australia, Canada, Denmark, Norway, Sweden, and the UK, 1995-2007 (the International Cancer Benchmarking Partnership): an analysis of population-based cancer registry data. *Lancet.* 2011;377(9760):127-138.

8. De Angelis R, Sant M, Coleman MP, et al; EUROCARE-5 Working Group. Cancer survival in Europe 1999-2007 by country and age: results of EUROCARE-5—a population-based study. *Lancet Oncol.* 2014. 15(1):23-34.

9. Rossouw JE, Anderson GL, Prentice RL, et al; Writing Group for the Women's Health Initiative Investigators. Risks and benefits of estrogen plus progestin in healthy postmenopausal women: principal results from the Women's Health Initiative randomized controlled trial. *JAMA.* 2002;288(3):321-333.

10. Iqbal J, Ginsburg O, Rochon PA, Sun P, Narod SA. Differences in breast cancer stage at diagnosis and cancer-specific survival by race and ethnicity in the united states. *JAMA.* 2015;313(2):165-173. Erratum in: *JAMA.* 2015; 313(22):2287.

11. Antoniou A, Pharoah PDP, Narod S, et al. Average risks of breast and ovarian cancer associated with *BRCA1* or *BRCA2* mutations detected in case series unselected for family history: a combined analysis of 22 studies. *Am J Hum Genet.* 2003;72(5):1117-1130. Erratum in: *Am J Hum Genet.* 2003;73(3):709.

12. Antoniou AC, Pharoah PDP, Easton DF, Evans DG. *BRCA1* and *BRCA2* cancer risks. *J Clin Oncol.* 2006;24(20):3312-3313.

13. Antoniou AC, Casadei S, Heikkinen T, et al. Breast-cancer risk in families with mutations in *PALB2*. *N Engl J Med.* 2014;371(6):497-506.

14. Chlebowski RT, Kuller LH, Prentice RL, et al; WHI Investigators. Breast cancer after use of estrogen plus progestin in postmenopausal women. *N Engl J Med.* 2009;360(6):573-587.

15. Chlebowski RT, Anderson GL. Menopausal hormone therapy and breast cancer mortality: clinical implications. *Ther Adv Drug Saf.* 2015;6(2):45-56.

16. Dignam JJ, Wieand K, Johnson KA, Fisher B, Xu L, Mamounas EP. Obesity, tamoxifen sse, and outcomes in women with estrogen receptor-positive early-stage breast cancer. *J Natl Cancer Inst.* 2003;95(19):1467-1476.

17. Eliassen A, Colditz GA, Rosner B, Willett WC, Hankinson SE. Adult weight change and risk of postmenopausal breast cancer. *JAMA.* 2006;296(2):193-201.

18. Ewertz M, Jensen M-B, Gunnarsdóttir KÁ, et al. Effect of besity on prognosis after early-stage breast cancer. *J Clin Oncol.* 2011;29(1):25-31.

19. Hancock SL, Tucker MA, Hoppe RT. Breast cancer after treatment of Hodgkin's disease. *J Natl Cancer Inst.* 1993;85(1):25-31.

20. Hill DA, Gilbert E, Dores GM, et al. Breast cancer risk following radiotherapy for Hodgkin lymphoma: modification by other risk factors. *Blood.* 2005;106(10):3358-3365.

21. Pharoah PD, Antoniou AC, Easton DF, Ponder BA. Polygenes, risk prediction, and targeted prevention of breast cancer. *N Engl J Med.* 2008;358(26):2796-2803.

22. White AJ, DeRoo LA, Weinberg CR, Sandler DP. Lifetime alcohol intake, binge drinking behaviors, and breast cancer risk. *Am J Epidemiol.* 2017;186(5):541-549.

23. Yang XR, Chang-Claude J, Goode EL, et al. Associations of breast cancer risk factors with tumor subtypes: a pooled analysis from the Breast Cancer Association Consortium studies. *J Natl Cancer Inst.* 2011;103(3):250-263.

24. Zhang SM, Lee IM, Manson JE, Cook NR, Willett WC, Buring JE. Alcohol consumption and breast cancer risk in the Women's Health Study. *Am J Epidemiol.* 2007;165(6):667-676.

25. Oeffinger KC, Fontham ET, Etzioni R, et al; American Cancer Society. Breast cancer screening for women at average risk: 2015 guideline update from the American Cancer Society. *JAMA.* 2015;314(15):1599-1614. Erratum in: *JAMA.* 2016;315(13):1406.

26. NCCN Clinical Practice Guidelines in Oncology. *Breast Cancer Screening and Diagnosis.* Version 3.2018. October 4, 2018. www.nccn.org/professionals/physician_gls/pdf/breast-screening.pdf. Accessed July 3, 2019.

27. Siu AL; US Preventive Services Task Force. Screening for breast cancer: US Preventive Services Task Force recommendation statement. *Ann Intern Med.* 2016;164(4):279-296. Erratum in: *Ann Intern Med.* 2016;164(6):448.

28. Kriege M, Brekelmans CT, Boetes C, et al. Efficacy of MRI and mammography for breast-cancer screening in women with a familial or genetic predisposition. *N Engl J Med.* 2004;351(5):427-437.

29. Plevritis SK, Kurian AW, Sigal BM, et al. Cost-effectiveness of screening *BRCA1/2* mutation carriers with breast magnetic resonance imaging. *JAMA.* 2006;295(20):2374-2384.

30. Phi XA, Saadatmand S, De Bock GH, et al. Contribution of mammography to MRI screening in *BRCA* mutation carriers by *BRCA* status and age: individual patient data meta-analysis. *Br J Cancer.* 2016;114(6):631-637.

31. Fisher B, Anderson S, Bryant J, et al. Twenty-year follow-up of a randomized trial comparing total mastectomy, lumpectomy, and lumpectomy plus irradiation for the treatment of invasive breast cancer. *N Engl J Med.* 2002;347(16):1233-1241.

32. Cao JQ, Olson RA, Tyldesley SK. Comparison of recurrence and survival rates after breast-conserving therapy and mastectomy in young women with breast cancer. *Curr Oncol.* 2013;20(6):e593-e601.

33. Dowsett M, Sestak I, Lopez-Knowles E, et al. Comparison of PAM50 risk of recurrence score with oncotype DX and IHC4 for predicting risk of distant recurrence after endocrine therapy. *J Clin Oncol.* 2013;31(22):2783-2790.

34. Sparano JA, Gray RJ, Makower DF, et al. Adjuvant chemotherapy guided by a 21-gene expression assay in breast cancer. *N Engl J Med.* 2018;379(2):111-121.

35. Giuliano AE, Connolly JL, Edge SB, et al. Breast cancer—major changes in the American Joint Committee on Cancer eighth edition cancer staging manual. *CA Cancer J Clin.* 2017;67(4):290-303. Erratum in: *CA Cancer J Clin.* 2017;67(4).345.

36. Blum JL, Flynn PJ, Yothers G, et al. Anthracyclines in early breast cancer: the ABC trials—USOR 06-090, NSABP B-46-I/USOR 07132, and NSABP B-49 (NRG oncology). *J Clin Oncol.* 2017;35(23):2647-2655.

37. Tolaney SM, Barry WT, Dang CT, et al. A phase II study of adjuvant paclitaxel (T) and trastuzumab (H) (APT trial) for node-negative, HER2-positive breast cancer (BC) [abstract]. *Cancer Res.* 2013;73(24 suppl). Abstract S1-04.

38. Romond EH, Perez EA, Bryant J, et al. Trastuzumab plus adjuvant chemotherapy for operable HER2-positive breast cancer. *N Engl J Med.* 2005;353(16):1673-1684.

39. Piccart-Gebhart MJ, Procter M, Leyland-Jones B, et al; Herceptin Adjuvant (HERA) Trial Study Team. Trastuzumab after adjuvant chemotherapy in HER2-positive breast cancer. *N Engl J Med.* 2005;353(16):1659-1672.

40. Mamounas EP, Anderson SJ, Dignam JJ, et al. Predictors of locoregional recurrence after neoadjuvant chemotherapy: results from combined analysis of national surgical adjuvant breast and bowel project B-18 and B-27. *J Clin Oncol.* 2012;30(32):3960-3966.

41. Fisher B, Bryant J, Wolmark N, et al. Effect of preoperative chemotherapy on the outcome of women with operable breast cancer. *J Clin Oncol.* 1998;16(8):2672-2685.

42. Fisher B, Brown A, Mamounas E, et al. Effect of preoperative chemotherapy on local-regional disease in women with operable breast cancer: findings from National Surgical Adjuvant Breast and Bowel Project B-18. *J Clin Oncol.* 1997;15(7):2483-2493.

43. Schneeweiss A, Chia S, Hickish T, et al. Pertuzumab plus trastuzumab in combination with standard neoadjuvant anthracycline-containing and anthracycline-free chemotherapy regimens in patients with HER2-positive early breast cancer: a randomized phase II cardiac safety study (TRYPHAENA). *Ann Oncol.* 2013;24(9):2278-2284.

44. Gianni L, Pienkowski T, Im YH, et al. Efficacy and safety of neoadjuvant pertuzumab and trastuzumab in women with locally advanced, inflammatory, or early HER2-positive breast cancer (NeoSphere): a randomised multicentre, open-label, phase 2 trial. *Lancet Oncol.* 2012;13(1):25-32.

45. von Minckwitz G, Huang CS, Mano MS, et al; KATHERINE Investigators. Tratsuzumab emtansine for residual invasive HER2-positive breast cancer. *New Engl J Med.* 2019;380(7):617-628.

46. Decker MR, Greenblatt DY, Havlena J, Wilke LG, Greenberg CC, Neuman HB. Impact of neoadjuvant chemotherapy on wound complications after breast surgery. *Surgery.* 2012;152(3):382-388.

47. Davies C, Pan H, Godwin J, Gray R, Peto R; ATLAS Collaborators Worldwide. ATLAS—10 v 5 years of adjuvant tamoxifen (TAM) in ER+ disease: effects on outcome in the first and in the second decade after diagnosis [abstract]. *Cancer Res.* 2012;72(24 suppl):89s. Abstract S1-2.

48. Burstein HJ, Temin S, Anderson H, et al. Adjuvant endocrine therapy for women with hormone receptor-positive breast cancer: American Society of Clinical Oncology Clinical Practice Guideline focused update. *J Clin Oncol.* 2014;32(21):2255-2269.

49. Davies C, Pan H, Godwin J, et al; Longer Against Shorter (ATLAS) Collaborative Group. Long-term effects of continuing adjuvant tamoxifen to 10 years versus stopping at 5 years after diagnosis of oestrogen receptor-positive breast cancer: ATLAS, a randomised trial. *Lancet.* 2013;381(9869):805-816.

50. Al-Mubarak M, Tibau A, Templeton AJ, et al. Extended adjuvant tamoxifen for early breast cancer: a meta-analysis. *PLoS One.* 2014;9(2):e88238.

51. Swain SM, Jeong JH, Geyer CE Jr, et al. Longer therapy, iatrogenic amenorrhea, and survival in early breast cancer. *N Engl J Med.* 2010;362(22):2053-2065.

52. Swain SM, Jeong JH, Wolmark N. Amenorrhea from breast cancer therapy—not a matter of dose. *N Engl J Med.* 2010;363(23):2268-2270.

53. Yang J, Neugut AI, Wright JD, Accordino M, Hershman DL. Nonadherence to oral medications for chronic conditions in breast cancer survivors. *J Oncol Pract.* 2016;12(8):e800-e809.

54. Colzani E, Liljegren A, Johansson AL, et al. Prognosis of patients with breast cancer: causes of death and effects of time since diagnosis, age, and tumor characteristics. *J Clin Oncol.* 2011;29(30):4014-4021.

55. Bordeleau L, Pritchard KI, Loprinzi CL, et al. Multicenter, randomized, cross-over clinical trial of venlafaxine versus gabapentin for the management of hot flashes in breast cancer survivors. *J Clin Oncol.* 2010;28(35):5147-5152.

56. Loprinzi CL, Kugler JW, Barton DL, et al. Phase III trial of gabapentin alone or in conjunction with an antidepressant in the management of hot flashes in women who have inadequate control with an antidepressant alone: NCCTG N03C5. *J Clin Oncol.* 2007;25(3):308-312.

57. Mortimer JE. Managing the toxicities of the aromatase inhibitors. *Curr Opin Obstet Gynecol.* 2010;22(1):56-60.

58. Crew KD, Greenlee H, Capodice J, et al. Prevalence of joint symptoms in postmenopausal women taking aromatase inhibitors for early-stage breast cancer. *J Clin Oncol.* 2007;25(25):3877-3883.

59. Niravath P. Aromatase inhibitor-induced arthralgia: a review. *Ann Oncol.* 2013;24(6):1443-1449.

60. Morales L, Pans S, Verschueren K, et al. Prospective study to assess short-term intra-articular and tenosynovial changes in the aromatase inhibitor-associated arthralgia syndrome. *J Clin Oncol.* 2008;26(19):3147-3152.

61. Sestak I, Sapunar F, Cuzick J. Aromatase inhibitor-induced carpal tunnel syndrome: results from the ATAC trial. *J Clin Oncol.* 2009;27(30):4961-4965.

62. Dhesy-Thind S, Fletcher GG, Blanchette PS, et al. Use of adjuvant bisphosphonates and other bone-modifying agents in breast cancer: a cancer care Ontario and American Society of Clinical Oncology clinical practice guideline. *J Clinl Oncol.* 2017;35(18):2062-2081.

63. Coleman R, Bundred N, Boer RD, et al. Impact of zoledronic acid in postmenopausal women with early breast cancer receiving adjuvant letrozole: Z-FAST, ZO-FAST, and E-ZO-FAST [abstract]. *Cancer Res.* 2009;69(24 suppl). Abstract 4082.

64. Early Breast Cancer Trialists' Collaborative Group (EBCTCG). Adjuvant bisphosphonate treatment in early breast cancer: meta-analyses of individual patient data from randomised trials. *Lancet.* 2015;386(10001):1353-1361. Erratum in: *Lancet.* 2016;387(10013):30.

65. Abdel-Qadir H, Austin PC, Lee DS, et al. A population-based study of cardiovascular mortality following early-stage breast cancer. *JAMA Cardiol.* 2017;2(1):88-93.

66. Goldvaser H, Barnes TA, Šeruga B, et al. Toxicity of extended adjuvant therapy with aromatase inhibitors in early breast cancer: a systematic review and meta-analysis. *J Natl Cancer Inst.* 2018;110(1):djx141.

67. Committee Opinion No. 601: Tomoxifen and uterine cancer. *Obstet Gynecol.* 2014;123(6):1394-1397.

68. Oberguggenberger A, Martini C, Huber N, et al. Self-reported sexual health: breast cancer survivors compared to women from the general population—an observational study. *BMC Cancer.* 2017;17(1):599.

69. Juliato PT, Rodrigues AT, Stahlschmidt R, Juliato CRT, Mazzola PG. Can polyacrylic acid treat sexual dysfunction in women with breast cancer receiving tamoxifen? *Climacteric.* 2017;20(1):62-66.

70. Goetsch MF, Lim JY, Caughey AB. Locating pain in breast cancer survivors experiencing dyspareunia: a randomized controlled trial. *Obstet Gynecol.* 2014;123(6):1231-1236.

71. Le Ray I, Dell'Aniello S, Bonnetain F, Azoulay L, Suissa S. Local estrogen therapy and risk of breast cancer recurrence among hormone-treated patients: a nested case-control study. *Breast Cancer Res Treat.* 2012;135(2):603-609.

72. O'Meara ES, Rossing MA, Daling JR, Elmore JG, Barlow WE, Weiss NS. Hormone replacement therapy after a diagnosis of breast cancer in relation to recurrence and mortality. *J Natl Cancer Inst.* 2001;93(10):754-761.

73. Committee on Practice Bulletins-Gynecology. Practice Bulletin No. 126: Management of gynecologic issues in women with breast cancer. *Obstet Gynecol.* 2012;119(3):666-682.

74. Caan BJ, Kwan ML, Weltzien E, et al. Weight gain after a breast cancer diagnosis and breast cancer outcomes [abstract]. *Cancer Res.* 2011; 71(8 suppl). Abstract 3722.

75. Dieli-Conwright CM, Wong L, Waliany S, Bernstein L, Salehian B, Mortimer JE. An observational study to examine changes in metabolic syndrome components in breast cancer patients receiving neoadjuvant or adjuvant chemotherapy. *Cancer.* 2016;122(17):2646-2653.

76. Demark-Wahnefried W, Peterson BL, Winer EP, et al. Changes in weight, body composition, and factors influencing energy balance among premenopausal breast cancer patients receiving adjuvant chemotherapy. *J Clin Oncol.* 2001;19(9):2381-2389.

77. Moyer VA; US Preventive Services Task Force. Screening for lung cancer: US Preventive Services Task Force recommendation statement. *Ann Intern Med.* 2014;160(5):330-338.

78. US Preventive Services Task Force; Bibbins-Domingo K, Grossman DC, et al. Screening for colorectal cancer: US Preventive Services Task Force recommendation statement. *JAMA.* 2016;315(23):2564-2575. Erratum in: *JAMA.* 2016;315(5):545; *JAMA.* 2017;317(21):2239.

79. Gail MH, Brinton LA, Byar DP, et al. Projecting individualized probabilities of developing breast cancer for white females who are being examined annually. *J Natl Cancer Inst.* 1989;81(24):1879-1886.

80. Boggs DA, Rosenberg L, Adams-Campbell LL, Palmer JR. Prospective approach to breast cancer risk prediction in African American women: the black women's health study model. *J Clin Oncol.* 2015;33(9):1038-1044.

81. Kuchenbaecker KB, Hopper JL, Barnes DR, et al. Risks of breast, ovarian, and contralateral breast cancer for *BRCA1* and *BRCA2* mutation carriers. *JAMA.* 2017;317(23):2402-2416.

82. Rebbeck TR, Kauff ND, Domchek SM. Meta-analysis of risk reduction estimates associated with risk-reducing salpingo-oophorectomy in *BRCA1* or *BRCA2* mutation carriers. *J Natl Cancer Inst.* 2009;101(2):80-87.

83. Rebbeck TR, Lynch HT, Neuhausen SL, et al; Prevention and Observation of Surgical End Points Study Group. Prophylactic oophorectomy in carriers of BRCA1 or BRCA2 mutations. N Engl J Med. 2002;346(21):1616-1622.

84. Kauff ND, Satagopan JM, Robson ME, et al. Risk-reducing salpingo-oophorectomy in women with a BRCA1 or BRCA2 mutation. N Engl J Med. 2002;346(21):1609-1615.

85. American Society of Clinical Oncology Clinical Practice Guideline Update on the use of pharmacologic interventions including tamoxifen, raloxifene, and aromatase inhibition for breast cancer risk reduction. J Oncol Pract. 2009;5(4):196-199.

86. Coopey SB, Mazzola E, Buckley JM, et al. The role of chemoprevention in modifying the risk of breast cancer in women with atypical breast lesions. Breast Cancer Res Treat.2012;136(3):627-633.

87. King M, Wieand S, Hale K, et al; National Surgical Adjuvant Breast and Bowel Project. Tamoxifen and breast cancer incidence among women with inherited mutations in BRCA1 and BRCA2: National Surgical Adjuvant Breast and Bowel Project (NSABP-P1) Breast Cancer Prevention Trial. JAMA. 2001;286(18):2251-2256.

88. Vogel VG, Costantino JP, Wickerham DL, et al; National Surgical Adjuvant Breast and Bowel Project (NSABP). Effects of tamoxifen vs raloxifene on the risk of developing invasive breast cancer and other disease outcomes: the NSABP Study of Tamoxifen and Raloxifene (STAR) P-2 trial. JAMA. 2006;295(23):2727-2741.

89. Goss PE, Ingle JN, Alés-Martínez JE, et al; NCIC CTG MAP.3 Study Investigators. Exemestane for breast-cancer prevention in postmenopausal women. N Engl J Med. 2011;364(25):2381-2391. Erratum in: N Engl J Med. 2011;365(14):1361.

90. Cuzick J, Sestak I, Forbes JF, et al; IBIS-II Investigators. Anastrozole for prevention of breast cancer in high-risk postmenopausal women (IBIS-II): an international, double-blind, randomised placebo-controlled trial. Lancet. 2014;383(9922):1041-1048. Erratum in: Lancet. 2014;383(9922):1040.

91. American Cancer Society. Key Statistics for Endometrial Cancer. Last revised January 4, 2018. www.cancer.org/cancer/endometrial-cancer/about/key-statistics.html. Accessed July 3, 2019.

92. Siegel RL, Miller KD, Jemal A. Cancer statistics, 2017. CA: Cancer J Clin. 2017;67(1):7-30.

93. Yap OW, Matthews RP. Racial and ethnic disparities in cancers of the uterine corpus. J Natl Med Assoc. 2006;98(12):1930-1933.

94. Martin JY, Schiff MA, Weiss NS, Urban RR. Racial disparities in the utilization of preventive health services among older women with early-stage endometrial cancer enrolled in Medicare. Cancer Med. 2017;6(9):2153-2163.

95. Rauh-Hain JA, Melamed A, Schaps D, et al. Racial and ethnic disparities over time in the treatment and mortality of women with gynecological malignancies. Gynecol Oncol. 2018;149(1):4-11.

96. Doll KM, Winn AN, Goff BA. Untangling the black-white mortality gap in endometrial cancer: a cohort simulation. Am J Obstet Gynecol. 2017;216(3):324-325.

97. Hensley ML, Barrette BA, Baumann K, et al. Gynecologic Cancer InterGroup (GCIG) consensus review: uterine and ovarian leiomyosarcomas. Int J Gynecol Cancer. 2014;24(9 suppl 3):561-566.

98. Bokhman JV. Two pathogenetic types of endometrial carcinoma. Gynecol Oncol. 1983;15(1):10-17.

99. Creasman W. Revised FIGO staging for carcinoma of the endometrium. Int J Gynaecol Obstet. 2009;105(2):109.

100. Levine RL, Cargile CB, Blazes MS, van Rees B, Kurman RJ, Ellenson LH. PTEN mutations and microsatellite instability in complex atypical hyperplasia, a precursor lesion to uterine endometrioid carcinoma. Cancer Res. 1998;58(15):3254-3258.

101. Emons G, Fleckenstein G, Hinney B, Huschmand A, Heyl W. Hormonal interactions in endometrial cancer. Endocr Relat Cancer. 2000;7(4):227-242.

102. Clement PB, Young RH. Non-endometrioid carcinomas of the uterine corpus: a review of their pathology with emphasis on recent advances and problematic aspects. Adv Anat Pathol. 2004;11(3):117-142.

103. Amant F, Moerman P, Neven P, Timmerman D, Van Limbergen E, Vergote I. Endometrial cancer. Lancet. 2005;366(9484):491-505.

104. Hamilton CA, Cheung MK, Osann K, et al. Uterine papillary serous and clear cell carcinomas predict for poorer survival compared to grade 3 endometrioid corpus cancers. Br J Cancer. 2006;94(5):642-646.

105. Leslie KK, Thiel KW, Goodheart MJ, De Geest K, Jia Y, Yang S. Endometrial cancer. Obstet Gynecol Clin North Am. 2012; 39(2):255-268.

106. Talhouk A, McAlpine JN. New classification of endometrial cancers: the development and potential applications of genomic-based classification in research and clinical care. Gynecol Oncol Res Pract. 2016;3:14.

107. Merisio C, Berretta R, De Ioris A, et al. Endometrial cancer in patients with preoperative diagnosis of atypical endometrial hyperplasia. Eur J Obstet Gynecol Reprod Biol. 2005;122(1):107-111.

108. Lacey JV Jr, Ioffe OB, Ronnett BM, et al. Endometrial carcinoma risk among women diagnosed with endometrial hyperplasia: the 34-year experience in a large health plan. Br J Cancer. 2008;98(1):45-53.

109. Lacey JV Jr, Sherman ME, Rush BB, et al. Absolute risk of endometrial carcinoma during 20-year follow-up among women with endometrial hyperplasia. J Clin Oncol. 2010;28(5):788-792.

110. Mariani A, Dowdy SC, Keeney GL, Long HJ, Lesnick TG, Podratz KC. High-risk endometrial cancer subgroups: candidates for target-based adjuvant therapy. Gynecol Oncol. 2004;95(1):120-126.

111. Felix AS, Weissfeld JL, Stone RA, et al. Factors associated with type I and type II endometrial cancer. Cancer Causes Control. 2010;21(11):1851-1856.

112. Morice P, Leary A, Creutzberg C, Abu-Rustum N, Darai E. Endometrial cancer. Lancet. 2016;387(10023):1094-1108.

113. Setiawan VW, Yang HP, Pike MC, et al. Type I and II endometrial cancers: have they different risk factors? J Clin Oncol. 2013;31(20):2607-2618.

114. Matsuzaki S, Fukaya T, Suzuki T, Murakami T, Sasano H, Yajima A. Oestrogen receptor alpha and beta mRNA expression in human endometrium throughout the menstrual cycle. Mol Hum Reprod. 1999;5(6):559-564.

115. Deroo BJ, Korach KS. Estrogen receptors and human disease. J Clin Invest. 2006;116(3):561-570.

116. Mishra GD, Cooper R, Tom SE, Kuh D. Early life circumstances and their impact on menarche and menopause. Womens Health (Lond). 2009;5(2):175-190.

117. Setiawan VW, Pike MC, Karageorgi S, et al; Australian National Endometrial Cancer Study Group. Age at last birth in relation to risk of endometrial cancer: pooled analysis in the Epidemiology of Endometrial Cancer Consortium. Am J Epidemiol. 2012;176(4):269-278.

118. Pocobelli G, Doherty JA, Voigt LF, et al. Pregnancy history and risk of endometrial cancer. Epidemiology. 2011;22(5):638-645.

119. Phipps AI, Doherty JA, Voigt LF, et al. Long-term use of continuous-combined estrogen-progestin hormone therapy and risks of endometrial cancer. Cancer Causes Control. 2011;22(12):1639-1646.

120. Weiderpass E, Brismar K, Bellocco R, Vainio H, Kaaks R. Serum levels of insulin-like growth factor-I, IGF-binding protein 1 and 3, and insulin and endometrial cancer risk. Br J Cancer. 2003;89(9):1697-1704.

121. Hill DA, Weiss NS, Beresford SA, et al. Continuous combined hormone replacement therapy and risk of endometrial cancer. Am J Obstet Gynecol. 2000;183(6):1456-1461.

122. Shang Y, Brown M. Molecular determinants for the tissue specificity of SERMs. Science. 2002;295(5564):2465-2468.

123. Polin SA, Ascher SM. The effect of tamoxifen on the genital tract. Cancer Imaging. 2008;8(1):135-145.

124. DeMichele A, Troxel AB, Berlin JA, et al. Impact of raloxifene or tamoxifen use on endometrial cancer risk: a population-based case-control study. J Clin Oncol. 2008;26(25):4151-4159.

125. Bulun SE, Chen D, Lu M, et al. Aromatase excess in cancers of breast, endometrium and ovary. J Steroid Biochem Mol Biol. 2007;106(1-5):81-96.

126. Wedrén S, Lovmar L, Humphreys K, et al. Estrogen receptor alpha gene polymorphism and endometrial cancer risk—a case-control study. BMC Cancer. 2008;8:322.

127. Lucenteforte E, Bosetti C, Talamini R, et al. Diabetes and endometrial cancer: effect modification by body weight, physical activity and hypertension. Br J Cancer. 2007;97(7):995-998.

128. Doll A, Abal M, Rigau M, et al. Novel molecular profiles of endometrial cancer—new light through old windows. *J Steroid Biochem Mol Biol.* 2008;108(3-5):221-229.

129. Lagarda H, Catasus L, Arguelles R, Matias-Guiu X, Prat J. K-ras mutations in endometrial carcinomas with microsatellite instability. *J Pathol.* 2001;193(2):193-199.

130. Scholten AN, Creutzberg CL, van den Broek LJ, Noordijk EM, Smit VT. Nuclear beta-catenin is a molecular feature of type I endometrial carcinoma. *J Pathol.* 2003;201(3):460-465.

131. Hinkula M, Pukkala E, Kyyrönen P, Kauppila A. Grand multiparity and incidence of endometrial cancer: a population-based study in Finland. *Int J Cancer.* 2002;98(6):912-915.

132. Li X, Qi X, Zhou L, et al. P2X(7) receptor expression is decreased in epithelial cancer cells of ectodermal, uro-genital sinus, and distal paramesonephric-duct origin. *Purinergic Signal.* 2009;5(3):351-368.

133. Czarnecka AM, Klemba A, Semczuk A, et al. Common mitochondrial polymorphisms as risk factor for endometrial cancer. *Int Arch Med.* 2009;2(1):33.

134. Himbert C, Delphan M, Scherer D, Bowers LW, Hursting S, Ulrich CM. Signals from the adipose microenvironment and the obesity-cancer link-a systematic review. *Cancer Prev Res (Phila).* 2017;10(9):494-506.

135. Allen NE, Key TJ, Dossus L, et al. Endogenous sex hormones and endometrial cancer risk in women in the European Prospective Investigation into Cancer and Nutrition (EPIC). *Endocr Relat Cancer.* 2008;15(2):485-497.

136. Calle EE, Kaaks R. Overweight, obesity and cancer: epidemiological evidence and proposed mechanisms. *Nat Rev Cancer.* 2004;4(8):579-591.

137. Lu L, Risch H, Irwin ML, et al. Long-term overweight and weight gain in early adulthood in association with risk of endometrial cancer. *Int J Cancer.* 2011;129(5):1237-1243.

138. Anveden Å, Taube M, Peltonen M, et al. Long-term incidence of female-specific cancer after bariatric surgery or usual care in the Swedish Obese Subjects Study. *Gynecol Oncol.* 2017;145(2):224-119.

139. Winder AA, Kularatna M, MacCormick AD. Does bariatric surgery affect the incidence of endometrial cancer development? A systematic review. *Obesity Surg.* 2018;28(5):1433-1440.

140. Furberg AS, Thune I. Metabolic abnormalities (hypertension, hyperglycemia and overweight), lifestyle (high energy intake and physical inactivity) and endometrial cancer risk in a Norwegian cohort. *Int J Cancer.* 2003;104(6):669-676. Erratum in: *Int J Cancer.* 2003;104(6):799.

141. Augustin LS, Dal Maso L, Franceschi S, et al. Association between components of the insulin-like growth factor system and endometrial cancer risk. *Oncology.* 2004;67(1):54-59.

142. Friberg E, Mantzoros CS, Wolk A. Diabetes and risk of endometrial cancer: a population-based prospective cohort study. *Cancer Epidemiol Biomarkers Prev.* 2007;16(2):276-280.

143. Moore SC, Gierach GL, Schatzkin A, Matthews CE. Physical activity, sedentary behaviours, and the prevention of endometrial cancer. *Br J Cancer.* 2010;103(7):933-938.

144. Arem H, Irwin ML, Zhou Y, Lu L, Risch H, Yu H. Physical activity and endometrial cancer in a population-based case-control study. *Cancer Causes Control.* 2011;22(2):219-226.

145. Seger HM, Soisson AP, Dodson MK, Rowe KG, Cannon-Albright LA. Familial clustering of endometrial cancer in a well-defined population. *Gynecol Oncol.* 2011;122(1):75-78.

146. Johnatty SE, Tan YY, Buchanan DD, et al. Family history of cancer predicts endometrial cancer risk independently of Lynch syndrome: implications for genetic counselling. *Gynecol Oncol.* 2017;147(2):381-387.

147. Kopciuk KA, Choi YH, Parkhomenko E, et al. Penetrance of HNPCC-related cancers in retrolective cohort of 12 large Newfoundland families carrying a MSH3 founder mutation: an evaluation using modified segregation models. *Hered Cancer Clin Pract.* 2009;7(1):16.

148. Wang Y, Wang Y, Li J, et al. Lynch syndrome related endometrial cancer: clinical significance beyond the endometrium. *J Hematol Oncol.* 2013;6:22.

149. Gayther SA, Pharoah PD. The inherited genetics of ovarian and endometrial cancer. *Curr Opin Genet Dev.* 2010;20(3):231-238.

150. Tan MH, Mester JL, Ngeow J, Rybicki LA, Orloff MS, Eng C. Lifetime cancer risks in individuals with germline *PTEN* mutations. *Clin Cancer Res.* 2012;18(2):400-407.

151. Setiawan VW, Monroe KR, Goodman MT, Kolonel LN, Pike MC, Henderson BE. Alcohol consumption and endometrial cancer risk: the multiethnic cohort. *Int J Cancer.* 2008;122(3):634-638.

152. Viswanathan AN, Feskanich D, De Vivo I, et al. Smoking and the risk of endometrial cancer: results from the Nurses' Health Study. *Int J Cancer.* 2005;114(6):996-1001.

153. Cui X, Rosner B, Willett WC, Hankinson SE. Antioxidant intake and risk of endometrial cancer: results from the Nurses' Health Study. *Int J Cancer.* 2011;128(5):1169-1178.

154. Burbos N, Musonda P, Giarenis I, et al. Age-related differential diagnosis of vaginal bleeding in postmenopausal women: a series of 3047 symptomatic postmenopausal women. *Menopause Int.* 2010;16(1):5-8.

155. Creasman WT, Morrow CP, Bundy BN, Homesley HD, Graham JE, Heller PB. Surgical pathologic spread patterns of endometrial cancer. A Gynecologic Oncology Group study. *Cancer.* 1987;60 (8 suppl):2035-2041.

156. Horn LC, Schnurrbusch U, Bilek K, Hentschel B, Einenkel J. Risk of progression in complex and atypical endometrial hyperplasia: clinicopathologic analysis in cases with and without progestogen treatment. *Int J Gynecol Cancer.* 2004;14(2):348-353.

157. Lai CH, Huang HJ. The role of hormones for the treatment of endometrial hyperplasia and endometrial cancer. *Curr Opin Obstet Gynecol.* 2006;18(1):29-34.

158. Gallos ID, Ganesan R, Gupta JK. Prediction of regression and relapse of endometrial hyperplasia with conservative therapy. *Obstet Gynecol.* 2013;121(6):1165-1171.

159. Wei J, Zhang W, Feng L, Gao W. Comparison of fertility-sparing treatments in patients with early endometrial cancer and atypical complex hyperplasia: a meta-analysis and systematic review. *Medicine (Baltimore).* 2017;96(37):e8034.

160. Randall TC, Kurman RJ. Progestin treatment of atypical hyperplasia and well-differentiated carcinoma of the endometrium in women under age 40. *Obstet Gynecol.* 1997;90(3):434-440.

161. Suh-Burgmann E, Hung YY, Armstrong MA. Complex atypical endometrial hyperplasia: the risk of unrecognized adenocarcinoma and value of preoperative dilation and curettage. *Obstet Gynecol.* 2009;114(3):523-529.

162. Chiva L, Lapuente F, González-Cortijo L, et al. Sparing fertility in young patients with endometrial cancer. *Gynecol Oncol.* 2008; 111(2 suppl):S101-S104.

163. Reed SD, Voigt LF, Newton KM, et al. Progestin therapy of complex endometrial hyperplasia with and without atypia. *Obstet Gynecol.* 2009;113(3):655-662.

164. Mariani A, Dowdy SC, Cliby WA, et al. Prospective assessment of lymphatic dissemination in endometrial cancer: a paradigm shift in surgical staging. *Gynecol Oncol.* 2008;109(1):11-18.

165. Frumovitz M, Slomovitz BM, Singh DK, et al. Frozen section analyses as predictors of lymphatic spread in patients with early-stage uterine cancer. *J Am Coll Surg.* 2004;199(3):388-393.

166. Cragun JM, Havrilesky LJ, Calingaert B, et al. Retrospective analysis of selective lymphadenectomy in apparent early-stage endometrial cancer. *J Clin Oncol.* 2005;23(16):3668-3675.

167. Case AS, Rocconi RP, Straughn JM Jr, et al. A prospective blinded evaluation of the accuracy of frozen section for the surgical management of endometrial cancer. *Obstet Gynecol.* 2006; 108(6):1375-1379.

168. Chan JK, Wu H, Cheung MK, Shin JY, Osann K, Kapp DS. The outcomes of 27,063 women with unstaged endometrioid uterine cancer. *Gynecol Oncol.* 2007;106(2):282-288.

169. Benedetti Panici P, Basile S, Maneschi F, et al. Systematic pelvic lymphadenectomy vs. no lymphadenectomy in early-stage endometrial carcinoma: randomized clinical trial. *J Natl Cancer Inst.* 2008;100(23):1707-1716.

170. Keys HM, Roberts JA, Brunetto VL, et al; Gynecologic Oncology Group. A phase III trial of surgery with or without adjunctive external pelvic radiation therapy in intermediate risk endometrial adenocarcinoma: a Gynecologic Oncology Group study. *Gynecol Oncol.* 2004;92(3):744-751. Erratum in: *Gynecol Oncol.* 2004;94(1):241-242.

171. ASTEC/EN.5 Study Group, Blake P, Swart AM, et al. Adjuvant external beam radiotherapy in the treatment of endometrial cancer (MRC ASTEC and NCIC CTG EN.5 randomized trials): pooled trial results, systematic review, and meta-analysis. *Lancet.* 2009;373(9658):137-146.

172. Nout RA, Smit VT, Putter H, et al; PORTEC Study Group. Vaginal brachytherapy versus pelvic external beam radiotherapy for patients with endometrial cancer of high-intermediate risk (PORTEC-2): an open-label, non-inferiority, randomised trial. *Lancet.* 2010;375(9717):816-823.

173. Nout RA, Putter H, Jürgenliemk-Schulz IM, et al. Quality of life after pelvic radiotherapy or vaginal brachytherapy for endometrial cancer: first results of the randomized PORTEC-2 trial. *J Clin Oncol.* 2009;27(21):3547-3456.

174. Bestvina CM, Fleming GF. Chemotherapy for endometrial cancer in adjuvant and advanced disease settings. *Oncologist.* 2016;21(10):1250-1259.

175. Barakat RR, Bundy BN, Spirtos NM, Bell J, Mannel RS; Gynecologic Oncology Group Study. Randomized double-blind trial of estrogen replacement therapy versus placebo in stage I or II endometrial cancer: a Gynecologic Oncology Group Study. *J Clin Oncol.* 2006;24(4):587-592.

176. Suriano KA, McHale M, McLaren CE, Li KT, Re A, DiSaia PJ. Estrogen replacement therapy in endometrial cancer patients: a matched control study. *Obstet Gynecol.* 2001;97(4):555-560.

177. Reid RL. Progestins in hormone replacement therapy: impact on endometrial and breast cancer. *J SOGC.* 2000;22(9):677-681.

178. Del Carmen MG, Rice LW. Management of menopausal symptoms in women with gynecologic cancers. *Gynecol Oncol.* 2017;146(2):427-435.

179. Anderson GL, Judd HL, Kaunitz AM, et al; Women's Health Initiative Investigators. Effects of estrogen plus progestin on gynecologic cancers and associated diagnostic procedures: the Women's Health Initiative randomized trial. *JAMA.* 2003;290(13):1739-1748.

180. Ferlay J, Soerjomataram I, Dikshit R, et al. Cancer incidence and mortality worldwide: sources, methods and major patterns in GLOBOCAN 2012. *Int J Cancer.* 2015;136(5):E359-E386.

181. Durson P, Gultekin M, Bozdag G, et al. Primary cervical lymphoma: report of two cases and review of the literature. *Gynecol Oncol.* 2005;98(3):484-489.

182. Wright JD, Rosenblum K, Huettner PC, et al. Cervical sarcomas: an analysis of incidence and outcome. *Gynecol Oncol.* 2005;99(2):348-351.

183. Tempfer CB, Tischoff I, Dogan A, et al. Neuroendocrine carcinoma of the cervix: a systematic review of the literature. *BMC Cancer.* 2018;18(1):530.

184. Plummer M, Schiffman M, Castle PE, Maucort-Boulch D, Wheeler CM; ALTS Group. A 2-year prospective study of human papillomavirus persistence among women with a cytological diagnosis of atypical squamous cells of undetermined significance or low-grade squamous intraepithelial lesion. *J Infect Dis.* 2007;195(11):1582-1589.

185. Schiffman M, Castle PE, Jeronimo J, Rodriguez AC, Wacholder S. Human papillomavirus and cervical cancer. *Lancet.* 2007;370(9590):890-907.

186. Watson RA. Human papillomavirus: confronting the epidemic—a urologist's perspective. *Rev Urol.* 2005;7(3):135-144.

187. Woodman CB, Collins S, Winter H, et al. Natural history of cervical human papillomavirus infection in young women: a longitudinal cohort study. *Lancet.* 2001;357(9271):1831-1836.

188. Plummer M, Herrero R, Franceschi S, et al; IARC Multi-Centre Cervical Cancer Study Group. Smoking and cervical cancer: pooled analysis of the IARC multi-centric case-control study. *Cancer Causes Control.* 2003;14(9):805-814.

189. Bleyer WA. Cancer in older adolescents and young adults: epidemiology, diagnosis, treatment, survival, and importance of clinical trials. *Med Pediatr Oncol.* 2002;38(1):1-10.

190. Hemminki K, Chen B. Familial risks for cervical tumors in full and half siblings: etiologic apportioning. *Cancer Epidemiol Biomarkers Prev.* 2006;15(7):1413-1414.

191. Wang Q, Zhang C, Walayat S, Chen HW, Wang Y. Association between cytokine gene polymorphisms and cervical cancer in a Chinese population. *Eur J Obstet Gynecol Reprod Biol.* 2011;158(2):330-333.

192. Nguyen ML, Flowers L. Cervical cancer screening in immunocompromised women. *Obstet Gynecol Clin North Am.* 2013;40(2):339-357.

193. Dugué PA, Rebolj M, Garred P, Lynge E. Immunosuppression and risk of cervical cancer. *Expert Rev Anticancer Ther.* 2013;13(1):29-42.

194. Holcomb K, Maiman M, Dimaio T, Gates J. Rapid progression to invasive cervix cancer in a woman infected with the human immunodeficiency virus. *Obstet Gynecol.* 1998;91(5 pt 2):848-850.

195. Dobbs SP, Asmussen T, Nunns D, Hollingworth J, Brown LJ, Ireland D. Does histological incomplete excision of cervical intraepithelial neoplasia following large loop excision of transformation zone increase recurrence rates? A six-year cytological follow up. *BJOG.* 2000;107(10):1298-1301.

196. Saslow D, Solomon D, Lawson HW, et al; American Cancer Society, American Society for Colposcopy and Cervical Pathology; American Society for Clinical Pathology. American Cancer Society, American Society for Colposcopy and Cervical Pathology, and American Society for Clinical Pathology screening guidelines for the prevention and early detection of cervical cancer. *Am J Clin Path.* 2012;137(4):516-524.

197. US Preventive Services Task Force, Curry SJ, Krist AH, et al. Screening for cervical cancer: US Preventive Services Task Force recommendation statement. *JAMA.* 2018;320(7):674-686.

198. Pecorelli S, Zigliani L, Odicino F. Revised FIGO staging for carcinoma of the cervix. *Int J Gynaecol Obstet.* 2009;105(2):107-108.

199. Walboomers JM, Jacobs MV, Manos MM, et al. Human papillomavirus is a necessary cause of invasive cervical cancer worldwide. *J Pathol.* 1999;189(1):12-19.

200. Papanikolau A, Kalogiannidis I, Misailidou D, et al. Results on the treatment of uterine cervix cancer: ten years experience. *Eur J Gynaecol Oncol.* 2006;27(6):607-610.

201. Shepherd JH, Spencer C, Herod J, Ind TE. Radical vaginal trachelectomy as a fertility-sparing procedure in women with early-stage cervical cancer—cumulative pregnancy rate in a series of 123 women. *BJOG.* 2006;113(6):719-724.

202. Suprasert P, Srisomboon J, Charoenkwan K, et al. Twelve years experience with radical hysterectomy and pelvic lymphadenectomy in early stage cervical cancer. *J Obstet Gynaecol.* 2010;30(3):294-298.

203. Landoni F, Colombo A, Milani R, Placa F, Zanagnolo V, Mangioni C. Randomized study between radical surgery and radiotherapy for the treatment of stage IB-IIA cervical cancer: 20-year update. *J Gynecol Oncol.* 2017;28(3):e34.

204. Shah CA, Beck T, Liao JB, Giannakopoulos NV, Veljovich D, Paley P. Surgical and oncologic outcomes after robotic radical hysterectomy as compared to open radical hysterectomy in the treatment of early cervical cancer. *J Gynecol Oncol.* 2017;28(6):e82.

205. Obermair A, Gebski V, Frumovitz M, et al. A phase III randomized clinical trial comparing laparoscopic or robotic radical hysterectomy with abdominal radical hysterectomy in patients with early stage cervical cancer. *J Minim Invasive Gynecol.* 2008;15(5):584-588.

206. Rotman M, Sedlis A, Piedmonte MR, et al. A phase III randomized trial of postoperative pelvic irradiation in stage IB cervical carcinoma with poor prognostic features: follow-up of a gynecology oncology group study. *Int J Radiat Oncol Biol Phys.* 2006;65(1):169-176.

207. Peters WA 3rd, Liu PY, Barrett RJ 2nd, et al. Concurrent chemotherapy and pelvic radiation therapy compared with radiation therapy alone as adjuvant therapy after radical surgery in high-risk early-stage cancer of the cervix. *J Clin Oncol.* 2000;18(8):1606-1613.

208. Green JA, Kirwan JM, Tierney JF, et al. Survival and recurrence after concomitant chemotherapy and radiotherapy for cancer of the uterine cervix: a systematic review and meta-analysis. *Lancet.* 2001;358(9284):781-786.

209. Monk BJ, Tewari KS, Koh WJ. Multimodality therapy for locally advanced cervical carcinoma: state of the art and future directions. *J Clin Oncol.* 2007;25(20):2952-2965.

210. Naga CH P, Gurram L, Chopra S, Mahantshetty U. The management of locally advanced cervical cancer. *Curr Opin Oncol.* 2018;30(5):323-329.

211. Green J, Kirwan J, Tierney J, et al. Concomitant chemotherapy and radiation therapy for cancer of the uterine cervix. *Cochrane Database Syst Rev.* 2005;(3):CD002225.

212. Peiretti M, Zapardiel I, Zanagnolo V, Landoni F, Morrow CP, Maggioni A. Management of recurrent cervical cancer: a review of the literature. *Surg Oncol.* 2012;21(2):e59-e66.

213. Tewari KS, Sill MW, Long HJ 3rd, et al. Improved survival with bevacizumab in advanced cervical cancer. *N Engl J Med.* 2014; 370(8):734-743.

214. Colombo N, Carinelli S, Colombo A, Marini C, Rollo D, Sessa C; ESMO Guidelines Working Group. Cervical cancer: ESMO clinical practice guidelines for diagnosis, treatment and follow-up. *Ann Oncol.* 2012;23(suppl 7):vii27-vii32.

215. Frenel JS, Le Tourneau C, O'Neil B, et al. Safety and efficacy of pembrolizumab in advanced, programmed death ligand 1-positive cervical cancer: results from the phase Ib KEYNOTE-028 trial. *J Clin Oncol.* 2017;35)36):4035-4041.

216. de Sanjose S, Quint WG, Alemany L et al; Retrospective International Survey and HPV Time Trends Study Group. Human papillomavirus genotype attribution in invasive cervical cancer: a retrospective cross-sectional worldwide study. *Lancet Oncol.* 2010;11(11):1048-1056.

217. Clifford GM, Smith JS, Plummer M, Muñoz N, Franceschi S. Human papillomavirus types in invasive cervical cancer worldwide: a meta-analysis. *Br J Cancer.* 2003;88(1):63-73.

218. McCormack PL. Quadrivalent human papillomavirus (types 6, 11, 16, 18) recombinant vaccine (Gardasil®): a review of its use in the prevention of premalignant anogenital lesions, cervical and anal cancers, and genital warts. *Drugs.* 2014;74(11):1253-1283.

219. Niccolai LM, Julian PJ, Meek JI, McBride V, Hadler JL, Sosa LE. Declining rates of high-grade cervical lesions in young women in Connecticut, 2008-2011. *Cancer Epidemiol Biomarkers Prev.* 2013;22(8):1446-1450.

220. Petrosky E, Bocchini JA Jr, Hariri S, et al; Centers for Disease Control and Prevention (CDC). Use of 9-valent human papillomavirus (HPV) vaccine: updated HPV vaccination recommendations of the advisory committee on immunization practices. *MMWR Morb Mortal Wkly Rep.* 2015;64(11):300-304.

221. Durham DP, Ndeffo-Mbah ML, Skrip LA, Jones FK, Bauch CT, Galvani AP. National- and state-level impact and cost-effectiveness of nonavalent HPV vaccination in the United States. *Proc Natl Acad Sci U S A.* 2016;113(18):5107-5112.

222. Torre LA, Trabert B, DeSantis CE, et al. Ovarian cancer statistics, 2018. *CA Cancer J Clin.* 2018;68(4):284-296.

223. Noone AM, Howlader N, Krapcho M, et al. SEER Cancer Statistics Review, 1975-2015. April 2017. Bethesda, MD: National Cancer Institute; 2018. Updated September 10, 2018. https://seer.cancer.gov/csr/1975_2015/. Accessed July 3, 2019.

224. Kurman RJ, Carcangiu ML, Herrington CS, Young RH, eds. *WHO Classification of Tumours of Female Reproductive Organs.* Vol 6. 4th ed. Lyon, France: International Agency for Research on Cancer; 2014.

225. Corzo C, Iniesta MD, Patrono MG, Lu KH, Ramirez PT. Role of fallopian tubes in the development of ovarian cancer. *J Minim Invasive Gynecol.* 2017;24(2):230-234.

226. Daly MB, Dresher CW, Yates MS, et al. Salpingectomy as a means to reduce ovarian cancer risk. *Cancer Prev Res (Phila).* 2015;8(5):342-348.

227. Oda K, Stokoe D, Taketani Y, McCormick F. High frequency of coexistent mutations of PIK3CA and PTEN genes in endometrial carcinoma. *Cancer Res.* 2005;65(23):10669-10673.

228. Chui MH, Gilks CB, Cooper K, Clarke BA. Identifying Lynch syndrome in patients with ovarian carcinoma: the significance of tumor subtype. *Adv Anat Pathol.* 2013;20(6):378-386.

229. Ye S, Yang J, Cao D, et al. Characteristic and prognostic implication of venous thromboembolism in ovarian clear cell carcinoma: a 12-year retrospective study. *PLoS One.* 2015;10(3):e0121818.

230. Lewin S, Dezube D, Guddati A, Mittal K, Muggia F, Klein P. Paraneoplastic hypercalcemia in clear cell ovarian adenocarcinoma. *Ecancermedicalscience.* 2012;6:271.

231. Borah T, Mahanta RK, Bora BD, Saikia S. Brenner tumor of ovary: an incidental finding. *J Midlife Health.* 2011;2(1):40-41.

232. Lancaster JM, Powell CB, Kauff ND, et al; Society of Gynecologic Oncologists Education Committee. Society of Gynecologic Oncologists Education Committee statement on risk assessment for inherited gynecologic cancer predispositions. *Gynecol Oncol.* 2007;107(2):159-162.

233. Rooth C. Ovarian cancer: risk factors, treatment and management. *Br J Nurs.* 2013;22(17):S23-S30.

234. Riman T, Nilsson S, Persson IR. Review of epidemiological evidence for reproductive and hormonal factors in relation to the risk of epithelial ovarian malignancies. *Acta Obstet Gynecol Scand.* 2004;83(9):783-795.

235. Jensen A, Sharif H, Frederiksen K, Kjaer SK. Use of fertility drugs and risk of ovarian cancer: Danish population-based cohort study. *BMJ.* 2009;338:b249.

236. Pearce CL, Templeman C, Rossing MA, et al; Ovarian Cancer Association Consortium. Association between endometriosis and risk of histological subtypes of ovarian cancer: a pooled analysis of case-control studies. *Lancet Oncol.* 2012;13(4):385-394.

237. Olsen CM, Nagle CM, Whiteman DC, et al; Ovarian Cancer Association Consortium. Obesity and risk of ovarian cancer subtypes: evidence from the Ovarian Cancer Association Consortium. *Endocr Relat Cancer.* 2013;20(2):251-262.

238. Robb K, Stubbings S, Ramirez A, et al. Public awareness of cancer in Britain: a population-based survey of adults. *Br J Cancer.* 2009;101(suppl 2):S18-S23.

239. Moss EL, Hollingworth J, Reynolds TM. The role of CA125 in clinical practice. *J Clin Pathol.* 2005;58(3):308-312.

240. Walker JL, Powell CB, Chen LM, et al. Society of Gynecologic Oncology recommendations for the prevention of ovarian cancer. *Cancer.* 2015;121(13):2108-2120.

241. Chang SJ, Bristow RE. Evolution of surgical treatment paradigms for advanced-stage ovarian cancer: redefining 'optimal' residual disease. *Gynecol Oncol.* 2012;125(2):483-492.

242. McGuire WP, Hoskins WJ, Brady MF, et al. Cyclophosphamide and cisplatin compared with paclitaxel and cisplatin in patients with stage III and stage IV ovarian cancer. *N Engl J Med.* 1996;334(1):1-6.

243. Vasey PA, Jayson GC, Gordon A, et al; Scottish Gynaecological Cancer Trials Group. Phase III randomized trial of docetaxel-carboplatin versus paclitaxel-carboplatin as first-line chemotherapy for ovarian carcinoma. *J Natl Cancer Inst.* 2004;96(22):1682-1691.

244. Parmar MK, Ledermann JA, Colombo N, et al; ICON and AGO Collaborators. Paclitaxel plus platinum-based chemotherapy versus conventional platinum-based chemotherapy in women with relapsed ovarian cancer: the ICON4/AGO-OVAR-2.2 trial. *Lancet.* 2003;361(9375):2099-2106.

245. Pfisterer J, Plante M, Vergote I, et al; AGO-OVAR; NCIC CTG; EORTC GCG. Gemcitabine plus carboplatin compared with carboplatin in patients with platinum-sensitive recurrent ovarian cancer: an intergroup trial of the AGO-OVAR, the NCIC CTG, and the EORTC GCG. *J Clin Oncol.* 2006;24(29):4699-4707.

246. Pujade-Lauraine E, Wagner U, Aavall-Lundqvist E, et al. Pegylated liposomal doxorubicin and carboplatin compared with paclitaxel and carboplatin for patients with platinum-sensitive ovarian cancer in late relapse. *J Clin Oncol.* 2010;28(20):3323-3329.

247. Markman M, Rothman R, Hakes T, et al. Second-line platinum therapy in patients with ovarian cancer previously treated with cisplatin. *J Clin Oncol.* 1991;9(3):389-393.

248. Gordon AN, Tonda M, Sun S, Rackoff W; Doxil Study 30-49 Investigators. Long-term survival advantage for women treated with pegylated liposomal doxorubicin compared with topotecan in a phase 3 randomized study of recurrent and refractory epithelial ovarian cancer. *Gynecol Oncol.* 2004;95(1):1-8.

249. Ferrandina G, Ludovisi M, Lorusso D, et al. Phase III trial of gemcitabine compared with pegylated liposomal doxorubicin in progressive or recurrent ovarian cancer. *J Clin Oncol.* 2008;26(6):890-896.

250. Lee P, Rosen DG, Zhu C, Silva EG, Liu J. Expression of progesterone receptor is a favorable prognostic marker in ovarian cancer. *Gynecol Oncol*. 2005;96(3):671-677.

251. Hatch KD, Beecham JB, Blessing JA, Creasman WT. Responsiveness of patients with advanced ovarian carcinoma to tamoxifen. A Gynecologic Oncology Group study of second-line therapy in 105 patients. *Cancer*. 1991;68(2):269-271.

252. Markman M, Webster K, Zanotti K, Rohl J, Belinson J. Use of tamoxifen in asymptomatic patients with recurrent small-volume ovarian cancer. *Gynecol Oncol*. 2004;93(2):390-393.

253. Van Der Velden J, Gitsch G, Wain GV, Friedlander ML, Hacker NF. Tamoxifen in patients with advanced epithelial ovarian cancer. *Int J Gynecol Cancer*. 1995;5(4):301-305.

254. Papadimitriou CA, Markaki S, Siapkaras J, et al. Hormonal therapy with letrozole for relapsed epithelial ovarian cancer. Long-term results of a phase II study. *Oncology*. 2004;66(2):112-117.

255. Gelmon KA, Tischkowitz M, Mackay H, et al. Olaparib in patients with recurrent high-grade serous or poorly differentiated ovarian carcinoma or triple-negative breast cancer: a phase 2, multicentre, open-label, non-randomised study. *Lancet Oncol*. 2011;12(9):852-861.

256. Swisher EM, Lin KK, Oza AM, et al. Rucaparib in relapsed, platinum-sensitive high-grade ovarian carcinoma (ARIEL2 Part 1): an international, multicentre, open-label, phase 2 trial. *Lancet Oncol*. 2017;18(1):75-87.

257. Mirza MR, Monk BJ, Herrstedt J, et al; ENGOT-OV16/NOVA Investigators. Niraparib maintenance therapy in platinum-sensitive, recurrent ovarian cancer. *N Engl J Med*. 2016;375(22):2154-2164.

258. Jemal A, Miller KD, Ma J, et al. Higher lung cancer incidence in young women than young men in the United States. *N Engl J Med*. 2018;378(21):1999-2009.

259. Barrera-Rodriguez R, Morales-Fuentes J. Lung cancer in women. *Lung Cancer Targets Ther*. 2012;3:79-89.

260. Lemjabbar-Alaoui H, Hassan O, Yang YW, Buchanan P. Lung cancer: biology and treatment options. *Biochim Biophys Acta*. 2015;1856(2):189-210.

261. Torre LA, Siegel RL, Jemal A. Lung cancer statistics. In: Ahmad A, Gadgeel S, eds. *Lung Cancer and Personalized Medicine: Current Knowledge and Therapies*. Advances in Experimental Medicine and Biology. Switzerland: Springer; 2015:1-19.

262. Kanwal M, Ding XJ, Cao Y. Familial risk for lung cancer. *Oncol Lett*. 2017;13(2):535-542.

263. Peto R, Darby S, Deo H, Silcocks P, Whitley E, Doll R. Smoking, smoking cessation, and lung cancer in the UK since 1950: combination of national statistics with two case-control studies. *BMJ*. 2000;321(7257):323-329.

264. Reid A, de Klerk N, Ambrosini GL, et al. The effect of asbestosis on lung cancer risk beyong the dose related effect of asbestos along. *Occup Environ Med*. 2005;62(12):885-889.

265. Hessel PA, Gamble JF, McDonald JC. Asbestos, asbestosis, and lung cancer: a critical assessment of the epidemiological evidence. *Thorax*. 2005;60(5):433-436.

266. Darby S, Hill D, Auvinen A, et al. Radon in homes and risk of lung cancer: collaborative analysis of individual data from 13 European case-control studies. *BMJ*. 2005;330(7485):223.

267. Barone-Adesi F, Chapman RS, Silverman DT, et al. Risk of lung cancer associated with domestic use of coal in Xuanwei, China: retrospective cohort study. *BMJ*. 2012;345:e5414.

268. Barcenas CH, Delcios GL, El-Zein R, Tortolero-Luna G, Whitehead LW, Spitz MR. Wood dust exposure and the association with lung cancer risk. *Am J Ind Med*. 2005;47(4):349-357.

269. Neugut AI, Robinson E, Lee WC, Murray T, Karwoski K, Kutcher GJ. Lung cancer after radiation therapy for breast cancer. *Cancer*. 1993;71(10):3054-3057.

270. Schoenfeld JD, Mauch PM, Das P, et al. Lung malignancies after Hodgkin lymphoma: disease characteristics, detection methods and clinical outcome. *Ann Oncol*. 2012;23(7):1813-1818.

271. Shan S, She J, Xue ZQ, Su CX, Ren SX, Wu FY. Clinical characteristics and survival of lung cancer patients associated with multiple primary malignancies. *PLoS One*. 2017;12(9):e0185485.

272. Hopkins RJ, Duan F, Chiles C, et al. Reduced expiratory flow rate among heavy smokers increases lung cancer risk. Results from the National Lung Screening Trial-American College of Radiology Imaging Network Cohort. *Ann Am Thorac Soc*. 2017;14(3):392-402.

273. Middha P, Weinstein SJ, Männistö S, Albanes D, Mondul AM. β-carotene supplementation and lung cancer incidence in the ATBC study: the role of tar and nicotine [published online ahead of print June 8, 2018]. *Nicotine Tob Res*.

274. National Lung Screening Trial Research Team, Aberle DR, Adams AM, et al. Reduced lung-cancer mortality with low-dose computed tomographic screening. *N Engl J Med*. 2011;365(5):395-409.

275. Chlebowski RT. Menopausal hormone therapy, hormone receptor status, and lung cancer in women. *Semin Oncol*. 2009;36(6):566-571.

276. Siegfried JM, Hershberger PA, Stabile LP. Estrogen receptor signaling in lung cancer. *Semin Oncol*. 2009;36(6):524-531.

277. Schwartz AG, Ray RM, Cote ML, et al. Hormone use, reproductive history, and risk of lung cancer: the Women's Health Initiative studies. *J Thorac Oncol*. 2015;10(7):1004-1013.

278. Chlebowski RT, Wakelee H, Pettinger M, et al. Estrogen plus progestin and lung cancer: follow-up of the Women's Health Initiative randomized trial. *Clin Lung Cancer*. 2016;17(1):10.e1-17.e1.

279. Ramchandran K, Patel JD. Sex differences in susceptibility to carcinogens. *Semin Oncol*. 2009;36(6):516-523.

280. Patel JD. Lung cancer: a biologically different disease in women? *Womens Health (Lond)*. 2009;5(6):685-691.

281. Cote ML, Yoo W, Wenzlaff AS, et al. Tobacco and estrogen metabolic polymorphisms and risk of non-small cell lung cancer in women. *Carcinogenesis*. 2009;30(4):626-635.

282. Bouchardy C, Benhamou S, Schaffer R, et al. Lung cancer mortality risk among breast cancer patients treated with anti-estrogens. *Cancer*. 2011;117(6):1288-1295.

283. Chia PL, Mitchell P, Dobrovic A, John T. Prevalence and natural history of ALK positive non-small cell lung cancer and the clinical impact of targeted thearpy with ALK inhibitors. *Clin Epidemiol*. 2014;6:423-432.

284. Dugay F, Llamas-Gutierrez F, Gournay M, et al. Clinicalpathological charateristincs of ROS1- and RET-rearranged NSCLC in caucasian patients: data from a cohort of 713 non-squamous NSCLC lacking KRAS/EGFR/HER2/BRAF/PIK3CA/ALK alterations. *Oncotarget*. 2017;8(32):53336-53351.

285. Kang JK, Lim HJ, Park JS, et al. Comparison of clinical characteristics between patients with ALK-positive and EGFR-positive lung adenocarcinoma. *Respir Med*. 2014;108(2):388-394.

286. Kim HR, Lim SM, Kim HJ, et al. The frequency and impact of ROS1 rearrangement on clinical outcomes in never smokers with lung adenocarcinoma. *Ann Oncol*. 2013;24(9):2364-2370.

287. Kim H, Chung JH. Overview of clinical pathologic features of ALK-reaaringed lung adenocarcinoma and current diagnositc testing for ALK rearrangement. *Transl Lung Cancer Res*. 2015;4(2):149-155.

288. Prabhakar CN. Epidermal growth factor receptor in non-small cell lung cancer. *Transl Lung Cancer Res*. 2015;4(2):110-118.

289. Reck M, Rodriguez-Abreu D, Robinson AG, et al; KEYNOTE-024 Investigators. Pembrolizumab versus chemotherapy for PD-L1-positive non-small-cell lung cancer. *N Engl J Med*. 2016;375(19):1823-1833.

290. Shigematsu H, Lin L, Takahashi T, et al. Clinical and biological features associated with epidermal growth factor receptor gene mutations in lung cancers. *J Natl Cancer Inst*. 2005;97(5):339-346.

291. Wang A, Wang HY, Liu Y, et al. The prognostic value of PD-L1 expression for non-small cell lung cancer patients: a meta-analysis. *Eur J Surg Oncol*. 2015;41(4):450-456.

292. Siegel RL, Miller KD, Fedewa SA, et al. Colorectal cancer statistics, 2017. *CA Cancer J Clin*. 2017;67(3):177-193.

293. Zauber AG. The impact of screening on colorectal cancer mortality and incidence: has it really made a difference? *Dig Dis Sci*. 2015;60(3):681-691.

294. American Cancer Society. Colorectal cancer. www.cancer.org/cancer/colon-rectal-cancer.html. Accessed July 3, 2019.

295. Bardou M, Barkun AN, Martel M. Republished: obesity and colorectal cancer. *Postgrad Med J*. 2013;89(1055):519-533.

296. Cho E, Lee JE, Rimm EB, Fuchs CS, Giovannucci EL. Alcohol consumption and the risk of colon cancer by family history of colorectal cancer. *Am J Clin Nutr*. 2012;95(2):413-419.

297. Doubeni CA, Major JM, Laiyemo AO, et al. Contribution of behavioral risk factors and obesity to socioeconomic differences in colorectal cancer. *J Natl Cancer Inst*. 2012;104(18):1353-1362.

298. Mills KT, Bellows CF, Hoffman AE, Kelly TN, Gagliardi G. Diabetes mellitus and colorectal cancer prognosis: a meta-analysis. *Dis Colon Rectum*. 2013;56(11):1304-1319.

299. Nimptsch K, Bernstein AM, Giovannucci E, Fuchs CS, Willett WC, Wu K. Dietary intake of red meat, poultry, and fish during high school and risk of colorectal adenomas in women. *Am J Epidemiol*. 2013;178(2):172-183.

300. Zgaga L, Agakov F, Theodoratou E, et al. Model selection approach suggests causal association between 25-hydroxyvitamin D and colorectal cancer. *PLoS One*. 2013;8(5):e63475.

301. Lagerstedt Robinson K, Liu T, Vandrovcova J, et al. Lynch syndrome (hereditary nonpolyposis colorectal cancer) diagnostics. *J Natl Cancer Inst*. 2007;99(4):291-299.

302. Lynch HT, Snyder CL, Shaw TG, Heinen CD, Hitchins MP. Milestones of Lynch syndrome: 1895-2015. *Nat Rev Cancer*. 2015;15(3):181-194.

303. Kohlmann W, Gruber SB. Lynch syndrome. In: Adam MP, Ardinger HH, Pagon RA, et al, eds *GeneReviews [Internet]*. Seattle, WA: University of Washington, Seattle; 1993-2018. Last revision April 12, 2018. www.ncbi.nlm.nih.gov/books/NBK1211/. Accessed July 3, 2019.

304. Lynch PM. When and how to perform genetic testing for inherited colorectal cancer syndromes. *J Natl Compr Canc Netw*. 2013;11(12):1577-1583.

305. Half E, Bercovich D, Rozen P. Familial adenomatous polyposis. *Orphanet J Rare Dis*. 2009;4:22.

306. Chan DS, Lau R, Aune D, et al. Red and processed meat and colorectal cancer incidence: meta-analysis of prospective studies. *PLoS One*. 2011;6(6):e20456.

307. Moghaddam AA, Woodward M, Huxley R. Obesity and risk of colorectal cancer: a meta-analysis of 31 studies with 70,000 events. *Cancer Epidemiol Biomarkers Prev*. 2007;16(12):2533-2547.

308. Wolin KY, Yan Y, Colditz GA, Lee IM. Physical activity and colon cancer prevention: a meta-analysis. *Br J Cancer*. 2009;100(4):611-616.

309. Larsson SC, Orsini N, Wolk A. Diabetes mellitus and risk of colorectal cancer: a meta-analysis. *J Natl Cancer Inst*. 2005;97(22):1679-1687.

310. Garland CF, Gorham ED. Dose-response of serum 25-hydroxyvitamin D in association with risk of colorectal cancer: a meta-analysis. *J Steroid Biochem Mol Biol*. 2017;168:1-8.

311. Wei MY, Garland CF, Gorham ED, Mohr SB, Giovannucci E. Vitamin D and prevention of colorectal adenoma: a meta-analysis. *Cancer Epidemiol Biomarkers Prev*. 2008;17(11):2958-2969.

312. Garland CF, Garland FC, Gorham ED, et al. The role of vitamin D in cancer prevention. *Am J Public Health*. 2006;96(2):252-261.

313. Baron JA, Barry EL, Mott LA, et al. A trial of calcium and vitamin D for the prevention of colorectal adenomas. *N Engl J Med*. 2015;373(16):1519-1530.

314. Rex DK, Boland CR, Dominitz JA, et al. Colorectal cancer screening: recommendations for physicians and patients from the U.S. Multi-Society Task Force on Colorectal Cancer. *Gastroenterology*. 2017;153(1):307-323.

315. Levin B, Lieberman DA, McFarland B, et al; American Cancer Society Colorectal Advisory Group; US Multi-Society Task Force; American College of Radiology Colon Cancer Committee. Screening and surveillance for the early detection of colorectal cancer and adenomatous polyps, 2008: a joint guideline from the American Cancer Society, the US Multi-Society Task Force on Colorectal Cancer, and the American College of Radiology. *CA Cancer J Clin*. 2008;58(3):130-160.

316. Bretthauer M, Kalager M, Weinberg DS. From colorectal cancer screening guidelines to headlines: beware! *Ann Intern Med*. 2018;169(6):405-406.

317. Tinmouth J, Lansdorp-Vogelaar I, Allison JE. Faecal immunochemical tests versus guaiac faecal occult blood tests: what clinicians and colorectal cancer screening programme organisers need to know. *Gut*. 2015;64(8):1327-1337.

318. Imperiale TF, Ransohoff DF, Itzkowitz SH, et al. Multitarget stool DNA testing for colorectal-cancer screening. *N Engl J Med*. 2014;370(14):1287-1297.

319. Arora G, Mannalithara A, Singh G, Gerson LB, Triadafilopoulos G. Risk of perforation from a colonoscopy in adults: a large population-based study. *Gastrointest Endosc*. 2009;69(3 pt 2):654-664.

320. Bielawska B, Day AG, Lieberman DA, Hookey LC. Risk factors for early colonoscopic perforation include non-gastroenterologist endoscopists: a multivariable analysis. *Clin Gastroenterol Hepatol*. 2014;12(1):85-92.

321. Zauber AG, Winawer SJ, O'Brien MJ, et al. Colonoscopic polypectomy and long-term prevention of colorectal-cancer deaths. *N Engl J Med*. 2012;366(8):687-696.

322. Winawer SJ, Stewart ET, Zauber AG, et al. A comparison of colonoscopy and double-contrast barium enema for surveillance after polypectomy. National Polyp Study Work Group. *N Engl J Med*. 2000;342(24):1766-1772.

323. Pickhardt PJ, Choi JR, Hwang I, et al. Computed tomographic virtual colonoscopy to screen for colorectal neoplasia in asymptomatic adults. *N Engl J Med*. 2003;349(23):2191-2200.

324. Iafrate F, Iussich G, Correale L, et al. Adverse events of computed tomography colonography: an Italian national survey. *Dig Liver Dis*. 2013;45(8):645-650.

325. Stoffel EM, Mangu PB, Gruber SB, et al; American Society of Clinical Oncology; European Society of Clinical Oncology. Hereditary colorectal cancer syndromes: American Society of Clinical Oncology Clinical Practice Guideline endorsement of the familial risk-colorectal cancer: European Society for Medical Oncology Clinical Practice Guidelines. *J Clin Oncol*. 2015;33(2):209-217.

326. Umar A, Boland CR, Terdiman JP, et al. Revised Bethesda guidelines for hereditary nonpolyposis colorectal cancer (Lynch syndrome) and microsatellite instability. *J Natl Cancer Inst*. 2004;96(4):261-268.

327. Sengupta N, Yee E, Feuerstein JD. Colorectal cancer screening in inflammatory bowel disease. *Dig Dis Sci*. 2016;61(4):980-989.

328. Beresford SA, Johnson KC, Ritenbaugh C, et al. Low-fat dietary pattern and risk of colorectal cancer: the Women's Health Initiative Randomized Controlled Dietary Modification Trial. *JAMA*. 2006;295(6):643-654.

329. Lanza E, Schatzkin A, Daston C, et al; PPT Study Group. Implementation of a 4-y, high-fiber, high-fruit-and-vegetable, low-fat dietary intervention: results of dietary changes in the Polyp Prevention Trial. *Am J Clin Nutr*. 2001;74(3):387-401.

330. Park Y, Hunter DJ, Spiegelman D, et al. Dietary fiber intake and risk of colorectal cancer: a pooled analysis of prospective cohort studies. *JAMA*. 2005;294(22):2849-2857.

331. Chan AT, Giovannucci EL. Primary prevention of colorectal cancer. *Gastroenterology*. 2010;138(6):2029-2043.

332. Longacre TA, Fenoglio-Preiser CM. Mixed hyperplastic adenomatous polyps/serrated adenomas. A distinct form of colorectal neoplasia. *Am J Surg Pathol*. 1990;14(6):524-537.

333. Lieberman DA, Rex DK, Winawer SJ, Giardiello FM, Johnson DA, Levin TR. Guidelines for colonoscopy surveillance after screening and polypectomy: a consensus update by the US Multi-Society Task force on Colorectal Cancer. *Gastroenterology*. 2012;143(3):844-857.

334. Nishihara R, Lochhead P, Kuchiba A, et al. Aspirin use and risk of colorectal cancer according to BRAF mutation status. *JAMA*. 2013;309(24):2563-2571.

335. Baron JA, Cole BF, Sandler RS, et al. A randomized trial of aspirin to prevent colorectal adenomas. *N Engl J Med*. 2003;348:891-899.

336. Chan AT, Ogino S, Fuchs CS. Aspirin and the risk of colorectal cancer in relation to the expression of COX-2. *N Engl J Med*. 2007;356(21):2131-2142.

337. Ishikawa H, Wakabayashi K, Suzuki S, et al. Preventive effects of low-dose aspirin on colorectal adenoma growth in patients with familial adenomatous polyposis: double-blind, randomized clinical trial. *Cancer Med*. 2013;2(1):50-56.

338. Steinbach G, Lynch PM, Phillips RK, et al. The effect of celecoxib, a cyclooxygenase-2 inhibitor, in familial adenomatous polyposis. *N Engl J Med*. 2000;342(26):1946-1952.

339. Giardiello FM, Hamilton SR, Krush AJ, et al. Treatment of colonic and rectal adenomas with sulindac in familial adenomatous polyposis. *N Engl J Med*. 1993;328(18):1313-1316.

340. Bibbins-Domingo K; US Preventive Services Task Force. Aspirin use for the primary prevention of cardiovascular disease and colorectal cancer: US Preventive Services Task Force recommendation statement. *Ann Intern Med*. 2016;164(12):836-845.

341. Razzak AA, Oxentenko AS, Vierkant RA, et al. Associations between intake of folate and related micronutrients with molecularly defined colorectal cancer risks in the Iowa Women's Health Study. *Nutr Cancer*. 2012;64(7):899-910.

342. Chlebowski RT, Wactawski-Wende J, Ritenbaugh C, et al; Women's Health Initiative Investigators. Estrogen plus progestin and colorectal cancer in postmenopausal women. *N Engl J Med*. 2004;350(10):991-1004.

343. Simon MS, Chlebowski RT, Wactawski-Wende J, et al. Estrogen plus progestin and colorectal cancer incidence and mortality. *J Clin Oncol*. 2012;30(32):3983-3990.

344. Domingo E, Church DN, Sieber O, et al. Evaluation of PIK3CA mutation as a predictor of benefit from nonsteroidal anti-inflammatory drug therapy in colorectal cancer. *J Clin Oncol*. 2013;31(34):4297-4305.

345. Sandler RS, Halabi S, Baron JA, et al. A randomized trial of aspirin to prevent colorectal adenomas in patients with previous colorectal cancer. *N Engl J Med*. 2003;348(10):883-890. Erratum in: *N Engl J Med*. 2003;348(19):1939.

346. Fadelu T, Zhang S, Niedzwiecki D, et al. Nut consumption and survival in stage III colon cancer: results from CALGB 89803 (Alliance). *J Clin Oncol*. 2018;36(11):1112-1120.

347. Xue L, Williamson A, Gaines S, et al. An update on colorectal cancer. *Curr Prob Surg*. 2018;55(3):76-116.

348. Glynne-Jones R, Wyrwicz L, Tiret E, et al; ESMA Guidelines Committee. Rectal cancer: ESMO clinical practice guidelines for diagnosis, treatment and follow-up. *Ann Oncol*. 2017;28(suppl 4):iv22-iv40.

349. Gong J, Cho M, Fakih M. RAS and BRAF in metastatic colorectal cancer management. *J Gastrointest Oncol*. 2016;7(5):687-704.

350. Rogers HW, Weinstock MA, Feldman SR, Coldiron BM. Incidence estimate of nonmelanoma skin cancer (keratinocyte carcinomas) in the US population, 2012. *JAMA Dermatol*. 2015;151(10):1081-1086.

351. Lee WW, Ashley W, Cotliar J, Jung J. Management of elderly patients with skin cancer. *J Geriatr Oncol*. 2016;7(1):7-9.

352. Roewert-Huber J, Stockfleth E, Kerl H. Pathology and pathobiology of actinic (solar) keratosis—an update. *Br J Dermatol*. 2007; 157(suppl 2):18-20.

353. Madan V, Lear JT, Szeimies RM. Non-melanoma skin cancer. *Lancet*. 2010;375(9715):673-685.

354. Kim RH, Armstrong AW. Nonmelanoma skin cancer. *Dermatol Clin*. 2012;30(1):125-139, ix.

355. Williams ML, Sagebiel RW. Melanoma risk factors and atypical moles. *West J Med*. 1994;160(4):343-350.

356. Ribero S, Glass D, Bataille V. Genetic epidemiology of melanoma. *Eur J Dermatol*. 2016;26(4):335-339.

357. Friedman RJ, Rigel DS, Kopf AW. Early detection of malignant melanoma: the role of physician examination and self-examination of the skin. *CA Cancer J Clin*. 1985;35(3):130-151.

358. Abbasi NR, Shaw HM, Rigel DS, et al. Early diagnosis of cutaneous melanoma: revisiting the ABCD criteria. *JAMA*. 2004; 292(22):2771-2776.

359. Ilyas M, Costello CM, Zhang N, Sharma A. The role of the ugly duckling sign in patient education. *J Am Acad Dermatol*. 2017;77(6):1088-1095.

360. Grob JJ, Bonerandi JJ. The "ugly duckling" sign: identification of the common characteristics of nevi in an individual as a basis for melanoma screening. *Arch Dermatol*. 1998;134(1):103-104.

361. Marsden JR, Newton-Bishop JA, Burrows L, et al; British Association of Dermatologists Clinical Standards Unit. Revised UK guidelines for the management of cutaneous melanoma 2010. *Br J Dermatol*. 2010;163(2):238-256.

362. Coit DG, Thompson JA, Algazi A, et al. Melanoma, version 2.2016, NCCN Clinical Practice Guidelines in Oncology. *J Natl Compr Canc Netw*. 2016;14(4):450-473.

363. Amber K, McLeod MP, Nouri K. The Merkel cell polyomavirus and its involvement in Merkel cell carcinoma. *Dermatol Surg*. 2013;39(2):232-238.

364. Heath M, Jaimes N, Lemos B, et al. Clinical characteristics of Merkel cell carcinoma at diagnosis in 195 patients: the AEIOU features. *J Am Acad Dermatol*. 2008;58(3):375-381.

365. Buck DW 2nd, Kim JY, Alam M, et al. Multidisciplinary approach to the management of dermatofibrosarcoma protuberans. *J Am Acad Dermatol*. 2012;67(5):861-866.

366. Criscione VD, Weinstock MA. Descriptive epidemiology of dermatofibrosarcoma protuberans in the United States, 1973 to 2002. *J Am Acad Dermatol*. 2007;56(6):968-973.

367. Ingraffea A. Benign skin neoplasms. *Facial Plast Surg Clin North Am*. 2013;21(1):21-32.

368. Hafner C, Vogt T. Seborrheic keratosis. [Article in English, German.] *J Dtsch Dermatol Ges*. 2008;6(8):664-677.

369. Praetorius C, Sturm RA, Steingrimsson E. Sun-induced freckling: ephelides and solar lentigines. *Pigment Cell Melanoma Res*. 2014;27(3):339-350.

370. Salam GA. Lipoma excision. *Am Fam Physician*. 2002;65(5):901-904.

371. Duncan DI, Palmer M. Fat reduction using phosphatidylcholine/sodium deoxycholate injections: standard of practice. *Aesthetic Plast Surg*. 2008;32(6):858-872.

372. Lanigan SW, Robinson TW. Cryotherapy for dermatofibromas. *Clin Exp Dermatol*. 1987;12(2):121-123.

373. Han TY, Chang HS, Lee JH, Lee WM, Son SJ. A clinical and histopathological study of 122 cases of dermatofibroma (benign fibrous histiocytoma). *Ann Dermatol*. 2011;23(2):185-192.

374. Kwok CS, Gibbs S, Bennett C, Holland R, Abbott R. Topical treatments for cutaneous warts. *Cochrane Database Syst Rev*. 2012;(9):CD001781.

Vitamins, Minerals, and Other Dietary Supplements

Government Regulation of Dietary Supplements

Modalities for treatment of menopause symptoms run the gamut from FDA-approved prescription drugs manufactured in tightly regulated factories by commercial pharmaceutical companies to "custom" prescription drugs that are prepared by compounding pharmacies from physician prescriptions for patients on an individualized basis when a commercially available drug product does not meet the patient's specific medical need, to over-the-counter (OTC) substances that can be purchased in a pharmacy, health-food store, or supermarket without a prescription and do not require physician supervision to use safely. There are many major nonprescription therapies considered for use by women at menopause, including vitamins, minerals, and other nonbotanical dietary supplements, all available over the counter.

Based in no small part on a recommendation made in the 2017 Hormone Therapy Position Statement from The North American Menopause Society that "treatment or preventive therapy is indicated for women aged 60 years or younger or within 10 years of menopause who have bothersome vasomotor symptoms or elevated risk for bone loss or fracture,"[1] it is a virtual certainty that many menopausal women are taking some of these nonprescription substances or products.

The words "substances or products" are used in the broadest possible way, because the spectrum of OTC products used by consumers for treatment of hundreds of medical conditions—among them menopause symptoms—is enormous, ranging from vitamins and minerals to herbal preparations of either western or eastern origin. All these OTC compounds may be lumped under the term "dietary supplements," defined as products in tablet, capsule, droplet, softgel, or gelcap form or products in conventional food form that are not represented as conventional foods and that were intended (or at least originally intended) to supplement the diet.[2] By statute, a substance may be considered a dietary supplement if it contains a vitamin, a mineral, an herb or other botanical, an amino acid, any dietary substance for use by humans to supplement the diet by increasing the total dietary intake, or any concentrate, constituent, extract, or combination thereof.

Making sense of all of the medical and legal nuances of dietary supplements for menopause-related symptoms (or almost any other medical condition for that matter) and how they are regulated may confuse consumers and even seasoned food-and-drug law experts. There are several reasons for this.

First, any discussion of dietary supplements and how to regulate them—if one believes they should be regulated at all—must take place in the context of the decades of mistrust, missteps, and misunderstandings by federal regulators (specifically, FDA), consumer health advocates, Congress, the medical profession, the food industry, and the producers of dietary supplements. It is no understatement to say that at times FDA has viewed dietary supplements and some of their associated health claims with barely concealed hostility.

The end result of this half-century of fighting among these groups was the passage in 1994 of the Dietary Supplement Health and Education Act (DSHEA),[3] a unique piece of legislation in which Congress stripped FDA of most of its regulatory authority over dietary supplements and that largely exempted this new legal class of food products from the normal statutory and legal restrictions that apply to prescription drugs, biologics, medical devices, and foods. It is important to note that even though the DSHEA greatly restricted FDA's authority over whether dietary supplements can be marketed without any proof of efficacy or safety, the DSHEA does not prevent FDA from determining that a dietary supplement is a drug—and intervening accordingly—if the manufacturer makes overt health-benefit claims (ie, a "drug claim") that have not been specifically approved by FDA.

Second, the role that dietary supplements play in the normal diet of US citizens, what falls under the current umbrella of the term "dietary supplement," and how these substances have been promoted to consumers has changed drastically since the 1938 Federal Food Drug and Cosmetic Act (FDCA) first enabled regulation of food and drugs.[4] The fact is that after the Depression, when the 1938 FDA-enabling statute was enacted, there were documented deficiencies in certain vitamins and minerals in the diet of many Americans and an identified health/medical need for dietary supplementation. The original intent of many of these substances was in fact to serve as supplemental foods to normal foodstuffs.

Although there remains a problem of poor nutrition and the need for supplementation for some, this is not the case for most Americans. There has been a perceptible increase in the types of products being marketed as dietary supplements and an expansion of the purported health benefits provided by these products. Coupled with the powerful tradition in the United States for empowerment of consumers to make their own choices about the benefits of healthcare programs and medications, as well as a tendency for FDA to view many of the stated benefits for dietary supplements, homeopathic remedies, and alternative medical therapies with a great deal of skepticism, dialogue about nonprescription treatments for menopause symptoms has an inherent political dimension even when physicians discuss the relative merits of dietary supplements in the women's health arena.

The controversy over medical merits aside, most consumers do believe that dietary supplements have substantive medical benefits, are for the most part safe (particularly if they have the word "natural" on the label), and are important in promoting better health. Even if there is little to no medical data to prove the claimed benefits of many of these products, nor any systematic collection of safe data to establish dosage or avoid potentially dangerous interactions with other drugs, there is no question that a substantial number of women use these OTC products for treatment of menopause symptoms instead of either commercially available prescription drugs or even compounded bioidentical hormone products. (See also "Estrogen Therapy and Estrogen-Progestogen Therapy" in Chapter 11.)

Third, although what constitutes a drug and what constitutes food are defined by statute in the FDCA, as amended, in the real world (that is, the world in which health products are directly advertised and promoted to consumers), FDA has long struggled to find the "bright line" that separates a food from a drug when health claims are made for what is essentially a food product.

If a product is classified as a drug, then the full regulatory apparatus of FDA may be brought to bear on its safety data, advertising, promotion, and indeed whether the drug actually does what it claims to do (ie, its efficacy); an otherwise OTC dietary supplement such as an herbal remedy would then move from the protection of the DSHEA into the category of a "new drug" and could be removed from the market if there were no data to prove it either worked or was safe. Obviously then, dietary-supplement producers want to avoid being classified as a drug despite the fact that the makers of these substances also want to be able to make claims about the health benefits of their products. Section 201 of the FDCA contains the definitions of what constitutes a drug as well as a food (Table 1).[4]

The DSHEA specifically modified the original FDCA definition of a drug to permit what are called "structure-function" claims. This is a critical core concept in understanding much of the advertising and content of labels for dietary substances. Manufacturers of dietary supplements must be careful, however. Even if the label that the dietary supplement manufacturer puts on a bottle specifically states that the tablets are not drugs, if the promotion (ie, labeling) of the products makes a drug claim (a therapeutic claim that the product is intended to prevent, treat, or cure a disease in man), the courts and FDA are likely to consider the product a drug. The problem is that under this framework, because of the vague and broad nature of the language "structure and function," dietary supplement claims that purportedly are just permissible structure and function claims sometimes cross the line and begin to sound like disease treatments. And, given the enormity of the dietary supplement industry, FDA simply lacks the resources to police the industry on all health claims being made for all of the products.

Finally, the health-claims issue is complicated further by the fact that FDA has a longstanding policy of allowing select health claims for some dietary supplements when there may be a clear relationship between the disease and the food supplement; any effort by FDA to restrict the manner in which manufacturers promote their products to consumers quickly runs into a First Amendment commercial speech area that has been a

Table 1. Federal Food Drug and Cosmetic Act Definitions of Food and Drug

The term *food* means

1. Article used for food or drink for man or other animals
2. Chewing gum
3. Articles used for components of any such article

The term *drug* means

1. Articles recognized in the official United States Pharmacopeia (USP), official Homeopathic Pharmacopeia of the United States, or official National Formulary, or any supplement to any of them
2. Articles intended for use in the diagnosis, cure, mitigation, treatment, or prevention of a disease in man or other animals
3. Articles (other than food) intended to affect the structure or any function of the body or man or other animals

1938 Federal Food Drug and Cosmetic Act.[4]

minefield for federal regulators. This is so even though the DSHEA specifically allows dietary-supplement manufacturers to make certain types of health-benefit statements without fear that FDA will consider them a drug claim.

For example, the claim that folic acid reduces the incidence of neural tube defects in newborns or that certain cereals promote cardiac health are permissible health claims. These two examples aside, to date FDA has approved no more than a dozen or so health claims for foods and dietary supplements, even though any perusal of the plethora of products on the health food store shelves quickly reveals many health claims that could easily be interpreted as more than simple structure and function claims and begin to approach more traditional drug claims for treatment, prevention, mitigation, or cure of disease.

The current regulatory approach to medical claims made for dietary supplements may be summarized by noting that federal courts have favored the placement of disclaimers on labels rather than risk suppression or restriction of health claims, even if it is possible that the purported medical benefits claimed might be slightly misleading. Protection of commercial speech under the First Amendment is considered more important than eliminating every structure and function claim that fails to have universal scientific agreement or that skirts the line on a traditional drug claim. The reliance

on disclaimers stating that the product has not been approved by FDA and that the product is not intended to "diagnose, treat, cure, or prevent any disease" and the ability of health consumers to navigate product information on internet, television, and the label itself are the preferred regulatory routes for dietary supplements.

These issues are exemplified by the array of products for treatment of menopause symptoms that are available in the women's health section of most pharmacies. Some indicate clearly that they are dietary supplements and have only a structure and function claim on the label, as in the case that the product supports "women's internal balance, digestive flora, and immune health." These nonspecific claims are clearly not drug claims and fall well within the structure and function claim permitted for a dietary supplement by the DSHEA.

Examination of some of the multiple "menopause relief" products is more problematic. The words "dietary supplement" may appear in much smaller letters in the lower right-hand corner of the label, and the front and back of the label may state that the product "helps reduce hot flashes and night sweats." This latter claim is unquestionably a drug claim for treatment of a disease or specific medical condition. Although there is a very small rectangular box on both the front and back of the package that contains the statement that the relief of night sweats claim has not been evaluated by FDA, the fact is that this treatment claim appears in much larger print and is not substantively different from similar claims made by manufacturers of commercially available drug products.

Current FDA regulations for dietary supplements in the United States and Canada concern essential information for healthcare professionals and patients, although both countries do regulate dietary supplements differently than prescription drugs with regard to allowed health claims. Safety may not be mentioned at all in a nonprescription product's advertising or label on the bottle, although the word *natural* is often used, and there may be an indication that the product has not been approved by FDA.

United States

Government regulations in the United States regarding whether a dietary supplement is effective and safe are so much less strict than those for prescription drugs that there is almost no way that the two sets of regulations can be compared. Although food-and-drug law attorneys, as well as manufacturers of medical products, are under no illusions about the more lenient regulatory framework for dietary supplements, some physicians and many consumers fail to appreciate how severely the DSHEA restricted the power of FDA to regulate the quality of dietary supplements or to intervene when a potential safety issue arises regarding a particular product.

Under the DSHEA, the manufacturer (not FDA) is responsible for determining whether any representations or claims made about its products are substantiated by adequate evidence to show that they are not false or misleading. Dietary supplement marketers can make health claims for so-called natural conditions (eg, hot flashes, age-related memory loss) without providing documentation for efficacy and safety to the government. However, they cannot claim that a product prevents, treats, or cures a disease (eg, prevents heart attacks or osteoporosis; cures depression) unless FDA approves the claim. Because of this prohibition, manufacturers find other ways to convey what their supplements might do. For example, a dietary supplement pill for men will claim to "enhance male potency," whereas sildenafil citrate claims to treat erectile dysfunction.

The DSHEA further states that the manufacturer (not FDA) is responsible for ensuring that labels on packages of dietary supplements are truthful and not misleading and requires that they contain enough information for consumers to make informed choices, that the serving size ("dose") is appropriate, and that all dietary ingredients in the product are accurately listed.

Because the normal regulations for new prescription drugs or OTC drugs do not apply to dietary supplements, the normal FDA rules require drug manufacturers to prove that their products are effective and safe for their intended use. Demonstrating product safety is not required before a dietary supplement is approved for sale. Under the DSHEA, dietary supplement manufacturers are responsible for substantiating the safety of the ingredients used in a product. FDA is responsible for taking action against any unsafe dietary supplement product after it reaches the market but can only intervene, if at all, if the degree of risk to public safety is significant or presents an unreasonable risk of illness or injury. FDA accomplishes its responsibilities through monitoring safety literature, dietary supplement adverse event (AE) reports, and product information.

Although a number of manufacturers employ rigorous quality-control (QC) measures, many products are not monitored for purity or level of active ingredient nor in fact do they have to be. As a result, strength and quality can be unpredictable. If a product is suspected of causing harm, FDA can halt sales and have it analyzed.

Botanicals (eg, soy, isoflavones, black cohosh) are classified by FDA as a food, drug, or dietary supplement, depending on the intended use of the product. There are numerous QC concerns with botanicals, including misidentification, "underlabeling" (ie, including prescription drugs in OTC products without listing them), adulteration, substitution, and contamination. In addition, analytic-method standards are lacking for many products, leading to difficulty when attempting to assess product quality. Marketers use different methods to determine the levels of active ingredient in their products.

To address these concerns, FDA established a rule in 2007 for good manufacturing practices for dietary supplements. This rule helps to ensure that these products are produced in a quality manner, do not contain contaminants or impurities, and are accurately labeled. Manufacturers are required to evaluate the identity, purity, strength, and composition of their dietary supplements and are required to report all serious AEs to FDA.

In the United States, the designations "USP" and "NSF" (National Sanitation Foundation) are generally reliable indicators of good QC in manufacturing. However, these designations do not indicate to consumers whether the products have actually been tested in clinical trials.

Canada

In Canada, the term *natural health product* is used in place of *dietary supplement* as defined by the Natural Health Products Regulations, which came into effect in 2004. Natural Health Products include vitamins and minerals, probiotics, and other products such as amino acids and essential fatty acids. Also classified as natural health products are herbal products, homeopathic medicines, and complementary and alternative medicines such as traditional Chinese medicine. The Canadian definition of what constitutes a dietary supplement appears to be more expansive than that of FDA's; for example, FDA has not completely addressed the regulation of Chinese medicines.

It is the role of the Natural and Non-prescription Health Products Directorate to ensure access to safe, effective, high-quality natural health products. The experience has been similar to that in the United States, with most of the responsibility placed on the government to prove that products were unsafe or ineffective. Canadian regulations require that all natural health products have a product license before they can be sold.

All licensed natural health products in Canada display a product identification number preceded by the prefix NPN (Natural Product Number) or DIN-HM (Drug Identification Number for homeopathic medicines), assigned once the product is authorized for sale. All manufacturers, packagers, labelers, and importers are required to obtain site licensing and practice product safety and quality. Standard labeling requirements ensure that customers can make informed choices. The Canadian adverse-reaction reporting system assists in issuing safety advisories to the public.

Canadian consumers are advised to purchase products displaying an NPN or DIN on their labels, which indicate that the product has undergone and passed a review of its formulation, labeling, and instructions for use.

Vitamins and Combination Multivitamin Supplements

Vitamins are various organic substances essential in small quantities to the nutrition of most animals and some plants. They act especially as coenzymes and precursors of coenzymes in the regulation of metabolic processes but do not provide energy or serve as building units. They are present in natural foodstuffs or sometimes are produced within the body.

The human body requires more than 45 vitamins and minerals to maintain health, and healthcare professionals prefer that these come from a balanced diet rich in fruits and vegetables. In some cases, the daily diet may not contain all the nutrients necessary for optimal health, and some women may benefit from a daily multivitamin and mineral supplement. The US Preventive Services Task Force (USPSTF) finds insufficient evidence for multivitamins or single-nutrient supplements to prevent cancer or cardiovascular disease (CVD)[5] but does not make a generalized suggestion for their use otherwise. Furthermore, β-carotene and vitamin E each may carry more risk than benefit with regards to cancer and CVD.

Nutrition science is difficult, and its evidence can be challenging. Many studies have evaluated whole diet patterns rather than focusing on specific foods for their effect on disease and prevention. The Mediterranean diet has perhaps the best evidence for its health benefits, including lowering risk of coronary heart disease (CHD),[6,7] improving cognition in some populations,[8] and preventing metabolic syndrome.[9] The Mediterranean diet also has been associated with reduced risk for breast and colorectal cancers.[10,11]

In the *Dietary Guidelines for Americans 2015-2020*, the US Department of Agriculture aligns with the vegetable-, fruit-, and whole grain-focused Healthy Eating Index-2015 (HEI2015).[12,13] The HEI2015 has been deemed a valid and accurate tool for assessing the overall health of a person's diet; however, health outcomes from higher HEI2015 scores are unreported.

Another healthy, well-researched dietary pattern is the Dietary Approaches to Stop Hypertension (DASH) diet, which promotes vegetables, fruit, low-fat dairy products, whole grains, chicken, fish, and nuts.[14] Intake of fat, meat, sweets, and sodas are minimized in DASH. Adherence to the DASH diet is associated with reduced rates of CHD, stroke, and colorectal cancer,[15-17] as well as improved metabolic outcomes in polycystic ovary syndrome[18] and nonalcoholic fatty liver disease.[19]

Several studies also have assessed food groups in relation to risk of disease. Higher fruit and vegetable intake has been shown to be associated with reduced CHD, cancer, and all-cause mortality.[20] In the Nurses' Health Study and the Health Professionals Follow-up Study, the quantity of fruit and vegetable intake was associated with a significantly lower risk of CHD.[21] Greater fruit and vegetable intake has been associated with decreased risk or outcomes of specific cancers, including pancreatic cancer,[22,23] bladder cancer,[24,25] breast cancer,[26] and colorectal cancer.[27]

Daily recommended dietary intakes

Since 1994, the National Academy of Sciences in the United States and Health Canada have collaborated on the revision of the dietary reference standards known as dietary reference intakes (DRI). This provides a set of four nutrient-based reference values designed to replace the recommended dietary allowances (RDA) in the United States and the recommended nutrient intakes in Canada. The DRI includes recommended intakes for individual persons, estimated average requirements, adequate intakes, and tolerable upper intake levels (UL) (Table 2).[12,28] These references apply to dietary and supplemental intake.

Many nutrients are taken in concentrated, supplemental form, often in excess of the DRI. Among the most popular are antioxidants (including vitamins A, C, and E), although their effects on disease are far from certain. Antioxidant supplements have not been shown to have any effect on mortality or disease prevention[29] nor on the incidence of major cardiovascular (CV) events, myocardial infarction (MI), stroke, total death, and cardiac death.[30,31]

A cross-sectional study using the National Health and Nutrition Examination Survey examined nutrient intake in relation to prevalence of peripheral artery disease (PAD) in the US population.[32] Higher consumption of specific nutrients, including antioxidants (vitamins A, C, and E), vitamin B_6, fiber, folate, and omega-3 fatty acids

Table 2. Dietary Reference Intakes: Recommended Dietary Allowance and Adequate Intake for Women Aged 50 Years and Older	
Type 1	
Vitamin A	700 µg
Vitamin B₁ (thiamin)	1.1 mg
Vitamin B₂ (riboflavin)	1.1 mg
Vitamin B₃ (niacin)	14 mg
Vitamin B₆ (pyridoxine)	1.5 mg
Vitamin B₉ (folate)	400 µg
Vitamin B₁₂ (cyanocobalamine)	2.4 µg
Vitamin C	75 mg
Vitamin D	Ages 51-70, 15 µg / Ages >70 y, 20 µg
Vitamin E (α-tocopherol)	15 mg
Minerals	
Calcium	1,200 mg
Magnesium	320 mg
Phosphorus	700 mg

US Department of Health and Human Services[12]; Institute of Medicine (US) Committee to Review Dietary Reference Intakes for Vitamin D and Calcium, Food and Nutrition Board.[28]

may have a significant protective effect, irrespective of traditional CVD risk factors. These findings suggest but are not definitive that specific dietary supplementation may afford additional protection, above traditional risk factor modification, for the prevention of PAD.

Antioxidants have also been evaluated for their role in cancer. The relationship between dietary intake of supplemental antioxidant nutrients and ovarian cancer was evaluated in 133,614 postmenopausal women enrolled in the Women's Health Initiative (WHI).[33] Intake of dietary antioxidants, carotenoids, and vitamin A were not associated with a reduction in ovarian cancer risk. These results were corroborated in a pooled analysis of more than 500,000 women.[34] In a meta-analysis of 3,832 participants, dietary intake of vitamin C and β-carotene was associated with reduced risk of colorectal adenoma; dietary intake of vitamins A and E was not.[35] The focus was on dietary and not supplemental intakes.

A review of 26 studies concluded that there was mixed evidence between vitamin supplementation and breast cancer prevention.[36] Another meta-analysis of 18 studies showed lycopene intake had marginal association with reduction in pancreatic cancer, but there was no effect from other antioxidants.[37]

The association between antioxidant vitamin intakes and cervical cancer risk was calculated for 144 patients with cervical cancer and 288 age-matched, hospital-based control patients.[38] Total intakes of vitamins A, C, and E were strongly and inversely associated with cervical cancer risk.

There is little evidence to support the use of antioxidant supplements for prevention of disease, and there is a potential for harm at high intakes. Although fruit and vegetable intake is seemingly protective against disease, this may be a marker of healthier lifestyles in general. The best advice to patients is probably to get nutrients from dietary sources as part of an overall healthy diet pattern.

Multivitamins

Multivitamin/Multimineral (MVM) supplements are among the most common natural products used by US consumers.[39] For people with restricted or insufficient diets, this may be appropriate. Again, nutrients should be obtained through intake of a variety of healthy foods whenever possible. Certain adult populations should be encouraged to consider a MVM supplement, including those with poor absorption, including older adults, those with known vitamin or mineral deficiency because of health status or medication use, and those on a restricted diet, including vegan.

Women who are planning pregnancy or who are pregnant need folate and should consider multivitamin supplementation. Postmenopausal women might consider MVM products containing calcium and vitamin D for bone health. Those taking multivitamins for prevention of chronic disease, however, should be reminded that evidence is insufficient to recommend multivitamins for the prevention of cancer and CVD.[40] In addition, the 41% of women taking multivitamins while participating in the WHI over 8 years did not demonstrate health benefits in regards to CVD, cancer, or mortality.[41] A cohort of women from the WHI who were diagnosed with invasive breast cancer and took multivitamins had lower breast cancer-specific mortality compared with those who did not.[42]

Some observational studies have raised concerns regarding disease risk associated with MVM use, particularly a widely publicized study in 35,000 women in Sweden taking MVM supplements who demonstrated an increased incidence of breast cancer.[43] No such association was found in a prospective study of 38,000 US women.[44] In the prospective Iowa Women's Health Study of 39,000 women followed for nearly 20 years, an association was made between MVM supplement use and increased mortality during the observation period.[45]

In order to assess potential benefits for MVM supplement use, it is best to understand the recommendations for and against its specific components.

Vitamin A

Vitamin A is necessary for the health of skin, vision, bone growth, and immune function. Vitamin A deficiency is associated with significant eye problems, including night blindness and conjunctival dryness. Vitamin A actually refers to a group of retinoids, not just one chemical. Two common forms of vitamin A are retinol, or preformed vitamin A, and the provitamin A carotenoids such as β-carotene.

The daily DRI of vitamin A for women aged older than 51 years is 700 µg (2,330 International Units [IU]) retinol activity equivalents (a measure of vitamin A activity based on the body's capacity to convert provitamin carotenoids into retinaldehyde). Populations at risk for vitamin A deficiency and malabsorption include those with pancreatic insufficiency, cystic fibrosis, or any condition in which fat malabsorption occurs. Absorption requires the presence of bile salts, pancreatic lipase, protein, and dietary fat. Medications such as orlistat can interfere with vitamin A absorption. Retinol is a form of vitamin A that is commonly used to treat acne, psoriasis, and other skin conditions; hypervitaminosis A is a risk in patients taking retinol-based medications. Food sources include liver, eggs, sweet potato, pumpkin, carrots, spinach, collards, kale, turnip greens, egg yolk, milk, cheese, and butter.

As a fat-soluble vitamin, oversupplementation can cause buildup, with potential for toxic effects. Prolonged high doses may cause bleeding from the gums, dry or sore mouth, or drying, cracking, or peeling of the lips. Excessive intake (>10,000 IU/d) may stimulate bone loss, counteract the effects of calcium supplements, and cause hypercalcemia, hair loss, and hepatoxicity. The UL for vitamin A is 3,000 µg retinol activity equivalents (10,000 IU) per day for adults aged older than 18 years.

Studies in postmenopausal women have shown that too much vitamin A intake from retinol may increase the risk of hip fracture.[46] Scientists believe that excessive amounts of vitamin A may trigger an increase in osteoclasts, which break down bone. It also may interfere with vitamin D, which helps preserve bone. Carotenoids (vegetable sources of vitamin A) may be associated with lower fracture risk[47] and are preferred over preformed animal sources of retinol.

There are limited data to support vitamin A supplementation for disease prevention. The USPSTF has issued a statement recommending against β-carotene for the prevention of CVD and cancer.[5] Supplemental β-carotene data has been inconsistent with regard to lung cancer risk reduction.[48] Dietary vitamin A and carotenoid levels, however, have been associated with a reduced risk of breast,[49] pancreatic,[50] bladder,[25] and brain cancers.[51]

B vitamins

Vitamin B_1 (thiamin), B_2 (riboflavin), B_3 (niacin), B_5 (pantothenic acid), B_6 (pyridoxine), B_9 (folic acid), and B_{12} (cyanocobalamin) are water-soluble vitamins. Supplements are available either in combination or individually.

Vitamin B_1 (thiamin)

Vitamin B_1 is a coenzyme in the metabolism of carbohydrates and branched-chain amino acids. Food sources include whole-grain products, meat, fish, and fortified foods. The recommended dietary allowance of thiamin for adult women is 1.1 mg, and there is no UL. Populations at risk for deficiency include those with chronic alcohol use, malnutrition, history of bariatric surgery, heart failure, and history of critical illness.[52] Deficiency is also seen in older adults. Thiamin deficiency is associated with dementia.[53,54]

Vitamin B_2 (riboflavin)

Vitamin B_2 is a coenzyme in numerous reactions necessary for energy production, cell function, and metabolism. It is also needed for activation of pyridoxine and for conversion of tryptophan to niacin. Food sources are eggs, meat, dairy, and fortified foods. The DRI of riboflavin for adult women is 1.1 mg. Excess riboflavin can cause the urine to turn bright yellow. Riboflavin deficiency is rare but can be seen in vegan and vegetarian diets and in pregnant women.

Vitamin B_3 (niacin, niacinamide)

Niacin, after conversion to niacinamide, is a component of the coenzymes necessary for tissue respiration, glycogenolysis, and lipid, amino acid, protein, and purine metabolism. Food sources of vitamin B$_3$ include meat, fish, poultry, enriched and whole-grain breads, and fortified cereals. The DRI of niacin for adult women is 14 mg.

Niacin is used to treat hyperlipidemia. It improves all major lipid parameters, reducing low-density lipoprotein cholesterol (LDL-C) and triglycerides and increasing high-density lipoprotein cholesterol (HDL-C). In a meta-analysis of five trials involving 432 patients, LDL-C and triglyceride reduction in women was greater than in men at all doses.[55] More recently, niacin's lack of evidence supporting prevention of CV events has deemed it less useful in clinical practice.[56]

Adverse events of niacin intake include flushing, itching, and gastrointestinal (GI) discomfort. These are more commonly experienced when therapeutic rather than nutritional doses are taken, especially when beginning therapy. Niacin should be taken with the evening meal. Flushing may be minimized by taking aspirin 1 hour earlier, by increasing the niacin dose gradually, or by using the extended-release form. Nonflushing niacin supplements typically contain little or no nicotinic acid and should be avoided if the therapeutic target is hyperlipidemia.

Vitamin B$_6$ (pyridoxine)

Vitamin B$_6$ is a group of six compounds that function as a coenzyme for many metabolic functions primarily affecting protein metabolism. It is involved in the conversion of tryptophan to niacin or serotonin and of glycogen to glucose, in the synthesis of γ-aminobutyric acid within the central nervous system, and in red blood cell synthesis.

Food sources of pyridoxine are fish, organ meats, potatoes, and fruit. The DRI of pyridoxine for adult women is 1.5 mg, with a UL of 100 mg. Adequate absorption of vitamin B$_6$ can be assessed by measuring pyridoxal 5' phosphate levels. Populations at risk for deficiency include those with chronic renal insufficiency, autoimmune disease, and alcohol use.

Recommended intakes may be increased if a woman is taking cycloserine, antiepileptics, or theophylline. Although it is generally nontoxic, high doses of pyridoxine (2-6 g/d) taken for several months have caused severe, dose-dependent sensory neuropathy with residual weakness.

Pyridoxine supplements have been used to treat a variety of conditions, including premenstrual syndrome, nausea in pregnancy, cancer, chemotherapy-induced AEs, and cognitive decline, with varied results. Many studies have also investigated the use of vitamin B$_6$ in combination with folate and vitamin B$_{12}$ for CVD.[57] These homocysteine-lowering interventions have not been shown to affect CV events or outcomes.

Vitamin B$_9$ (folate, folic acid)

Vitamin B$_9$ is converted in the liver and plasma into its metabolically active form, tetrafolic acid, in the presence of ascorbic acid. This vitamin is necessary for normal erythropoiesis, synthesis, and metabolism of various amino acids and for other metabolic processes. Folate is a water-soluble B vitamin that plays a critical role in DNA synthesis, methylation, and repair.

Folate occurs naturally in food. Dietary sources include vegetables, particularly dark leafy greens, nuts, seafood, and fortified foods. Folic acid is the synthetic form of folate that is found in supplements and added to fortified foods. Folic acid is almost completely absorbed, primarily in the upper duodenum.

Folic acid supplements are routinely recommended preconception and during pregnancy because this nutrient reduces the incidence of neural tube defects in the newborn.[58]

The DRI of vitamin B$_9$ in adult women is 400 µg dietary folate equivalents. The UL is 1,000 µg dietary folate equivalents. Requirements may be increased in those receiving estrogen-containing contraceptives. Absorption is impaired in malabsorption syndromes, and chronic alcohol use puts people at risk for deficiency.

Deficiency may produce megaloblastic and macrocytic anemias. Higher doses than the DRI are generally not recommended until a diagnosis of pernicious anemia has been ruled out, because higher doses correct the hematologic manifestations of pernicious anemia while allowing neurologic damage to progress irreversibly. Excessive folate states have also been implicated in promoting cancer tissue growth.[59]

Folate has been associated with a slightly reduced colon cancer risk.[60] It has been studied in reducing CVD but is no longer recommended.[57] Adequate folate also is proposed to decrease risk of dementia[61] and improve treatment of depression.[62]

Vitamin B$_{12}$ (cyanocobalamin)

Vitamin B$_{12}$ acts as a coenzyme for various metabolic functions.[63] It is necessary for erythropoiesis, nerve function, and DNA synthesis. Dietary vitamin B$_{12}$ is released from the proteins to which it is bound by gastric acid and pancreatic proteases, then bound to intrinsic factor and absorbed from the lower half of the ileum.

Food sources are fish, seafood, egg yolk, milk, and fermented cheeses. Bacteria found on vegetables may be a source of vitamin B_{12} for vegans. Ordinary cooking temperatures will not cause loss of vitamin B_{12} from foods, but extreme heating should be avoided to maintain vitamin B_{12} levels.

Deficiency may lead to macrocytic and megaloblastic anemias and possible irreversible neurologic damage, with pernicious anemia caused by either lack of or inhibition of intrinsic factor. Deficiency may be the result of inadequate nutrition or intestinal malabsorption. It can occur in vegans, because vitamin B_{12} is found in animal protein and not in vegetables. Additional causes of deficiency are alcoholism, gastritis with achlorhydria, lack of intrinsic factor, and gastrectomy. Deficiency is increased in older adults.

The oral route is useful for treating nutritional vitamin B_{12} deficiency when absorption is normal, but it is not useful in small-bowel disease, in malabsorption syndromes, or after total gastrectomy or ileal resection. For treating deficiency resulting from lack of absorption, vitamin B_{12} is given by injection (either intramuscularly or deep subcutaneously). It is also available in a sublingual dosage form. Vitamin B_{12} plasma concentration determination is recommended before treatment of deficiency.

The DRI of B_{12} in adult women is 2.4 µg. Recommended intakes may need to be increased by those taking medications, most notably prolonged use of metformin[64] and proton pump inhibitors.[65] Patients aged older than 50 years and strict vegetarians should consider consuming foods fortified with vitamin B_{12} and vitamin B_{12} supplements rather than attempting to get vitamin B_{12} strictly from dietary sources.[63]

Health benefits of vitamin B_{12} classically include improved energy and reversal of cognitive decline. However, there is insufficient evidence to support the role of vitamin B_{12} repletion in treating cognitive disorders.[66] Low-quality evidence exists for the association between B_{12} deficiency and cognitive decline, and moderate-quality evidence that vitamin B_{12} depletion does not improve cognition.[67] Similarly, limited evidence exists to address the question of the role of vitamin B_{12} supplementation for fatigue.

Vitamin C

Ascorbic acid, a water-soluble vitamin, is needed for collagen formation and tissue repair as well as for metabolism of folic acid, iron, phenylalanine, tyrosine, norepinephrine, and histamine; use of carbohydrates; synthesis of lipids and proteins; immune function; hydroxylation of serotonin; and preservation of blood vessel integrity. Ascorbic acid enhances absorption of nonheme iron. Ascorbic acid is an essential dietary vitamin in that it cannot be manufactured in the body. It is absorbed from the jejunum.

Dietary sources include citrus fruits; vegetables such as peppers, broccoli, and cabbage; tomatoes, and potatoes. Vitamin C supplements gradually lose potency with storage, and in foods, vitamin C is rapidly destroyed by exposure to air, by drying or salting, and by up to 50% through ordinary cooking.

The DRI of vitamin C for adult women is 75 mg and 110 mg in smokers. Populations at risk for deficiency include smokers, those exposed to secondhand smoke, people with extremely restricted diets, and those with malabsorption syndromes. The UL for vitamin C is 2,000 mg.

Vitamin C is important to overall health; dietary sources such as fruits and vegetables should be promoted to reach the DRI. A severe deficiency in vitamin C can cause scurvy, a disease that results in extreme weakness, lethargy, easy bruising, and bleeding. The role of vitamin C in chronic diseases requires further study.

Excessive supplemental vitamin C has been associated with an increased risk of kidney stones. High-dose ascorbic acid (but not sodium ascorbate) may decrease urine pH, causing renal tubular reabsorption of oxalate, with the possibility of precipitation of oxalate stones in the urinary tract. High doses also may cause diarrhea. Another hypothetical concern with excess vitamin C is iron overload or exacerbation of hemochromatosis, although this has not been a problem clinically.[68]

Vitamin C and cancer

The relationship between vitamin C and cancer is complex. A meta-analysis of 785 trials including 62,000 participants revealed no association with an overall reduction in cancer of all types.[69] In pancreatic cancer, vitamin C intake has shown mixed data, with reduced risk[37,70] and no effect.[71] Vitamin C has been associated with a reduced risk for cervical,[72] esophageal,[73] renal cell,[74] and primary brain[75] cancers.

The role for vitamin C treatment in breast cancer remains controversial. A meta-analysis of 10 studies involving more than 17,000 women with breast cancer showed a significant reduction in all-cause and breast cancer-specific mortality in participants taking higher amounts of dietary vitamin C or oral vitamin C supplements (400-1,000 mg).[76] (See also "Breast Cancer" in Chapter 9.)

Vitamin C and cardiovascular disease

Vitamin C as an antioxidant has been proposed as having a role in the reduction of CVD. No evidence has been shown to support vitamin C preventing development of cardiac disease.[77] In a population-based prospective cohort study, women aged 40 to 75 years at baseline were followed for 12 years, with a strong inverse association shown between plasma vitamin C level and a 62% reduction in type 2 diabetes mellitus (DM) risk.[78] (See also Chapter 8, "Cardiometabolic Disorders Midlife Women.")

Vitamin C and the common cold

Using vitamin C for prevention and treatment of the common cold was popularized in the 1970s by Linus Pauling. Subsequently, a Cochrane review of more than 11,000 participants demonstrated no protective effect in the general population but significant reduction in marathon runners, skiers, and soldiers.[79] Studies examining vitamin C's effect on the duration of symptoms have shown inconsistent results.[80]

Vitamin D

Vitamin D is a sterol-like compound synthesized in nature by interaction between 7-dehydrocholesterol and ultraviolet light that, by a photochemical reaction, opens up the B ring of the steroid molecule. Typically, this synthesis takes place in the skin of many animals, including humans. This compound—also called vitamin D_3 or cholecalciferol—is biologically inactive.

After synthesis in the skin, vitamin D (as cholecalciferol) is transported to the liver and hydroxylated to 25-hydroxycholecalciferol, also called 25-hydroxyvitamin D (25[OH]D). The 25(OH)D is measurable in serum, and as such it serves as the functional indicator for vitamin D status.[81]

The final hydroxylation in the kidney produces 1,25-dihydroxycholecalciferol, or calcitriol. Calcitriol is instrumental in calcium metabolism and balance.

Another form of vitamin D is a similar compound, ergocalciferol, or vitamin D_2, which in experimental animals has an ability to prevent rickets in a way roughly similar to that of cholecalciferol. Ergocalciferol is produced synthetically by irradiation of a product of ergot mold.

Both forms of vitamin D (vitamin D_2 and D_3) are measured in IUs, with 1 µg of cholecalciferol being equivalent to 40 IU. These forms had been considered to be equipotent, but it is now commonly believed that vitamin D_3 is substantially more potent than vitamin D_2 by a factor of at least 4.[82]

Vitamin D is essential for the efficient intestinal absorption of calcium and thus for bone health. In women with a severe vitamin D deficiency, gross absorption of dietary calcium is no more than 10%, and net absorption may be zero or even negative. Calcium absorption, bone mineral density (BMD), and other bone health benefits plateau at a serum 25(OH)D level of 50 nmol/L (20 ng/mL).[83,84]

In a population-based study of National Health and Nutrition Examination Survey III data, BMD improved as vitamin D status improved up to levels above 80 nmol/L (32 ng/mL).[85,86] Studies have found that vitamin D (≥600 IU/d for ages 1-70 y, and 800 IU/d for ages older than 70 y) with supplemental calcium can reduce the rate of postmenopausal bone loss, especially in older women.[83] Results from the WHI found that participants taking calcium (1,000 mg/d) plus vitamin D (400 IU/d) had a small but significant 1% improvement in hip BMD.[87] Meta-analyses of randomized, controlled trials (RCTs) in postmenopausal women (mean age, 71-85 y) show that vitamin D doses of 700 IU to 800 IU per day were associated with significant reductions in the risk of hip and nonvertebral fractures.[88] No significant changes were found in outcomes for either of those fracture sites in trials that used fewer than 700 IU per day.

A subsequent National Osteoporosis Foundation (NOF) meta-analysis reported a 15% reduction in total fracture and 30% reduction in hip fracture in women taking calcium and vitamin D.[89] A USPSTF meta-analysis also supported the protective effect of calcium and vitamin D,[90] although the independent effect of vitamin D alone is less certain. High doses (>800-1,000 IU daily) are recommended in patients who already have a diagnosis of osteoporosis with low vitamin D levels (below 20-30 ng/dL).[91] (See also Chapter 7, "Osteoporosis.")

Some uncertainty remains with respect to the utility and optimal level of serum 25(OH)D. Some promote the bottom end of a healthy range of 30 ng/mL to 32 ng/mL (75-80 nmol/L). Still, many experts believe there is a threshold at approximately 20 ng/mL (50 nmol/L), with minimal additional benefit above this level.[83,92]

In 2011, the Institute of Medicine (IOM) set the UL of vitamin D at 4,000 IU per day, which correlates with 25(OH)D levels of 125 nmol/L (50 ng/mL).[83] The IOM did not recommend increasing sun exposure to achieve adequate 25(OH)D levels and based the dietary guidelines on an assumption of minimal to no sun exposure. For the typical fair-skinned person living in the Northeast United States, sunlight exposure of 5 to 15 minutes on the arms and legs between the hours of 10 AM and 3 PM two to three times a week has been proposed by some. Women with darker skin may require as much as 5 to 10 times longer skin exposure because their skin pigment markedly reduces vitamin D production from sunlight. Moreover, solar radiation is classified as a carcinogen, so the recommendation to increase sun exposure to raise vitamin D levels is controversial. Wearing a sunscreen with a sun protection factor of 8 or more blocks the skin's ability to produce vitamin D by 95%. (See also "Skin Changes" in Chapter 2 and "Skin Cancer" in Chapter 9.)

The IOM's RDA of 600 IU per day of vitamin D for all people aged up to 70 years and 800 IU per day for those aged 71 years and older are public health guidelines for a generally healthy population (Table 3).[83] The IOM has acknowledged that some people may have greater requirements. The NOF recommends 800 IU to 1,000 IU per day of vitamin D for women aged 50 years and older.[93]

Canada's Food Guide agrees with the IOM's RDA of vitamin D for its citizens.[94] It also recommends that all Canadians aged older than 2 years, including pregnant and lactating women, consume 500 mL (two cups) of vitamin D-fortified milk or soy beverages daily. Health Canada recommends a vitamin D DRI for adults aged younger than 70 years of 600 IU and 800 IU for those aged older than 70 years. Health Canada also sets a UL for both groups at 4,000 IU.

The actual requirement for additional oral intake will vary from person to person, although it will be similar within various age and ethnic groups. Although the optimal range for 25(OH)D levels continues to be debated, expert opinion holds fairly consistently to a minimum level of 20 ng/mL to 30 ng/mL (50-80 nmol/L)[95] and an optimal level of 30 ng/mL to 44 ng/ml (75-110 nmol/L).[96] The upper end of the therapeutic target level is less certain, although levels above 60 ng/mL are seemingly without additional benefit.

As a rough guide, the serum 25(OH)D level, under steady-state dosing, will rise by about 1 nmol/L per µg cholecalciferol per day. Thus, a person with a serum 25(OH)D value of 50 nmol/L (20 ng/mL) may need at least 30 µg of additional vitamin D_3 per day (1,200 IU) to reach a level of 80 nmol/L (32 ng/mL)—or, to use the

Table 3. Institute of Medicine Committee to Review Dietary Reference Intakes for Vitamin D and Calcium RDAs, by Life Stage

Life-stage group, age and sex	Vitamin D		Calcium	
	RDA, IU/d[a]	UL, IU/d[a]	RDA, mg/d[a]	UL, mg/d[b]
1-3 y M+F	600	2,500	700	2,500
4-8 y M+F	600	3,000	1,000	2,500
9-13 y M+F	600	4,000	1,300	3,000
14-18 y M+F	600	4,000	1,300	3,000
19-30 y M+F	600	4,000	1,000	2,500
31-50 y M+F	600	4,000	1,000	2,500
51-70 y M	600	4,000	1,000	2,000
51-70 y F	600	4,000	1,200	2,000
71+ y M+F	800	4,000	1,200	2,000
Pregnant or lactating F				
14-18 y	600	4,000	1,300	3,000
19-50 y	600	4,000	1,000	2,500
Infants				
0-6 mo M+F		1,000		1,000
6-12 mo M+F		1,500		1,500

Abbreviations: F, female; IU, international unit; M, male; RDA, recommended dietary allowance; UL, tolerable upper intake level.
[a]Intake that covers the needs of ≥97.5% of population.
[b]Not intended as a target intake (no consistent evidence of greater benefit at intake levels above the RDA).
Adapted from Institute of Medicine (US) Committee to Review Dietary Reference Intakes for Vitamin D and Calcium, Food and Nutrition Board.[83]

units commonly reported in the United States, serum 25(OH)D will rise by about 1 ng/mL for every 100 IU per day of additional cholecalciferol.

An estimated 60% of people—whether institutionalized or free living, using common vitamin D supplements or not—have serum 25(OH)D values less than 80 nmol/L (32 ng/mL).[97,98] Vitamin D insufficiency is highly prevalent in people aged older than 90 years.[99] Postmenopausal women have a high prevalence of vitamin D inadequacy and deficiency, which varies among the seasons.[100]

A few food sources of vitamin D are available—primarily oily fish such as salmon and mackerel, eggs, and fortified foods. Wild-caught fish, deriving their vitamin D from ingested phytoplankton, are good sources; farm-raised fish have far less vitamin D. Fish liver oil has long been the classic source of vitamin D, and years ago cod and halibut liver oils were used as mainstays in the prevention of rickets in children. For decades, milk has been fortified with a small amount of vitamin D (100 IU/8-oz serving), and more recently some orange juices have been fortified to the same level. Small amounts of vitamin D have been added to certain ready-to-eat cereals.

Women aged older than 70 years who have little or no sun exposure and rely on diet alone for vitamin D intake are likely to have suboptimal 25(OH)D levels. Daily requirements can usually be met with cholecalciferol 600 IU to 800 IU vitamin D plus dietary intake. Taking vitamin D at the same time as a calcium supplement is not necessary. However, many calcium supplements contain vitamin D, providing the convenience of obtaining both nutrients in a single-dose form.

The principal high-potency form of vitamin D available to clinicians was once 50,000 IU of ergocalciferol (vitamin D_2) as an oral prescription product. However, there are several OTC products containing 1,000 IU to 50,000 IU cholecalciferol (vitamin D_3) per dose, allowing consumers to replete vitamin D without a prescription. In some populations, such as those with chronic kidney disease, cholecalciferol is preferred.[101]

Other than metabolic bone disease, several associations have been made between vitamin D and health conditions, although most have been controversial. Vitamin D's role in cancer development includes the knowledge that deficiency states are associated with an increased risk of colon and breast cancer, whereas elevated levels have been associated with an increased risk of pancreatic cancer.[102] A large RCT (VITAL) of 25,871 participants, however, showed that supplemental vitamin D_3 did not result in a lower incidence of invasive cancer or cardiovascular events compared with placebo.[103]

Vitamin E

Much like vitamin A, vitamin E represents a combination of compounds. These tocopherols and tocotrienols are fat-soluble antioxidants that protect polyunsaturated fatty acids in various cell structures and red blood cells from hemolysis. Deficiency of this vitamin is rare.

Food sources include nuts, seeds, vegetable oil, vegetables, and wheat germ. The DRI of vitamin E for adult women is 15 mg (22.5 IU), based on α-tocopherol because it is the most available form. Populations at risk for deficiency are very few, limited to those with extremely limited diets or fat malabsorption.

The UL for vitamin E is 1,500 IU (1,000 mg/d). However, the Physicians' Health Study found an increased risk of hemorrhagic stroke at 400 IU vitamin E every other day.[104] Moreover, a meta-analysis of 19 trials of patients with chronic diseases found a significant deleterious relationship between high-dosage (defined as ≥400 IU/d) vitamin E and all-cause mortality, although the trials were often small.[104] The USPSTF has recommended against the use of vitamin E for cancer or CVD prevention.[5]

General guidelines caution that vitamin E doses higher than 400 IU per day are to be avoided in people taking medications that increase risk of bleeding.

The Heart Outcomes Prevention Evaluation (HOPE) trial, designed to assess angiotensin-converting enzyme-inhibitor effect in participants at high risk for heart disease, also examined the effect of vitamin E supplementation.[106] The study demonstrated that vitamin E had no apparent protective benefit from cardiac events. The HOPE extension trial examined the effects of long-term vitamin E 400 IU daily on CV events and cancer. Study participants were aged 55 years and older and had a history of CHD or PAD, stroke, or DM plus one other CVD risk factor. Results demonstrated no significant difference in the primary outcomes of MI, stroke, or CV death.

Vitamin E had no effect on occurrence of cancer. In postmenopausal women, the Women's Angiographic Vitamin and Estrogen study showed no vascular benefit with the addition of vitamins E and C, but participants in this group did have increased mortality.[107]

The Women's Health Study evaluated vitamin E for primary prevention of CVD and cancer.[108] The study randomized 39,876 women (aged ≥45 y) to receive 600 IU of vitamin E or placebo and aspirin or placebo on alternate days. After 10 years' follow-up, there was no significant difference in CVD or cancer incidence between those who were and were not taking vitamin E, but there was a reduction in CV mortality in the vitamin E group. The same study assessed venous thromboembolism and showed a 21% hazard reduction in those taking vitamin E and a 49% hazard reduction in women with either factor V Leiden or prothrombin or methylenetetrahydrofolate reductase mutations taking vitamin E.[109]

Dietary vitamin E intake has been associated with a reduced risk of lung cancer.[110] More research is needed to best understand the role vitamin E plays in disease prevention, but for now, very little supports the clinical use of high-dose vitamin E supplements.

Vitamin K

Vitamin K is a group of fat-soluble compounds required for protein metabolism, most notably functioning in coagulation and bone formation. It is found naturally as phylloquinone (vitamin K_1), for which sources include green leafy vegetables, and menaquinone (vitamin K_2), for which sources include meat, eggs, dairy, and fermented soy.

Given lack of data, there is no estimated average requirement of vitamin K. Instead, the recommended adequate intake of vitamin K for adult women is 90 µg. Vitamin K deficiency is uncommon and most commonly detected by a prolonged prothrombin time on laboratory evaluation. Patients with fat malabsorption may be at risk for deficiency. Vitamin K supplements are contraindicated in women taking warfarin and other vitamin K-dependent anticoagulants.

Vitamin K supplements have become popular in products marketed for bone health, although the science for efficacy is mixed. In observational studies including nearly 81,000 women, dietary vitamin K_1 was associated with a 22% reduction in fracture (relative risk [RR], 0.78; 95% confidence interval [CI], 0.56-0.99).[111] Meta-analysis of 19 RCTs involving nearly 7,000 women using vitamin K_2 demonstrated benefit in osteocalcin metabolism, without an associated reduction in fracture or improvement in BMD, and a concurrent increase in minor AEs (nausea and abdominal pain).[112]

In the European Prospective Incidence of Cancer and Nutrition study, 24,340 participants aged 35 to 64 years were followed for cancer incidence and mortality in relation to dietary intake.[113] In an analysis of the effect of ingesting foods rich in vitamin K, dietary intake of vitamin K_2 was associated with a reduced risk of incident and fatal cancer, mainly prostate and lung. However, there is also evidence suggesting that vitamin K antagonists may have a protective effect against prostate cancer.[114] Clearly, further research is needed, as with many vitamins, to better understand these associations.

Mineral Supplements

Trace elements and metals in biologic fluids are essential nutrients for humans. They act as "biochemical triggers," some forming complexes with enzymes and helping in the binding of biologic ligands.

Calcium

Calcium, a divalent, cationic element, is the fifth most abundant element in the earth's crust, present in pearls and marble, ivory and antlers, and corals and bone. Calcium is also the most abundant mineral in the human body. An adult human body contains 1,000 g to 1,200 g of calcium, 99% of which is in bones and teeth. As an element, calcium can neither be synthesized nor degraded as it moves through the processes of cellular- and organ-level metabolism.

Calcium requirements for skeletal maintenance fluctuate throughout a woman's life (Table 4).[28] During the teen years, calcium requirements are high because of the demands of a rapidly growing skeleton. Peak acquisition of bone mineral content occurs at about 12 years of age in girls, about a year after the average peak height velocity occurs.[115] All but one of nine RCTs of calcium supplementation in youth found a small but consistent positive effect on BMD or bone mineral content accrual as measured by dual-energy x-ray absorptiometry (DXA). The average increment in bone density in the calcium group compared with the placebo group was from 0.57% to 5.8%, depending on the skeletal site.[89]

During a woman's reproductive years, less calcium is required for bone health as bone turnover stabilizes at a low level and peak adult bone mass is achieved and maintained (Table 3).[28] Calcium requirements remain stable until menopause, when the bone resorption rate increases because of the decrease in ovarian estrogen production. Calcium needs rise at that time because of decreased efficiency in the use of dietary calcium. This is largely because of estrogen-related shifts in intestinal calcium absorption and renal conservation.

Fractional calcium absorption is affected by the amount of calcium consumed and reaches a peak of about 35% at an intake of about 400 mg, and then falls off as intake

Table 4. Institute of Medicine Dietary Reference Intakes for Calcium by Life Stage

Life-stage group, age (sex)	RDA, mg/d	UL, mg/d
1-3 y (m/f)	700	2,500
4-8 y (m/f)	1,000	2,500
9-18 y (m/f)	1,300	3,000
19-50 y (m/f)	1,000	2,500
51-70 y (m)	1,000	2,000
51-70 y (f)	1,200	2,000
≥71 y (m/f)	1,200	2,000

RDA indicates the intake level that covers the needs of ≥97.5% of the population.
Abbreviations: f, female; m, male; RDA, recommended dietary allowance, UL, tolerable upper intake level.
Adapted from Institute of Medicine Committee to Review Dietary Reference Intakes for Vitamin D and Calcium.[28]

increases further to a level of 20%, with an intake of approximately 1,000 mg.[116] The amount of calcium needed also is affected by the decrease in intestinal absorption that occurs with age. An age-related decrease in calcium absorption has been shown in postmenopausal women in addition to the decline that occurs at menopause. This decrease could be because of a decline in either the active calcium transport or diffusion component of the calcium absorption system.[117] Declines in estradiol, as occur in menopause, are associated with declines in calcium absorption.[118] One factor that may limit active calcium absorption is reduced vitamin D resulting from age-related declines in several functions, including ingestion, cutaneous synthesis of the parent vitamin, renal synthesis of the active form of the vitamin (1,25-dihydroxyvitamin D), and intestinal responsiveness.[119] In addition, aging reduces the expression of two key intestinal calcium transporters, TRPV6 and calbindin-D9k.[120]

Dietary survey data have shown that calcium intakes for most groups are far below recommended amounts, especially in older adults and in those with lower income levels.[121,122]

Dietary factors limiting calcium absorption include consumption of oxalic acid (found in spinach, rhubarb, and certain other green vegetables), grains that contain large amounts of phytates (eg, wheat bran, soy protein isolates), and possibly tannins (found in tea). Evidence indicates that other dietary components such as fat, phosphorus, magnesium, and caffeine have negligible effects on calcium absorption at generally prevalent intake levels. Other factors that can decrease calcium absorption include vitamin D deficiency, estrogen deficiency, decreased gastric acid production, and malabsorptive disorders.[123]

Calcium plus vitamin D has been shown to reduce bone loss in healthy postmenopausal women and in postmenopausal women with substantial bone loss or previous fracture, especially in the 5 or more years after menopause.[124-126] A benefit of calcium on bone mass has been shown.[127]

Calcium and vitamin D supplementation can lead to modest reductions in all fractures and specifically hip fracture[125,128,129]; however, significant efficacy of daily oral calcium supplements alone in preventing fracture has not been shown.

Baseline calcium intake and treatment adherence need to be considered when evaluating calcium and vitamin D supplementation trials. In fact, one review of trials that used a per-protocol analysis showed that calcium and vitamin D supplementation resulted in a significant 15% reduced risk of total fractures (summary RR estimate [SRRE], 0.85; 95% CI, 0.73-0.98) and a 30% reduced risk of hip fractures (SRRE, 0.70; 95% CI, 0.56-0.87), using subgroup analysis from the WHI.[89]

Calcium may potentiate the effect of exercise on peak bone mass, primarily in those with higher daily calcium intake. For peak bone mass, three of four RCTs of calcium and exercise combined found that the combined intervention had a significantly greater effect on bone accrual as assessed by DXA than either exercise or calcium alone.[89]

Calcium, either alone or with vitamin D, is not as effective for fracture prevention as pharmacotherapy with menopause estrogen-alone therapy (ET), estrogen-progestogen therapy (EPT), an estrogen agonist/antagonist, or a bisphosphonate. However, supplemental calcium substantially improves the efficacy of these agents in reducing menopause-related bone loss.[130,131] Because of the well-established need for adequate calcium intake, all key clinical trials with either an estrogen agonist/antagonist or a bisphosphonate have provided supplemental calcium to treatment and placebo arms. Although it is likely that calcium potentiates the positive BMD effects of an estrogen agonist/antagonist and bisphosphonates as it does for ET and EPT, this conclusion can only be surmised.

The importance of an adequate calcium intake for skeletal health is well established. Calcium also has been associated with beneficial effects in several nonskeletal disorders, primarily colorectal cancer and hypertension, although the extent of those effects has not been fully elucidated.[132]

There has been debate as a result of several studies, including two meta-analyses and two large Scandinavian longitudinal studies, about the possible causal association between calcium supplementation and increased CV risk. These studies suggested that calcium supplements were associated with a higher risk of MI.[133-136] However, subsequent studies did not find increased risk, including an NOF study in which a dose-response relationship could not be found between dietary or total calcium intake and the risk of CVD.[137] A statement was issued by the NOF and the American Society for Preventive Cardiology in 2016 indicating that calcium intake, either from diet or from supplements, has no apparent effect on the risk of CVD or cerebrovascular disease.[138]

Serum calcium is not an accurate biomarker of calcium nutritional status, intake, or stores, because serum calcium does not fluctuate with changes in dietary calcium intake.[139]

Serum calcium is maintained in the normal range in most cases, even in the presence of severe deficiency. Some combination of a history of low calcium intake, coupled with decreased bone mass for age, increased bone-remodeling indices, and high serum parathyroid hormone (PTH), will usually be characteristic of calcium deficiency; however, each of these associated changes can be produced by other causes.

Most women need to consume more dietary calcium. In fact, calcium is considered a shortfall nutrient in women, with more than half of the US population regularly having intakes below the DRI.[12,140] Also, women with low 25(OH)D levels are unlikely to absorb calcium optimally. Given the fact that low serum vitamin D levels are linked to calcium deficiency, laboratory tests for vitamin D are being used.

Several organizations have published calcium-intake guidelines. The last International Osteoporosis Foundation (IOF) guideline concluded that calcium and vitamin D supplementation (but not calcium alone) leads to modest reduction in fracture risk and that CV concerns associated with calcium supplements are not convincingly supported by current evidence.[141] The NOF recommends that women follow the IOF calcium DRI (women aged ≤50 y consume 1,000 mg calcium/d, and women aged ≥51 y consume 1,200 mg calcium/d) and promote food as the best source of calcium.[142] The 2016 NOF/American Society for Preventive Cardiology guideline on the safety and benefit of calcium supplementation stated that calcium intake below the UL (2,000-2,500 mg/d) is not associated with CVD risk in generally healthy adults.[137,138] However, this report also suggests that obtaining calcium from food is preferred to the use of calcium supplements to correct shortfalls in dietary intake. (See also Chapter 7, "Osteoporosis.")

Recommended intakes for calcium are probably sufficient for most people to maintain skeletal mass during the peak adult years and to minimize age-related bone loss during involution (Table 3),[28] again noting that dietary calcium intake is preferable to supplementation.[138]

It is difficult to pin down the calcium-intake status of the population because of the rapidly changing environment with respect to food fortification and supplement use. From food sources alone, median calcium intakes for women aged 40 to 60 years are less than 600 mg per day and have been approximately stable at that level for many years, despite education and other campaigns to improve calcium intake.[28,143] This leaves a substantial gap that ranges from 400 mg to 900 mg per day to be filled by fortified foods, supplements, or both. Specific populations of postmenopausal women at extra risk for inadequate calcium intake include women who are lactose intolerant, who follow a pure vegetarian diet (typically getting only 250 mg/d of calcium), or who have poor eating habits. Women tend to find nutritional advice from their clinicians more credible than the comparable advice they get from all other sources, so it is critically important that clinicians continue to emphasize the importance of adequate calcium intake.

Dietary sources are the preferred means of obtaining adequate calcium intake because there are other essential nutrients in high-calcium foods. For most US residents, dairy products (milk, cheese, yogurt, ice cream) are the major contributors of dietary calcium, providing approximately 70% of the total calcium intake of postmenopausal women aged 60 years and older. An 8-oz serving of milk or yogurt or a 1-oz to 1.5-oz cube of hard cheese contains about 300 mg of calcium. All other (nondairy) foods combined contribute only 150 mg to 250 mg calcium to a typical adult diet. Hence, meeting current intake recommendations from commonly available foods generally requires consumption of approximately three servings of dairy food per day. Reduced-fat or low-fat products contain at least as much calcium per serving as high-fat dairy products, and they offer alternatives for women concerned about body weight and lipid profiles.

Because many people are not able to achieve the recommended three dairy servings a day, food manufacturers have introduced a variety of calcium-fortified products, including fruit juices, breakfast cereals, and breads. These foods are not equally well engineered because the added calcium may exhibit reduced bioavailability or such poor physical properties so that the fortificant settles into the bottom of the carton (as with soy beverages requiring shaking of the carton before pouring). Thus, although calcium fortification of foods is a welcome improvement in the nutritional value of available foods, it still functions in a climate of "buyer beware," and the consumer would be well advised to read labels carefully. The best way to understand the calcium content of a tablet or food item is to look at the label. A 100% daily calcium value is 1,000 mg, so if the label shows that the item contains 40% of the daily value, the amount of calcium is 400 mg.

Lactose intolerance is a real and important clinical syndrome, but its true prevalence is not known.[144] An estimate of self-reported prevalence of lactose intolerance in Canada resulted in 16%.[145] Most people with lactose malabsorption do not have clinical lactose intolerance and are unlikely to be lactose malabsorbers. Many persons with real or perceived lactose intolerance avoid dairy and ingest inadequate amounts of calcium and vitamin D, which may predispose them to decreased bone accrual, osteoporosis, and other adverse health outcomes. In most cases, persons do not need to eliminate dairy consumption completely.[144] Lactase nonpersistence is more common in people of East Asian, African, and South American descent.[121] Other GI problems (celiac disease, irritable bowel syndrome, Crohn disease, infection) or their treatment with intestinal antibiotics can cause temporary or permanent lactose intolerance. Many women with lactase nonpersistence can tolerate milk normally if they have never stopped drinking it since youth or if they increase intake gradually, thereby conditioning their intestinal flora to produce lactase. To increase tolerance, the National Medical Association has issued a consensus report recommending three servings of dairy per day for all African Americans.[146] Those few who remain intolerant may substitute yogurt and lactase-treated milk. True milk intolerance or allergy is rare. Calcium supplements or calcium-fortified foods should be considered if dietary preferences or lactase nonpersistence restricts consumption of dairy foods.

Calcium supplements offer a convenient alternative to women unable to consume enough calcium from diet alone. Their use should be confined to what their name denotes, supplementing an already nearly adequate diet. Dependence on supplements for basal intake is not wise and probably not effective, because a low calcium intake is commonly a marker for a globally poor diet, and fixing only the calcium component is not an adequate response to a woman's need. Nevertheless, calcium supplements do play an important role, particularly as adjuvants in the treatment of existing disease such as osteoporosis. It is important to stress that any use of calcium supplements should take into account dietary calcium intake and only use as much of a supplement as needed to bring total intake (diet and supplements) to 1,000 mg to 1,200 mg.

As with food fortification, not all supplements are engineered equally. In the past, some calcium tablets did not disintegrate in the body to release the nutrient. Because calcium supplements (like calcium-fortified foods) are not regulated as drugs, caution is advised. Brands that have demonstrated calcium bioavailability are the best choices. Calcium supplements vary in type of calcium salt (and hence calcium content), formulation, price, and to some extent, absorbability.

The two most-often used calcium supplement types contain either calcium carbonate or calcium citrate, but a wide variety of calcium salts are found in calcium supplements, including calcium acetate, calcium citrate malate, calcium gluconate, calcium lactate, calcium lactogluconate, and calcium phosphate (the latter being a collective term that describes supplements consisting of either the monobasic, dibasic, or tribasic phosphate salt of calcium). Calcium is also available in bone meal (basically, calcium phosphate) as well as in dolomite or oyster shell (both basically calcium carbonate) supplements. In the past, some of these have contained toxic contaminants, especially lead; however, analyses of the most commonly used brands did not reveal toxic levels of contaminants.

Different calcium salts contain different percentages of calcium. Calcium carbonate provides the highest percentage (40%); thus 1,250 mg of calcium carbonate provides 500 mg of calcium. Calcium citrate (tetrahydrated form) contains 21% calcium; 2,385 mg of calcium citrate therefore provides 500 mg of calcium. All marketed calcium supplements list the actual calcium content, and this value needs to be taken into consideration when calculating daily intake.

Various formulations of calcium supplements are available, including oral tablets, chewable tablets, dissolvable oral tablets, and liquids. Another formulation for women with difficulty swallowing is an effervescent calcium supplement, typically calcium carbonate combined with materials such as citric acid that facilitate dissolving in water or orange juice.

Absorbability is also a concern. Contrary to popular belief, calcium carbonate and calcium citrate are equally well absorbed if taken with meals, the normal way of assimilating any nutrient. Calcium citrate malate is highly bioavailable, as are supplements containing calcium that is chelated to an amino acid (eg, bisglycinocalcium), but these lesser-used supplements are typically more expensive than calcium carbonate. Studies comparing various commonly used calcium compounds found little differences in their bioavailability when supplements were taken with food. Calcium absorption is optimized if taken with meals and intake is spread out over the day. When taken without food, calcium citrate may be more bioavailable than calcium carbonate. Pharmaceutical formulation of the supplement (ie, the other ingredients in the tablet and how they are packed together) actually makes more of a difference in absorbability than does the chemical nature of the calcium salt.[147] For example, two different calcium carbonate tablets may differ in absorbability by as much as 2-fold.

The AE profile from recommended levels of calcium intake is insignificant, but in one trial, the risk of nephrolithiasis was 17% higher with calcium-vitamin D supplements than with placebo.[148] This risk may be greater with long-term supplementation in healthy women; one review concluded that calcium supplements may slightly increase the risk of nephrolithiasis.[149] Some women have reported difficulty swallowing a large tablet or have adverse GI events. Tolerability can be addressed by getting most or all of a requirement from food or by switching the type of calcium or reducing the dose. Adverse GI events are often related to a woman's taking more calcium than required, not dividing doses, not consuming enough water, or perhaps confusing supplemental intake with recommended total daily intake.

There are no reported cases of calcium toxicity from food calcium sources, even in pastoral populations whose calcium intake may be in excess of 6,000 mg per day (almost entirely from dairy sources). All reported

cases of calcium intoxication have come from the prolonged use of calcium supplement sources, principally calcium carbonate. Even from this source, intakes associated with toxicity have usually been more than 4,500 mg per day, taken over prolonged periods. Intake of more than 2,500 mg per day (the upper limit for healthy adults set by the IOM) can increase the risk of hypercalcemia, which in extreme cases can lead to kidney damage. It is not necessary to measure urine calcium excretion before increasing calcium intake to recommended levels in women who have not had a renal calculus, but a woman diagnosed with renal calculi should not consume calcium supplements more than the level recommended for her age (Table 3)[28] until the specific cause of the stone has been determined.

Chromium

Chromium helps to maintain normal blood glucose levels. No DRI of chromium for women aged 51 to 70 years has been established; the adequate intake established by the National Academy of Sciences for women aged 50 years and older is 20 µg per day.[150]

Food sources include cereals, meats, poultry, fish, and beer. Promotion of high doses of chromium supplements for weight loss has become popular, but valid trials of safety and efficacy are lacking. The role of chromium supplements in patients with chromium deficiency or glucose intolerance has not been defined.

Iron

Iron serves numerous important functions in the body relating to the metabolism of oxygen, not the least of which is its role in hemoglobin transport of oxygen to tissues. Almost two-thirds of iron in the body is found in hemoglobin.

Excess iron results in cellular dysfunction, leading to toxicity and even death. Although earlier research linked high iron stores with increased rates of MI in men, more recent studies have not supported such an association.

A reduction in iron negatively affects the function of oxygen transport in red blood cells. In 2011, almost 500 million nonpregnant women were anemic.[151] Iron deficiency severity ranges from iron depletion, which yields little physiologic damage, to iron deficiency anemia, which can affect the function of numerous organ systems. Anemia also can result in reduced work productivity, which is likely because of the reduced oxygen-carrying capacity in a person's blood.[152] Iron deficiency contributes to 50% of all anemia.[153] In one analysis, anemia prevalence was approximately 40% in countries with a high infection burden and 12% and 7% in countries with moderate and low infection burdens, respectively.[154]

The most common causes of iron deficiency anemia are GI bleeding or excess menstrual flow. During perimenopause, women experiencing prolonged or repeated heavy uterine bleeding may need additional iron if they develop iron deficiency anemia. After menopause, most women should not choose a multivitamin or mineral supplement containing iron, because iron is no longer lost through menstrual bleeding. The DRI of elemental iron for menstruating women is 18 mg per day; after menopause, 8 mg per day is sufficient. Women who use multivitamins should be advised to use an appropriate formulation.

In addition to GI bleeding and excess menstrual flow, other conditions associated with a high risk of developing iron deficiency anemia include end-stage kidney failure; chronic infectious, inflammatory, or malignant disorders; and GI malabsorption diseases (celiac disease and Crohn disease). Not all these conditions will respond to iron supplementation. Many persons (particularly menstruating women and vegetarians) who engage in regular, intense exercise have marginal or inadequate iron status requiring iron supplementation. Signs of iron deficiency anemia include fatigue and weakness, decreased work performance, difficulty maintaining body temperature, decreased immune function, and glossitis (inflamed tongue).

Iron is readily available in food (eg, organ meats, beef, turkey, clams, oysters, oatmeal, beans) and fortified foods (eg, breakfast cereals). When iron deficiency anemia is diagnosed, OTC or prescription oral iron supplements are often recommended.

Supplemental iron is available in two forms: ferrous and ferric. Ferrous iron salts (ferrous fumarate, ferrous sulfate, and ferrous gluconate) are the best-absorbed forms of iron supplements. *Elemental iron* is the amount of iron in a supplement that is available for absorption.

Prescription intravenous iron therapy may be called for in severe anemia or in persons unable to adequately absorb oral iron supplements. Total dietary iron intake in vegetarian diets may meet recommended levels; however, the iron is less available for absorption compared with diets that include meat.[155]

Magnesium

Magnesium is a divalent, cationic element, and like calcium, it is relatively abundant in the earth's crust. The normal adult human body contains approximately 1,000 mmol/L of magnesium (22-26 g).[156] Approximately 99% of total body magnesium is intracellular, stored predominantly in bone (85%), muscle, and soft tissues, with only 1% in the extracellular space.[157] Up to 70% of serum magnesium exists in the ionized (free), physiologically active form, which is important for physiological processes including neuromuscular transmission and CV tone. The normal total serum magnesium in adults ranges between 0.70 mmol/L and 1.10 mmol/L, with a typical reference range for serum ionized magnesium concentration of 0.54 mmol/L to 0.67 mmol/L.

Magnesium is a necessary cofactor for numerous cellular enzymes involved in intermediary and energy metabolism. In magnesium deficiency, global cellular functions are impaired, although there is no discrete disease syndrome that is characteristic of magnesium deficiency. Magnesium is said to function as a physiologic calcium channel blocker, modulating the entry of calcium into the cytosol of various functioning tissues. When magnesium is deficient, cell calcium rises, with resultant hypertonia, muscle cramps, and elevated vascular tone.

Magnesium absorption from the diet is much more efficient than that of calcium, with net absorption usually in the range of 40% to 60% of ingested intake. Urinary magnesium can be reduced sharply with inadequate intake but may rise substantially in uncontrolled DM and with certain diuretics.

With severe magnesium deficiency, calcium homeostasis is disrupted. The parathyroid glands cannot respond to hypocalcemia by secretion of PTH, and the bone-resorptive apparatus is not able to respond to PTH; therefore, hypocalcemia, refractory to intervention other than magnesium repletion, ensues. Clinically recognizable magnesium deficiency occurs when there is excessive electrolyte loss through the intestine (eg, intestinal fistulae and hypersecretory malabsorption syndromes), as well as during recovery from alcoholism. Milder degrees of deficiency, to the extent they occur, are presumably because of either inadequate dietary intake or are hypermagnesiuria induced, for example, by DM or diuretics. The full extent of the clinical expression of magnesium deficiency is uncertain, but seems to include a higher risk of hypertensive CVD, excessive platelet aggregation, platelet-induced thrombosis, and at least in some persons, osteoporosis.

Magnesium is sometimes mentioned as a necessary supplement for the protection of bone health, for absorption of calcium, or both. However, in most trials focused on BMD or osteoporotic fracture, benefits of calcium were observed without magnesium supplements. There are, however, two lines of evidence suggesting that subclinical magnesium deficiency may contribute to bone loss in certain women.

Celiac disease is a syndrome of malabsorption and can result in excess electrolyte loss through the intestine. A nonnegligible fraction of women with osteoporosis have silent celiac disease as a cause or contributor. These women clearly need calcium supplementation, but available evidence suggests that they benefit from magnesium supplementation as well. Women with osteoporosis, even though they lack overt intestinal symptoms and nevertheless have positive tissue transglutaminase antibodies would not be harmed by magnesium supplementation and might be helped.

A second line of evidence derives from the fact that many women with vitamin D deficiency fail to show the expected PTH response to inefficient calcium absorption.[158] These women have presumptive magnesium deficiency by virtue of a positive magnesium tolerance test and PTH response to supplementation with magnesium citrate. The cause of the magnesium deficiency in these women is unknown, and the significance of their silent magnesium deficiency remains unclear.

The DRI for magnesium is 320 mg per day for women. The evidence supporting this recommendation is weak because there are no generally agreed-on indicators of optimal magnesium status. For the most part, this estimate is based on the amount of ingested magnesium needed to maintain zero magnesium balance, which, as with other nutrients, is a weak criterion.

Magnesium is considered a shortfall nutrient in women, with more than half of the US population regularly having intakes below the DRI.[12] This ostensible shortfall is about as large as the intake gap for calcium and vitamin D, but its clinical significance is much less clear. Until firmer evidence becomes available, it would seem both prudent and safe to attempt to improve magnesium intake status for most adults.

Magnesium is fairly widely distributed in a variety of foods, the richest sources being nuts, certain seeds, legumes, and various marine fish. Dairy foods are also good sources of magnesium and in typical diets will often be the major source of magnesium. If a woman reaches the target figure for calcium (three servings of dairy/d), she would automatically receive from that source alone roughly 40% of her DRI of magnesium.

Women with Crohn disease, celiac disease, or a history of intestinal bypass surgery are at increased risk of magnesium deficiency, as are women with DM and alcoholism and older women with poor diets.[159] Magnesium supplementation would be appropriate in these women; however, in the general population, it would be better to promote a diet high in vegetables, fruits, legumes, and whole grains rather than use magnesium supplements.

There are no known cases of magnesium toxicity from food sources. Magnesium taken by mouth as various salts tends to have a cathartic effect, and one such preparation (magnesium citrate) has routinely been used as a means of cleaning out the GI tract before endoscopy or surgery. Anything that represents more than modest supplementation with magnesium salts is likely to elicit some degree of catharsis. The UL published by the IOM for magnesium applies only to supplemental sources and not to food sources.[160] That value has been set at 350 mg of supplemental magnesium per day.

Zinc

Found in almost every cell, zinc is an essential mineral that stimulates the activity of approximately 100 enzymes. Zinc is involved in nucleic acid and protein synthesis and degradation, is needed for DNA synthesis and wound healing, supports the immune system, and helps maintain the senses of taste and smell. The DRI of zinc for women aged 51 to 70 years zinc is 8 mg.[150]

Zinc is found in a wide variety of foods such as oysters, red meat, poultry, beans, nuts, seafood, and dairy. Zinc absorption is greater from a diet high in animal protein than a diet rich in plant proteins. Vegetarians may need as much as 50% more zinc than nonvegetarians because of the lower absorption of zinc from plant foods.

Women who experience chronic diarrhea should be careful to add sources of zinc to their daily diet and may benefit from zinc supplementation. Anyone who has had GI surgery or digestive disorders that result in malabsorption, Crohn disease, or short-bowel syndrome are at greater risk of zinc deficiency and should be evaluated for a zinc supplement if diet alone fails to maintain normal zinc levels.

The effect of zinc treatments on the severity or duration of cold symptoms is controversial. A meta-analysis indicated that OTC zinc lozenges decreased the duration of colds by 33%, and there is no evidence that zinc doses of more than 100 mg per day might lead to greater efficacy in the treatment of the common cold.[161,162]

Iron fortification programs for iron deficiency anemia may affect the absorption of zinc and other nutrients. Fortification of foods with iron does not significantly affect zinc absorption, but large amounts of iron supplements (>25 mg) may decrease zinc absorption. Taking iron supplements between meals will help decrease its effect on zinc.

Other minerals

For most people, some other additional vitamins or minerals will be present in a wholesome diet that includes five or more servings of fruits and vegetables per day. However, supplementation may be required.

Boron

Boron acts as a cofactor in magnesium metabolism and thus helps in bone regulation. There is no DRI for boron. Food sources are potatoes, legumes, milk, avocado, and peanuts. A daily MVM supplement containing 3 mg to 9 mg is adequate. Overdose can cause nausea, vomiting, and diarrhea.

Copper

Copper is a component of enzymes involved in iron metabolism. The DRI of copper for women aged 51 to 70 years is 900 µg.[150] Food sources include organ meats, seafood, nuts, seeds, wheat bran, whole-grain products, and cocoa.

Manganese

Manganese is involved in bone formation as well as in enzymes in amino acid, cholesterol, and carbohydrate metabolism. Adequate intake is 1.8 mg daily.[150]

Phosphorus

Phosphorus is an important mineral for bones, with too much or too little resulting in bone loss. One symptom of phosphorus deficiency is bone pain. Low phosphorus levels can result from excessive urinary loss, poor diet, intestinal malabsorption, and excessive use of antacids that bind to phosphorus. Food sources include milk, yogurt, ice cream, cheese, peas, meat, eggs, some cereals, and breads. Soft drinks are an additional source. The DRI of phosphorus for women aged 50 years and older is 700 mg, with the UL set at 4,000 mg per day for those aged 50 to 70 years and 3,000 mg per day for women aged older than 70 years.[160]

Selenium

Selenium acts to defend against oxidative stress and the reduction and oxidation of vitamin C and other substances and in the regulation of thyroid hormone action. Food sources include organ meats, seafood, and plants (depending on soil content). The DRI of selenium for women aged 51 to 70 years is 55 µg.[163] Overdose results in hair and nail brittleness and loss. In addition, higher selenium levels in the environment were associated with increased stroke risk, and the hazard ratio for the fourth quartile compared with the first quartile was 1.33 (95% CI, 1.09-1.62).[164] In a meta-analysis, selenium supplementation did not lead to a significant risk reduction in cause-specific death, CVD, or cancer.[165]

Other Dietary Supplements

Popular nonbotanical dietary supplements in the United States and natural health products in Canada do not have direct menopause-related symptom relief but are used for general health benefits by midlife women.

Coenzyme Q10

Coenzyme Q10 —also called CoQ10 or ubiquinone—is a fat-soluble, vitamin-like compound that is found in humans and other mammals. CoQ10 is a cofactor in energy-production reactions, particularly adenosine triphosphate, and functions as an antioxidant, protecting against free radical damage within mitochondria. It is found in all cells in the human body, with the highest concentrations in the heart, kidney, liver, and pancreas. Of note, the body is able to make its own CoQ10, so it is not essential to obtain from the diet or supplements for most healthy adults.

CoQ10 as oral tablets and capsules is marketed in the United States and Canada as a dietary supplement and a natural health product, respectively; they are not regulated as drugs. As such, evidence for safety and efficacy is limited. Most information available is from anecdotal reports, case reports, and uncontrolled clinical studies.

Widely used throughout Europe and Asia, CoQ10 is claimed to be of benefit in CVD, including angina, congestive heart failure, and hypertension, as well as musculoskeletal disorders, DM, and obesity. However, study results are mixed.

Congestive heart failure

CoQ10 supplementation is commonly used by patients with congestive heart failure in an attempt to replace levels lost in myocardial cells. The extent of CoQ10 deficiency correlates with the severity of heart failure. A meta-analysis of 13 trials showed significant improvement in the ejection fraction with the use of CoQ10 compared with controls when used in the short term (≤28 wk).[166] More clinical trials evaluating objective measures of cardiac performance, as well as clinical outcomes in diverse populations over longer durations, are needed.

Encouraging results were seen in a trial of 443 older Swedish citizens with the use of combined selenium and CoQ10 supplementation. Over a follow-up of 5.2 years, a significant reduction in CV mortality occurred in the treatment arm compared with placebo.[167] The large Q-Symbio trial of 420 participants showed no significant short-term (16 wk) effects on cardiac health.[168] Compared with placebo plus standard therapy, supplementation of CoQ10 100 mg three times a day plus standard therapy showed significant improvement in long-term (2 y) primary endpoints, including the New York Heart Association 6-minute walk test and levels of N-terminal pro-B type natriuretic peptide. Cardiovascular mortality, all-cause mortality, and incidence of hospital stays for heart failure were all lower in the treatment group. CoQ10 has not been recommended as a therapy for heart failure by the American College of Cardiology or the American Heart Association.

Hypertension

CoQ10 has been shown to reduce blood pressure without significant AEs, and it appears effective as an adjunctive therapy for hypertension; however, it remains unclear whether CoQ10 should be used as an antihypertensive agent on its own.[169,170] A review of two trials showed no significant effects on diastolic blood pressure, with only one of the studies showing statistically significant effects on systolic blood pressure (mean difference, –15.00 mm Hg; 95% CI, –19.06, –10.94).[171] (See also "Hypertension" in Chapter 8.)

Statin-induced myopathies

It has been proposed that CoQ10 depletion may be a contributing factor for statin-induced myopathies. Although statins have been shown to reduce serum CoQ10 levels by blocking the synthesis of mevalonic acid (a precursor of CoQ10), studies on the effects of CoQ10 supplementation on statin-induced myalgias have been inconsistent.[172-174] In a meta-analysis and systematic review of six RCTs with 302 participants, no significant benefit of supplementation with CoQ10 in preventing statin-induced myopathies was shown.[175]

Migraine

CoQ10 may prevent migraines by improving oxidative phosphorylation in the mitochondria.[176] In a small RCT of 42 participants with migraine, CoQ10 was shown to be superior to placebo for attack frequency, headache days, and days with nausea at doses of 100 mg three times daily.[177] It can take up to 3 months to see benefit.[178] In another small RCT on prophylaxis of migraine headaches, 36 participants treated with supplemental CoQ10 versus 37 baseline-matched controls had a significant decrease in migraine attacks per month and severity of headaches.[179] (See also "Headache" in Chapter 5.)

Breast cancer

Interest in the potential effect of CoQ10 in cancer began after lesser amounts were noted in the blood of patients with breast cancer. Studies of CoQ10 in patients with cancer are limited. One clinical trial found no improvement in treatment-induced fatigue in newly diagnosed patients with breast cancer using standard doses of CoQ10.[180] An RCT of 57 participants did show significant improvement in global and worst level of cancer-related fatigue in the intervention group taking an amino acid jelly with CoQ10 and L-carnitine compared with controls taking placebo. It did not find significant difference in average level of fatigue.[181]

Dosing

Dosing recommendations for CoQ10 range from 30 mg to 300 mg per day, depending on the indication. Doses higher than 100 mg should be taken in divided doses (2 or 3 times/d). Patients should be advised to take it with food. As a fat-soluble supplement, absorption is likely increased with foods that have some fat.

Adverse events

CoQ10 is relatively safe, with a low incidence of AEs.[182] Adverse events include nausea, epigastric pain, heartburn, headache, and fatigue.

Interactions

Because CoQ10 can lower blood pressure, caution should be taken when using in combination with antihypertensives or at the same time as herbal medications or supplements with additive hypotensive effects.[170] Smoking has been shown to decrease CoQ10 levels.[183]

Fish oil/Omega-3 and omega-6 fatty acids

Essential nutrients for humans include the parent fatty acids of the omega-3 and omega-6 families of polyunsaturated fatty acids. Omega-3 fatty acids are polyunsaturated fats and include the three major dietary fatty acids: α-linolenic acid, eicosapentaenoic acid, and docosahexaenoic acid.[184] Fish oil and algae are composed of eicosapentaenoic acid and docosahexaenoic acid, whereas plants such as flaxseeds and walnuts are the main source of α-linolenic acid. Although the human body can convert a very small amount of eicosapentaenoic acid and docosahexaenoic acid from α-linolenic acid, it cannot otherwise produce omega-3 fatty acids, so they must be ingested in diet or taken as supplements.

Omega-6 fatty acids are polyunsaturated fatty acids and include linoleic acid, γ-linoleic acid, and arachidonic acid. Sources of linoleic acid include plant-based oils such as corn, safflower, soybean, and evening primrose seed. Omega-6 fatty acids may compete for common enzymatic processes with omega-3 fatty acids.[185] Most American diets provide at least 10 times more omega-6 than omega-3 fatty acids. It is not known whether a desirable ratio of omega-6 to omega-3 fatty acids exists or to what extent high intakes of omega-6 fatty acids interfere with any benefits of omega-3 fatty acid consumption.

These fatty acids are associated with CV and other health benefits; however, most of the CV and triglyceride-lowering benefits have been seen specifically with omega-3 fatty acids from fish oils (eicosapentaenoic acid and docosahexaenoic acid).[186] The body's conversion of α-linolenic acid into eicosapentaenoic acid and docosahexaenoic acid is inefficient, so nutritional sources must be relied on for an optimal level.

The most abundant sources of docosahexaenoic acid and eicosapentaenoic acid are fatty fish such as salmon, sardines, herring, mackerel, black cod, and bluefish. The α-linolenic acid is found in oils from vegetables and legumes such as canola, soy, walnuts, and especially flaxseed, as well as in dairy products and some red meat.

Dietary intake of omega-3 fatty acids in foods is best, as with all nutrients, but supplementation may be beneficial in a variety of conditions. These include CVD, asthma, dementia and cognitive performance with aging, multiple sclerosis, Parkinson disease, premenstrual syndrome, rheumatoid arthritis, systemic lupus erythematosus, irritable bowel disease, renal disease, and various skin conditions. As with many supplements, the quality of studies varies, and study results have been either insignificant or inconclusive.

Cardiovascular disease

Omega-3 fatty acids from fish oils have a number of reported benefits on CVD risk factors, including lowering triglyceride levels, improving blood pressure, preventing arrhythmias, and decreasing platelet aggregation.[184] When considering fish oil for treatment of dyslipidemia, it is important to note that the greatest effect on lowering triglycerides has been in patients with very high baseline levels, and it does not affect HDL-C.[187] (See also "Nutrition" in Chapter 8.)

Prospective cohort studies have indicated a lower risk of fatal CHD in primary prevention in those who consume fish once or twice a week.[188] Several prospective clinical trials have shown positive results with omega-3 fatty acids for the secondary prevention of cardiac events.[189-191] One RCT did find a decrease in CV events and death from CV events in those receiving eicosapentaenoic acid plus statin early after an MI compared with controls who only received a statin.[192] Other trials have failed to replicate these findings,[193,194] and several meta-analyses have concluded that even though omega-3 fatty acid supplementation may protect against vascular events, there is no clear effect on CV death or major CV events.[195-198] A large RCT (VITAL) showed that supplementation with omega-3 fatty acids did not result in a lower incidence of cardiovascular events than placebo.[199]

Ongoing trials, including the REDUCE-IT trial and the STRENGTH trial, will evaluate whether omega-3 fatty acid supplementation in high-risk patients with elevated triglycerides treated with statins has an effect on primary prevention of heart disease.

Alzheimer disease

Epidemiologic data have indicated that dietary use of omega-3 fatty acids, specifically docosahexaenoic acid, may be protective against Alzheimer disease. A small trial showed improvement in memory function in 36 older patients with mild cognitive impairment over 12 months with the use of fish oils.[200] Another small trial in 34 participants with Alzheimer disease showed less cognitive and function decline in those taking omega-3 plus α-lipoic acid compared with controls.[201] Based on a Cochrane review of three RCTs with 632 participants over 6, 12, and 18 months, there remain no data for the use of omega-3 fatty acid supplements for the treatment of mild to moderate Alzheimer disease.[202] Larger and longer clinical trials are required.

Depression

Numerous studies have been published on the use of omega-3 fatty acids in depression with varying results.[203] Several meta-analyses have found a benefit of omega-3 fatty acids in treating depression and augmenting the effects of antidepressants[204,205]; however, a recent meta-analysis found that efficacy became nonsignificant with the inclusion of other published trials.[206]

Dosing

Fish oil capsules containing varying amounts of omega-3 and omega-6 fatty acids are available as OTC dietary supplements in the United States and natural health products in Canada. The US government has approved a prescription form of omega-3 fatty acids (omega-3 acid ethyl ester concentrate), with higher concentrates of docosahexaenoic acid and eicosapentaenoic acid than standard fish oil, as an adjunct to the diet for the treatment of very high triglycerides. The American Heart Association advises that treating hypertriglyceridemia should be done under a clinician's care.

Fish oils are well tolerated at doses of 4 g or less daily. Dosing recommendations vary from 1 g to 4 g per day, depending on the indication. Doses of 3 g to 4 g per day are required for triglyceride lowering. Standard fish oil contains 120 mg docosahexaenoic acid and 180 mg eicosapentaenoic acid in a 1-g capsule. Omega-3 fatty acid supplements containing varying docosahexaenoic acid and eicosapentaenoic acid concentrations are also available.

Adverse events

Fish oil supplements can produce heartburn, nausea, dyspepsia, loose stools, and bad breath, as well as a fishy aftertaste. Fish oil supplements are generally derived from small pelagic fish or from formulations produced by algae; furthermore, mercury is tightly bound to fish proteins instead of fatty acid, therefore, fish oil supplements contain little to no mercury.[207,208]

Interactions

Supplements of fish oil greater than 3 g per day have the potential to slow blood clotting and increase bleeding by decreasing platelet aggregation.[209] Caution should be used when taking other herbal medications or drugs that have antiplatelet effects as well as anticoagulants such as warfarin. For this reason, patients are generally advised to stop using fish oil supplements before surgical procedures. Fish oils may also decrease blood pressure and may have additive effects with blood pressure medications.

Glucosamine and chondroitin

Glucosamine is an amino monosaccharide that is present in almost all human tissues, especially cartilaginous tissues. Chondroitin is a complex carbohydrate that helps cartilage retain water.

These agents have been promoted for pain relief, primarily in osteoarthritis (OA). They are sometimes taken individually but primarily in combination and are used as alternatives or along with analgesics and nonsteroidal anti-inflammatory drugs (NSAIDs). In the United States and Canada, glucosamine and chondroitin are sold as dietary supplements and as natural health products, respectively; thus, they are not regulated as drugs.

Glucosamine is stabilized as one of two salts, glucosamine sulfate or glucosamine hydrochloride, and also is available as N-acetyl glucosamine. The sulfate form has been the most studied, and it is unknown whether the hydrochloride salt or N-acetyl glucosamine are as effective. Persons may respond differently to the two salts. Chondroitin is available as a sulfate salt.

Glucosamine sulfate (alone and with chondroitin sulfate) has been shown to be symptomatically effective in a number of studies and may have a structure-modifying effect on knee OA.

Clinical studies have been conducted on glucosamine sulfate for OA for more than 20 years, primarily in Europe, where it is available by prescription. Systematic reviews, one a Cochrane review, have found clinical trial evidence supporting the safety and efficacy of glucosamine sulfate for relieving pain and improving function in patients with OA.[210-212] The Cochrane review identified 25 RCTs evaluating oral glucosamine in OA.[211]

In several placebo-controlled trials, oral glucosamine sulfate was found to be superior to placebo in most but not all trials. In five trials comparing glucosamine sulfate and NSAIDs, glucosamine was superior in two of the trials and equivalent in two trials. Glucosamine and chondroitin were found to have a small but significant effect on radiographic joint space measurement when taking consistently for 3 and 2 years, respectively.[212]

Chondroitin is used in an attempt to influence cartilage loss, with the assumption that because it is partially absorbed in the intestine, some of it may reach joints. Few studies have been done examining the effect on joint space; more have looked at pain relief. An RCT of 217 healthy adults showed lower levels of high-sensitivity C-reactive protein and prostaglandin estradiol metabolite for high users of glucosamine and/or chondroitin compared to nonusers.[213] Another RCT of 18 healthy adults showed significant decrease in C-reactive protein in patients taking glucosamine hydrochloride plus chondroitin compared with placebo over 1 month.[214]

There was no decrease in interleukin 6, soluble tumor necrosis factor receptors I or II, urinary inflammation biomarker, prostaglandin estradiol-metabolite, or urinary oxidative stress biomarker F2-isoprostane. In vitro studies suggest that chondroitin may inhibit some of the cartilage-degrading enzymes. The results of a meta-analysis of available trials suggest that the benefit of chondroitin on OA symptoms may be minimal.[215]

The Glucosamine/chondroitin Arthritis Intervention Trial, the first such large-scale US multicenter clinical trial, examined the combination of glucosamine hydrochloride and chondroitin sulfate for relief of mild pain in knee OA.[216] In this 6-month study, these substances were compared separately or in combination with each other, with celecoxib, and with placebo. Glucosamine hydrochloride and chondroitin sulfate together or alone did not provide statistically significant pain relief for the group as a whole (which included those with any level of symptomatic knee osteoarthritis); however, patients with *moderate to severe* pain did have a significantly higher rate of response in the combination group compared with placebo.

A meta-analysis of 54 studies reviewing the effects of glucosamine, chondroitin, the two in combination, and celecoxib in the treatment of OA of the knee found that, compared with placebo, glucosamine plus chondroitin, glucosamine alone, and celecoxib were all superior in both relief of pain and improvement of function.[217] Only glucosamine plus chondroitin showed significant improvement from baseline function.

Several trials have assessed the structure-modifying effect of glucosamine sulfate and chondroitin sulfate using plain radiography to measure joint-space narrowing.[218-220] In two earlier trials, glucosamine had positive effects on the rate of progression of the disease on knee OA,[218,219] as well as preventing total joint replacement.[221]

Results from the Glucosamine/chondroitin Arthritis Intervention Trial showed glucosamine (alone and with chondroitin) had no effect on overall progression of knee OA at 2 years.[222] However, a subset of patients with grade 2 OA showed a nonstatistically significant trend toward improvement. A meta-analysis of six RCTs showed that glucosamine sulfate may delay the radiologic progression of knee OA over 2 to 3 years, and another meta-analysis of 10 trials found no effect of glucosamine sulfate supplementation on joint space narrowing.[212,223] In a review of seven studies evaluating effect on structure, both glucosamine alone and chondroitin alone reduced joint space narrowing compared with placebo.[217] Thus, the structure-modifying effect of glucosamine remains unclear.

In two cohorts, including the Nurses' Health study and Health Professionals Follow-up Study, participants were assessed for regular use of glucosamine and chondroitin.[224] Those who regularly used them together were found to have significant reduction in relative risk for colorectal cancer. However, randomized trials are needed to support a causal effect.

Dosing
Nearly all trials used glucosamine at doses of 500 mg three times daily or 1,500 mg once a day. Chondroitin has been typically studied at a dose of 400 mg three times daily.

Adverse events
Glucosamine and chondroitin are considered to be safe, and no serious AEs have been reported. In a Cochrane review, the reported AEs for glucosamine were similar to placebo, although some studies noted GI complaints and sleepiness.[211] In a meta-analysis, there were no significant differences in AEs among placebo, glucosamine alone, chondroitin alone, or glucosamine plus chondroitin.[217]

Glucosamine used in supplements is obtained from chitin, extracted from marine exoskeletons. Thus, for women with shellfish allergies, this supplement should be used with caution, depending on the severity of the allergy.

Interactions
Concerns have been raised that glucosamine and chondroitin may interfere with glycemic control in women with type 2 DM because animal models have demonstrated such effects; however, animals may handle glucosamine differently than humans do. A trial of 35 patients with type 2 DM showed no changes in glycemic control from daily therapy with 1,500 mg glucosamine sulfate and 1,200 mg chondroitin sulfate.[225] Glucosamine alone or in combination with chondroitin may increase the anticoagulation effects of warfarin. Patients on warfarin should be advised to avoid glucosamine and chondroitin or have their international normalized ratio (INR) closely monitored.[226]

Inferior oral supplements of glucosamine (alone and with chondroitin) also may contain a large quantity of sodium chloride or potassium chloride or both, unneeded but less-expensive "salts." These products should be avoided.

S-Adenosylmethionine
S-Adenosylmethionine (SAM-e) is a metabolite of folate that can be found in all living cell. Via enzymatic transmethylation, it plays a role in the formation, activation, or metabolism of neurotransmitters, hormones, proteins,

and phospholipids. It is available as an oral supplement and marketed as a dietary supplement in the United States and as a natural health product in Canada. In some European countries, SAM-e is a prescription drug. SAM-e has been studied for treatment of depression and OA and for prevention of liver disease.

Depression

Several systematic reviews and meta-analyses have found SAM-e to be well tolerated and effective for the treatment of mild to moderate depression.[203,227] However, a systematic review of eight RCTs including 934 adults showed no strong evidence of change in depressive symptoms from baseline when comparing SAM-e with placebo.[228] These results were reportedly based on very low-quality evidence. In comparing effects of SAM-e with imipramine, there was no significant difference, whereas compared with escitalopram, there was little evidence of a difference. SAM-e does appear to be superior to placebo when added to selective serotonin-reuptake inhibitors (SSRIs), but again, the quality of evidence is low. Compared with conventional antidepressant therapy, SAM-e has been found to be equivalent to tricyclic antidepressants; however, few studies have compared SAM-e to antidepressants from other classes.

SAM-e has not been well studied in severe depression, although preliminary data have suggested that SAM-e may be effective as adjunctive therapy to antidepressants, especially in those patients who were not responders to selective SSRIs.[229] Dosage for depression is 800 mg to 1,600 mg per day.

Osteoarthritis

A number of clinical trials have been completed assessing the use of SAM-e for pain relief in OA.[230] In all trials, SAM-e was more effective than placebo in decreasing the pain of OA and equally effective as NSAIDs. A Cochrane review found a small clinical effect with SAM-e in improving OA pain and function; however, studies were not adequately sized and were too heterogeneous to make conclusions.[231] Dosage for OA is 1,200 mg per day.

Liver disease

Even though SAM-e has been studied in a range of chronic liver disease, the greatest interest has been with intrahepatic cholestasis, although studies have been found to be inadequate to make comparisons with prescription therapies. A Cochrane review found no evidence to support the use of SAM-e for alcoholic liver disease.[232] A meta-analysis

of 11 RCTs with 705 patients showed significant decreases in total bilirubin and aspartate transaminase levels but not alanine transaminase levels in patients with chronic liver disease.[233] The authors suggest that data remain limited with regard to effect and cannot yet suggest SAM-e for use in clinical practice. Dosages used in studies for liver disorders are 200 mg to 400 mg per day.

Adverse events

Supplementation with SAM-e is well tolerated, with an AE profile that includes occasional GI upset, nausea, dry mouth, headache, dizziness, restlessness, and insomnia.[229]

Melatonin

Melatonin (N-acetyl-5-methoxytryptamine), an endogenous pineal gland hormone, regulates the rest-activity cycles.[234] It is produced from its precursor, tryptophan, with the process regulated by the suprachiasmatic nucleus of the hypothalamus, the site of the body's circadian "central clock." Endogenous melatonin levels are highest in childhood, drop significantly during puberty, and decline steadily thereafter throughout life.

From a circadian perspective, light suppresses melatonin secretion during the day to a level that is virtually unmeasurable.[235] Melatonin blood levels begin to increase in the evening and peak between midnight and 3:00 AM, resulting in a direct sedative effect and drop in body temperature, thus promoting sleep. In postmenopausal versus premenopausal women under consistent routine conditions, melatonin was shown to peak earlier in the night without differences in time of melatonin onset or amplitude.

Although melatonin is a hormone, it is regulated in the United States only as a dietary supplement and as a natural health product in Canada, not as a drug. Melatonin is available over the counter in most pharmacies and health food stores. However, the lack of regulation and its availability in small doses with increased vehicle-to-drug ratio increases the likelihood of misformulation and poor release of melatonin.

Melatonin has been widely used by women, but its effects on sleep and behavioral sedation are inconsistent in studies.

Circadian rhythm sleep disorders

Melatonin supplementation may shift the circadian rhythm and has been proposed for circadian rhythm sleep disorders (ie, shift work) and to prevent or treat jet lag, particularly in those who have crossed several time zones.[236,237] Additionally, melatonin has been evaluated in conditions with circadian rhythm disturbances, such as in dementia.[238]

Insomnia

Some studies have shown melatonin beneficial in improving sleep latency and sleep duration, especially in older persons, although most studies have been small and of short duration. A meta-analysis of 19 trials concluded that melatonin had a modest but significant improvement in sleep latency, total sleep time, and sleep quality; however, this effect may be smaller than what has been shown for other sleep medications.[239] The dose range of melatonin in these studies varied from 0.3 mg to 5 mg, and duration of use ranged from 7 days to 126 days. A greater effect on sleep latency and total sleep time was seen in studies using higher doses and longer durations, but there was no effect on sleep quality with dose or duration.

A postmarketing surveillance study of prolonged-release melatonin evaluated its effects on 653 patients showed improvement in mean sleep quality and morning alertness after 3 weeks of therapy and up to 2 weeks after stopping the supplement.[240] Rebound insomnia was seen only in 2.0% of participants 2 weeks after stopping treatment.

There are limited data showing that melatonin provides relief from menopause-related sleep disturbances or that melatonin retards aging. A meta-analysis of nine studies demonstrated that melatonin was effective for delayed sleep-phase disorder.[241] Dose range was 0.3 mg to 5 mg, with 5 mg being the most commonly used. Duration was 10 days to 4 weeks, but dose and duration were not considered in this analysis. (See also "Sleep Disturbance" in Chapter 5.)

Nocturnal blood pressure

Studies have evaluated the effects of melatonin on nocturnal blood pressure, with inconsistent results. A recent meta-analysis showed that controlled-release melatonin may significantly reduce nocturnal blood pressure, but this same effect was not observed with immediate-release formulations.[242] One 3-week trial of 97 retired home-dwelling older volunteers aged 63 to 91 years showed a 1.5-mg supplement of melatonin significantly decreased systolic and diastolic nocturnal blood pressure measurements compared with controls.[243]

Benzodiazepine withdrawal

Similar to benzodiazepines, melatonin augments γ-aminobutyric acid receptors and may be useful in weaning patients from long-term benzodiazepine use. In one study, discontinuation of benzodiazepine therapy in patients with insomnia was achieved using a 2-mg controlled-release melatonin formulation for 6 weeks, with good sleep quality preserved at 6 months.[244] In another study, melatonin improved sleep quality in patients undergoing benzodiazepine withdrawal,[245] although in a systematic review of six trials with 322 participants, melatonin did not have a significant effect on benzodiazepine discontinuation.[246]

Dosing

The optimal dose of melatonin for long-term safety is not known. For sleep disorders, it has been used in doses varying from 0.5 mg to 5 mg daily, taken approximately 1.5 to 2 hours before going to bed. It is generally regarded as safe for short-term use (≤3 months).[247] Melatonin is available in two formulations: quick release and sustained release. Because melatonin has a short half-life of approximately 30 to 60 minutes, the quick release may be preferable for initiating sleep, whereas a sustained-release formulation is likely beneficial to sustain sleep. Studies using sustained-release formulations have had better outcomes on sleep parameters.[248,249]

Adverse events

Adverse effects such as abdominal cramps, hangover effects, dizziness, fatigue, irritability, and impaired balance are associated with high doses (>3 mg/d) of melatonin. High doses also exacerbate depression; its use is best avoided in women with a history of mental illness.

Interactions

Melatonin should be used cautiously with other central nervous system depressants (sedatives, anxiolytics) because there may be an additive effect. Melatonin may impair the antihypertensive effect of the calcium channel blocker nifedipine.[250] Data regarding its use in postmenopausal women with DM are conflicting because there have been reports of increased insulin resistance with melatonin.[251]

REFERENCES

1. The NAMS 2017 Hormone Therapy Position Statement Advisory Panel. The 2017 hormone therapy position statement of The North American Menopause Society. *Menopause.* 2017;24(7):728-753.

2. Pendergast WR, Walman BP, Wertzberger MS. Dietary supplements. Chapter 6. In: Adams DG, Cooper RM, Hahn MJ, Kahan JS; Food and Drug Law Institute, eds. Food and Drug Law and Regulation. 3rd ed. Washington, DC: Food and Drug Law Institute; 2015:185-228.

3. Dietary Supplement Health and Education Act of 1994. Pub L No. 103-417, 108 Stat 4325 (October 25, 1994).

4. 1938 Federal Food Drug and Cosmetic Act. Pub L No. 75-717, 52 Stat 1040 (1938).

5. Moyer VA; US Preventive Services Task Force. Vitamin, mineral, and multivitamin supplements for the primary on of cardiovascular disease and cancer: US Preventive Services Task Force recommendation statement. *Ann Intern Med.* 2014;160(8):558-564.

6. Mente A, de Koning L, Shannon HS, Anand SS. A systematic review of the evidence supporting a causal link between dietary factors and coronary heart disease. *Arch Intern Med.* 2009;169(7):659-669.

7. Liyanage T, Ninomiya T, Wang A, et al. Effects of the Mediterranean diet on cardiovascular outcomes—a systematic review and meta-analysis. *PLoS One.* 2016;11(8):e0159252.

8. Aridi YS, Walker JL, Wright ORL. The association between the Mediterranean dietary pattern and cognitive health: a systematic review. *Nutrients.* 2017;9(7). pii: E674.

9. Godos J, Zappalà G, Bernardini S, Giambini I, Bes-Rastrollo M, Martinez-Gonzalez M. Adherence to the Mediterranean diet is inversely associated with metabolic syndrome occurrence: a meta-analysis of observational studies. *Int J Food Sci Nutr.* 2017;68(2):138-148.

10. Toledo E, Salas-Salvadó J, Donat-Vargas C, et al. Mediterranean diet and invasive breast cancer risk among women at high cardiovascular risk in the PREDIMED trial: a randomized clinical trial. *JAMA Intern Med.* 2015;175(11):1752-1760.

11. Schoenberg MH. Physical activity and nutrition in primary and tertiary prevention of colorectal cancer. *Visc Med.* 2016;32(3):199-204.

12. US Department of Health and Human Services, US Department of Agriculture. *2015-2020 Dietary Guidelines for Americans.* 8th ed. December 2015. https://health.gov/dietaryguidelines/2015/resources/2015-2020_Dietary_Guidelines.pdf. Accessed July 11, 2019.

13. Reedy J, Lerman JL, Krebs-Smith SM, et al. Evaluation of the Healthy Eating Index-2015. *J Acad Nutr Diet.* 2018;118(9):1622-1633.

14. Appel LJ, Moore TJ, Obarzanek E, et al. A clinical trial of the effects of dietary patterns on blood pressure. DASH Collaborative Research Group. *N Engl J Med.* 1997;336(16):1117-1124.

15. Fung TT, Chiuve SE, McCullough ML, Rexrode KM, Logroscino G, Hu FB. Adherence to a DASH-style diet and risk of coronary heart disease and stroke in women. *Arch Intern Med.* 2008;168(7):713-720. Erratum in: *Arch Intern Med.* 2008;168(12):1276.

16. Salehi-Abargouei A, Maghsoudi Z, Shirani F, Azadbakht L. Effects of Dietary Approaches to Stop Hypertension (DASH)-style diet on fatal or nonfatal cardiovascular diseases—incidence: a systematic review and meta-analysis on observational prospective studies. *Nutrition.* 2013;29(4):611-618.

17. Fung TT, Hu FB, Wu K, Chiuve SE, Fuchs CS, Giovannucci E. The Mediterranean and Dietary Approaches to Stop Hypertension (DASH) diets and colorectal cancer. *Am J Clin Nutr.* 2010;92(6):1429-1435.

18. Azadi-Yazdi M, Karimi-Zarchi M, Salehi-Abargouei A, Fallahzadeh H, Nadjarzadeh A. Effects of Dietary Approach to Stop Hypertension diet on androgens, antioxidant status and body composition in overweight and obese women with polycystic ovary syndrome: a randomised controlled trial. *J Hum Nutr Diet.* 2017;30(3):275-283.

19. Razavi Zade M, Telkabadi MH, Bahmani F, Salehi B, Farchbaf S, Asemi Z. The effects of DASH diet on weight loss and metabolic status in adults with non-alcoholic fatty liver disease: a randomized clinical trial. *Liver Int.* 2016;36(4):563-571.

20. Aune D, Giovannucci E, Boffetta P, et al. Fruit and vegetable intake and the risk of cardiovascular disease, total cancer and all-cause mortality—a systematic review and dose-response meta-analysis of prospective studies. *Int J Epidemiol.* 2017;46(3):1029-1056.

21. Bhupathiraju SN, Wedick NM, Pan A, et al. Quantity and variety in fruit and vegetable intake and risk of coronary heart disease. *Am J Clin Nutr.* 2013;98(6):1514-1523.

22. Jansen RJ, Robinson DP, Stolzenberg-Solomon RZ, et al. Nutrients from fruit and vegetable consumption reduce the risk of pancreatic cancer. *J Gastrointest Cancer.* 2013;44(2):152-161.

23. Wu QJ, Wu L, Zheng LQ, Xu X, Ji C, Gong TT. Consumption of fruit and vegetables reduces risk of pancreatic cancer: evidence from epidemiological studies. *Eur J Cancer Prev.* 2016;25(3):196-205.

24. Park SY, Ollberding NJ, Woolcott CG, Wilkens LR, Henderson BE, Kolonel LN. Fruit and vegetable intakes are associated with lower risk of bladder cancer among women in the Multiethnic Cohort Study. *J Nutr.* 2013;143(8):1283-1292.

25. Al-Zalabani AH, Stewart KF, Wesselius A, Schols AM, Zeegers MP. Modifiable risk factors for the prevention of bladder cancer: a systematic review of meta-analyses. *Eur J Epidemiol.* 2016;31(9):811-851.

26. He J, Gu Y, Zhang S. Consumption of vegetables and fruits and breast cancer survival: a systematic review and meta-analysis. *Sci Rep.* 2017;7(1):599. Erratum in: *Sci Rep.* 2018;8(1):8693.

27. Ben Q, Zhong J, Liu J, et al. Association between consumption of fruits and vegetables and risk of colorectal adenoma: a PRISMA-compliant meta-analysis of observational studies. *Medicine (Baltimore).* 2015;94(42):e1599.

28. Institute of Medicine Committee to Review Dietary Reference Intakes for Vitamin D and Calcium. Food and Nutrition Board. *Dietary Reference Intakes for Calcium and Vitamin D.* Ross AC, Taylor CL, Yaktine AL, Del Valle HB, eds. Washington DC: National Academies Press; 2011.

29. Bjelakovic G, Nikolova D, Gluud LL, Simonetti RG, Gluud C. Antioxidant supplements for prevention of mortality in healthy participants and patients with various diseases. *Cochrane Database Syst Rev.* 2012;(3):CD007176.

30. Ye Y, Li J, Yuan Z. Effect of antioxidant vitamin supplementation on cardiovascular outcomes: a meta-analysis of randomized controlled trials. *PloS One.* 2013;8(2):e56803.

31. Myung SK, Ju W, Cho B, et al; Korean Meta-Analysis Study Group. Efficacy of vitamin and antioxidant supplements in prevention of cardiovascular disease: systematic review and meta-analysis of randomised controlled trials. *BMJ.* 2013;346:f10.

32. Lane JS, Magno CP, Lane KT, Chan T, Hoyt DB, Greenfield S. Nutrition impacts the prevalence of peripheral arterial disease in the United States. *J Vasc Surg.* 2008;48(4):897-904.

33. Thomson CA, Neuhouser ML, Shikany JM, et al. The role of antioxidants and vitamin A in ovarian cancer: results from the Women's Health Initiative. *Nutr Cancer.* 2008;60(6):710-719.

34. Koushik A, Wang M, Anderson KE, et al. Intake of vitamins A, C, and E and folate and the risk of ovarian cancer in a pooled analysis of 10 cohort studies. *Cancer Causes Control.* 2015;26(9):1315-1327.

35. Xu X, Yu E, Liu L, et al. Dietary intake of vitamins A, C, and E and the risk of colorectal adenoma: a meta-analysis of observational studies. *Eur J Cancer Prev.* 2013;22(6):529-539.

36. Misotti AM, Gnagnarella P. Vitamin supplement consumption and breast cancer risk: a review. *Ecancermedicalscience.* 2013;7:365.

37. Chen J, Jiang W, Shao L, Zhong D, Wu Y, Cai J. Association between intake of antioxidants and pancreatic cancer risk: a meta-analysis. *Int J Food Sci Nutr.* 2016;67(7):744-753.

38. Kim J, Kim MK, Lee JK, et al. Intakes of vitamin A, C, and E, and beta-carotene are associated with risk of cervical cancer: a case-control study in Korea. *Nutr Cancer.* 2010;62(2):181-189.

39. Bailey RL, Gahche JJ, Lentino CV, et al. Dietary supplement use in the United States: 2003-2006. *J Nutr.* 2011;141(2):261-266.

40. Fortmann SP, Burda BU, Senger CA, Lin JS, Whitlock EP. Vitamin and mineral supplements in the primary prevention of cardiovascular disease and cancer: an updated systematic evidence review for the US Preventive Services Task Force. *Ann Intern Med.* 2013;159(12):824-834.

41. Neuhouser ML, Wassertheil-Smoller S, Thomson C, et al. Multivitamin use and risk of cancer and cardiovascular disease in the Women's Health Initiative cohorts. *Arch Intern Med.* 2009;169(3):294-304.

42. Wassertheil-Smoller S, McGinn AP, Budrys N, et al. Multivitamin and mineral use and breast cancer mortality in older women with invasive breast cancer in the Women's Health Initiative. *Breast Cancer Res Treat.* 2013;141(3):495-505.

43. Larsson SC, Akesson A, Bergkvist L, Wolk A. Multivitamin use and breast cancer incidence in a prospective cohort of Swedish women. *Am J Clin Nutr.* 2010;91(5):1268-1272.

44. Ishitani K, Lin J, Manson JE, Buring JE, Zhang SM. A prospective study of multivitamin supplement use and risk of breast cancer. *Am J Epidemiol.* 2008;167(10):1197-1206.

45. Mursu J, Robien K, Harnack LJ, Park K, Jacobs DR Jr. Dietary supplements and mortality rate in older women: the Iowa Women's Health Study. *Arch Intern Med.* 2011;171(18):1625-1633.

46. Wu AM, Huang CQ, Lin ZK, et al. The relationship between vitamin A and risk of fracture: meta-analysis of prospective studies. *J Bone Miner Res.* 2014;29(9):2032-2039.

47. Xu J, Song C, Song X, Zhang X, Li X. Carotenoids and risk of fracture: a meta-analysis of observational studies. *Oncotarget.* 2017;8(2):2391-2399.

48. Fritz H, Kennedy D, Fergusson D, et al. Vitamin A and retinoid derivatives for lung cancer: a systematic review and meta analysis. *PLoS One.* 2011;6(6):e21107.

49. Fulan H, Changxing J, Baina WY, et al. Retinol, vitamins A, C, and E and breast cancer risk: a meta-analysis and meta-regression. *Cancer Causes Control.* 2011;22(10):1383-1396.

50. Zhang T, Chen H, Qin S, et al. The association between dietary vitamin A intake and pancreatic cancer risk: a meta-analysis of 11 studies. *Biosci Rep.* 2016;36(6).

51. Lv W, Zhong X, Xu L, Han W. Association between dietary vitamin A intake and the risk of glioma: evidence from a meta-analysis. *Nutrients.* 2015;7(11):8897-8904.

52. Frank LL. Thiamin in clinical practice. *JPEN J Parenter Enteral Nutr.* 2015;39(5):503-520.

53. National Institutes of Health. Office of Dietary Supplements. Thiamin: Fact Sheet for Health Professionals. https://ods.od.nih.gov/factsheets/Thiamin-HealthProfessional/#h5. Last updated August 22, 2018. Accessed July 9, 2019.

54. DiNicolantonio JJ, Liu J, O'Keefe JH. Thiamine and cardiovascular disease: a literature review. *Prog Cardiovasc Dis.* 2018;61(1):27-32.

55. Goldberg AC. A meta-analysis of randomized controlled studies on the effects of extended-release niacin in women. *Am J Cardiol.* 2004;94(1):121-124.

56. Garg A, Sharma A, Krishnamoorthy P, et al. Role of niacin in current clinical practice: a systematic review. *Am J Med.* 2017;130(2):173-187.

57. Marti-Carvajal AJ, Solà I, Lathyris D, Karakitsiou DE, Simancas-Racines D. Homocysteine-lowering interventions for preventing cardiovascular events. *Cochrane Database Syst Rev.* 2013;(1):CD006612.

58. De-Regil LM, Peña-Rosas JP, Fernández-Gaxiola AC, Rayco-Solon P. Effects and safety of periconceptional oral folate supplementation for preventing birth defects. *Cochrane Database Syst Rev.* 2015;(12):CD007950.

59. National Institutes of Health. Office of Dietary Supplements. *Folate: Fact Sheet for Health Professionals.* https://ods.od.nih.gov/factsheets/Folate-HealthProfessional/. Last updated October 4, 2018. Accessed July 9, 2019.

60. Liu Y, Yu Q, Zhu Z, et al. Vitamin and multiple-vitamin supplement intake and incidence of colorectal cancer: a meta-analysis of cohort studies. *Med Oncol.* 2015;32(1):434.

61. Cooper C, Sommerlad A, Lyketsos CG, Livingston G. Modifiable predictors of dementia in mild cognitive impairment: a systematic review and meta-analysis. *Am J Psychiatry.* 2015;172(4):323-334.

62. Bender A, Hagan KE, Kingston N. The association of folate and depression: a meta-analysis. *J Psychiatr Res.* 2017;95:9-18.

63. National Institutes of Health. Office of Dietary Supplements. *Vitamin B12: Fact Sheet for Health Professionals.* https://ods.od.nih.gov/factsheets/VitaminB12-HealthProfessional/. Last update November 29, 2018. Accessed July 9, 2019.

64. Chapman LE, Darling AL, Brown JE. Association between metformin and vitamin B12 deficiency in patients with type 2 diabetes: a systematic review and meta-analysis. *Diabetes Metab.* 2016;42(5):316-327.

65. Lam JR, Schneider JL, Zhao W, Corley DA. Proton pump inhibitor and histamine 2 receptor antagonist use and vitamin B12 deficiency. *JAMA.* 2013;310(22):2435-2442.

66. Malouf R, Areosa Sastre A. Vitamin B12 for cognition. *Cochrane Database Syst Rev.* 2003;(3):CD004326.

67. Health Quality Ontario. Vitamin B12 and cognitive function: an evidence-based analysis. *Ont Health Technol Assess Ser.* 2013;13(23):1-45.

68. National Institutes of Health. Office of Dietary Supplements. *Vitamin C: Fact Sheet for Health Professionals.* https://ods.od.nih.gov/factsheets/VitaminC-HealthProfessional/. Last updated September 18, 2018. Accessed July 9, 2019.

69. Lee B, Oh SW, Myung SK. Efficacy of vitamin C supplements in prevention of cancer: a meta-analysis of randomized controlled trials. *Korean J Fam Med.* 2015;36(6):278-285.

70. Fan H, Kou J, Han D, et al. Association between vitamin C intake and the risk of pancreatic cancer: a meta-analysis of observational studies. *Sci Rep.* 2015;5:13973.

71. Hua YF, Wang GQ, Jiang W, Huang J, Chen GC, Lu CD. Vitamin C intake and pancreatic cancer risk: a meta-analysis of published case-control and cohort studies. *PLoS One.* 2016;11(2):e0148816.

72. Cao D, Shen K, Li Z, Xu Y, Wu D. Association between vitamin C Intake and the risk of cervical neoplasia: a meta-analysis. *Nutr Cancer.* 2016;68(1):48-57.

73. Bo Y, Lu Y, Zhao Y, et al. Association between dietary vitamin C intake and risk of esophageal cancer: a dose-response meta-analysis. *Int J Cancer.* 2016;138(8):1843-1850.

74. Jia L, Jia Q, Shang Y, Dong X, Li L. Vitamin C intake and risk of renal cell carcinoma: a meta-analysis. *Sci Rep.* 2015;5:17921.

75. Zhou S, Wang X, Tan Y, Qiu L, Fang H, Li W. Association between vitamin C intake and glioma risk: evidence from a meta-analysis. *Neuroepidemiology.* 2015;44(1):39-44.

76. Harris HR, Orsini N, Wolk A. Vitamin C and survival among women with breast cancer: a meta-analysis. *Eur J Cancer.* 2014;50(7):1223-1231.

77. Al-Khudairy L, Flowers N, Wheelhouse R, et al. Vitamin C supplementation for the primary prevention of cardiovascular disease. *Cochrane Database Syst Rev.* 2017;3:CD011114.

78. Harding AH, Wareham NJ, Bingham SA, et al. Plasma vitamin C level, fruit and vegetable consumption, and the risk of new-onset type 2 diabetes mellitus: the European prospective investigation of cancer—Norfolk prospective study. *Arch Intern Med.* 2008;168(14):1493-1499.

79. Hemilä H, Chalker E. Vitamin C for preventing and treating the common cold. *Cochrane Database Syst Rev.* 2013;(1):CD000980.

80. Hemilä H. Vitamin C and infections. *Nutrients.* 2017;9(4): doi 3390/nu9040339.

81. Standing Committee on the Scientific Evaluation of Dietary Reference Intakes. Food and Nutrition Board Institute of Medicine. Vitamin D. In: *Dietary Reference Intakes: Calcium, Phosphorus, Magnesium, Vitamin D, and Fluoride.* Washington, DC: National Academy Press; 1997:250-287.

82. Armas LA, Hollis BW, Heaney RP. Vitamin D2 is much less effective than vitamin D3 in humans. *J Clin Endocrinol Metab.* 2004;89(11):5387-5391.

83. Institute of Medicine (US) Committee to Review Dietary Reference Intakes for Vitamin D and Calcium, Food and Nutrition Board. Overview of vitamin D. In: Ross AC, Taylor CL, Yaktine AL, Del Valle HB, eds. *Dietary Reference Intakes for Calcium and Vitamin D.* Washington, DC: National Academies Press; 2011:75-124.

84. Ross AC, Manson JE, Abrams SA, et al. The 2011 report on dietary reference intakes for calcium and vitamin D from the Institute of Medicine: what clinicians need to know. *J Clin Endocrinol Metab.* 2011;96(1):53-58.

85. Bischoff-Ferrari HA, Dietrich T, Orav EJ, Dawson-Hughes B. Positive association between 25-hydroxy vitamin D levels and bone mineral density: a population-based study of younger and older adults. *Am J Med.* 2004;116(9):634-639.

86. Bischoff-Ferrari HA, Dietrich T, Orav EJ, et al. Higher 25-hydroxyvitamin D concentrations are associated with better lower-extremity function in both active and inactive persons aged ≥60 y. *Am J Clin Nutr.* 2004;80(3):752-758.

87. Jackson RD, LaCroix AZ, Gass M, et al; Women's Health Initiative Investigators. Calcium plus vitamin D supplementation and the risk of fractures. *N Engl J Med.* 2006;354(7):669-683. Erratum in: *N Engl J Med.* 2006;354(10):1102.

88. Bischoff-Ferrari HA, Willett WC, Wong JB, Giovannucci E, Dietrich T, Dawson-Hughes B. Fracture prevention with vitamin D supplementation: a meta-analysis of randomized controlled trials. *JAMA.* 2005;293(18):2257-2264.

89. Weaver CM, Alexander DD, Boushey CJ, et al. Calcium plus vitamin D supplementation and risk of fractures: an updated meta-analysis from the National Osteoporosis Foundation. *Osteoporos Int.* 2016;27(1):367-376. Erratum in: *Osteoporosis Int.* 2016;27(8):2643-2646.

90. Chung M, Lee J, Terasawa T, Lau J, Trikalinos TA. Vitamin D with or without calcium supplementation for prevention of cancer and fractures: an updated meta-analysis for the US Preventive Services Task Force. *Ann Intern Med.* 2011.155(12):827-823. Erratum in: *Ann Intern Med.* 2014;161(8):615-616.

91. Brincat M, Gambin J, Brincat M, Calleja-Agius J. The role of vitamin D in osteoporosis. *Maturitas.* 2015;80(3):329-332.

92. Lips P. Which circulating level of 25-hydroxyvitamin D is appropriate? *J Steroid Biochem Mol Biol.* 2004;89-90(1-5):611-614.

93. Cosman F, de Beur SJ, LeBoff MS, et al; National Osteoporosis Foundation. Clinician's guide to prevention and tratment of osteoporosis. *Osteoporosis Int.* 2014;25(10):2359-2381.

94. Health Canada. Eating Well With Canada's Food Guide. 2007. www.canada.ca/content/dam/hc-sc/migration/hc-sc/fn-an/alt_formats/hpfb-dgpsa/pdf/food-guide-aliment/print_eatwell_bienmang-eng.pdf. Accessed July 9, 2019.

95. Dawson-Hughes B, Heaney RP, Holick MF, Lips P, Meunier PJ, Vieth R. Estimates of optimal vitamin D status. *Osteoporos Int.* 2005;16(7):713-716.

96. Bischoff-Ferrari HA, Shao A, Dawson-Hughes B, Hathcock J, Giovannucci E, Willett WC. Benefit-risk assessment of vitamin D supplementation. *Osteoporos Int.* 2010;21(7):1121-1132.

97. Looker AC, Dawson-Hughes B, Calvo MS, Gunter EW, Sahyoun NR. Serum 25-hydroxyvitamin D status of adolescents and adults in two seasonal subpopulations from NHANES III. *Bone.* 2002;30(5):771-777.

98. Lappe JM, Davies KM, Travers-Gustafson D, Heaney RP. Vitamin D status in a rural postmenopausal female population. *J Am Coll Nutr.* 2006;25(5):395-402.

99. Passeri G, Pini G, Troiano L, et al. Low vitamin D status, high bone turnover, and bone fractures in centenarians. *J Clin Endocrinol Metab.* 2003;88(11):5109-5115.

100. Kuchuk NO, van Schoor NM, Pluijm SM, Chines A, Lips P. Vitamin D status, parathyroid function, bone turnover, and BMD in postmenopausal women with osteoporosis: global perspective. *J Bone Miner Res.* 2009;24(4):693-701.

101. Mangoo-Karim R, Da Silva Abreu J, Yanev GP, Perez NN, Stubbs JR, Wetmore JB. Ergocalciferol versus cholecalciferol for nutritional vitamin D replacement in CKD. *Nephron.* 2015;130(2):99-104.

102. Bjelakovic G, Gluud LL, Nikolova D, et al. Vitamin D supplementation for prevention of cancer in adults. *Cochrane Database Syst Rev.* 2014;(6):CD007469.

103. Manson JE, Cook NR, Lee IM, et al; VITAL Research Group. Vitamn D supplements and prevention of cancer and cardiovascular disease. *N Engl J Med.* 2019;380(1):33-44.

104. Sesso HD, Buring JE, Christen WG, et al. Vitamins E and C in the prevention of cardiovascular disease in men: the Physicians' Health Study II randomized controlled trial. *JAMA.* 2008;300(18):2123-2133.

105. Miller ER 3rd, Pastor-Barriuso R, Dalal D, Riemersma RA, Appel LJ, Guallar E. Meta-analysis: high-dosage vitamin E supplementation may increase all-cause mortality. *Ann Intern Med.* 2005;142(1):37-46.

106. Lonn E, Bosch J, Yusuf S, et al; HOPE and HOPE-TOO Trial Investigators. Effects of long-term vitamin E supplementation on cardiovascular events and cancer: a randomized controlled trial. *JAMA.* 2005;293(11):1338-1347.

107. Waters DD, Alderman EL, Hsia J, et al. Effects of hormone replacement therapy and antioxidant vitamin supplements on coronary atherosclerosis in postmenopausal women: a randomized controlled trial. *JAMA.* 2002;288(19):2432-2440.

108. Lee IM, Cook NR, Gaziano JM, et al. Vitamin E in the primary prevention of cardiovascular disease and cancer: the Women's Health Study: a randomized controlled trial. *JAMA.* 2005;294(1):56-65.

109. Glynn RJ, Ridker PM, Goldhaber SZ, Zee RY, Buring JE. Effects of random allocation to vitamin E supplementation on the occurrence of venous thromboembolism: report from the Women's Health Study. *Circulation.* 2007;116(13):1497-1503.

110. Zhu YJ, Bo YC, Liu XX, Qiu CG. Association of dietary vitamin E intake with risk of lung cancer: a dose-response meta-analysis. *Asia Pac J Clin Nutr.* 2017;26(2):271-277.

111. Hao G, Zhang B, Gu M, et al. Vitamin K intake and the risk of fractures: a meta-analysis. *Medicine (Baltimore).* 2017;96(17):e6725.

112. Huang ZB, Wan SL, Lu YJ, Ning L, Liu C, Fan SW. Does vitamin K2 play a role in the prevention and treatment of osteoporosis for postmenopausal women: a meta-analysis of randomized controlled trials. *Osteoporos Int.* 2015;26(3):1175-1186.

113. Nimptsch K, Rohrmann S, Kaaks R, Linseisen J. Dietary vitamin K intake in relation to cancer incidence and mortality: results from the Heidelberg cohort of the European Prospective Investigation into Cancer and Nutrition (EPIC-Heidelberg). *Am J Clin Nutr.* 2010;91(5):1348-1358.

114. Pottegård A, Friis S, Hallas J. Cancer risk in long-term users of vitamin K antagonists: a population-based case-control study. *Int J Cancer.* 2013;132(11):2606-2612.

115. McCormack SE, Cousminer DL, Chesi A, et al. Association between linear growth and bone accrual in a diverse cohort of children and adolescents. *JAMA Pediatr.* 2017;171(9):e171769.

116. World Health Organization and Food and Agriculture Organization of the United Nations. Calcium. In: *Vitamin and Mineral Requirements in Human Nutrition.* 2nd ed. Geneva: World Health Organization; 2004:59-93.

117. Nordin BE, Need AG, Morris HA, O'Loughlin PD, Horowitz M. Effect of age on calcium absorption in postmenopausal women. *Am J Clin Nutr.* 2004;80(4):998-1002.

118. Shapses SA, Sukumar D, Schneider SH, et al. Hormonal and dietary influences on true fractional calcium absorption in women: role of obesity. *Osteoporos Int.* 2012;23(11):2607-2614.

119. Pattapaungkul S, Riggs BL, Yegey AL, Viera AL, O'Fallon WM, Khosla S. Relationship of intestinal calcium absorption to 1,25-dihydroxyvitamin D [1,25(OH)2D] levels in young versus elderly women: evidence for age-related intestinal resistance to 1,25(OH)2D action. *J Clin Endocrinol Metab.* 2000;85(11):4023-4027.

120. Christakos S, Dhawan P, Porta A, Mady LJ, Seth T. Vitamin D and intestinal calcium absorption. *Mol Cell Endocrinol.* 2011;347(1-2):25-29.

121. Bailey RK, Fileti CP, Keith J, Tropez-Sims S, Price W, Allison-Ottey SD. Lactose intolerance and health disparities among African Americans and Hispanic Americans: an updated consensus statement. *J Natl Med Assoc.* 2013;105(2):112-127.

122. Adatorwovor R, Roggenkamp K, Anderson JJ. Intakes of calcium and phosphorus and calculated calcium-to-phosphorus ratios of older adults: NHANES 2005-2006 data. *Nutrients.* 2015;7(11):9633-9639.

123. Wilczynski C, Camacho P. Calcium use in the management of osteoporosis: continuing questions and controversies. *Curr Osteoporos Rep.* 2014;12(4):396-402.

124. Shea B, Wells G, Cranney A, et al; Osteoporosis Methodology Group and the Osteoporosis Research Advisory Group. Meta-analyses of therapies for postmenopausal osteoporosis. VII. Meta-analysis of calcium supplementation for the prevention of postmenopausal osteoporosis. *Endocr Rev.* 2002;23(4):552-559.

125. Tang BM, Eslick GD, Nowson C, Smith C, Bensoussan A. Use of calcium or calcium in combination with vitamin D supplementation to prevent fractures and bone loss in people aged 50 years and older: a meta-analysis. *Lancet.* 2007;370(9588):657-666. Erratum in: *Lancet.* 2012;380(9844):806.

126. Khan B, Nowson CA, Daly RM, et al. Higher dietary calcium intakes are associated with reduced risks of fractures, cardiovascular events, and mortality: a prospective cohort study of older men and women. *J Bone Miner Res.* 2015;30(10):1758-1766.

127. Tai V, Leung W, Grey A, Reid IR, Bolland MJ. Calcium intake and bone mineral density: systematic review and meta-analysis. *BMJ.* 2015;351:h4183.

128. Bolland MJ, Leung W, Tai V, et al. Calcium intake and risk of fracture: systematic review. *BMJ.* 2015;351:h4580.

129. DIPART (Vitamin D Individual Patient Analysis of Randomized Trials) Group. Patient level pooled analysis of 68 500 patients from seven major vitamin D fracture trials in US and Europe. *BMJ.* 2010;340:b5463.

130. Nieves JW, Komar L, Cosman F, Lindsay R. Calcium potentiates the effect of estrogen and calcitonin on bone mass: review and analysis. *Am J Clin Nutr.* 1998;67(1):18-24.

131. New SA, Banjour J-P, Nieves J, Cosman F. The treatment of osteoporosis and interaction of medications with nutrition. In: Lanham-New SA, Banjour J-P, eds. *Nutritional Aspects of Bone Health.* London: Royal Society of Chemistry;2003:565-588.

132. Cormick G, Ciapponi A, Cafferata ML, Belizán JM. Calcium supplementation for prevention of primary hypertension. *CochraneDatabaseSystRev.* 2015;(6):CD010037.

133. Bolland MJ, Avenell A, Baron JA, et al. Effect of calcium supplements on risk of myocardial infarction and cardiovascular events: meta-analysis. *BMJ.* 2010;341:c3691.

134. Bolland MJ, Grey A, Avenell A, Gamble GD, Reid IR. Calcium supplements with or without vitamin D and risk of cardiovascular events: reanalysis of the Women's Health Initiative limited access dataset and meta-analysis. *BMJ.* 2011;342:d2040.

135. Michaëlsson K, Melhus H, Warensjö Lemming E, Wolk A, Byberg L. Long term calcium intake and rates of all cause and cardiovascular mortality: community based prospective longitudinal cohort study. *BMJ.* 2013;346:f228.

136. Pentti K, Tuppurainen MT, Honkanen R, et al. Use of calcium supplements and the risk of coronary heart disease in 52-62-year-old women: the Kuopio Osteoporosis Risk Factor and Prevention Study. *Maturitas.* 2009;63(1):73-78.

137. Chung M, Tang AM, Fu Z, Wang DD, Newberry SJ. Calcium intake and cardiovascular disease risk: an updated systematic review and meta-analysis. *Ann Intern Med.* 2016;165(12):856-866.

138. Kopecky SL, Bauer DC, Gulati M, et al. Lack of evidence linking calcium with or without vitamin D supplementation to cardiovascular disease in generally healthy adults: a clinical guideline from the National Osteoporosis Foundation and the American Society for Preventive Cardiology. *Ann Intern Med.* 2016;165(12):867-868.

139. Beto JA. The role of calcium in human aging. *Clin Nutr Res.* 2015;4(1):1-8.

140. Bailey RL, Akabas SR, Paxson EE, Thuppal SV, SaklaniS, Tucker KL. Total usual intake of shortfall nutrients varies with poverty among US adults. *J Nutr Educ Behav.* 2017;49(8):639.e3-646.e3.

141. Harvey NC, Biver E, Kaufman JM, et al. The role of calcium supplementation in healthy musculoskeletal ageing: an expert consensus meeting of the European Society for Clinical and Economic Aspects of Osteoporosis, Osteoarthritis and Musculoskeletal Diseases (ESCEO) and the International Foundation for Osteoporosis (IOF). *Osteoporos Int.* 2017;28(2):447-462.

142. National Osteoporosis Foundation. *Calcium/Vitamin D.* www.nof.org/patients/treatment/calciumvitamin-d/. Last updated February 26, 2018. Accessed July 9, 2019.

143. Office of the Surgeon General (US). *Bone Health and Osteoporosis: A Report of the Surgeon General.* Rockville, MD: Office of the Surgeon General (US); 2004.

144. Suchy FJ, Brannon PM, Carpenter TO, et al. NIH consensus development conference statement: lactose intolerance and health. *NIH Consens State Sci Statements.* 2010;27(2):1-27.

145. Barr SI. Perceived lactose intolerance in adult Canadians: a national survey. *Appl Physiol Nutr Metab.* 2013;38(8):830-835.

146. National Medical Association. Lactose intolerance and African Americans: implications for the consumption of appropriate intake levels of key nutrients. *J Natl Med Assoc.* 2009;101(10 suppl):5S-23S.

147. Rafferty K, Walters G, Heaney RP. Calcium fortificants: overview and strategies for improving calcium nutriture of the US population. *J Food Sci.* 2007;72(9):R152-158.

148. Wallace RB, Wactawski-Wende J, O'Sullivan MJ, et al. Urinary tract stone occurrence in the Women's Health Initiative (WHI) randomized clinical trial of calcium and vitamin D supplements. *Am J Clin Nutr.* 2011;94(1):270-277.

149. Kozyrakis D, Paridis D, Karatzas A, Soukias G, Dailiana Z. Do calcium supplements predispose to urolithiasis? *Current Urol Rep.* 2017;18(3):17.

150. Institute of Medicine Panel on Micronutrients. *Dietary Reference Intakes for Vitamin A, Vitamin K, Arsenic, Boron, Chromium, Copper, Iodine, Iron, Manganese, Molybdenum, Nickel, Silicon, Vanadium, and Zinc.* Washington, DC: National Academies Press; 2001.

151. World Health Organization. The global prevalence of anaemia in 2011. Geneva: World Health Organization; 2015.

152. Haas JD, Brownlie T 4th. Iron deficiency and reduced work capacity: a critical review of the research to determine a causal relationship. *J Nutr.* 2001;131(2S-2):676S-688S.

153. Wirth JP, Woodruff BA, Engle-Stone R, et al. Predictors of anemia in women of reproductive age: Biomarkers Reflecting Inflammation and Nutritional Determinants of Anemia (BRINDA) project. *Am J Clin Nutr.* 2017;106(suppl 1):416S-427S.

154. Kassebaum NJ, Jasrasaria R, Naghavi M, et al. A systematic analysis of global anemia burden from 1990 to 2010. *Blood.* 2014;123(5):615-624.

155. Camaschella C. Iron-deficiency anemia. *N Engl J Med.* 2015;372(19):1832-1843.

156. Saris NE, Mervaala E, Karppanen H, Khawaja JA, Lewenstam A. Magnesium. An update on physiological, clinical and analytical aspects. *Clin Chim Acta.* 2000;294(1-2):1-26.

157. Konrad M, Schlingmann KP, Gudermann T. Insights into the molecular nature of magnesium homeostasis. *Am J Physiol Renal Physiol.* 2004;286(4):F599-F605.

158. Sahota O, Mundey MK, San P, Godber IM, Hosking DJ. Vitamin D insufficiency and the blunted PTH response in established osteoporosis: the role of magnesium deficiency. *Osteoporos Int.* 2006;17(7):1013-1021.

159. Nieves JW. Bone. Maximizing bone health—magnesium, BMD and fractures. *Nat Rev Endocrinol.* 2014;10(5):255-256.

160. Institute of Medicine Standing Committee on the Scientific Evaluation of Dietary Reference Intakes. *Dietary Reference Intakes for Calcium, Phosphorus, Magnesium, Vitamin D, and Fluoride.* Washington, DC: National Academies Press; 1997.

161. Hemilä H. Zinc lozenges and the common cold: a meta-analysis comparing zinc acetate and zinc gluconate, and the role of zinc dosage. *JRSM Open.* 2017;8(5):2054270417694291.

162. Caruso TJ, Prober CG, Gwaltney JM Jr. Treatment of naturally acquired common colds with zinc: a structured review. *Clin Infect Dis.* 2007;45(5):569-574.

163. Institute of Medicine Health and Medicine Division. *Dietary Reference Intakes for Vitamin C, Vitamin E, Selenium, and Carotenoids.* Washington, DC: National Academies Press; 2000.

164. Merrill PD, Ampah SB, He K, et al. Association between trace elements in the environment and stroke risk: the reasons for geographic and racial differences in stroke (REGARDS) study. *J Trace ElementsMed Biol.* 2017;42:45-49.

165. Schwingshackl L, Boeing H, Stelmach-Mardas M, et al. Dietary supplements and risk of cause-specific death, cardiovascular disease, and cancer: a systematic review and meta-analysis of primary prevention trials. *Adv Nutrl.* 2017;8(1):27-39.

166. Fotino AD, Thompson-Paul AM, Bazzano LA. Effect of coenzyme Q10 on heart failure: a meta-analysis. *Am J Clin Nutr.* 2013;97(2):268-275.

167. Alehagen U, Johansson P, Björnstedt M, Rosén A, Dahlström U. Cardiovascular mortality and N-terminal-proBNP reduced after combined selenium and coenzyme Q10 supplementation: a 5-year prospective randomized double-blind placebo-controlled trial among elderly Swedish citizens. *Int J Cardiol.* 2013;167(5):1860-1866.

168. Mortensen SA, Rosenfeldt F, Kumar A, et al; Q-SYMBIO Study Investigators. The effect of coenzyme Q10 on morbidity and mortality in chronic heart failure: results from Q-SYMBIO: a randomized double-blind trial. *JACC Heart Fail.* 2014;2(6):641-649.

169. Hodgson JM, Watts GF, Playford DA, Burke V, Croft KD. Coenzyme Q10 improves blood pressure and glycaemic control: a controlled trial in subjects with type 2 diabetes. *Eur J Clin Nutr.* 2002;56(11):1137-1142.

170. Rosenfeldt FL, Haas SJ, Krum H, et al. Coenzyme Q10 in the treatment of hypertension: a meta-analysis of the clinical trials. *J Hum Hypertens.* 2007;21(4):297-306.

171. Flowers N, Hartley L, Todkill D, Stranges S, Rees K. Co-enzyme Q10 supplementation for the primary prevention of cardiovascular disease. *Cochrane Database Syst Rev.* 2014;(12):CD010405.

172. Bookstaver DA, Burkhalter NA, Hatzigeorgiou C. Effect of coenzyme Q10 supplementation on statin-induced myalgias. *Am J Cardiol.* 2012;110(4):526-529.

173. Young JM, Florkowski CM, Molyneux SL, et al. Effect of coenzyme Q(10) supplementation on simvastatin-induced myalgia. *Am J Cardiol*. 2007;100(9):1400-1403.

174. Marcoff L, Thompson PD. The role of coenzyme Q10 in statin-associated myopathy: a systematic review. *J Am Coll Cardiol*. 2007;49(23):2231-2237.

175. Banach M, Serban C, Sahebkar A, et al; Lipid and Blood Pressure Meta-analysis Collaboration Group. Effects of coenzyme Q10 on statin-induced myopathy: a meta-analysis of randomized controlled trials. *Mayo Clin Proc*. 2015;90(1):24-34.

176. Rozen TD, Oshinsky ML, Gebeline CA, et al. Open label trial of coenzyme Q10 as a migraine preventive. *Cephalalgia*. 2002;22(2):137-141.

177. Sándor PS, Di Clemente L, Coppola G, et al. Efficacy of coenzyme Q10 in migraine prophylaxis: a randomized controlled trial. *Neurology*. 2005;64(4):713-715.

178. Pringsheim T, Davenport W, Mackie G, et al; Canadian Headache Society Prophylactic Guidelines Development Group. Canadian Headache Society guideline for migraine prophylaxis. *Can J Neurol Sci*. 2012;39 (2 suppl 2):S1-S59.

179. Shoeibi A, Olfati N, Soltani Sabi M, Salehi M, Mali S, Akbari Oryani M. Effectiveness of coenzyme Q10 in prophylactic treatment of migraine headache: an open-label, add-on, controlled trial. *Acta Neurol Belg*. 2017;117(1):103-109.

180. Lesser GJ, Case D, Stark N, et al; Wake Forest University Community Clinical Oncology Program Research Base. A randomized, double-blind, placebo-controlled study of oral coenzyme Q10 to relieve self-reported treatment-related fatigue in newly diagnosed patients with breast cancer. *J Support Oncol*. 2013;11(1):31-42.

181. Iwase S, Kawaguchi T, Yotsumoto D, et al. Efficacy and safety of an amino acid jelly containing coenzyme Q10 and L-carnitine in controlling fatigue in breast cancer patients receiving chemotherapy: a multi-institutional, randomized, exploratory trial (JORTC-CAM01). *Support Care Cancer*. 2016;24(2):637-646.

182. Hidaki T, Fujii K, Funahashi I, Fukutomi N, Hosoe K. Safety assessment of coenzyme Q10 (CoQ10). *BioFactors*. 2008;32(1-4):199-208.

183. Elsayed NM, Bendich A. Dietary antioxidants: potential effects on oxidative products in cigarette smoke. *Nutr Res*. 2001;21(3):551-567.

184. Harris WS, Miller M, Tighe AP, Davidson MH, Schaefer EJ. Omega-3 fatty acids and coronary heart disease risk: clinical and mechanistic perspectives. *Atherosclerosis*. 2008;197(1):12-24.

185. Riediger ND, Othman RA, Suh M, Moghadasian MH. A systematic review of the roles of n-3 fatty acids in health and disease. *J Am Diet Assoc*. 2009;109(4):668-679.

186. Lee JH, O'Keefe JH, Lavie CJ, Marchioli R, Harris WS. Omega-3 fatty acids for cardioprotection. *Mayo Clin Proc*. 2008;83(3):324-332. Erratum in: *Mayo Clin Proc*. 2008;83(6):730.

187. McKenney JM, Sica D. Role of prescription omega-3 fatty acids in the treatment of hypertriglyceridemia. *Pharmacotherapy*. 2007;27(5):715-728.

188. Zheng J, Huang T, Yu Y, Hu X, Yang B, Li D. Fish consumption and CHD mortality: an updated meta-analysis of 17 cohorts. *Public Health Nutr*. 2012;15(4):725-737.

189. Burr ML Fehily AM, Gilbert JF, et al. Effects of changes in fat, fish, and fibre intakes on death and myocardial reinfarction: diet and reinfarction trial (DART). *Lancet*. 1989;2(8666):757-761.

190. Marchioli R, Barzi F, Bomba E, et al; GISSI-Prevenzione Investigators. Early protection against sudden death by n-3 polyunsaturated fatty acids after myocardial infarction: time-course analysis of the results of the Gruppo Italiano per lo Studio della Sopravvivenza nell'Infarto Miocardico (GISSI)-Prevenzione. *Circulation*. 2002;105(16):1897-1903.

191. Yokoyama M, Origasa H, Matsuzaki M, et al; Japan EPA Lipid Intervention Study (JELIS) Investigators. Effects of eicosapentaenoic acid on major coronary events in hypercholesterolaemic patients (JELIS): a randomised open-label, blinded endpoint analysis. *Lancet*. 2007;369(9567):1090-1098.

192. Nosaka K, Miyoshi H, Iwamoto M, et al. Early initiation of eicosapentaenoic acid and statin treatment is associated with better clinical outcomes than statin alone in patients with acute coronary syndromes: 1-year outcomes of a randomized controlled study. *Int J Cardiol*. 2017;228:173-179.

193. Kromhout D, Giltay EJ, Geleijnse JM; Alpha Omega Trial Group. n-3 fatty acids and cardiovascular events after myocardial infarction. *N Engl J Med*. 2010:363(21):2015-2026.

194. Galan P, Kesse-Guyot E, Czernichow S, Briancon S, Blacher J, Hercberg S; SU.FOL.OM3 Collaborative Group. Effects of B vitamins and omega 3 fatty acids on cardiovascular disease: a randomized placebo controlled trial. *BMJ*. 2010;341:c6273

195. Kotwal S, Jun M, Sullivan D, Perkovic V, Neal B. Omega 3 fatty acids and cardiovascular outcomes: systematic review and meta-analysis. *Circ Cardiovasc Qual Outcomes*. 2012;5(6):808-818.

196. Kwak SM, Myung SK, Lee YJ, Seo HG; Korean Meta-analysis Study Group. Efficacy of omega-3 fatty acid supplements (eicosapentaenoic acid and docosahexaenoic acid) in the secondary prevention of cardiovascular disease: a meta-analysis of randomized, double-blind, placebo-controlled trials. *Arch Intern Med*. 2012;172(9):686-694.

197. Rizos EC, Ntzani EE, Bika E, Kostapanos MS, Elisaf MS. Association between omega-3 fatty acid supplementation and risk of major cardiovascular disease events: a systematic review and meta-analysis. *JAMA*. 2012;308(10):1024-1033.

198. Aung T, Halsey J, Kromhout D, et al; Omega-3 Treatment Trialists' Collaboration. Associations of omega-3 fatty acid supplement use with cardiovascular disease risks: meta-analysis of 10 trials involving 77 917 individuals. *JAMA Cardiol*. 2018;3(3):225-234.

199. Manson JE, Cook NR, Lee IM, et al; VITAL Research Group. Marine n-3 fatty acids and prevention of cardiovascular disease and cancer. *N Engl J Med*. 2019;380(1):23-32.

200. Lee LK, Shahar S, Chin AV, Yusoff NA. Docosahexaenoic acid-concentrated fish oil supplementation in subjects with mild cognitive impairment (MCI): a 12-month randomised, double-blind, placebo-controlled trial. *Psychopharmacology (Berl)*. 2013;225(3):605-612.

201. Shinto L, Quinn J, Montine T, et al. A randomized placebo-controlled pilot trial of omega-3 fatty acids and alpha lipoic acid in Alzheimer's disease. *J Alzheimers Dis*. 2014;38(1):111-120.

202. Burckhardt M, Herke M, Wustmann T, Watzke S, Langer G, Fink A. Omega-3 fatty acids for the treatment of dementia. *Cochrane Database Syst Rev*. 2016;4:CD009002.

203. Ravindran AV, Lam RW, Filtreau MJ, et al; Canadian Network for Mood and Anxiety Treatments (CANMET). Canadian Network for Mood and Anxiety Treatments (CANMET) clinical guidelines for the management of major depressive disorders in adults. V. Complementary and alternative medicine treatments. *J Affect Disord*. 2009;117(suppl 1):S54-S64.

204. Appleton KM, Hayward RC, Gunnell D, et al. Effects of n-3 long-chain polyunsaturated fatty acids on depressed mood: systematic review of published trials. *Am J Clin Nutr*. 2006;84(6):1308-1316.

205. Lin PY, Su KP. A meta-analytic review of double-blind, placebo controlled trials of antidepressant efficacy of omega-3 fatty acids. *J Clin Psychiatry*. 2007;68(7):1056-1061.

206. Bloch MH, Hannestad J. Omega-3 fatty acids for the treatment of depression: systematic review and meta-analysis. *Mol Psychiatry*. 2012;17(12):1272-1282.

207. Foran SE, Flood JG, Lewandrowski KB. Measurement of mercury levels in concentrated over-the-counter fish oil preparations: is fish oil healthier than fish? *Arch Pathol Lab Med*. 2003;127(12):1603-1605.

208. Mozaffarian D, Rimm EB. Fish intake, contaminants, and human health: evaluating the risks and the benefits. *JAMA*. 2006;296(15):1885-1899. Erratum in: *JAMA*. 2007;297(6):590.

209. Zucker ML, Bilyeu DS, Helmkamp GM, Harris WS, Dujovne CA. Effects of dietary fish oil on platelet function and plasma lipids in hyperlipoproteinemic and normal subjects. *Atherosclerosis*. 1988;73(1):13-22.

210. Poolsup N, Suthisisang C, Channark P, Kittikulsuth W. Glucosamine long-term treatment and the progression of knee osteoarthritis: systematic review of randomized controlled trials. *Ann Pharmacother*. 2005;39(6):1080-1087.

211. Towheed TE, Maxwell L, Anastassiades TP, et al. Glucosamine therapy for treating osteoarthritis. *Cochrane Database Syst Rev*. 2005;(2):CD002946.

212. Lee YH, Woo JH, Choi SJ, Ji JD, Song GG. Effect of glucosamine or chondroitin sulfate on the osteoarthritis progression: a meta-analysis. *Rheumatol Int*. 2010;30(3):357-363.

213. Kantor ED, Lampe JW, Navarro SL, Song X, Milne GL, White E. Associations between glucosamine and chondroitin supplement use and biomarkers of systemic inflammation. *J Altern Complement Med.* 2014;20(6):479-485.

214. Navarro SL, White E, Kantor ED, et al. Randomized trial of glucosamine and chondroitin supplementation on inflammation and oxidative stress biomarkers and plasma proteomics profiles in healthy humans. *PloS One.* 2015;10(2):e0117534.

215. Reichenbach S, Sterchi R, Scherer M, et al. Meta-analysis: chondroitin for osteoarthritis of the knee or hip. *Ann Intern Med.* 2007;146(8):580-590.

216. Clegg DO, Reda DJ, Harris CL, et al. Glucosamine, chondroitin sulfate, and the two in combination for painful knee osteoarthritis. *N Engl J Med.* 2006;354(8):795-808.

217. Zeng C, Wei J, Li H, et al. Effectiveness and safety of Glucosamine, chondroitin, the two in combination, or celecoxib in the treatment of osteoarthritis of the knee. *Sci Rep.* 2015;5:16827.

218. Pavelká K, Gatterová J, Olejarová M, Machacek S, Giacovelli G, Rovati LC. Glucosamine sulfate use and delay of progression of knee osteoarthritis: a 3-year, randomized, placebo-controlled, double-blind study. *Arch Intern Med.* 2002;162(18):2113-2123.

219. Reginster JY, Deroisy R, Rovati LC, et al. Long-term effects of glucosamine sulphate on osteoarthritis progression: a randomized, placebo controlled trial. *Lancet.* 2001;357(9252):251-256.

220. Rozendaal RM, Koes BW, van Osch G, et al. Effect of glucosamine on hip osteoarthritis: a randomized trial. *Ann Intern Med.* 2008; 148(4):268-277.

221. Bruyere O, Pavelka K, Rovati LC, et al. Total joint replacement after glucosamine sulphate treatment in knee osteoarthritis: results of a mean 8-year observation of patients from two previous 3-year, randomised, controlled trials. *Osteoarthritis Cartilage.* 2008;16(2):254-260.

222. Sawitzke AD, Shi H, Finco MF, et al. The effect of glucosamine and/or chondroitin sulphate on the progression of knee osteoarthritis: a report from the Glucosamine/chondroitin Arthritis Intervention Trial. *Arthritis Rheum.* 2008;58(10):3183-3191.

223. Wandel S, Jüni P, Tendal B, et al. Effects of glucosamine, chondroitin, or placebo in patients with osteoarthritis of hip or knee: network meta-analysis. *BMJ.* 2010;341:c4675.

224. Kantor ED, Zhang X, Wu K, et al. Use of glucosamine and chondroitin supplements in relation to risk of colorectal cancer: results from the Nurses' Health Study and Health Professionals follow-up study. *Int J Cancer.* 2016;139(9):1949-1957.

225. Marshall PD, Poddar S, Tweed EM, Brandes L. Clinical inquiries: Do glucosamine and chondroitin worsen blood sugar control in diabetes? *J Fam Pract.* 2006;55(12):1091-1093.

226. Knudsen JF, Sokol GH. Potential glucosamine-warfarin interaction resulting in increased international normalized ratio: case report and review of the literature and MedWatch database. *Pharmacotherapy.* 2008;28(4):540-548.

227. Carpenter DJ. St John's wort and S-adenosyl methionine as "natural" alternatives to conventional antidepressants in the era of the suicidality boxed warning: what is the evidence for clinically relevant benefit? *Altern Med Rev.* 2011;16(1):17-39.

228. Galizia I, Oldani L, Macritchie K, et al. S-adenosyl methionine (SAMe) for depression in adults. *Cochrane Database Syst Rev.* 2016;10:CD011286.

229. Papakostas GI. Evidence for S-adenosyl-L-methionine (SAM-e) for the treatment of major depressive disorder. *J Clin Psychiatry.* 2009;70(suppl 5):18-22.

230. De Silva V, El-Metwally A, Ernst E, Lewith G, Macfarlane GJ; Arthritis Research UK Working Group on Complementary and Alternative Medicines. Evidence for the efficacy of complementary and alternative medicines in the management of osteoarthritis: a systematic review. *Rheumatology (Oxford).* 2011;50(5):911-920.

231. Rutjes AW, Nüesch E, Reichenbach S, Jüni P. S-Adenosylmethionine for osteoarthritis of the knee or hip. *Cochrane Database Syst Rev.* 2009;(4):CD007321.

232. Rambaldi A, Gluud C. S-adenosyl-L-methionine for alcoholic liver disease. *Cochrane Database Syst Rev.* 2006;(2):CD002235.

233. Guo T, Chang L, Xiao Y, Liu Q. S-adenosyl-L-methionine for the treatment of chronic liver disease: a systematic review and meta-analysis. *PloS One.* 2015;10(3):e0122124.

234. Claustrat B, Brun J, Chazot G. The basic physiology and pathophysiology of melatonin. *Sleep Med Rev.* 2005;9(1):11-24.

235. Rohr UD, Herold J. Melatonin deficiencies in women. *Maturitas.* 2002;41(suppl 1):S85-S104.

236. Bjortvatn B, Pallesen S. A practical approach to circadian rhythm sleep disorders. *Sleep Med Rev.* 2009;13(1):47-60.

237. Herxheimer A, Petrie KJ. Melatonin for the prevention and treatment of jet lag. *Cochrane Database Sys Rev.* 2002;(2):CD001520.

238. de Jonghe A, Korevaar JC, van Munster BC, de Rooij SE. Effectiveness of melatonin treatment on circadian rhythm disturbances in dementia. Are there implications for delirium? A systematic review. *Int J Geriatr Psychiatry.* 2010;25(12):1201-1208.

239. Ferracioli-Oda E, Qawasmi A, Bloch MH. Meta-analysis: melatonin for the treatment of primary sleep disorders. *PLoS One.* 2013;8(5):e63773.

240. Hajak G, Lemme K, Zisapel N. Lasting treatment effects in a postmarketing surveillance study of prolonged-release melatonin. *Int Clin Psychopharmacol.* 2015;30(1):36-42.

241. van Geijlswijk IM, Korzilius HP, Smits MG. The use of exogenous melatonin in delayed sleep phase disorder: a meta-analysis. *Sleep.* 2010;33(12):1605-1614.

242. Grossman E, Laudon M, Zisapel N. Effect of melatonin on nocturnal blood pressure: meta-analysis of randomized controlled trials. *Vasc Health Risk Manag.* 2011;7:577-584.

243. Gubin DG, Gubin GD, Gapon LI, Weinert D. Daily melatonin administration attenuates age-dependent disturbances of cardiovascular rhythms. *Curr Aging Sci.* 2016;9(1):5-13.

244. Garfinkel D, Zisapel N, Wainstein J, Laudon M. Facilitation of benzodiazepine discontinuation by melatonin: a new clinical approach. *Arch Intern Med.* 1999;159(20):2456-2460.

245. Peles E, Hetzroni T, Bar-Hamburger R, Adelson M, Schreiber S. Melatonin for perceived sleep disturbances associated with benzodiazepine withdrawal among patients in methadone maintenance treatment: a double-blind randomized clinical trial. *Addiction.* 2007;102(12):1947-1953.

246. Wright A, Diebold J, Otal J, et al. The effect of melatonin on benzodiazepine discontinuation and sleep auality in adults attempting to discontinue benzodiazepines: a systematic review and meta-analysis. *Drugs Aging.* 2015;32(12):1009-1018.

247. Buscemi N, Vandermeer B, Hooton N, et al. Efficacy and safety of exogenous melatonin for secondary sleep disorders and sleep disorders accompanying sleep restriction: meta-analysis. *BMJ.* 2006;332(7538):385-393.

248. Luthringer R, Muzet M, Zisapel N, Staner L. The effect of prolonged-release melatonin on sleep measures and psychomotor performance in elderly patients with insomnia. *Int Clin Psychopharmacol.* 2009;24(5):239-249.

249. Wade A, Downie S. Prolonged-release melatonin for the treatment of insomnia in patients over 55 years. *Expert Opin Investig Drugs.* 2008;17(10):1567-1572.

250. Lusardi P, Piazza E, Fogari R. Cardiovascular effects of melatonin in hypertensive patients well controlled by nifedipine: a 24-hour study. *Br J Clin Pharmacol.* 2000;49(5):423-427.

251. Cagnacci A, Arangino S, Renzi A, et al. Influence of melatonin administration on glucose tolerance and insulin sensitivity of postmenopausal women. *Clin Endocrinol (Oxf).* 2001;54(3):339-346.

11

Prescription Therapies

Prescription hormone drugs—including contraceptives, hormone therapy (HT), androgens, and estrogen agonists/antagonists—and nonprescription, over-the-counter (OTC) hormones are among the treatments considered for women during perimenopause and beyond. Almost all are government approved for the indication (or indications) for which they are most commonly prescribed, whereas some are prescribed off-label (used for an indication other than what is FDA approved).

Those with premature or early menopause (natural, induced, or surgical) should be considered for HT until the average age of menopause to prevent the health consequences of loss of estrogen at an early age. Numerous clinical trials have shown the effectiveness of HT to prevent osteoporosis and reduce the risk of fractures. Extended duration can be considered for women with persistent hot flashes who elect to continue very-low doses and longer-term use to relieve menopause symptoms, prevent bone loss, and improve quality of life (QOL).

For women who need relief from the progressive symptoms of the genitourinary syndrome of menopause (GSM), low-dose vaginal estrogen (cream, ring, or tablet) or intravaginal dehydroepiandrosterone (DHEA) can be used at any age with benefit and minimal risk without the need for opposing progestogen therapy, based on 1 to 3 years' clinical data. The use of testosterone therapy, either alone or with HT, has been used in selected postmenopausal women with sexual interest/arousal disorder, but there are no FDA-approved testosterone therapies in the United States or Canada. Compounded, non–FDA-approved or monitored therapies are not recommended if there are FDA-approved therapies because of the lack of rigorous safety and efficacy testing, lack of government regulation, concern about batch standardization,

overdosing or underdosing, and purity and sterility concerns. (See also "Bioidentical Hormone Therapy" in this chapter.)

Contraceptives

Despite a decline in fertility during perimenopause, pregnancy is still possible until menopause is reached. (See also "Decline in Fertility With Reproductive Aging" in Chapter 5.) Perimenopausal women who wish to avoid pregnancy should be counseled regarding various birth control methods. However, this population has special characteristics that influence contraceptive choice. Women of older reproductive age may be experiencing perimenopause symptoms that could be managed with contraceptives, but these women may have concomitant medical conditions that would make certain contraceptive methods inappropriate. Women aged older than 40 years also are more likely to desire long-acting or permanent contraception. Women of older reproductive age have lower rates of contraceptive failure than do younger women because of lower fecundity, less frequent sexual intercourse, and higher compliance with contraceptive regimens.[1] Hormone contraceptives (HCs), with and without estrogen, and intrauterine devices (IUDs) offer effective options for perimenopausal women.

For any woman who desires long-term protection from pregnancy, long-acting, reversible contraceptive methods, which include the copper IUD, the four levonorgestrel-releasing intrauterine systems (LNG-IUS), and the etonogestrel subdermal implant, provide superior contraceptive effectiveness, high user satisfaction, and easy placement in an office or clinic setting.[2] For women who have completed their childbearing, long-acting reversible contraceptive methods are convenient and less expensive and invasive than surgical sterilization.

The Centers for Disease Control and Prevention (CDC) has issued evidence-based guidelines, facilitating contraceptive provision and clinical decision making: the *US Selected Practice Recommendations for Contraceptive Use* (*SPR*) and the *US Medical Eligibility Criteria for Contraceptive Use* (*MEC*).[3,4] The *SPR* explains how to safely initiate contraceptive methods at any time during the menstrual cycle and when it is necessary to perform a pelvic examination before contraceptive initiation (ie, only before intrauterine contraception [IUC]). The *MEC* categorizes contraceptive methods according to their safety when used in women with a variety of medical conditions. (Both these CDC documents are available together on the free *CDC Contraception* app for Iphone and Android.) For each condition, eligibility for the use of each contraceptive method is categorized into one of four categories: 1) a condition for which there is no restriction for use; 2) a condition for which the advantages generally outweigh the theoretical or proven risks; 3) a condition for which the theoretical or proven risks usually outweigh the advantages; and 4) a condition that represents an unacceptable health risk if the method is used.

According to the *MEC* guidelines, there are no contraceptive methods that are contraindicated on the basis of age alone (Table 1).[4] However, some medical conditions more common in older women may make some contraceptive methods inappropriate (Table 2; Table 3). Clinical judgment will be required to balance the risks and benefits when a woman has multiple medical conditions.

The availability of safe, effective methods, including IUDs and implants, suggests that use of estrogen-containing methods should increasingly be used with caution in older women with cardiovascular (CV) risk factors. It also is important for perimenopausal women to be aware that use of oral contraceptive (OC) pills or any other hormone or IUD method does not reduce the risk of sexually transmitted infections. Accordingly, women at risk should protect themselves through use of safer sex practices. (See also "Sexually Transmitted Infections" in Chapter 6.)

Concomitant administration of St. John's wort and some enzyme-inducing drugs (including certain anticonvulsants and the antibiotic rifampicin) may reduce plasma progestin levels and thus the effectiveness of some HCs, including combined HCs, the progestin-only pill, the etonogestrel implant, and emergency contraception.[3] Switching to methods such as an IUD and depot medroxyprogesterone acetate (DMPA), for which efficacy is not affected by enzyme-inducing drugs, or using condoms for added protection are options for women taking medications that may impair the efficacy of an HC.

Intrauterine contraception

Intrauterine contraception offers perimenopausal women safe, highly effective, convenient, and long-term contraception.[5] The use of IUDs has increased in the United States from 5.6% in 2008 to 11.8% in 2014.[6] Intrauterine contraception may be a particularly desirable alternative for midlife women, including those considering surgical sterilization.

One IUD method government approved for 5 years' contraception in the United States and Canada is the 52-mg LNG-IUS. It remains highly effective for up to 7 years.[7] In the United States, there is a second 52-mg LNG-IUS available, FDA-approved for up to 5 years' use.[8] Irregular uterine bleeding and spotting are the most commonly reported adverse events (AEs). These nuisances subside as women develop either light cyclical menses or amenorrhea (19% of users become amenorrheic at 1 y, and 37% at 3 y).[9] A few women continue to have ongoing, unpredictable light uterine bleeding or spotting.

Use of the 52-mg LNG-IUS reduces menstrual blood loss.[10] The 52-mg LNG-IUS was approved in the United States and Canada in 2009 to treat heavy menstrual bleeding in women desiring to use IUDs. For perimenopausal women considering surgery to treat heavy menstrual bleeding, the high endometrial progestin levels associated with this device reduces blood loss as effectively as endometrial ablation, thereby allowing many women to avoid surgery.[11] This approach may not be effective for heavy endometrial bleeding in women with uterine fibroids with distortion or enlargement of the uterine cavity. Use of this IUS is as effective as gonadotropin-releasing hormone agonists in the off-label treatment of pain associated with endometriosis.[12] (See also "Abnormal Uterine Bleeding" in Chapter 5.)

A third, noncontraceptive use of the 52-mg LNG-IUS is to prevent bleeding and endometrial hyperplasia in postmenopausal women using estrogen therapy (ET), which is an off-label use in the United States and Canada.[13]

In 2013, a second, smaller 13.5-mg LNG-IUS received US and Canadian approval for up to 3 years' use and provides highly effective contraception. Because of its smaller dimensions, it can be an appropriate choice for nulliparous or other women with a smaller cervix or uterine cavity desiring IUDs.[14] Because of its lower dose of LNG, it has a lower rate of amenorrhea at 1 year (13%).[15] In 2016, a 19.5-mg LNG-IUS with the same dimensions

Table 1. US Medical Eligibility Criteria for Contraceptive Use Categories, Based on Age

Method	Age, y	Category
Estrogen-containing contraception	≥40	Benefits outweigh risks
POP	≥40	No restriction
Progestin implant	≥40	No restriction
DMPA	≥40 to 45	No restriction
	>45	Benefits outweigh risks
Cu-IUD	≥40	No restriction
LNG-IUS	≥40	No restriction

Abbreviations: Cu-IUD, copper intrauterine device; DMPA, depot medroxyprogesterone acetate; LNG-IUS, levonorgestrel intrauterine system; POP, progestin-only pill.
Curtis KM, et al.[4]

as the 13.5-mg device was approved in the United States and Canada for up to 5 years' use. The amenorrhea rate for the 19.5 mg LNG-IUS is 19% at 1 year.

Another IUD method available in the United States is the nonhormone copper T 380A IUD, which is approved for 10 years' contraception but remains highly effective for at least 12 years.[16] Canada has multiple approved copper IUDs, providing between 5 and 10 to 12 years' contraception, depending on the type. The principal AEs associated with use of the copper IUD are increased cramping and menstrual flow, especially in the first few months.[17] Accordingly, the copper IUD may not be an optimal choice for women who have problems with dysmenorrhea or heavy menstrual bleeding at baseline.

Placement of an IUD is an office-based procedure, but the insertion procedure is different for each type. The risk of uterine perforation is approximately 1 per 1,000 insertions, with a 6-fold increased risk in women who are breastfeeding.[18] Cumulative expulsion rates can be as high as 10% over 3 years' use.[19] Experienced clinicians have the lowest rate of uterine perforations.[18]

Progestin-only contraceptives
Progestin-only contraceptives can be used by most perimenopausal women for whom contraceptive doses of estrogen are contraindicated (Table 3).[4] Progestin-only contraceptives provide a safer alternative for cigarette smokers aged 35 years or older, women with hypertension (HTN; controlled and uncontrolled), and those with a history of venous thromboembolism (VTE). Contraindications include a history of hormone-dependent cancer (breast, endometrial).

Progestin-only contraceptives are available through several routes of delivery: IUD, subdermal implant,

injection, and OCs. These methods also offer noncontraceptive advantages such as decreased menstrual bleeding and decreased menstrual-related disorders (eg, menstrual migraines, dysmenorrhea) because of suppression of menses (less so with the progestin-only OC pill [sometimes called the mini-pill]). Although bleeding or spotting is commonly irregular, the amount and the days of bleeding are decreased overall.

Implant progestin-only contraceptives
An etonogestrel subdermal contraceptive implant (available in the United States only) consists of one toothpick-sized polymer capsule placed under the skin of the inner arm by a healthcare professional. It is approved for 3 years' use but offers highly effective contraception for up to 5 years.[20] The implant is radio-opaque in order to be located by X-ray and packaged in a preloaded inserter designed to facilitate superficial subdermal placement. Irregular bleeding, spotting, or amenorrhea commonly occurs throughout implant use.[21]

Injectable progestin-only contraceptives
Depot MPA provides highly effective contraception when the hormone is administered suspended in an injectable solution ("depot").[22] Intramuscular DMPA is available in the United States and Canada. The 150-mg dose is injected into either the buttock or upper arm every 3 months and does not need to be adjusted for body weight. Some call DMPA "the birth control shot." Although DMPA contraception is reversible, return of fertility after cessation of therapy could be delayed 12 to 18 months.[23] Some DMPA users report weight gain.

A DMPA version containing 31% less progestin (104 mg) is available in the United States but not in Canada.[24] The

Table 2. US Medical Eligibility Criteria for Contraceptive Use Categories for the Use of Estrogen-Containing Contraception, According to Condition

Condition	Category
Smoking age ≥35	
<15 cigarettes/d	Risks outweigh benefits
≥15 cigarettes/d	Unacceptable risk
Obesity	
BMI ≥30	Benefits outweigh risks
Hypertension	
Controlled hypertension	Risks outweigh benefits
Elevated BP	
Systolic >140-159 mm Hg or diastolic >90-99 mm Hg	Risks outweigh benefits
Systolic ≥160 mm Hg or diastolic ≥100 mm Hg	Unacceptable risk
Vascular disease	Unacceptable risk
DM	
No vascular disease	Benefits outweigh risks
Vascular disease or DM >20 years' duration	Either risks outweigh benefits or unacceptable risk (based on severity of condition)
Stroke	**Unacceptable risk**
Current or history of ischemic heart disease	Unacceptable risk
Multiple risk factors for CVD (older age, smoking, obesity, DM, hypertension)	**Either risks outweigh benefits or unacceptable risk (based on severity of condition)**

Abbreviations: BMI, body mass index; BP, blood pressure; CVD, cardiovascular disease; DM, diabetes mellitus.
Curtis KM, et al.[4]

dose is injected subcutaneously into the anterior thigh or abdomen every 3 months, using a smaller needle than for intramuscular administration, which may cause less pain. This subcutaneous DMPA formulation is also FDA approved for the treatment of endometriosis-related pain.

Initially, irregular bleeding or spotting is common with use of an injectable progestin-only contraceptive. After four or more injections, at least one-half of users will experience amenorrhea.[21] Use of injectable progestin suppresses ovarian estradiol production, which can reversibly lower bone mineral density (BMD).[25] Two case-control studies suggest that DMPA was associated with an increased risk of fracture.[26] However, a retrospective cohort study found that although DMPA users have a higher risk of fracture than nonusers, it might be because women who had an elevated fracture risk at baseline chose to use DMPA for contraception, a factor that was not controlled for in previous studies.[27]

Oral progestin-only contraceptives

A progestin-only OC formulated with norethindrone 0.35 mg provides effective contraception for perimenopausal women. This formulation needs to be taken at the same time every day for maximum efficacy, because after 24 hours, drug levels return to low levels.[3] There are no hormone-free (inactive) pills. Unscheduled bleeding is common and can be decreased by taking the pills at the same time every day. Amenorrhea is less common than with other progestin-only contraceptives.

Combination (estrogen-progestin) contraceptives

Combination contraceptives (containing estrogen and progestin) include many oral formulations and two nonoral contraceptives: the transdermal patch and the vaginal ring.

Labeling for all combination contraceptives in the United States and Canada includes a boxed warning that cigarette smoking increases the risk of serious CV AEs from HC use and that this risk increases with age and with heavy smoking (≥15 cigarettes/d). This risk is significant in women aged 35 years or older. Estrogen-containing contraceptives are generally contraindicated in women aged 35 years and older who smoke.[3]

Obesity is a relative contraindication for combination contraceptives in perimenopausal women. Combination contraceptives increase the risk of VTE, and although the incidence of VTE is very low in reproductive-aged women, the risk increases with age and BMI.[28,29] Guidance from the CDC suggests that the benefits of combination contraceptives outweigh risks in women aged 35 years and older who are obese.[4] Nevertheless, it may be prudent to prescribe a lower-dose formulation (with <30 μg ethinyl estradiol) for older women with a BMI greater than 30.[30]

Combination contraceptives are safe, effective birth-control options for midlife women who are healthy, lean, and do not smoke. Combination OCs also provide important noncontraceptive benefits for such women, including regulation of irregular uterine bleeding,

Table 3. US Medical Eligibility Criteria for Contraceptive Use Categories for the Use of Progestin-Only Methods of Contraception, According to Condition

Condition	POP	DMPA	Implant	LNG-IUS
Smoking age ≥35	No restriction	No restriction	No restriction	No restriction
Obesity	No restriction	No restriction	No restriction	No restriction
Hypertension				
Controlled hypertension	No restriction	Benefits outweigh risks	No restriction	No restriction
Elevated BP				
Systolic >140-159 mm Hg or diastolic >90-99 mm Hg	No restriction	Benefits outweigh risks	No restriction	No restriction
Systolic ≥160 mm Hg or diastolic ≥95 mm Hg	Benefits outweigh risks	Risks outweigh benefits	Benefits outweigh risks	Benefits outweigh risks
Vascular disease	Benefits outweigh risks	Risks outweigh benefits	Benefits outweigh risks	Benefits outweigh risks
DM				
No vascular disease	Benefits outweigh risks	Benefits outweigh risks	Benefits outweigh risks	Benefits outweigh risks
Vascular disease or DM >20 y duration	Benefits outweigh risks	Risks outweigh benefits	Benefits outweigh risks	Benefits outweigh risks
Stroke	I: Benefits outweigh risks C: Risks outweigh benefits	Risks outweigh benefits	I: Benefits outweigh risks C: Risks outweigh benefits	Benefits outweigh risks
Current or history of ischemic heart disease	I: Benefits outweigh risks C: Risks outweigh benefits	Risks outweigh benefits	I: Benefits outweigh risks C: Risks outweigh benefits	I: Benefits outweigh risks C: Risks outweigh benefits
Multiple risk factors for CVD (older age, smoking, obesity, diabetes, hypertension)	Benefits outweigh risks	Risks outweigh benefits	Benefits outweigh risks	Benefits outweigh risks

Abbreviations: BP, blood pressure; C, continuation; CVD, cardiovascular disease; DM, diabetes mellitus; DMPA, depot medroxyprogesterone acetate; I, initiation; LNG-IUS, levonorgestrel intrauterine system; POP, progestin-only pill.
Curtis KM, et al.[4]

reduction of vasomotor symptoms (VMS), decreased risk of ovarian and endometrial cancer, and maintenance of bone density (with a potential for decreased risk of postmenopausal osteoporotic fractures).[31] The incidence of CV events (VTE, myocardial infarction [MI], stroke) is rare in combination OC users who are appropriate candidates for combination contraceptives. Although some large studies suggest that long-term use does not affect the risk of breast cancer,[32] others suggest the possibility of a small elevation in risk.[33] When counseling midlife women regarding contraceptive options, the possibility that combination OCs might elevate the risk of breast cancer to a modest degree should be weighed against the well-established benefits of such contraceptives, including prevention of ovarian and endometrial cancer. These observations likely apply for nonoral combination contraceptives as well.

Oral combination contraceptives

Oral combination contraceptives are the most commonly used combination contraceptive, and dozens are available in North America. Many refer to an OC as "the pill."

Newer OC formulations use shorter or no hormone-free intervals. Several OC formulations are based on a 24/4 regimen (24 active pills followed by 4 inactive pills) rather than the traditional 21/7 cycle and contain ultralow doses.[34,35] These formulations may have a better bleeding profile despite their ultralow doses of ethinyl estradiol, although studies are lacking in perimenopausal women. In addition, with the shorter hormone-free interval of 4 days compared with 7 days, ovarian follicular activity is better suppressed.[36,37] This enhanced follicular suppression has the potential to lead to increased efficacy, as shown in one study.[38] Some perimenopausal women may note the occurrence of bothersome VMS or other symptoms during the hormone-free interval. Use of continuous hormonally active OC tablets or formulations with shorter or no hormone-free intervals often reduces such symptoms.

Drospirenone differs from other synthetic progestins in that it is derived from 17α-spironolactone. The ethinyl estradiol plus drospirenone OC has similar efficacy to other low-dose OCs, and one formulation is government approved for the treatment of symptoms of premenstrual dysphoric disorder.[39,40] Drospirenone has mild antimineralocorticoid effects, including the potential for hyperkalemia in high-risk patients.[41] The diuretic effect of drospirenone has not been found to cause sustained weight loss.

Because of conflicting data and interpretation, there has been controversy over the possibility that the risk of VTE in women using drospirenone-containing OCs may be higher than in women using OCs formulated with other progestins.[42] In 2013, FDA revised the label of drospirenone-containing products to say that there may be an increased risk of VTE and that some studies reported as high as a 3-fold increase in the risk of blood clots compared with products containing LNG or other progestins,[43] but some studies found no additional risk. A 2014 large prospective study (N >85,000) conducted in the United States and six European countries found that the risk of VTE associated with the 24/4 drospirenone OC formulation is similar to that of OCs formulated with other progestins.[44]

An OC containing estradiol valerate and dienogest has been government approved in the United States and Canada for contraception and treatment of heavy menstrual bleeding.[45] Before the availability of this formulation, the estrogen component of all low-dose OCs available in the United States had been ethinyl estradiol. Ethinyl estradiol is a potent synthetic estrogen with similar metabolic effects (eg, liver protein production)

regardless of the route of administration because of its long half-life and slow metabolism. In contrast, estradiol valerate is a synthetic hormone that is extensively metabolized to estradiol and valeric acid before reaching the systemic circulation.[46] Data from menopause use have shown that transdermally and vaginally administered estradiol is not associated with an increased production of liver proteins and therefore has a lower theoretical risk for thrombosis.[47] A daily dose of 2-mg estradiol valerate has biologic effects on the uterus, ovary, and hypothalamic-pituitary-ovarian axis similar to those of a 20-μg dose of ethinyl estradiol. Whether the estradiol valerate and dienogest OC will be safer than those formulated with ethinyl estradiol with respect to thromboembolism risk is unknown.

Use of extended OC formulations results in withdrawal bleeding less often than monthly. Evidence has consistently shown that these regimens are equivalent to traditional cyclic regimens in terms of contraceptive efficacy and safety, and patients on continuous regimens report fewer menstrual symptoms (eg, headaches, genital irritation, fatigue, bloating, withdrawal bleeding, and cramping).[48] Combination OCs packaged in extended regimens include 84 active tablets and seven inactive tablets. Scheduled withdrawal bleeding occurs every 3 months.

Unscheduled bleeding is common with the use of extended OC. In women using formulations with 84 tablets that contain estrogen and progestin, the addition of seven tablets with 10 μg of ethinyl estradiol at the time of the seven inactive tablets seems to reduce the occurrence of unscheduled bleeding.[49,50] Yet another strategy to reduce unscheduled bleeding persisting for more than 7 days in women using extended OC is to discontinue active tablets for 3 days. In women needing contraception, this strategy should only be employed after at least 21 days of continuous active tablets.[51] Use of continuous-combination OC does not cause weight gain or headaches.

Nonoral combination contraceptives

Government-approved nonoral combination contraceptives include a vaginal ring and a weekly patch, both approved to be used for 3 of 4 weeks. The ring releases ethinyl estradiol and etonogestrel, and the patch delivers ethinyl estradiol and norelgestromin.[52-54] Etonogestrel and norelgestromin are the biologically active metabolites of desogestrel and norgestimate, respectively, both of which are progestins used in commonly prescribed combination OCs. As with combination OCs, cyclic use of either the ring or patch results in monthly scheduled bleeding. Because these methods are longer acting, patient adherence (and therefore contraceptive efficacy) may be higher than with OCs. Although AEs and contraindications are in general similar to those for combination OCs, breast tenderness is more common with initial use of the patch, and increased physiologic vaginal discharge is more common with the ring.[55]

Studies indicate that women using the patch are exposed to about 60% more estrogen than with a typical OC containing 35 μg of ethinyl estradiol.[56] As a result, labeling for the patch contains a warning that its risk of VTE may be higher than with other combination contraceptives. One epidemiologic study found that VTE risk was similar to that of combination OCs, and another study found the risk was two times higher with the patch.[57] Because age is itself an independent risk factor for VTE, some experts believe that the ring and OCs are more appropriate choices for perimenopausal women than the patch.[58] The possibly elevated risk of VTE (compared with OC use) contrasts with low-dose estrogen HT formulations in which the transdermal route of estrogen administration may be associated with a lower risk of VTE compared with the oral route. Whereas the contraceptive patch releases a relatively high dose of ethinyl estradiol, transdermal estrogen formulations used in treating menopausal women release relatively low doses of estradiol.[59]

Emergency contraception

Emergency contraception refers to contraceptive measures that, if taken after sex, may prevent pregnancy. It may be appropriate after unprotected sexual intercourse, condom failure, an IUD partially or totally expelled, or if one or more OC active pills have been missed. Because other contraceptive methods are more reliable, it is meant only for occasional use, when primary means of contraception fail. This pill is often referred to as "the morning-after pill," but this phrase is figurative inasmuch as these products are licensed for use 72 to 120 hours after sexual intercourse. It is also important to remember that the most effective form of emergency contraception is the copper IUD, which is more than 99% effective when used as emergency contraception.[60] In this context, the copper IUD may inhibit fertilization and implantation and then can remain in place as long-acting reversible contraception.

Because emergency contraception methods act before fertilization, they are medically and legally considered forms of contraception according to the International Federation of Gynecology and Obstetrics and the US government.[61] These pills are not to be confused with "the abortion pill" (RU486 or mifepristone).

The progestin-only emergency contraception formulation, approved in the United States and in Canada, uses LNG as two 0.75-mg tablets taken 12 hours apart or as a single 1.5-mg dose. The government labeling states that this reduces the risk of pregnancy by 88%. In other words, if taken within 72 hours after coitus, seven of eight women who would have become pregnant will not.[62] Efficacy is increased if taken within the first 24 hours after coitus.[63] Persons of any age can now purchase this without a prescription in the United States. In Canada, it is available without a prescription, except in Quebec.

Ulipristal acetate (UPA), approved in the United States and Canada, is to be used as soon as possible and up to 5 days after unprotected sex. It is available by prescription only. Ulipristal is a progesterone receptor (PR) modulator. It is more effective than progestin-only emergency contraception when used within 24 hours or up to 5 days after unprotected sex. One meta-analysis showed that UPA almost halved the risk of pregnancy compared with LNG in women who received emergency contraception within 120 hours after sexual intercourse.[64] Furthermore, when emergency contraception was used within 24 hours of unprotected sex, the risk of pregnancy was reduced by almost two-thirds with UPA compared with LNG. In addition, UPA is more effective than LNG in women who are obese.[65]

Emergency contraception is not effective in women who are already pregnant. Inadvertent ingestion of emergency contraception during pregnancy, however, is not known to be harmful to the woman or her fetus.

Noncontraceptive benefits of hormone contraceptives

Perimenopause use of combined OCs for contraception has been associated with many noncontraceptive benefits (Table 4)[31]; these benefits may also apply to vaginal ring and transdermal estrogen-progestin contraceptives. Hormone contraceptives (including extended-use combination OCs, injectable progestin, and the LNG-IUS) are often used to reduce the frequency and amount of uterine bleeding or eliminate bleeding entirely. The use of OCs reduces risk of epithelial ovarian cancer in carriers of the BRCA mutation as well as in women at average risk for this malignancy.[66] Published reports are mixed with respect to

Table 4. Noncontraceptive Benefits of Combined Oral Contraceptives for Perimenopausal Women

- Restoration of regular menses
- Decreased dysmenorrhea
- Reduced heavy menstrual bleeding
- Reduced pain associated with endometriosis (continuous use of oral contraceptives)
- Suppression of VMS
- Enhanced BMD and possible prevention of osteoporotic fractures
- Decreased need for biopsies for benign breast disease
- Prevention of epithelial ovarian and endometrial malignancies
- Improvements in acne that may flare up with perimenopause

Abbreviations: BMD, bone mineral density; VMS, vasomotor symptoms.
Allen R, et al.[31]

whether use of OCs may elevate risk of breast cancer in *BRCA1* and *BRCA2* mutation carriers.[67] (See also "Breast Cancer" and "Ovarian Cancer" in Chapter 9.) Accordingly, mutation carriers will need to weigh the clear risk reduction for ovarian cancer associated with OC use against a possible increased risk of breast cancer.

Transitioning from hormone contraception to hormone therapy

For those women who choose to use HT, the challenge is determining when to make the transition from the use of HC to the lower-dose hormone formulations for menopause. Making the transition too soon may expose a perimenopausal woman to the risk of unintended pregnancy and result in irregular bleeding. However, once it can be assured that menopause has been reached, the transition to HT is advised so that hormone-related risks are minimized through use of lower-dose hormone formulations.

Historically, monitoring follicle-stimulating hormone levels (FSH) has been used to determine when menopause is reached. However, using FSH to determine when menopause has occurred in combination-contraceptive users may not be accurate.[3] The CDC, the American College of Obstetricians and Gynecologists, and The North American Menopause Society all recommend that HCs be used in a woman until she has reached an age at which she is statistically likely to be postmenopausal. In nonsmoking women, the median age of menopause is approximately 52 years—meaning that 50% of nonsmoking 52-year-old women have not reached menopause. About 90% of women will have reached menopause by

age 55. Therefore, clinicians may continue contraception for women who are appropriate candidates until they are in their mid-50s. With this approach, women who choose to transition from HC to HT can accomplish this without any hormone-free days. Women who have other means of contraception (tubal ligation or partner vasectomy) can discontinue contraceptive medication. Such women, along with their healthcare providers, can then determine whether they wish to initiate HT.

Estrogen Therapy and Estrogen-Progestogen Therapy

There is convincing clinical evidence that has documented the low absolute risks and favorable benefit-risk profile for prescription HT when used for symptomatic women in early menopause for relief of VMS (hot flashes, night sweats, and sleep disturbance) and for the prevention of bone loss in women at elevated risk of osteoporosis.[68] A variety of FDA-approved HT formulations are available that allows individualization of HT to maximize benefits and reduce risk. These include lower doses, different types, a nonprogestogen therapy for women with a uterus, and transdermal routes of delivery.

Estrogen

Terminology

The term *estrogen* describes a variety of related chemical compounds that have varying affinities for estrogen receptor (ER)-α and ER-β (not included here are estrogen agonists/antagonists, which also have affinity for these receptors).

Estrogen-containing drugs for menopause symptom use are divided into three categories: ET, combined estrogen-progestogen therapy (EPT), and ET combined with an estrogen agonist/antagonist.

Estrogen therapy is unopposed estrogen prescribed for postmenopausal women who have had a hysterectomy. Close surveillance is required if ET is prescribed for women with a uterus who are intolerant of progestogens because of estrogen stimulation of the endometrial lining.

Estrogen-progestogen therapy is a combination of estrogen and progestogen (either progesterone or progestin, synthetic forms of progesterone). Although the available data suggest that the benefits of EPT are almost exclusively because of the estrogen, progestogen reduces the risk of endometrial adenocarcinoma in women with a uterus, a risk that is significantly increased in women using unopposed estrogen.

Estrogen therapy combined with an estrogen antagonist/agonist is a progestogen-free combination for women with a uterus.

Hormone therapy encompasses ET, EPT, progestogen alone (usually taken with estrogen), and estrogen combined with an estrogen antagonist/agonist.

Previously, the terms *estrogen replacement therapy* and *hormone replacement therapy* were used. However, *replacement* is a misnomer because postmenopause estrogen levels are low in all women. That is the norm. It is not a deficiency state for which replacement is required. Women have high levels of estradiol and other hormones for a period of approximately 40 years for purposes of reproduction. Prepuberty and postmenopause levels are low, suggesting that those phases in a woman's life are not the optimal time for conception. Use of HT after menopause is considered therapeutic for menopause symptoms, not replacement for a deficiency state except in early or premature menopause.

Estrogen types

Estrogens can be divided into six main types:

Human estrogens. The estrogens produced in the human body are estrone, 17β-estradiol (often called estradiol), and estriol. Estradiol is the most biologically active, whereas estrone is 50% to 70% less active, and estriol, a weaker estrogen produced during pregnancy, is only 10% as active as estradiol. Estradiol, the principal estrogen secreted by the ovaries, is metabolized to estrone; estradiol and estrone can be metabolized to estriol. Exogenous estriol cannot be converted. Among the human estrogens, only 17β-estradiol is available in a government-approved, single-estrogen product.

Animal-derived estrogens. Nonhuman estrogens refer to conjugated equine estrogens (CEE), a mixture of at least 10 active estrogens obtained from natural sources (ie, the urine of pregnant mares), occurring as the sodium salts of water-soluble estrogen sulfates. Conjugated equine estrogens contain the sulfate esters of the ring B saturated estrogens—estrone (about 45%), 17β-estradiol, and 17α-estradiol—and the ring B unsaturated estrogens—equilin (about 25%), 17β-dihydroequilin, 17α-dihydroequilin, equilenin, 17β-dyhydroequilenin, 17α-dihydroequilenin,

and $\Delta^{8,9}$-estrone (ie, $\Delta^{8,9}$-dehydroestrone sulfate). The biologic effects of conjugated estrogens (CE) are a result of the sum of activities of these estrogens.

Synthetic estrogens. The two types of government-approved synthetic mixtures are esterified estrogens (which contain 75-85% sodium estrone sulfate) and synthetic CE. There are two designations of synthetic CE: synthetic CE-A (with a mixture of nine of the estrogens found in CE) and synthetic CE-B (including the estrogens found in synthetic CE-A plus $\Delta^{8,9}$-dehydroestrone sulfate—the 10 active estrogens found in CE).

Synthetic estrogen analogs with a steroid molecular structure. These compounds include ethinyl estradiol and estropipate (formerly called *piperazine estrone sulfate*).

Synthetic estrogen analogs without a steroid skeleton. These stilbesterol derivatives are not used for menopause-related therapy.

Plant-based estrogens without a steroid skeleton. Also known as *phytoestrogens*, plant-based estrogens can have weak estrogenic as well as antiestrogenic properties, depending on the target tissue. These are not prescription products.

Clinical pharmacology

Estrogen receptors are ubiquitous and present in almost all cells in the body. Thus, estrogens have an effect on most tissues. Estrogens are largely responsible for the development and maintenance of the female reproductive system and secondary sex characteristics. By direct action on ERs, they cause growth and development of the uterus, fallopian tubes, and vagina. Along with other hormones, such as pituitary hormones and progesterone, they cause enlargement of the breasts through promotion of ductal growth, stromal development, and the accretion of fat. Estrogens are intricately involved with other hormones, especially progesterone, in the processes of the ovulatory menstrual cycle and pregnancy and affect the release of pituitary gonadotropins. Estrogens stimulate bone growth during puberty and also close the bony epiphyses. They also contribute to the maintenance of tone and elasticity of urogenital structures and pigmentation of the nipples and genitals.

Circulating estrogens regulate the pituitary secretion of the gonadotropins, luteinizing hormone, and FSH through a negative-feedback mechanism. Estrogen therapy acts to reduce the elevated levels of these hormones in postmenopausal women.

Estrogens act by regulating the transcription of a number of genes. Estrogens readily diffuse through cell membranes, distribute themselves through the cell, and bind to ER-α or ER-β. This complex then interacts with chaperone proteins (ie, coregulators) to bind to the hormone response element and then initiate DNA transcription followed by protein synthesis and biologic effects.

The transcriptional responses to estrogen signaling depend on ligand identity and availability, the cellular concentration and localization of ERs, the presence of various coregulator proteins, and other signal transduction components. Estrogen receptor-α and ER-β exhibit distinct as well as overlapping functions at the level of DNA binding. In women, ERs have been identified in all tissues, including the reproductive tract, breast, brain, bone, and skin. Recently, nongenomic actions (those too rapid to be compatible with transcriptional activation and protein synthesis) of estrogen have been identified. There is strong evidence that the nongenomic estrogen activity is activated through membrane-associated ERs.

Estrogens occur naturally in several forms. The primary source of estrogen in normally cycling adult women is the ovarian follicle, which secretes 70 μg to 500 μg of estradiol daily, depending on the phase of the menstrual cycle. This is converted primarily to estrone, which circulates in roughly equal proportion to estradiol and to barely detectable amounts of estriol.

After menopause, most endogenous estrogen is produced by conversion of androstenedione (secreted by the adrenal cortex) to estrone by peripheral tissues through aromatase activity present in peripheral tissues. Thus, estrone and the sulfate conjugated form, estrone sulfate, are the most abundant circulating endogenous estrogens in postmenopausal women.

Although circulating estrogens exist in a dynamic equilibrium of metabolic interconversions, estradiol is the principal intracellular human estrogen and is substantially more potent than estrone or estriol at the receptor. Estriol is the major estrogen in pregnancy.

Estetrol is a natural estrogen synthesized exclusively during pregnancy by the human fetal liver and considered a very weak estrogen, with dose-dependent estrogenic effects on endocrine parameters, bone turnover markers, and lipids and lipoproteins.[69] Clinical studies have shown agonist effects on relief of menopause symptoms, bone, vagina, arteries, and uterus (both endometrium and myometrium). Estetrol appears to be highly tissue selective, with minimal effects on coagulation. However, it is an agonist in the uterus, and as such, needs to be combined with a progestogen to protect the uterus

if developed as HT. It is not FDA approved for use in the United States.

Pharmacokinetics

Estrogens used in oral ET are well absorbed from the gastrointestinal (GI) tract. Maximal plasma concentrations are attained 4 to 10 hours after oral administration. Estrogens are also well absorbed through the skin and mucous membranes. When applied transdermally or topically in higher doses (ie, 0.025-0.1 mg/d), absorption is usually sufficient to cause systemic effects. In contrast, low-dose ET (4-10 μg/d) administered locally in the vagina is associated with minimal systemic absorption.

Although naturally occurring estrogens circulate in the blood largely bound to sex hormone-binding globulin (SHBG) and albumin, only unbound estrogens enter target tissue cells. The half-life of the different estrogens in CE ranges from 10 to 25 hours; the half-life of estradiol is approximately 16 hours (oral) and 4 to 8 hours (transdermal). After removal of transdermal patches, serum estradiol levels decline in about 12 to 24 hours to preapplication levels.

Sex hormone-binding globulin binds DHEA with greater affinity than testosterone. Both androgens are more strongly bound than estradiol or estrone. Variations in SHBG concentration influence the ratio of bound to unbound steroids. Only free or unbound steroids bind to androgen receptors. Increasing SHBG leads to reduced available or free sex steroid levels, particularly free testosterone and free DHEA. Sex hormone-binding globulin is increased with oral estrogen, tamoxifen, and oral thyroxine. Conversely, oral testosterone, glucocorticosteroid therapy, a high-fructose diet, insulin resistance, and central visceral obesity lead to lower SHBG and an increase in free testosterone and dihydrotestosterone.[70]

Oral estrogen and combined oral-androgen therapy affect levels of endogenous sex hormones of testosterone, SHBG, DHEA, and androstenedione. Exogenous oral estrogen alone increases SHBG and decreases free testosterone. Combined oral estrogen-androgen treatment has the opposite effect, reducing SHBG levels but slightly increasing free testosterone. Findings across studies indicate that androgens are important for female sexual functioning.[69]

When orally administered, naturally occurring estrogens and their esters are rapidly metabolized in both the gut and the liver before reaching the general circulation through a metabolic process called the *first-pass effect*. This significantly decreases the amount of estrogen (primarily estrone sulfate) available for circulation.

In addition, the first pass through the liver affects other liver functions and is presumed to be one of the reasons various routes of administration affect lipid profiles differently. Synthetic estrogens (ie, ethinyl estradiol) are degraded very slowly in the liver and other tissues, which accounts for their high potency.

Systemic estrogens administered by nonoral routes are not subject to first-pass metabolism, but they do undergo significant hepatic uptake, metabolism, and enterohepatic recycling.

Timed-release transdermal and topical preparations cause less variability in blood levels than oral preparations at steady state and exhibit near zero-order pharmacokinetics. However, there may be substantial patient variability in blood levels because of differences in absorption. Transdermal and topical administrations produce therapeutic plasma levels of estradiol with lower circulating levels of estrone and estrone conjugates and require smaller total doses than oral therapy.

Marketed estrogens

Estrogens are available in many prescription preparations, including as single agents in oral preparations; transdermal patch, gel, or topical emulsion preparations; vaginal preparations; combination (EPT) preparations; and CE combined with bazedoxifene (BZA). Clinicians should refer to product labeling before prescribing.

All government-approved estrogen-containing products that achieve systemic levels at recommended doses in the United States and in Canada are approved for the treatment of moderate to severe VMS. All approved local vaginal ETs are used in treating moderate to severe vaginal dryness and symptoms of GSM, although their labels may say that they are for treatment of atrophic vaginitis because of menopause or for relief of moderate to severe dyspareunia, a symptom of GSM. Vaginal products—CE (Premarin) and estradiol (Estrace) vaginal cream; 10-µg vaginal estradiol tablets (Vagifem, Yuvafem); a 3-month vaginal estradiol ring (Estring); and a vaginal estradiol insert (Imvexxy)—are often used to treat pain with intercourse because of GSM. One product (Estring) is also indicated for urinary urgency and dysuria. Only one vaginal product, Femring, delivers systemic doses and thus also is approved for VMS. Femring should be used with a concomitant progestin for endometrial protection.

When prescribing solely to treat GSM, vaginal preparations should be considered. (See also "Genitourinary Syndrome of Menopause" in Chapter 4.) One oral estrogen, Enjuvia, is approved for the treatment of pain with intercourse.

Some estrogen-containing systemic products have government approval for the prevention of postmenopausal osteoporosis, based primarily on studies demonstrating preservation of BMD. Not all marketers of estrogen-containing products have funded the large, long-term trials necessary to prove efficacy. Some estrogen-containing products had been approved for the treatment of postmenopausal osteoporosis, but this indication was withdrawn from all such products by the government because the required fracture trials of women with documented osteoporosis had not been conducted.

Conjugated estrogens. Most clinical studies have used CEE. As a result, more is known about their efficacy and safety than any other estrogen product. Although Premarin has been on the US market for more than 65 years, no generic equivalent has been approved. The standard CEE oral dose has been 0.625 mg daily, based on bone protection studies. Studies have shown that many women receive substantial benefit from lower doses (0.45 or 0.3 mg/d), although some women require higher doses (0.9 mg, 1.25 mg) for symptom relief or osteoporosis prevention.[71]

In a 10.7-year follow-up study of surviving participants after completion of the Women's Health Initiative (WHI) Estrogen-Alone trial, a decreased risk of breast cancer was seen in CE users compared with placebo, with health benefits in general seen in younger women,[72] but findings from a 13-year follow-up and an 18-year follow-up from the WHI do not support the use of ET for chronic disease prevention.[73,74]

Conjugated equine estrogens are available combined with synthetic MPA. Major brand names of CEE in combination with MPA include continuous-combined Prempro and cyclic Premphase in the United States; Premplus in Canada.

Synthetic conjugated estrogens. Two types of synthetic CE mixtures are available as oral tablets—synthetic CE-A (with 9 estrogens) and synthetic CE-B (with 10 estrogens). The synthetic CE-A available in the United States is Cenestin (Congest, C.E.S., and PMS-Conjugated in Canada). The synthetic CE-B is Enjuvia, available in the United States but not in Canada. The government does not view Cenestin or Enjuvia as generic equivalents to Premarin, although Enjuvia contains the primary 10 estrogens included in Premarin. Both are available in multiple doses, including 0.3-mg, 0.45-mg, 0.625-mg, 0.9-mg, and 1.25-mg strengths. In Canada, C.E.S. has been approved as a generic equivalent to Premarin since 1963, although at least one study shows that it is not bioequivalent.[75]

No synthetic CE product is government approved for osteoporosis.

Estradiol. Initially, 17β-estradiol (or simply *estradiol*) could be administered only by injection because it was not absorbed from the GI tract. After micronization was developed, oral products (Estrace, Gynodiol, Innofem) were marketed; various oral generics are also available. Doses include 0.5 mg, 1 mg, or 2 mg of micronized estradiol (ME) per tablet. Subsequently, transdermal estradiol delivery systems were developed in which estradiol is impregnated into the adhesive. There are also transdermal estradiol alcohol-based gels (Divigel, Estrogel, Elestrin), a transdermal spray (Evamist), and a topical emulsion of estradiol hemihydrate (Estrasorb) available as options.

Vaginal forms of estradiol (Estrace vaginal cream, Estring vaginal ring) are available, as well as the estradiol acetate vaginal ring (Femring) that exerts systemic effects and estradiol hemihydrate vaginal tablets (Vagifem, Yuvafem) and estradiol inserts (Imvexxy) that exert local effects. Oral estradiol valerate is widely used in Europe, but it is available in the United States only in an injectable formulation not used for HT. Estradiol also is used in EPT products. Estradiol is the most widely used estrogen in Europe. It is the one estrogen available commercially in government-approved formulations that can be considered bioidentical.

Numerous studies have used lower doses of oral and transdermal estradiol for the treatment of VMS and for the prevention of bone loss. Ultralow-dose 0.25 mg oral micronized 17β-estradiol and 0.014 mg transdermal 17β-estradiol per day also have significantly increased spine and hip BMD compared with placebo.[76,77]

Ultralow-dose 0.014 mg per day transdermal 17β-estradiol, a product approved for prevention of osteoporosis, has been shown to be significantly more effective than placebo in reducing the frequency and severity of moderate and severe hot flashes, demonstrating that lower doses than were used in the past may be effective for many women.[78]

Esterified estrogens. Esterified estrogens (Menest in the United States; Neo-Estrone in Canada) are oral products of synthetic estrogen mixtures containing 75% to 85% sodium estrone sulfate. They are not indicated for osteoporosis.

Estropipate. Formerly called *piperazine estrone sulfate*, this is an oral form of estrone sulfate that has been solubilized and stabilized by piperazine. It is marketed as Ogen in the United States and as Ortho-Est in Canada, as well as in generic formulations. Ogen is approved for the prevention of postmenopausal osteoporosis.

Ethinyl estradiol. This synthetic steroid is widely used in combination contraceptives. It is also available in one oral estrogen-progestogen product (Femhrt in the United States; femHRT in Canada).

Dose equivalencies

Measuring estrogen potency presents a challenge because estrogens vary in their dose equivalency and in their effects on various target tissues (Table 5). Oral ME 1.0 mg is equivalent to CE 0.625 mg with respect to effects on liver function; whereas oral micronized estradiol 0.5 mg produces changes in bone density equivalent to CE 0.625 mg.

Very few head-to-head trials have compared different estrogens. Clinicians tend to view estrogen products as equivalent on a dose-for-dose basis, although data do not support this assumption; metabolic pathways and AEs can vary in general and from woman to woman. As for most medications, type, dose, formulation, and route of administration of HT must always be tailored to provide symptom relief for the individual woman.

Routes of administration

Estrogen can be administered orally, transdermally, topically, or vaginally. Intramuscular preparations are not recommended for HT because serum estrogen levels associated with injections rise to very high levels after administration and may increase risk for deep vein thrombosis.

Oral. Oral ET remains the most widely used formulation in North America (Table 6). With all oral estrogen products, estrone will be the predominant estrogen in the circulation because of the first-pass uptake and metabolism in the GI tract and the liver.

The hepatic effect with oral ET results in greater stimulation of certain proteins compared with transdermal therapy, including lipoproteins such as high-density lipoprotein cholesterol (HDL-C). Oral estrogen also is associated with about a 25% increase in triglycerides (TG), increasing the risk of pancreatitis in women who already have hypertriglyceridemia. Oral ET stimulates hepatic globulins, coagulation factors, and some inflammatory markers such as C-reactive protein and matrix metallopeptidase 9, with implications for coronary heart disease (CHD).[79,80] There also may be differences in glucose-insulin metabolism, but these data are less clear cut. Other

Table 5.	Approximate Equivalent Estrogen Doses for Postmenopause Use	
Oral		
CE	0.625 mg	
SCE	0.625 mg	
Esterified estrogens	0.625 mg	
Estropipate (0.75 mg)	0.625 mg	
Ethinyl estradiol	0.005-0.015 mg	
17β-estradiol	1.0 mg	
Transdermal/Topical		
Estradiol patch	0.05 mg	
Estradiol gel	1.5 mg/2 metered doses Divigel 0.1 mg/day	
Vaginal		
CE	0.3125 mg	
17β-estradiol	0.5 mg	

Abbreviations: CE, conjugated estrogens; SCE, synthetic conjugated estrogens.

important inflammatory markers such as E-selectin decrease with both modes of administration.

Transdermal/Topical. Estrogen delivered transdermally or topically can be prescribed in lower doses than oral administration because they are not dependent on GI absorption or subjected to first-pass hepatic metabolism. There is variation in absorption in transdermal and topical estrogens, depending on how the patches or gels are applied and the carrier vehicle (Table 7).

In contrast to oral ET, transdermal and topical administration of estrogen have the advantage of not increasing TG but the disadvantage of not increasing HDL-C. Because of less liver exposure, transdermal and topical ET may have less of an effect on gallbladder disease and coagulation factors.

Transdermal-patch ET is associated with relatively stable serum levels, unlike fluctuating serum levels found with oral estrogen. Thus, when stable estrogen levels are required, transdermal ET is a better choice than oral ET. Transdermal estrogen has minimal effects on SHBG and thus less negative effect on sexual functioning.[70] Transdermal estrogen may be the clinical choice because the controlled-release methods of administration may result in fewer migraines, for example.

Estraderm was the first transdermal patch approved for use in the United States and Canada; it administered estradiol from a reservoir patch. Other transdermal patches are available, each delivering estradiol from a matrix patch. Patch adhesives differ in product formulation. In addition, a transdermal gel, transdermal spray, and topical emulsion are available. The spray, gel, and emulsion formulations have the advantage over patches in that they are less likely to cause skin irritation, but the gel and emulsion products have the disadvantage that skin-to-skin contact within 2 hours after application can lead to person-to-person transfer of small amounts of estradiol. Also, sunscreen application shortly before applying transdermal and topical products may substantially increase estradiol exposure. When sunscreen is applied before the spray, there is no significant change in estradiol absorption or exposure. Use of sunscreen on the same area after application of transdermal estradiol has both increased and decreased estradiol absorption.

The multicenter, case-control Estrogen and Thromboembolism Risk trial suggested that oral ET but not transdermal ET is associated with an increase of VTE.[81] In a very large, population-based study, participants receiving an estradiol transdermal system had a significantly lower incidence of VTE than participants receiving oral ET.[82] Oral HT but not low-dose transdermal HT increased the risk of stroke in one nested case-control observational study.[83]

The 4-year, multicenter, Kronos Early Estrogen Prevention Study of 727 healthy women within 3 years of menopause is the first and only randomized, controlled trial (RCT) that compared the differential effects of oral versus transdermal estrogen on various health outcomes. Stroke and VTE events were comparable across oral, transdermal, and placebo groups.

Vaginal. There are several different ways to deliver estrogen vaginally—creams, rings, tablets, and inserts (Table 8). Vaginal estrogen cream has been available for decades; the tablet, ring, and insert products are newer. Small amounts of estrogen administered locally are effective for treating vaginal atrophy. Labeling for vaginal estrogen products often includes the same warnings, contraindications, and AEs as labeling for systemic estrogen products, despite the fact that low-dose vaginal ET does not typically result in significant systemic estrogen levels.[84]

Except for the estradiol acetate vaginal ring (Femring), vaginal estrogens are not used for systemic effects (eg, hot flashes). In general, estradiol levels vary according to the dose of the product but are all in the postmenopause range. Some women may report breast tenderness when initiating therapy, suggesting that low levels of systemic

Table 6. Oral Estrogen Therapy Products for Postmenopause Use in the United States and Canada

Composition	Product name	Dosages, mg/d
Conjugated estrogen	Premarin	0.3, 0.45,[a] 0.625, 0.9,[a] 1.25
Synthetic conjugated estrogen[a]	Cenestin[a]	0.3. 0.45, 0.625, 0.9, 1.25
	Congest[b]	0.3, 0.625, 0.9, 1.25, 2.5
	C.E.S.[b]	0.3, 0.625, 0.9, 1.25
	PMS-Conjugated[b]	0.3, 0.625, 0.9, 1.25
Synthetic conjugated estrogen[b]	Enjuvia[a]	0.3, 0.45, 0.625, 0.9, 1.25
Esterified estrogen	Menest[a]	0.3, 0.625, 1.25, 2.5
17β-estradiol	Estrace, various generics Gynodiol, Innofem	0.5, 1.0, 2.0
Estradiol acetate	Femtrace[a]	0.45, 0.9, 1.8
Estropipate	Ortho-Est[a]	0.625 (0.75 estropipate), 1.25 (1.5), 2.5 (3.0), 5.0 (6.0)
	Ogen	0.625 (0.75), 1.25 (1.5), 2.5 (3.0)
	Various generics	0.625 (0.75), 1.5 (3.0), 5.0 (6.0)

Estradiol-containing products are considered bioidentical.
Products not noted are available in the United States and in Canada.
[a]Available in the United States but not Canada.
[b]Available in Canada but not the United States.

absorption and adjustments in dose may be needed. No significant differences in AEs were reported among the different methods of vaginal delivery.

Adding a progestogen to low-dose vaginal ET is not typically recommended, based on 1-year endometrial safety data.[85] However, a progestogen is recommended with Femring or higher doses of other vaginal ET because of systemic effects leading to an increased risk of endometrial cancer if estrogen is used unopposed.

A woman's individual needs and preferences should be the primary factors in determining the estrogen delivery route. In some women, medical factors may be the determinant (eg, vaginal administration to treat GSM or transdermal administration for women with hypertriglyceridemia). Other factors include cost and insurance coverage.

Estrogen had been the only pharmacologic therapy government approved in the United States and in Canada for treating menopause symptoms until 2013, when FDA approved paroxetine 7.5 mg.[86,87] (See also "Treatment" in Chapter 3.)

Progestogen

Progestogen therapy can be an option to treat hot flashes and other conditions of women at menopause and beyond, but its primary use in menopause treatment is to reduce the risk of endometrial cancer associated with unopposed estrogen. (See also "Endometrial Cancer" in Chapter 7.)

Terminology

The term *progestogen* includes progesterone and the synthetic progestational compounds termed *progestins*, a wide range of hormones with the properties of the naturally occurring progesterone.

Progesterone. Progesterone is the steroid hormone produced by the ovary after ovulation and by the placenta during pregnancy. Exogenous progesterone is a compound identical to endogenous progesterone. Advances have allowed progesterone crystals to be micronized, resulting in improved oral absorption. Prometrium and its generic are the only FDA-approved bioidentical progestogens. Before micronization, the rapid inactivation and poor bioavailability of orally administered progesterone led to the development in the 1950s of progestins.

Progestin. Progestins are synthetic products that have progesterone-like activity but are not identical to the progesterone produced in the human body. Progestins can be classified as those more closely resembling in chemical structure of either progesterone or testosterone (also called

19-nortestosterone derivatives). In general, these progestins have a 10- to 100-fold greater progestational activity than natural progesterone.

Progestins structurally related to progesterone are further classified into two groups:

1. *Pregnane derivatives* (acetylated): MPA, megestrol acetate, cyproterone acetate, and chlormadinone acetate; and pregnane derivatives (nonacetylated) dydrogesterone and medrogestone.

2. *9-norpregnane derivatives* (acetylated): nomegestrol and nestorone; and 9-norpregnane derivatives (nonacetylated): demegestone, trimegestone, and promegestone.

Progestins structurally related to testosterone are further classified into two groups:

1. *Ethinylated*, which include estranges, norethindrone (also called norethisterone), norethindrone acetate, norethynodrel, lynestrenol, and ethynodiol diacetate, and 18-ethylgonanes LNG, norgestrel, desogestrel, gestodene, and norgestimate.

2. *Nonethinylated* dienogest and drospirenone.

Mode of action

In humans, two PR proteins, PR-A and PR-B, have been identified. Whether the available progestogen therapies preferentially bind to PR-A or PR-B is unclear. The primary actions of progestogens have been characterized in most detail in the uterus. In this target tissue, progestogens function primarily as antiestrogens, decreasing the number of nuclear ERs, most likely through downregulation of ERs. In the endometrium, progestogens increase the activity of 17β-hydroxysteroid dehydrogenase, resulting in conversion of estradiol to estrone, a biologically weaker estrogen. These changes result in less estrogen-induced endometrial stimulation.

Table 7. Transdermal Estrogen Therapy Products for Postmenopause Use in the United States and Canada

Composition	Product name	Dosage, mg
17β-estradiol matrix patch	Alora[a]	0.025, 0.05, 0.075, 0.1 twice/wk
	Climar[a]	0.025, 0.0375,[a] 0.05, 0.075, 0.1 once/wk
	Esclim[a]	0.025, 0.0375, 0.05, 0.075, 0.1 twice/wk
	Estradot[b]	0.025, 0.0375, 0.05, 0.075, 0.1 twice/wk
	Fempatch	0.025 once/wk
	Menostar[a]	0.014 once/wk
	Minivelle	0.025, 0.0375, 0.05, 0.075, 0.1 twice/wk
	Oesclim[b]	0.05, 0.1 twice/wk
	Vivelle[a]	0.025, 0.0375, 0.05, 0.075, 0.1 twice/wk
	Vivelle-Dot[a]	0.025, 0.0375, 0.05, 0.075, 0.1 twice/wk
	Various generics	0.1, 0.05 once or twice/wk
17β-estradiol reservoir patch	Estraderm	0.025,[b] 0.05,[a] 0.1 twice/wk
17β-estradiol transdermal gel	EstroGel,[a] Estrogel[b]	0.035/d
	Elestrin[a]	0.0125/d
	Divigel[a]	0.25, 0.5, and 1.0 g/d
17β-estradiol topical emulsion	Estrasorb[a]	0.05/d (2 packets)
17β-estradiol topical emulsion (estradiol hemihydrate 2.5 mg/g)		
17β-estradiol transdermal spray	Evamist[a]	0.021/90 μL/d (increase to 1.5/90 μL/d if needed)

Estradiol-containing products are considered bioidentical.
Products not noted are available in the United States and in Canada.
[a]Available in the United States but not Canada.
[b]Available in Canada but not the United States.

Table 8. Vaginal Estrogen Therapy Products for Postmenopause Use in the United States and Canada

Composition	Product name	Dosage
Vaginal creams		
17β-estradiol[a]	Estrace Vaginal Cream[b]	Initial: 2-4 g/d for 1-2 wk. Maintenance: 1 g 1-3x/wk. (0.1 mg active ingredient/g)
		Clinical use :1 g daily for 1-2 wk. Maintenance: 0.5-1 g 1-3 x /wk.
Conjugated estrogens[a]	Premarin Vaginal Cream	For GSM: 0.5-2 g/d for 21 d, then off 7 d. For dyspareunia: 0.5 g/d for 21 d, then off 7 d, or twice/wk (0.625 mg active ingredient/g)
		Clinical use: 0.5 g/d for 2 wk, then 0.5 g/d 2-3 x/wk.
Esterone	Estragyn Vaginal Cream[c]	2-4 g/d (1 mg active ingredient/g)
Vaginal rings		
17β-estradiol	Estring	Device containing 2 mg releases 7.5 µg/d for 90 d (for GSM).
Estradiol acetate	Femring[b]	Device containing 12.4 mg or 24.8 mg estradiol acetate releases 0.05 mg/d or 0.10 mg/d estradiol for 90 days. Both doses release systemic levels for treatment of GSM and VMS. (Progestogen recommended.)
Vaginal tablet/insert		
Estradiol	Imvexxy	4 µg and 10 µg
		Initial: 1 insert/d for 2 wk Maintenance: 1 tablet 2x/wk
Estradiol hemihydrate	Vagifem	Initial: 1 tablet/d for 2 wk. Maintenance: 1 tablet 2 x/wk
	Vagifem generic	(tablet containing 10 µg of estradiol hemihydrate, equivalent to 10 µg estradiol; for GSM)

Estradiol-containing products are considered bioidentical.
Products not noted are available in the United States and in Canada.
Abbreviations: GSM, genitourinary syndrome of menopause; VMS, vasomotor symptoms.
[a]Higher doses of vaginal estrogen are systemic and meant to relieve hot flashes as well as GSM; lower doses are intended for vaginal symptoms only, even though a small amount does get absorbed.
[b]Available in the United States but not Canada.
[c]Available in Canada but not the United States.

Marketed progestogens

A wide variety of progestogen types, modes of administration, and dosage regimens are available, each having distinct AEs as well as different actions on the endometrium and other organ systems (Table 9). Very few clinical trials have evaluated the relative potencies of progestogens.

The progestogen product most structurally related to progesterone is micronized progesterone (MP), available in an oral form as Prometrium or its generic. Generally speaking, progestins structurally related to testosterone are more potent than those related to progesterone and MPA.

The most commonly used progestogen formulation for endometrial protection in US women has been the oral progestin MPA, either alone or in combination with CE. It is also the most widely studied progestogen for postmenopause use. Other progestins are combined with other estrogens in several oral and transdermal EPT products. Low doses of transdermal progestogens (ie, norethindrone) should have metabolic advantages over higher doses of oral therapy because they avoid the first-pass hepatic effect; however, data on this are limited.

Anecdotal data and results from the Postmenopausal Estrogen/Progestin Interventions (PEPI) trial suggest that women who experience AEs, especially mood changes, with a synthetic progestin sometimes respond more favorably to progesterone.[88] Before the late 1990s, North

American women seeking progesterone products had to rely on custom-compounded formulations. Prometrium, an oral capsule containing MP, was first approved in Canada, then in the United States. Prometrium or its generic should never be used by a woman allergic to peanuts because the active ingredient is suspended in peanut oil. In addition, a small percentage of women may experience extreme dizziness or drowsiness during initial therapy, so women should use caution when driving or operating machinery.

Oral progesterone has mildly sedating effects, reducing wakefulness without affecting daytime cognitive functions, possibly through a γ-aminobutyric acid-agonistic effect,[89] and thus bedtime dosing is advised.[90] Micronized progesterone 300 mg nightly significantly decreases VMS compared with placebo and improves sleep.[91] Synthetic progestins have also shown benefit in studies. No long-term study results are available.

Micronized progesterone formulations (cream, lotion, gel, oral capsule, suppositories) are available by prescription through custom-compounding pharmacies.

Topical cream or gel preparations with progesterone, obtained either OTC or custom compounded from a prescription, will not exert sufficient activity to protect the endometrium from unopposed estrogen. There are insufficient progesterone levels to induce the secretory changes in the endometrium. Thus, these products should not be used for this purpose until optimum therapeutic doses for the various formulations are established.

Because vaginal administration at typical doses avoids systemic effects, vaginal progestogen is an attractive option. The vaginal bioadhesive gel containing 4% or 8% MP provides sustained and controlled delivery of progesterone to the vaginal tissue. In a trial using cyclic administration of the gel in women with secondary amenorrhea, no

Table 9. Progestogens Available in the United States and Canada

Composition	Product name	Dosage/d
Oral tablet: progestin		
MPA	Provera, various generics	2.5 mg, 5 mg, 10 mg
Norethindrone	Micronor,[a] Nor-QD,[a,b] various generics	0.35 mg
NETA	Aygestin,[a,b] various generics	5 mg
Megestrol acetate	Megace,[a] various generics	20 mg,[b] 40 mg, 40-mg suspension
Oral capsule: progesterone		
Micronized progesterone (in peanut oil)	Prometrium, generic	100 mg, 200 mg[b]
Intrauterine system: progestin		
Levonorgestrel	Mirena[a]	20 µg/d approx release rate (52 mg has 5-y use)
	Skyla	6 µg /d release rate (13.5 mg has 3-y use)
		Liletta: 19.5 µg /d release rate; 17 µg /d at 1 y (52 mg has 5-y use)
		Kyleena: 17.5 µg/d release rate (19.5 µg has 5-y use)
Vaginal gel		
Progesterone	Crinone[a] 4%,[b] 8%	45- or 90-mg applicator
Vaginal tablet		
Progesterone	Endometrin[a]	100 mg

Progesterone-containing products are considered bioidentical.
Abbreviations: MPA, medroxyprogesterone acetate; NETA, norethindrone acetate.
[a]Not approved by FDA for hormone therapy.
[b]Available in the United States but not Canada.

hyperplasia was observed after 3 months.[92] A 100-mg progesterone vaginal insert (Endometrin) has been approved for luteal phase support for assisted reproductive technology but not for EPT, although some practitioners use it off-label for vaginal progestogen.

The use of a progestin-releasing IUS to protect the endometrium is appealing because it delivers the progestin in the highest concentration precisely where it is needed. Mirena, an LNG-IUS available in the United States and Canada, is not approved for endometrial protection, although there are small studies suggesting that it is effective and effectiveness shown with regression of endometrial hyperplasia.[93] There is some systemic absorption of LNG with Mirena. Its relatively low dose (20 µg/d) and 5-year life span make it an attractive alternative for perimenopausal women. The 3-year Skyla is lower dose (6 µg/d), smaller and might be easier to insert for a postmenopause uterus, but there are no data on its endometrial protection. Two other progestin IUS include Liletta (19.5 µg/d release rate), with 5-year use, and Kyleena with a 17.5 µg per day release rate and 5-year use.

Estrogen-progestogen therapy

All government-approved progestogen formulations will provide endometrial protection if the dose and duration are adequate. Combined estrogen-progestogen products are available. Although these are convenient, and many women prefer to take one pill or use one patch, they do reduce dosing flexibility. All combined estrogen-progestogen products in the United States and in Canada are government approved for postmenopause use (Table 10).

Many regimens are used when prescribing EPT, and descriptive terminology is often inconsistent. The clinical goal of an EPT regimen is to provide uterine protection, maintain estrogen benefits, and minimize AEs (particularly uterine bleeding, which is annoying to many women and often reduces compliance), although there is no consensus on how to accomplish this goal. (See also "Abnormal Uterine Bleeding" in Chapter 5.) Regimens may be classified as continuous-cyclic sequential, continuous cyclic long-cycle, continuous-combined, and intermittent-combined (Table 11).

Continuous-cyclic (sequential) estrogen-progestogen therapy

In this regimen, estrogen is used every day with progestogen added cyclically for 12 to 14 days during each month. The combination oral EPT product Premphase uses a sequential regimen of estrogen for 14 days followed by estrogen and progestin for 14 days, similar to oral contraceptives dose packs. In a typical continuous-cyclic regimen, progestogen is started on the first or fifteenth day of the month. Starting on the first day of the month makes it easier for some women to track their uterine bleeding because the cycle day corresponds with the day of the month. (See also "Abnormal Uterine Bleeding" in Chapter 5.)

If women are on standard doses of estrogen (CE 0.625 mg/d or ME 1 mg/d), uterine bleeding occurs in about 80% of women when the progestogen is withdrawn, although it sometimes starts 1 or 2 days earlier, depending on the dose and type of progestogen used.

Continuous-cyclic (sequential) long-cycle estrogen-progestogen therapy

To lessen the exposure to progestogen and the incidence of uterine bleeding, modified continuous-cyclic EPT regimen of daily estrogen with cyclic progestogen given at longer intervals has been suggested. Although this regimen reduces the number of withdrawal bleeding episodes, it has resulted in heavier and longer bleeding episodes. The effect on endometrial protection is undetermined. (See also "Abnormal Uterine Bleeding" in Chapter 5.)

Two studies did not find evidence of endometrial hyperplasia after 1 year in women using estrogen at standard doses (CE 0.625 mg/d) or one-half standard doses (CE 0.3 mg/d), with MPA administered either quarterly or every 6 months.[94,95] However, the Scandinavian Long Cycle Study, which used 2 mg per day of 17β-estradiol (twice the standard dose) with a progestin administered quarterly, was stopped after 3 of 5 scheduled years because of an increased incidence of hyperplasia compared with a monthly progestogen regimen.[96]

Two-hundred eighteen women in the Estrogen in the Prevention of Atherosclerosis Trial or the Women's Estrogen-Progestin Lipid-Lowering Hormone Atherosclerosis Regression Trial randomly assigned to either 1 mg of micronized 17 beta-estradiol (n=96) or placebo (n=122) up to 3 years found that nine (9.4%) patients (95% confidence interval [CI], 3.6%-15.2%) in the estradiol group developed hyperplasia, of which eight were simple without atypia.[97] However, those on estradiol alone compared with placebo over 3 years of follow-up were more likely to have uterine bleeding (67% vs 11% at 3 y, respectively; $P<.001$) and an endometrial biopsy (48% vs 4% at 3 y; $P<.001$). Those with a body mass index greater than 30 kg/m² had a significantly higher risk of bleeding than those with a body mass index of 25 kg/m² or less (odds ratio, 3.7; 95% CI, 1.2-11.8). Thus, even with lower doses, by 3 years a higher risk of hyperplasia and bleeding was seen with 1 mg of estradiol.

Table 10. Combination Estrogen-Progestogen Therapy Products for Postmenopause Use in the United States and Canada

Composition	Product name	Dosage, mg/d
Oral continuous-cyclic regimen		
CE (E) + MPA (P)	Premphase[a]	0.625 mg E + 5.0 mg P (2 tablets: E and E + P) (E alone for days 1-14, followed by E + P on days 15-28)
Oral continuous-combined regimen		
17 β-estradiol (E) + progesterone	Bijuva	1 mg E + 100 mg P
CE (E) + MPA (P)	Prempro[a]	0.625 mg E + 2.5 or 5.0 mg P (1 tablet); 0.3 or 0.45 mg E + 1.5 mg P (1 tablet)
Ethinyl estradiol (E) + NETA (P)	Femhrt,[a] femHRT[b]	2.5 µg E + 0.5 mg P (1 tablet); 5 µg E + 1 mg P (1 tablet)
17β-estradiol (E) + NETA (P)	Activella[a]	0.5 mg E + 0.1 mg P (1 tablet); 1 mg E + 0.5 mg P (1 tablet)
	Activelle LD[b]	0.5 mg E + 0.1 mg P (1 tablet)
	Activelle[b]	1 mg E + 0.5 mg P (1 tablet)
17β-estradiol (E) + drospirenone (P)	Angeliq	0.5 mg E + 0.25 mg P (1 tablet)[a]; 1 mg E + 0.5 mg P (1 tablet)[b]
Oral intermittent-combined regimen		
17β-estradiol (E) + norgestimate (P)	Prefest[a]	1 mg E + 0.09 mg P (2 tablets: E and E + P) (E alone for 3 d, followed by E+P for 3 d, repeated continuously)
Transdermal continuous-combined regimen		
17β-estradiol (E) + NETA (P)	CombiPatch,[a] Estalis[b]	0.05 mg E + 0.14 mg P (9 cm2 patch, twice/wk); 0.05 mg E + 0.25 mg P (16 cm^2 patch, twice/wk)
17β-estradiol (E) + LNG (P)	Climara Pro	0.045 mg E + 0.015 mg P (22 cm^2 patch, once/wk)

Products not noted are available in the United States and in Canada.
Abbreviations: CE, conjugated estrogens; LNG, levonorgestrel; MPA, medroxyprogesterone acetate; NETA, norethindrone acetate.
[a]Available in the United States but not Canada.
[b]Available in Canada but not the United States.

Until more data are available, the continuous-cyclic (sequential) long-cycle regimen is not recommended as standard therapy when using standard doses of estrogen (CE 0.625 mg/d or ME 1 mg/d). If the long-cycle regimen is used, endometrial monitoring is mandatory. Some clinicians use the high negative-predictive value of a thin, distinct endometrial echo (<4 mm) on transvaginal ultrasound in women who wish to pursue such a regimen. Even if long-cycle regimens are used with low- or ultralow-dose estrogens, careful monitoring of the endometrium is advised, particularly with longer-term use.

Continuous-combined estrogen-progestogen therapy

These regimens were developed to address withdrawal uterine bleeding, which is a major reason for discontinuing EPT. In this regimen, a woman uses estrogen and progestogen every day. Within several months, the endometrium can become atrophic, and amenorrhea results.

Rates of endometrial hyperplasia are low, generally less than 1% in women using continuous-combined EPT preparations, based on short-term studies (usually ≤1 y).[98] Such studies are not considered long enough to

Table 11. Estrogen-Progestogen Therapy Regimens, Terminology

Regimen	Estrogen	Progestogen
Continuous-cyclic (sequential)	Daily	12-14 d/mo
Continuous-cyclic (sequential) long cycle	Daily	14 d q 2-6 mo
Continuous-combined	Daily	Daily
Intermittent-combined (pulsed-progestogen; continuous pulsed)	Daily	Repeated cycles, 3 d on, 3 d off

assess endometrial cancer risk. The continuous-combined regimen has been the predominant regimen used in North America. Micronized progesterone needs to be adequately dosed for endometrial protection. Improperly formulated or dosed or delivery issues with estrogen plus MP combinations have the potential of an increased risk of endometrial hyperplasia.[68,99]

Intermittent-combined estrogen-progestogen therapy

This regimen (also called *pulsed-progestogen* or *continuous-pulsed EPT*) uses estrogen daily with the progestogen dose intermittently administered in cycles of 3 days on and 3 days off, which is then repeated without interruption. This regimen, used in only one product (Prefest), was designed to lower the incidence of uterine bleeding while avoiding the downregulation of PRs that continuous progestogen can produce, a mechanism that theoretically may not fully protect the endometrium. By interrupting the progestogen for 3 of every 6 or 7 days, upregulation of PRs occurs intermittently.[100]

In clinical trials, pulsed regimens have shown amenorrhea rates of 80% after 1 year, with favorable endometrial hyperplasia safety profiles.[101] However, almost all prospective studies of this regimen were only 1-year long. Longer-term surveillance of endometrial effects will be needed to more fully ascertain efficacy and safety.

Clinical goal of estrogen-progestogen therapy

The clinical goal of progestogen in EPT is to provide endometrial protection while maintaining estrogen benefits and minimizing unwanted progestogen-induced effects, as well as minimizing progestogen exposure. Research is insufficient to recommend one regimen over another.

For the postmenopausal woman using systemic ET, adding progestogen reduces the risk of endometrial cancer induced by ET to the level found in women not taking hormones. Data from the PEPI trial showed that women who used unopposed ET during the 3-year trial had a significantly increased risk of hyperplasia (34%), whereas those using EPT had a risk of only 1%.[102] Cyclic progesterone added to ET also has been shown to inhibit the development of endometrial hyperplasia. In the PEPI trial, combining CE 0.625 mg per day with progesterone 200 mg per day for 12 days of the month over a 3-year follow-up did not produce an increase in endometrial hyperplasia compared with placebo. Progestogen does not totally eliminate endometrial cancer risk because there is an intrinsic risk independent of hormone use. (See also "Endometrial Cancer" in Chapter 7.)

Epidemiologic studies of continuous-combined EPT indicate no increased risk and may even suggest some added protection against endometrial cancer. A cohort study in more than 200,000 women in Finland compared the risk of endometrial cancer in HT users for at least 6 months with that in the general population.[103] The use of continuous-combined EPT for at least 3 years was associated with a 76% reduction in endometrial cancer. The use of sequential EPT for at least 5 years was associated with varying degrees of increased risk, depending on the progestogen interval used. (See also "Endometrial Cancer" in Chapter 7.)

Studies have provided data regarding the necessary dose and duration of the progestogen course to oppose the estrogen-induced risk of endometrial hyperplasia and adenocarcinoma (Table 12).[104] A progestin-containing IUD and a progesterone vaginal gel offer other possible options for endometrial protection, although long-term efficacy data and FDA approval are lacking regarding endometrial cancer protection.[13,105]

Uterine bleeding with estrogen-progestogen therapy

Various regimens have been designed to decrease bleeding during use of HT. (See also "Abnormal Uterine Bleeding" in Chapter 5.) Two types of bleeding are commonly seen: withdrawal uterine bleeding—bleeding that results from progestogen cessation (or withdrawal), and breakthrough uterine bleeding—irregular bleeding that may occur with regimens using continuous progestogen.

Breakthrough uterine bleeding has been observed in 40% of women on a continuous-combined regimen during the first 3 to 6 months.[98] The probability of achieving

Table 12. Minimum Progestogen Dosing Requirements for Endometrial Protection With Standard Estrogen Dosing

	Continuous-cyclic EPT (daily, 12-14 d/mo)	Continuous-combined EPT (daily)
Oral tablets		
Medroxyprogesterone acetate	5 mg	2.5 mg
Norethindrone	0.35 mg-0.7 mg	0.35 mg
Norethindrone acetate	2.5 mg	0.5 mg-1 mg
Micronized progesterone	200 mg	100 mg
Intrauterine system		
Levonorgestrel[a]	—	20 µg/d or 6 µg /d
Vaginal		
Progesterone gel[a]	45 mg	45 mg

Progesterone-containing products are considered bioidentical.
Standard estrogen dosing is 0.625 mg conjugated estrogens, 1 mg oral estradiol, 0.05 mg patch, or the equivalent.
Abbreviations: EPT, estrogen-progestogen therapy; ET, estrogen therapy.
[a]Not FDA approved for endometrial protection with ET.

amenorrhea is greater if EPT is started 12 months or more after menopause; women who are recently postmenopausal exhibit more breakthrough bleeding. Because of this observation, some clinicians start with a cyclic regimen for 1 year and then switch to continuous combined EPT. Most (75-89%) women who start with continuous-combined therapy become amenorrheic within 12 months. However, irregular bleeding may persist intermittently for months or years. Persistent breakthrough bleeding with continuous-combined EPT may necessitate switching to another regimen.

A study comparing two continuous-combined regimens—0.625 mg CE plus 2.5 mg MPA per day and 17β-estradiol 1 mg plus norethisterone acetate (NETA) 0.5 mg per day—found that within 3 months, 71.4% of the estradiol-NETA users experienced amenorrhea compared with 40.0% of the CE-MPA users, but after 6 months, the differences were not statistically significant.[106] This study confirmed other findings that recently postmenopausal women (within 1-2 y of last menses) experienced more breakthrough bleeding than women more than 3 years postmenopausal. Treatment with one of the 19-nortestosterone derivatives (norethindrone, NETA, LNG, norgestimate) or oral MP tends to produce less breakthrough uterine bleeding during the first few months of use.

In women using EPT beyond 2 years, those using a continuous-combined regimen have a lower rate of breakthrough uterine bleeding and fewer endometrial biopsies than those using the cyclic regimen.[99]

Extrauterine effects of progestogens

Progestogens exhibit effects on organ systems other than the endometrium. These effects vary depending on the progestogen type, dose, route of administration, and the EPT regimen.

For women with type 2 diabetes mellitus (DM), transdermal ET may offer advantages over the oral route because serum TG and other thrombotic factors are not increased further in patients with type 2 DM.

Progestogen has limited effect on the bone-enhancing action of ET. Although adding MPA 2.5 mg or NETA 1 mg to ET slightly enhances estrogen's ability to prevent BMD loss in early postmenopausal women, estrogen alone is adequate to maintain BMD. Estrogen-progestogen therapy reduces spine and hip fractures, but the role of progestogen in this effect is not known. The decision to add progestogen to ET should not be based on its skeletal effect.

Breast cancer risk is not decreased when progestogen is added to ET, and data indicate an increased risk with standard doses, particularly synthetic progestins.[107-109] Mammographic density is increased with progestogen use, with varying effects, depending on type of progestogen, although this effect will reverse with discontinuation. Breast discomfort and pain may increase with progestogen use, and new-onset breast tenderness (vs no breast tenderness) after initiation of CEE plus MPA therapy has been associated with increased risk of breast cancer.[110] It is not clear whether there is a class effect from progestogen or whether a certain type of progestogen can influence breast cancer risk. (See also "Breast Cancer" in Chapter 7.)

In the large French E3N Cohort case-control study, MP was not associated with an elevated risk of breast cancer as opposed to combinations using MPA or NETA.[109] Another case-control study showed no increase in breast cancer with MP compared with an increase with other progestogens and a higher risk with combined-continuous regimens versus sequential regimens.[111] The study has significant limitations because of confounding by socioeconomic status and the usual healthy-user bias. The differential effects of progestogens on breast cancer require further confirmation.

Some progestogens may negatively affect mood, particularly in women with a history of mood disorders. Data are inadequate to recommend specific progestogens or EPT regimens for minimal AEs. In general, the AEs of added progestogen are mild, although they may be severe in a small percentage of women.

For women who are sensitive to the mood changes with progestogens, a discussion of prescribing less progestogen or even unopposed ET for women with an intact uterus is an option. However, there is insufficient evidence regarding endometrial safety to recommend long-cycle progestogen (ie, progestogen for 12-14 d/3-6 mo), and there is clear evidence of endometrial cancer risk with use of unopposed estrogen. Using lower doses of estrogen should decrease the risk of endometrial cancer and allow for lower doses of progestogen.

Estrogen therapy combined with an estrogen antagonist/agonist

In October 2013, FDA approved a medication called a *tissue-selective estrogen complex* (TSEC; marketed as Dua-Vee), which pairs BZA 20 mg, a selective estrogen-receptor modulator (SERM), with CEE 0.45 mg for the treatment of moderate to severe VMS and for the prevention of osteoporosis in postmenopausal women with a uterus (Table 13). Endometrial safety, bleeding profile, breast tenderness, and breast density was comparable with placebo, with cumulative amenorrhea of more than 83%, similar to placebo. This will offer women another option instead of using EPT.[112-115]

Estrogen therapy and estrogen-progestogen therapy contraindications and warnings

The package insert list of ET and EPT contraindications is the same for all HT, whether their effects are systemic or local (Table 14). Refer to current product labeling before prescribing any hormone regimen.

Systemic and local ET and EPT therapy products marketed in the United States have "class labeling," which includes a boxed warning (indicating that the warning is significant) saying that ET increases the risk of

Table 13. Tissue Selective Estrogen Receptor Complex

Components	Dose	Brand names
0.45 mg CEE + 20 mg bazedoxifene (SERM)	Oral daily dose	Duavee; Duavive

Abbreviations: CEE, conjugated equine estrogens; SERM, selective estrogen receptor modulator.
Available in US and Canada.

endometrial cancer. Progestogen is advised when prescribing systemic ET for women with an intact uterus unless the combination CEE/BZA is used.

In the boxed warning of all systemic ET and EPT products (and some local ET products), the government requires the notation that the WHI found increased risks of stroke and deep vein thrombosis. The label further states that ET or EPT should not be used for the prevention of cardiovascular disease (CVD) or dementia. Also noted is that the WHI Memory Study, a substudy of the WHI, reported an increased risk of developing probable dementia in postmenopausal women aged 65 years or older during 5.2 years of treatment with oral CE 0.625 mg per day alone and during 4 years of treatment with oral CEE 0.625 mg per day combined with MPA 2.5 mg per day relative to placebo.[116,117] It is unknown whether this finding applies to younger women.

The labeling also states that other doses of CE and MPA and other combinations and dosage forms of ET and EPT were not studied in the WHI and that in the absence of comparable data, these risks should be assumed to be similar. Close clinical surveillance of all women using ET or EPT is important and should include endometrial sampling when indicated. There is no evidence that the use of compounded ET or EPT formulations will result in a different risk profile than FDA-approved ET and EPT formulations of equivalent dose with unique safety concerns raised by compounding.

Although not in the boxed warning, labeling also warns of an increased risk of breast cancer with ET and EPT. When compared with placebo, the WHI found fewer breast cancers with ET alone.[73] Refer to the labeling for additional warnings for various ET and EPT products before prescribing. (See also "Breast Cancer" in Chapter 7.)

Estrogen therapy and estrogen-progestogen therapy adverse events

A number of AEs are associated with ET and EPT (Table 15), although these vary depending on route of administration, type of progestogen, and dose (see labeling for specific products before prescribing). Although not life threatening, these AEs have a negative effect on QOL and often lead to discontinuation of therapy.

Women using EPT often experience uterine bleeding. Some women regard this EPT-induced bleeding as an unacceptable nuisance, although the bleeding often decreases or stops over time. Adjusting doses and evaluating for other causes of bleeding is indicated. In studies using ultralow-dose EPT (CE 0.30 mg-0.45 mg or equivalent), bleeding is a less common AE.

In some women, EPT causes fluid retention in the hands and feet or abdominal bloating with gaseous distention. A few women experience GI irritation and nausea from oral EPT administration. An analysis from the Nurses' Health Study showed that the risk of gastroesophageal reflux symptoms significantly increased with increasing dose and length of exposure to HT.[117] A prospective cohort study involving 31,494 postmenopausal women from the Swedish Mammography Cohort found that HT was associated with an increase in acute pancreatitis.[118]

Scientific evidence has found no association of EPT with weight gain.[68]

The most common AE of transdermal-patch ET or EPT is skin irritation at the patch application site. This can sometimes be alleviated by rotating the patch, putting it on the buttock, and ensuring that the site is very clean. Using OTC hydrocortisone cream can help, as well as switching to a different ET or EPT patch that may have a different type of adhesive that will not be as irritating. Using talcum powder around the patch edge can prevent formation of dirt rings (dirt rings can be cleaned with mineral oil).

Although the vaginal estrogen ring is generally well tolerated, headache, abdominal pain, and vaginal pain, irritation, and erosion have been reported. If the ring falls out, it can be rinsed off and reinserted. The ring does not usually interfere with sexual intercourse, although it can be removed if it is uncomfortable for either partner.

Estrogen vaginal creams are considered messy by some women. Estrogen cream should not be used as a lubricant at the time of intercourse.

A number of strategies exist for dealing with AEs of ET and EPT (Table 16). Although there is limited scientific evidence to support these tips, clinical experience has determined that they are helpful for some women.

An important principle to keep in mind when prescribing HT, and especially when managing AEs, is that each woman is an individual with her own psychology

---

Table 14. Contraindications for Estrogen Therapy or Estrogen-Progestogen Therapy

- Undiagnosed abnormal genital bleeding
- Known, suspected, or history of breast cancer, except in appropriately selected patients being treated for metastatic disease or with oncology involvement
- Known or suspected estrogen-dependent neoplasia
- Active or history of deep vein thrombosis, pulmonary embolism
- Active or recent (within the past year) arterial thromboembolic disease (eg, stroke, myocardial infarction)
- Liver dysfunction or disease
- Known or suspected pregnancy
- Known hypersensitivity to ET or EPT
- Porphyria cutanea tardis

Abbreviations: EPT, estrogen-progestogen therapy; ET, estrogen therapy.

---

and physiology. Each woman should be advised that it may take time to find the best regimen for her and that regular reevaluation with attempts to taper the dose are important. Sometimes it may take more than one or two products or regimens to find the appropriate one for an individual woman. A certain amount of the search is trial and error.

Women should be counseled not to expect immediate results. Clinical data suggest that relief of VMS with low-dose ET or EPT is not fully evident until 8 to 12 weeks of use. Similarly, improvement in GSM symptoms with local vaginal estrogen may require 8 to 12 weeks. Setting realistic expectations about outcomes with scientific support will help prevent disappointment.

Timing of initiation

The WHI investigators did not expect the timing of HT to affect the results. That concept was not appreciated when the trial was planned. Post hoc analyses revealed that the timing of HT initiation in naturally menopausal women is important.[120] For example, the absolute risk of CHD was lower in the younger, recently postmenopausal women in the WHI than in the older group.

In the WHI, heart attack risk increased during the first year of EPT use in older women but not in younger women. Many experts believe that HT may have beneficial effects in women whose arteries are still healthy, regardless of age. The *timing hypothesis* suggests that there may be less risk and potential CHD benefit when HT is initiated closer to the time of menopause, whereas starting HT further from menopause may be harmful.[74] In support of this hypothesis, in the WHI, the use

Table 15. Potential Adverse Events of Estrogen Therapy or Estrogen-Progestogen Therapy

- Uterine bleeding (starting or returning)
- Breast tenderness (sometimes enlargement)
- Nausea
- Abdominal bloating
- Fluid retention in extremities
- Changes in the shape of the cornea (sometimes leading to contact lens intolerance)
- Headache (sometimes migraine)
- Dizziness
- Mood changes with EPT, particularly with progestin
- Angioedema
- Gallstones, pancreatitis

Abbreviations: EPT, estrogen-progestogen therapy; ET, estrogen therapy

of hormones closer to the onset of menopause (within 10 y) demonstrated a trend toward lower risk of CHD compared with women who began therapy further from menopause (≥20 y) for both the ET and the EPT trials. The 13-year and 18-year comprehensive analyses of the WHI found that women aged 50 to 59 years in the ET arm had significantly more favorable all-cause mortality and fewer MIs.[73,74]

To evaluate the timing hypothesis, two smaller RCTs used surrogate CVD markers, including carotid intimal media thickness and coronary artery calcification. Neither the Kronos Early Estrogen Prevention Study (n=720)[121] or the Early Versus Late Intervention Trial With Estradiol (ELITE; n=504)[122] found increased CVD surrogate markers when HT was started closer to menopause, providing support for safety of HT use earlier in menopause. ELITE found a beneficial effect on atherosclerosis progression (as assessed by carotid intimal media thickness) when HT was started within 6 years of menopause onset but not when started after 10 years. In addition, the finding of fewer AEs in younger women further supports the safety of HT for symptomatic women in the perimenopause transition and early stages of menopause.[123]

Weighing benefits and risks of hormone therapy

The overall benefits and risks from both the ET and EPT trials from the WHI do not support the use of HT for chronic disease prevention.[74]

Some observational studies have shown that ET has beneficial effects on atherosclerosis, vasodilation, plasma lipids, arterial response to injury, and insulin sensitivity.[124-130] Adding progestogens may diminish these beneficial effects, but they generally do not eliminate them. All progestogens negate the beneficial effect of estrogen on blood flow. Selecting a metabolically neutral progestogen such as MP or norgestimate for EPT is recommended to maintain higher plasma levels of HDL-C. In animal studies, progestins with a higher androgenic potency reduce more of the beneficial effects of estrogens on vasodilation; progesterone and 19-norpregnane derivatives have less of an AE profile. These beneficial end points do not outweigh the overall lack of CVD benefit reported in RCTs. Evidence indicates that HT has been found to be safe and effective when initiated in women aged younger than 60 years or within 10 years of menopause to treat menopause symptoms or prevent bone loss. It is not recommend solely for coronary protection.

A meta-analysis of RCTs found no increased risk of stroke in women who began HT when aged younger than 60 years or within 10 years of menopause onset,[126] whereas observational study findings are mixed. In subgroup analysis of the WHI, the ET and EPT arms found a rare, absolute risk of stroke (<1/1,000 woman-years) in women who initiated HT when aged younger than 60 years but an increase in women taking CE alone who were within 10 years of menopause onset.[73] An increased risk of stroke, however, was seen in a meta-analysis of RCTs in women who initiated HT aged 60 years or older or who were more than 10 years from menopause onset.[126] Observational studies across all ages, including meta-analyses, suggest that compared with standard-dose oral HT, lower-dose oral as well as lower-dose transdermal therapy have less effect on risk of stroke.[81,126,131]

Premature menopause (at age <40 y) and primary ovarian insufficiency are conditions associated with a lower risk of breast cancer but an increased risk of persistent VMS, bone loss, VVA, mood changes, and increased risk of heart disease, dementia, stroke, Parkinson disease, ophthalmic disorders, and overall mortality.[132] Early initiation of ET in these women, with endometrial protection if the uterus is preserved, reduces risk for osteoporosis and related fractures, GSM, and dyspareunia, with benefit seen in observational studies for atherosclerosis and CVD, cognition, and dementia. Younger women may require higher doses for symptom relief or protection against bone loss.

After the July 2002 announcement of the first WHI results with CE plus MPA in predominantly asymptomatic postmenopausal women (mean age, 63 y), use of all systemic HT for any indication declined significantly, no doubt because clinicians and their patients were concerned about the risks identified in this study and the fact that HT was not demonstrated to be the preventive therapy people were expecting. Since that time, different methods of analyzing these data and information from other trials have reduced some of these concerns. In addition, lower-dose products are available that may offer similar benefits with fewer risks.

Leading healthcare organizations and medical societies support the use of HT in appropriate situations.[133] Use of HT should be consistent with treatment goals, benefits, and risks for the individual woman, taking into account the cause of menopause (natural, surgical), time since menopause, symptoms, and domains (ie, sexuality and sleep) that may have an effect on QOL and the underlying risk of CVD, stroke, VTE, type 2 DM, and other conditions.[134]

It may be helpful when reviewing risks with women considering HT to put them into perspective. Overall, these risks are rare (<1 event/1,000 woman-years) and even rarer when initiated in women aged younger than 60 years or within 10 years of menopause. Understanding risk is crucial in counseling and educating women about the role of HT and individualizing therapy.

The effects of ET or EPT on risks of breast cancer, CHD, stroke, total CVD, and osteoporotic fracture in perimenopausal women with moderate to severe menopause symptoms have not been established in clinical trials. The findings from trials in different populations should, therefore, be extrapolated with caution.

Different estrogens, progestogens, and routes of administration offer potential advantages for some women. In the absence of clinical trial data for each estrogen and progestogen, clinical trial results for one agent can be generalized to all agents within the same family. Caution is advised when considering custom-compounded HT products. Women being prescribed these products need to be informed of the risks.

There is strong evidence of the efficacy of ET or EPT in reducing the risk of postmenopausal fracture through long-term treatment. (In the WHI, daily oral CE 0.625 mg with or without MPA 2.5 mg was used; fracture protection with other HT or in lower doses still remains to be determined.) For women who require drug therapy for prevention of osteoporosis (including women at high risk of fracture during the next 5-10 y), HT can be considered as an option. The risks and benefits of HT, as well as those of other government-approved therapies, must be weighed. No HT products have been approved by FDA for treatment of osteoporosis, only for prevention.

Table 16. Coping Strategies for Estrogen Therapy or Estrogen-Progestin Therapy Adverse Events

Adverse event	Strategy
Fluid retention	Restrict salt; maintain adequate water intake; exercise; try a mild prescription diuretic.
Bloating	Switch to low-dose nonoral continuous estrogen; lower progestogen dose to a level that still protects the uterus; switch to another progestin or to micronized progesterone.
Breast tenderness	Lower estrogen dose; switch to another estrogen; restrict salt; switch to another progestin; cut down on caffeine and chocolate.
Headaches	Switch to nonoral continuous estrogen; lower dose of estrogen or progestogen or both; switch to a continuous-combined regimen; switch to progesterone or a 19-norpregnane derivative; ensure adequate water intake; restrict salt, caffeine, and alcohol.
Mood changes	Investigate preexisting depression or anxiety; lower progestogen dose; switch progestogen; switch from systemic progestin to the progestin intrauterine system; change to a continuous-combined EPT regimen; ensure adequate water intake; restrict salt, caffeine, and alcohol.
Nausea	Advise taking oral estrogen tablets with meals or before bed; switch to another oral estrogen; switch to nonoral estrogen; lower estrogen or progestogen dose.
Bleeding	Lower dose of estrogen or progestogen, switch to nonprogestogen combined therapy.

Abbreviation: EPT, estrogen-progestogen therapy.

Extended use of the lowest effective dose of systemic HT is acceptable under several circumstances, provided that the woman is well aware of the potential risks and benefits and that there is clinical supervision:
1. In the woman for whom, in her opinion, the benefits of menopause symptom relief outweigh risks, preferably after an attempt to stop HT has failed.

Use of Hormone Therapy in Menopausal Women
(from the 2017 Position Statement of The North American Menopause Society)

The recommendation that HT be used for the "lowest dose for the shortest period of time," as previously recommended, may be harmful for some women. Providers should determine the appropriate type, dose, formulation, route of administration, and duration of therapy on the basis of a woman's individual health characteristics and treatment goals.

On the basis of good observational evidence, those with premature or early menopause (natural, induced, or surgical) can be considered for HT until the average age of menopause to prevent the health consequences of loss of estrogen at an early age. Numerous clinical trials have shown the effectiveness of HT to prevent osteoporosis and reduce the risk for fractures. Extended duration of treatment can be considered for women with persistent hot flashes who elect to continue with very-low doses and longer-term use to relieve menopause symptoms, prevent bone loss, or improve QOL. For women who need relief of the progressive symptoms of GSM, low-dose vaginal estrogen (cream, ring, or tablet) can be used at any age with benefit and minimal risk and without the need for opposing progestogen therapy, based on 1-year RCT data.

Recommendations

- Hormone therapy is the most effective treatment for VMS and GSM and has been shown to prevent bone loss and fracture.

- Risks of HT differ for women, depending on type, dose, duration of use, route of administration, timing of initiation, and whether a progestogen is needed. Treatment should be individualized using the best available evidence to maximize benefits and minimize risks, with periodic reevaluation for the benefits and risks of continuing HT.

- For women aged younger than 60 years or who are within 10 years of menopause onset and have no contraindications, the benefit-risk ratio appears favorable for treatment of bothersome VMS and for those at elevated risk of bone loss or fracture. Longer duration may be more favorable for ET than for EPT, based on the WHI RCTs.

- For women who initiate HT more than 10 or 20 years from menopause onset or when aged 60 years or older, the benefit-risk ratio appears less favorable than for younger women because of greater absolute risks of CHD, stroke, VTE, and dementia.

- For GSM not relieved with OTC or other therapies, low-dose vaginal ET can be used.

2. In women who are at high risk of osteoporotic fracture and also have moderate to severe menopause symptoms.
3. For further prevention of bone loss in the woman with established reduction in bone mass when alternate therapies are not appropriate for that woman, or cause AEs, or when the outcomes of the extended use of alternate therapies are unknown.

When considering HT, various modes of administration are associated with different pros and cons (Table 17).

Monitoring therapy

Clinical monitoring of women using HT includes ongoing evaluation for potential AEs. At least yearly return visits are recommended, during which time the woman and her clinician should review any new medical problems and her decision to use HT, including a discussion of any new research findings. More frequent visits may be required, especially for women just starting HT or for those having bothersome AEs. Annual mammography is recommended for safety. Endometrial surveillance is not required for women using systemic ET and adequate progestogen unless postmenopausal bleeding develops. Data are insufficient to recommend annual endometrial surveillance in asymptomatic women using low-dose vaginal ET for treatment of GSM. If a woman is at high risk for endometrial cancer, using a higher dose of vaginal ET, or is having symptoms (spotting, breakthrough bleeding), closer surveillance may be required. The clinical goal is to use the most appropriate dose, duration, regimen, and route of administration for an individual woman with periodic reevaluation.

Stopping hormone therapy

When a decision is made to discontinue systemic HT, there are scarce data to inform the choice of abrupt cessation versus tapering the dose. In a Swedish trial of 81 women, there was no difference in the number or severity of hot flashes, QOL, or resumption of HT over 3 months, regardless of mode of cessation.[135] There seems to be little difference in terms of return of menopause symptoms. Approximately 50% of women experience a recurrence of symptoms when therapy is discontinued, independent of age and duration of HT use.[136] The decision to continue HT should be individualized on the basis of severity of symptoms and risk-benefit ratio considerations, provided that the woman (in consultation with her healthcare provider) believes that continuation of therapy is warranted.

Low-dose vaginal ET is generally recommended for postmenopausal women whose only menopause symptom is VVA. For symptomatic VVA that does not respond to nonhormone vaginal lubricants and moisturizers, low-dose vaginal ET is effective and well tolerated, and systemic absorption is limited. Progestogen is generally not indicated, but RCT endometrial safety data do not extend beyond 1 year. A large prospective observational study from the WHI found no increased risk of endometrial neoplasia for women using low-dose vaginal ET, as well as no increased risk of CVD, cancer, and other outcomes, and supports findings from earlier epidemiologic and pharmacokinetic reports that low-dose vaginal ET has primarily local vaginal estrogen effects without significant endometrial or systemic effect.[137]

Table 17. Pros and Cons of Hormone Therapy Routes of Administration

Oral estrogen	Vaginal (local) estrogen
Pros	*Pros*
• Familiar, easy	• Vaginal benefit at lower dose
• Beneficial effect on HDL-C, LDL-C, and total cholesterol	• Low-dose therapy typically avoids adverse systemic effects
• Large amount of data	*Cons*
• Usually relatively low cost	• Increase in vaginal discharge
Cons	• Some may consider less convenient to use
• Risk of thrombosis, stroke	• Lack of long-term uterine safety data for low-dose products
• Increase in triglycerides, C-reactive protein, other hepatic proteins	
• Risk of reduced libido through increased SHBG	
• Gallstones, pancreatitis	
Transdermal or topical estrogen	**Progestogens**
Pros	*Pros*
• Avoids hepatic first-pass effect	• Reduced AEs of estrogen on endometrium
• Less increase of triglycerides than oral ET	• Some progestogens reduce AEs of oral estrogen on triglycerides
• Less effect on C-reactive protein than oral ET	• Progesterone dosed at night can decrease insomnia, improve sleep
• Less risk of reducing libido than oral ET	*Cons*
• Fewer GI AEs than oral ET	• Some progestogens may increase risk of breast cancer
• Topical emulsion is moisturizing	• Some progestogens may reduce beneficial effect of oral estrogen on HDL-C
• Perhaps less risk of thrombosis than oral ET	• AEs such as bloating
Cons	• Dysphoric effect for some women
• Patch-adhesive sensitivity/residue	
• Patch is less private	
• Usually relatively higher cost	
• Gels, creams can possibly transfer to others	

Abbreviations: AEs, adverse events; ET, estrogen therapy; GI, gastrointestinal; HDL-C, high-density lipoprotein cholesterol; HT, hormone therapy; LDL-C, low-density lipoprotein cholesterol; SBHG, sex hormone-binding globulin.

Low-dose, local ET should be continued so long as distressing vaginal symptoms remain. For women treated for nonhormone-dependent cancers, management of vaginal atrophy is similar to that for women without a cancer history. For women with a history of hormone-dependent cancer, management recommendations depend on each woman's preference in consultation with her oncologist.

Bioidentical Hormone Therapy

The term *bioidentical hormone therapy* means different things to different people. To some scientists and health-care professionals, bioidentical hormones are those that are chemically identical to the hormones produced by women (primarily in the ovaries) during their reproductive years. To others, the term *bioidentical* is used to refer to custom-compounded HT that is not manufactured by a commercial pharmaceutical company but rather custom crafted for a particular patient by a compounding pharmacy. FDA has stated that the term *bioidentical hormone replacement therapy* is a marketing term not recognized by FDA.[138] The term *bioidentical hormones* refers to all hormones that are identical to those made in the human body.

A woman's body makes various estrogens (such as 17β-estradiol, estrone, and estriol) as well as progesterone, testosterone, and other hormones. Thus, bioidentical HT can mean a medication that provides one or more of these hormones as the active ingredient.[139]

Custom-compounded hormone drugs

Some well-tested, government-approved, brand-name prescription hormones meet the definition of bioidentical as currently used. Several government-approved drugs in the United States and Canada contain 17β-estradiol, and those that are not taken orally remain in the body as 17β-estradiol. There also are government-approved progesterone products, such as oral capsules, 4% and 8% vaginal gels, and a vaginal insert, that meet the definition of bioidentical.

For decades, pharmacists have custom compounded various drug formulations for individual patients as prescribed by their clinicians. Custom compounding of HT allows individualized dosing and combinations of therapy, depending on the prescribing healthcare provider's and a woman's preference or tolerance. It also allows for different modes of administration of hormones, including subdermal implants, sublingual tablets, rectal suppositories, and nasal sprays. Products can be prepared without the binders, fillers, dyes, preservatives, or adhesives that are found in patented, commercially available products. To a large extent, compounding was intended for the patient whose needs were not being met by FDA-approved products.

Hormone drugs that are custom compounded from a prescription are legal but have not gone through the rigorous testing and quality control that determines the safety and efficacy required for FDA approval. Often, third-party payers do not reimburse prescription costs for custom-compounded formulations because they are viewed as experimental drugs.[140,141]

Before an oral capsule MP product was marketed in the United States, oral MP USP was a frequently prescribed custom compound. Custom products are still used and may be especially appropriate for women with peanut allergies (oral capsule MP contains progesterone that is suspended in peanut oil). A 100-mg dose of MP USP is equivalent to about 2.5 mg MPA.

Custom topical preparations of progesterone are also available, although the strength typically used is available in OTC products. Over-the-counter hormone treatments are classified in the United States as either *dietary supplements* (*natural health products* in Canada) or *drugs*, depending on their intended use. As dietary supplements or natural health products, they are approved and regulated differently than are prescription drugs.

Topical progesterone products have not been shown to achieve adequate serum levels to counter the stimulatory effect of ET on the uterus. The dosing of compounded progesterone is particularly difficult to assess because it is not well absorbed through the skin, and levels in serum, saliva, and tissue may be quite different.[142] Custom-compounded formulations should be used with caution and only with informed patient consent.[143] There are women for whom the positives outweigh the negatives, but for most women, government-approved hormone products provide the appropriate therapy without assuming the risks and cost of custom preparations.

It is the stated position of the pharmacy industry that a compounded prescription drug product is not appropriate for a patient for whom there exists a commercially available prescription drug that matches the patient's medical need. More research is needed to sort out the risk-benefit ratio of using compounded hormones. In September 2018, FDA announced an agreement with the National Academies of Science, Engineering, and Medicine and expanded agreements with the University of Maryland and Johns Hopkins University Centers for

Regulatory Science and Innovation to conduct research to help inform the public and the agency's policies regarding compounded drugs.[144]

Concerns regarding custom-compounded formulations

Hormone drugs that are custom compounded for a patient on the basis of an individual prescription are not required to be approved by FDA before they are sold or marketed to women, even though some active ingredients in these compounded prescription drug products meet the specifications of the *United States Pharmacopeia (USP)*. Because pharmacy compounding of custom or individualized medications is part of the routine practice of a pharmacy, the regulation of such prescription medications is generally done by state medical or pharmacy boards, not the federal government, unless 1) the medications being compounded are an exact copy of a commercially available drug product (in which case the compounding pharmacy is acting as a manufacturer and thus subject to FDA jurisdiction), or 2) the compounded prescription drugs pose a substantial and significant risk to patient safety or public health (for example, the 2012 episode of multiple patient deaths from intrathecal injection of a compounded drug product made by a compounding pharmacy in Massachusetts).

Transdermal creams and pills of many varieties are compounded. Some of the most widely used custom estrogen products contained estriol, a weak estrogen having 5% to 10% of the effect of estradiol. Limited data show that oral estriol helps to relieve hot flashes. Estriol alone or in an oral mixture of two estrogens (either 80% estriol and 20% estradiol or 50% each) or three estrogens (usually 80% estriol, 10% estrone, and 10% estradiol) was often promoted as providing the benefits of government-approved estrogen products without increasing the risk of breast or endometrial cancer. Although estriol is a weak estrogen, it will have a stimulatory effect on the breast and endometrium. Claims supporting estriol or any compounded or bioidentical formulation as safer than the government-approved formulations have not been substantiated by any well-designed clinical trials.[145,146]

Although estriol was initially banned without obtaining an investigational new drug application for its use, a report based on an informal email reported that FDA indicated that drug products containing estriol could be compounded in accordance with Section 503A by a licensed pharmacist pursuant to a patient-specific prescription.[147] This was based on estriol being the subject of an applicable *USP* monograph.

In the wake of the WHI findings, compounding became much more popular because symptomatic women had concerns about pharmaceutical-grade HT. Women were led to believe that bioidentical compounded HT products were safer and more effective than government-evaluated and government-approved medications, even though they had not been tested for effectiveness and safety. Bioidentical compounded HT safety information is often not provided to women because there is no standard label or standard patient package insert, and information given to a patient by a compounding pharmacy or a prescribing healthcare provider may vary greatly. As a result, many women are unaware of potential risks and are often surprised to learn that the active hormones are produced in a laboratory. A US survey of compounded HT reported substantial use of these products and suggested the possibility of higher rates of endometrial AEs.[148]

In November 2013, FDA clarified its role in compounded drugs by passing the H.R.3204 Drug Quality and Security Act that created a new category of compounders called *outsourcing facilities*. Large-scale nationwide pharmacy compounders and distributers were provided with a framework to compound drugs for patients when FDA-approved drugs are not available, with the goal of meeting the clinical needs of patients with nongovernment-approved compounded products.

Compounded products pose greater risk for patients because they have not undergone premarket review for safety, efficacy, and certain manufacturing controls. FDA's Compounding Policy Priorities Plan will include how to "address quality standards for outsourcing facilities; regulate compounding from bulk drug substances; restrict compounding of drugs that are essentially copies of FDA-approved drugs; solidify the FDA's partnership with state regulatory authorities; and provide guidance on other activities that compounders undertake."[149]

FDA has stated that compounding pharmacies have made claims about the safety and effectiveness of bioidentical HT unsupported by clinical trial data and thus considered to be false and misleading, but in the absence of recognized jurisdiction over compounding pharmacies, it is unclear what effect, if any, FDA statements will have on either compounding pharmacy practices or their advertising and promotional claims about their products. Pharmacies continue to be monitored by their state boards but now have the option to be credentialed if they meet certain quality and safety standards through the Pharmacy Compounding Accreditation Board. The 2016 interim guidance from FDA on compounding safety and quality control of compounded HT and the 2018 Compounding Policy Priorities Plan will hopefully lead to improved safety of compounding.[149,150]

Several organizations, including The North American Menopause Society, FDA, the American College of Obstetricians and Gynecologists, the Society of Obstetricians and Gynaecologists of Canada, the Endocrine Society, the American Medical Association, and the American Cancer Society, agree that the benefits and risks of compounded bioidentical HT are not different from their government-approved counterparts. In addition, there is not enough evidence to support the health benefit claims or the safety claims made by bioidentical compounded HT promoters.

Selective Estrogen Receptor Modulators

Estrogen receptors are ubiquitous and present in almost all tissues. Selective estrogen-receptor modulators (SERMs) are compounds that were originally developed to block the action of estrogen at its receptor. However, in humans, these agents can exhibit both agonist and antagonist properties, depending on the available target tissue(s); thus they also are called estrogen receptor agonists/antagonists. Knowing how SERMs may vary from one another in specific tissues helps to optimize treatment choices. Additionally, the available SERM-estrogen combination offers benefits to some persons in lieu of traditional HT.

The ideal SERM for menopausal women would require the SERM to have estrogenic action in bone and brain tissue, preventing osteoporosis and hot flashes. In other tissues, the SERM should be neutral or antiestrogenic, preventing endometrial proliferation, VTE, and breast cancer. Although this ideal SERM does not exist, healthcare providers must understand the basic characteristics of available SERMs and their potential benefits and limitations to optimize treatment of women's symptoms while minimizing risks.

Molecular characteristics of selective estrogen receptor modulators

All estrogens and SERMs have lipid-soluble properties and bind to two specific hormone receptors, ER-α and ER-β, either on the cell surface or inside the cell. Estrogen receptors are present in many tissues, including in the vascular system, heart, brain, breast, lung, liver, bone, skin, and uterus. At the molecular level, SERMs bind to the ER to form a complex that combines with the estrogen response element on DNA.

Chaperone proteins, called *coactivators* and *corepressors*, attach to this receptor complex, which then binds to the estrogen response element and is transcribed into messenger RNA. For each tissue type, there can be different transcriptional coactivators and corepressors that distinctively influence the transcriptional efficacy of the HR complex, thereby modifying the transcriptional efficiency and the downstream protein synthesis within the target tissue. Additional tissue response may be influenced by the ratio of α to β ERs.[151,152]

Naturally occurring SERMs, often referred to as phytoestrogens or xenoestrogens, are nonsteroidal compounds with 3-dimensional structural similarities to 17-β estradiol but exhibit both estrogenic and antiestrogenic properties.[153] These compounds are broadly classified as isoflavones, coumestans, and prenylflavonoids and are considered dietary estrogens. Most phytoestrogens have an increased binding affinity for ER-β relative to ER-α.[154] Food sources that are rich in phytoestrogens include nuts, oil-containing seeds (flaxseed), legumes, and soy-containing products (tofu).

Currently available synthetic SERMs can be grouped into three different classes. Tamoxifen, toremifene, and ospemifene (a toremifene derivative) are triphenylethylenes; raloxifene is a benzothiophene; and BZA is an indole derivative.

Selective estrogen receptor modulators in clinical practice

Tamoxifen

In 1978, tamoxifen was approved by FDA for the adjuvant treatment of ER-positive breast cancer in premenopausal and postmenopausal women because it is a potent antiestrogen in breast tissue. Tamoxifen has been widely used for this indication.[155] Tamoxifen was approved for the primary prevention of breast cancer in high-risk premenopausal and postmenopausal women on the basis of the results of the Breast Cancer Prevention Trial, which demonstrated that tamoxifen can reduce the risk of invasive ER-positive breast cancer in high-risk women by 49%.[156]

In other tissues such as bone, liver, and uterus, tamoxifen behaves as an estrogenic agonist. For example, acting in the liver, tamoxifen decreases low-density lipoprotein cholesterol (LDL-C) levels and increases HDL-C levels. In bone, tamoxifen decreases bone mineral turnover and loss in postmenopausal women. In the uterus, tamoxifen is estrogenic and increases the risk of endometrial polyps and cancer. Similar to estrogen, women on tamoxifen are at increased risk for VTE and pulmonary embolism.

Although tamoxifen acts as an estrogen agonist in the bone and has been shown to prevent bone loss in the lumbar spine and hip in postmenopausal women, it is not as effective as estrogen alone and is not FDA approved for this indication.[157]

Up to 50% of women taking tamoxifen had reported hot flashes after starting the medication.[158] For providers monitoring high-risk women on tamoxifen for breast cancer chemoprophylaxis, it is important to consider periodic screening for endometrial hyperplasia and endometrial cancer.[159]

Raloxifene

Raloxifene is a second-generation SERM originally developed to treat osteoporosis as an estrogenic agonist. It has minimal effects on the uterine endometrium and exerts estrogenic action on bone and antiestrogenic effects on breast. In the Multiple Outcomes of Raloxifene Evaluation (MORE) trial, a double-blind, placebo-controlled study of postmenopausal women with osteoporosis, raloxifene increased BMD in the spine and reduced the risk of vertebral fracture but had little effect on hip or nonvertebral fractures.[160] The dual energy X-ray absorptiometry-determined increase in lumbar spine and femoral neck BMD with raloxifene therapy was conserved after 2, 3, and 4 years of treatment; however, because bone turnover is slower in the femur, the BMD femoral neck changes were modest.[161] The study demonstrated an increased risk of VTE (relative risk [RR], 3.1; 95% CI, 1.5-6.2) The trial led to FDA approval of raloxifene 60 mg per day for the prevention and treatment of postmenopausal osteoporosis.

An important ancillary observation of the MORE trial was that the incidence of invasive breast cancer with raloxifene was reduced by 76% after 3 years and 72% after 4 years.[162,163] In further follow-up of MORE trial participants, the risk of invasive breast cancer with raloxifene was significantly reduced by 59% after 8 years (hazard ratio, 034; 95% CI, 0.18-0.66).[163]

These results from the MORE trial were further investigated in a head-to-head trial comparing tamoxifen and raloxifene for breast cancer prevention, the National Surgical Adjuvant Breast and Bowel Project Study of Tamoxifen and Raloxifene trial.[164] This multicenter, randomized study demonstrated that both tamoxifen and raloxifene decreased the risk of breast cancer by approximately 50% in postmenopausal women at risk for the disease. This study also showed that women who took raloxifene (vs tamoxifen) had lower risks of AEs. Over the 4 years of the study, the raloxifene group had fewer uterine cancers (RR, 0.62; 95% CI, 0.35-1.08) and

thromboembolic events (RR, 0.70; 95% CI, 0.54-0.91). Other AEs also were lower with raloxifene, including decreased risk of uterine cancer, VTE, and cataracts. Hot flashes were observed with raloxifene but appeared to be less intense than with tamoxifen. After this study, raloxifene was FDA approved for the prevention of invasive breast cancer in high-risk postmenopausal women.

Raloxifene, when used alone, does not have any effect on GSM and has no effect on the vaginal maturation index. Women on raloxifene may have improvement of VVA with the use of local vaginal estrogen cream or an estrogen ring as an off-label combination.[165] Clinicians should not use raloxifene in combination with systemic estrogen because of increased endometrial stimulation and its subsequent risks.

Bazedoxifene

Bazedoxifene is a third-generation SERM that was developed as an estrogen agonist to treat osteoporosis. It is available in the United States only as DuaVee (CEE 0.45 mg/BZA 20 mg). In breast and endometrial tissues, it is an estrogen antagonist. In a 3-year RCT, BZA 20 mg or 40 mg per day alone significantly improved BMD and reduced bone marker levels compared with placebo ($P<.001$).[166] Similar to raloxifene, BZA also significantly reduced the risk of new vertebral fractures in postmenopausal women with osteoporosis ($P<.05$). In addition, BZA reduced the risk of nonvertebral fracture in patients at high fracture risk.

Bazedoxifene is approved for the treatment of osteoporosis in Europe and Japan at a 20-mg per day dose.[167] Use of this compound is associated with mild hot flashes and an increase in VTE but does not increase endometrial thickness, breast tenderness, or risk of breast cancer.[168] It also has no effect on symptoms of GSM.

Ospemifene

Ospemifene received FDA approval in 2013 for the treatment of moderate to severe dyspareunia. In two 12-week clinical trials, ospemifene 60 mg per day decreased the vaginal pH, improved vaginal dryness, and shifted the vaginal maturational index toward superficial cells.[87,169] Adverse events included a modest increase in hot flashes compared with placebo (9.6% vs 3.4%).[169]

Women taking ospemifene demonstrated estrogenic-type responses in the uterus and had more uterine polyps (5 vs 1 with placebo), actively proliferative endometrium (41 patients taking ospemifene vs 12 with placebo), and an increase in endometrial thickness greater than 5 mm (51 patients taking ospemifene vs 12 taking placebo) during the 1-year trial.[170]

Endometrial cancer or hyperplasia were not seen in women taking ospemifene, although this has not been assessed beyond 1 year of use.[170] Ospemifene also is associated with a slight increase in hemorrhagic (not thrombotic) stroke and VTE.[171] Thus, ospemifene labeling contains a black box warning regarding concerns for endometrial stimulation, VTE, and stroke.

Ospemifene was originally developed to prevent and treat osteoporosis, but to date no large human trials have been performed to evaluate its effectiveness for this indication. Preclinical data in a mouse model noted reduced bone turnover and increased bone strength.[172]

Toremifene

Toremifene is related to tamoxifen and is a triphenylethylene-derived SERM. It is FDA approved to treat advanced estrogen-sensitive breast cancer and as adjuvant treatment of early breast cancer at a dose of 60 mg per day. In contrast with tamoxifen, toremifene demonstrates a weaker effect on the uterine compartment because there is lower risk of endometrial cancer.[173] The risk of VTE also appears to be lower than with tamoxifen. FDA has placed a warning that it may prolong the QT interval in the heart, which may lead to ventricular arrhythmia.[174] Toremifene has favorable effects on BMD and results in favorable lipid profiles similar to that of tamoxifen.

Bazedoxifene and conjugated equine estrogen combination

Therapeutic approaches aimed at optimizing the desirable properties of receptor modulation combine an estrogen with a SERM forming a TSEC have been developed. Conceptually, this combination allows for the benefits of ET while minimizing the withdrawal endometrial bleeding effects in women with a uterus. Understanding the different tissue effects of each SERM within the TSEC concept helps to guide their use in menopause management.

The goal for developing TSECs was to eliminate the need for a combination EPT in women with VMS who had not had a hysterectomy. Clinical experience demonstrates that with combination EPT there is an increase in unscheduled bleeding requiring additional endometrial diagnostic procedures, breast pain/tenderness, and increased mammographic breast density that can lead to additional breast imaging.[175] These undesired effects have spurred the need to develop improved forms of HT.

The TSEC takes advantage of the tissue selective properties of the SERM by pairing a *specific* SERM with a *specific* estrogen by taking advantage of the estrogen-antagonistic properties of the SERM while offering the benefits of ET.

In 2013, FDA approved 20 mg BZA combined with 0.45 mg CEE to relieve hot flashes and prevent osteoporosis. Based on dose-response studies during drug development, 20 mg BZA per day was selected as the SERM because it demonstrated sufficient antagonist effect on endometrial tissue to be paired with a CEE. This is an important point, because clinicians should not combine other SERMs with other estrogens at varying doses in an off-label fashion.

The TSEC concept was established by a series of phase 3 studies called the Selective Estrogens, Menopause, and Response to Therapy (SMART) trials. Each SMART trial was designed to evaluate different menopause end points. The SMART 2 trial focused on VMS and evaluated 332 women aged 40 to 65 years with a uterus who had at least 50 hot flashes a week of moderate or severe intensity.[176] Bazedoxifene 20 mg/CEE 0.45 mg significantly reduced the number and severity of hot flashes at 4 and 12 weeks (P<.001). At week 12, BZA/CEE reduced hot flashes from baseline by 74% (from 10.3 hot flashes/wk to 2.8) compared with a 51% reduction with placebo (10.5 vs 5.4). There was also a significant reduction in the severity of hot flashes with BZA/CEE compared with placebo (37% vs 17%). The safety parameters were similar between BZA/CEE and placebo.[177]

In the SMART 3 study, vaginal health was evaluated in 664 healthy postmenopausal women aged 40 to 65 years with VVA for changes in vaginal maturation, vaginal pH, and severity of the most bothersome symptom of VVA at 4 and 12 weeks of treatment.[178] Bazedoxifene/CEE stimulated an estrogenic change in the vaginal mucosa, with significantly increased superficial cells and decreased parabasal cells, reduced vaginal pH, vaginal dryness, and the most bothersome VVA symptom (P<.05).

Osteoporosis prevention and other clinically relevant end points were evaluated in the SMART 1, 4, and 5 studies.[177] Dual-energy X-ray absorptiometry-derived lumbar spine and total hip BMD measurements increased significantly from baseline at years 1 and 2 with BZA/CEE compared with placebo (P<.001).[179]

SMART 5 noted similar rates of amenorrhea, breast tenderness, and AEs between BZA/CEE and placebo.[114] Assessment of the endometrial compartment noted a very low incidence of endometrial hyperplasia (<1%), endometrial proliferation, asymptomatic endometrial polyps, and endometrial thickening.

Although these trials were not powered to assess the effect on breast cancer, the incidence of breast cancer at 5 years of exposure was no different between BZA/CEE and placebo.[177] SMART-study participants reported a low incidence of breast pain or tenderness and a high rate of amenorrhea; they exhibited a low incidence of endo-metrial hyperplasia and no changes in mammographic breast density. This latter finding of lack of change in breast density is an important surrogate marker for esti-mating the risk of breast cancer.

Bazedoxifene/CEE is a good option for women taking ET for the treatment of VMS who do not tolerate proges-terone therapy or who have a history of irregular bleed-ing associated with a thickened endometrial stripe. For symptomatic menopausal women with a uterus who have hot flashes or GSM and do not want monthly vaginal bleeding, BZA/CEE can be considered for initial therapy.

A future selective estrogen receptor modulator: lasofoxifene

Lasofoxifene is a third-generation SERM that was originally developed for the prevention and treatment of osteoporosis.[180] Clinical observations during phase 3 trials suggested a weak estrogenic effect on the vaginal mucosa associated with increased vaginal moisture and a possible treatment for VVA in postmenopausal women. Lasofoxifene was effective at a dose of 0.5 mg per day for reduction of vertebral fractures by 42% (P<.001) and nonvertebral fractures by 24% (P=.002) at 5 years. Addi-tional assessments of the vaginal compartment showed an improvement in vaginal pH and increased superficial cells and maturation compared with placebo. Further tri-als with lasofoxifene were abandoned because of concern for increased endometrial thickness, even though there was no increase in endometrial hyperplasia or cancer in postmenopausal women treated with lasofoxifene.[181]

Guidelines for Prescribing Statin Therapy in Postmenopausal Women

Heart disease is the leading cause of death in US women. In 2015, women represented approximately 50% of all CVD deaths.[182] Although the leading cause of death for men is also heart disease, the risk factors of CVD can differ between sexes and age groups. The presence of risk factors dictates the onset of CVD for both men and women.

Men with CVD often present about a decade earlier than women, which has been attributed to the protec-tive effects of endogenous estrogen in women. Thus, pre-menopause, menopause, and postmenopause are the time periods of important risk factor modification and assess-ment. Additionally, stroke is emerging as a significant CV risk in women, particularly older women. In 2015, women comprised 58.5% of all stroke deaths. Annually, 55,000 more women than men will suffer from a stroke.[182]

The risk factors for CVD can be targeted through preven-tive strategies such as lifestyle modification and preven-tive medications, one of which is statin therapy.

Dyslipidemia: a risk factor for cardiovascular disease

Dyslipidemia, defined as elevated levels of total cholesterol (TC), LDL-C, and non-HDL-C, is a powerful risk factor for atherosclerotic CVD (ASCVD). A large case-control study performed in 52 countries identified dyslipidemia as one of nine modifiable risk factors that contributed to more than 90% of population-associated risk of a first MI.[183] Thus, screening for dyslipidemia for early detec-tion and management is a major component of reducing ASCVD risk. (See also "Hyperlipidemia" in Chapter 8.)

Treatment of dyslipidemia with statin therapy has become the number-one guideline-recommended therapy, because a number of large RCTs on statin use have dem-onstrated that lowering LDL-C with statins reduces the risk of CV AEs. Guideline recommendations for the use of lipid-lowering therapies are now provided in the con-text of an assessment of one's risk of "hard" ASCVD end points: fatal and nonfatal MI and stroke through a pooled-cohort equation that estimates 10-year ASCVD risk. The pooled-cohort equation was created from five prospective community-based studies that represented the US popu-lation from which the race- and sex-specific estimates are best validated in non-Hispanic white and non-Hispanic blacks aged from 40 to 75 years. (See also "Hyperlipidemia" in Chapter 8.) The pooled cohort equation incorporates traditional risk factors for CVD, including age, tobacco use, blood pressure, race, serum TC, HDL-C, and the presence or absence of DM.[184] The American College of Cardiology (ACC) created the ASCVD Risk Estimator Plus, an online calculator tool also available as an app that computes ASCVD scores. (See Figure 4 in Chapter 8, "Cardiometa-bolic Disorders in Midlife Women.")

Statin clinical trial data in women

The mechanism of action of statins is competitive inhibi-tion of the rate-limiting step of cholesterol synthesis in the liver. Statins are 3-hydroxy-3-methylglutaryl-coenzyme A (HMG-CoA) reductase inhibitors that prevent the forma-tion of mevalonate, which ceases cholesterol production. Hepatic maintenance of cholesterol homeostasis causes upregulation of LDL-C receptors, resulting in an increase in LDL-C uptake by hepatocytes and reduction in circulat-ing LDL-C in the blood. Collectively, statins lower LDL-C levels and TC and have pleiotropic effects such as plaque stabilization and anti-inflammatory properties.[185]

Statins as a class of drugs vary in their intensity of lipid lowering and can be categorized as low-, medium-, or high-intensity.[184] (See Table 10 in Chapter 8, "Cardiometabolic Disorders in Midlife Women.")

Primary prevention data

The US Preventive Services Task Force (USPSTF) commissioned a systematic review to analyze 19 RCTs to investigate the effects of statin therapy versus placebo or no statins in adults aged 40 to 75 years with an elevated ASCVD risk without known CVD.[186] In these trials, statin therapy was associated with a significant reduction in all-cause mortality (pooled RR, 0.86; 95% CI, 0.80-0.93), CV mortality (pooled RR, 0.69; 95% CI, 0.54-0.88), ischemic stroke (pooled RR, 0.71; 95% CI, 0.62-0.82), and heart attack (pooled RR, 0.64; 95% CI, 0.57-0.71). Predefined subgroup analysis of sex was evaluated in six trials and found no sex-specific difference in risk estimates for CVD. This remained true for other predefined subgroups such as race, age, and clinical characteristics. One consistent finding was that the degree of clinical benefit was proportional to the degree of underlying clinical risk.

The recommendations for statin use for primary prevention recommended by the USPSTF is based on one's estimated 10-year ASCVD risk event calculated from the pooled cohort equation described in the 2013 ACC/American Heart Association (AHA) cholesterol guidelines.[187] The USPSTF summarizes a recommendation of "moderate certainty" for the use of low- to moderate-intensity statin therapy in adults aged 40 to 75 years who have an ASCVD risk greater than 10% and one or more risk factors for CVD, including HTN, DM, dyslipidemia, or tobacco use.[188] However, the recommendation of low- to moderate-intensity statin therapy is less certain when the 10-year ASCVD risk falls between 7.5% and 10% because the likelihood of benefit is smaller as the risk of disease declines, thus the recommendation is left to the clinician's discretion. Therefore, a woman without underlying CVD should be assessed by her age, the presence of at least one CVD risk factor, and her 10-year ASCVD risk score to determine whether she should be initiated on statin therapy for primary prevention.

Secondary prevention data

Despite the compelling evidence for the use of statin therapy in secondary prevention, the unequal representation of women in statin clinical trials has challenged the evidence base for this treatment in women.

The Scandinavian Simvastatin Survival Trial was a large RCT that investigated the effect of simvastatin therapy on morbidity and mortality in patients with CVD.[189] On a background of a lipid-lowering diet, 4,444 patients were randomized to placebo versus simvastatin therapy and followed over a median of 5.4 years. The trial demonstrated that the RR of death with simvastatin compared with placebo was 0.70 (95% CI, 0.58-0.85; P=.0003), and the RR of coronary death was 0.58 (95% CI, 0.46-0.73) with simvastatin compared with placebo. This study included a protocol-specified subgroup of women that demonstrated a RR of 0.65 (95% CI, 0.47-0.90; P=.010) for a coronary event in the simvastatin group compared with placebo. Despite the limitation of less statistical power, the coronary-risk reduction in this subgroup supports the evidence for the use of statin therapy for women with dyslipidemia with established CVD.

The Cholesterol and Recurrent Events Trial was another large RCT trial that investigated the role of pravastatin therapy on recurrent CV events in women with average cholesterol levels after MI.[190] This trial randomized 576 postmenopausal women (mean age, 61 y) 3 and 20 months after MI with total cholesterol levels less than 240 mg/dL and LDL-C levels of 115 mg/dL to 174 mg/dL to 40 mg pravastatin per day versus placebo. The primary trial end point of coronary death or nonfatal MI was decreased by 43% (P=.035), and stroke was reduced by 56% (P=.07). Although men experienced a reduction in the primary end point as well, sex comparison revealed that women demonstrated a greater magnitude of benefit. Additionally, the treatment curve revealed that the greatest benefit began at 1 year. The results of the Cholesterol and Recurrent Events trial show the benefit of statin therapy in the reduction of recurrent CV events and stroke for women with average cholesterol levels.

Guidelines

The ACC/AHA completely revised their 2013 guidelines on the management of blood cholesterol in November 2018.[184] The 2013 guidelines introduced the pooled cohort equation and the concept of ASCVD risk evaluation.

As with prior cholesterol guidelines, the 2013 recommendations were written with the goal of reducing the risk of ASCVD. These guidelines were written using only high-quality data (RCTs and high-quality systematic reviews and meta-analyses) as the evidence base to specifically define which lipid-modulating strategies were most effective at reducing hard CV outcomes such as MI, stroke, and CV death. These guidelines concluded that the most powerful strategy with the greatest evidence base is statin therapy. Although prior guidelines offered several options for pharmacotherapies to reduce cholesterol, these guidelines state that at the time of writing, statins were by far the best evidence-based ASCVD risk-reducing therapies. These guidelines categorize patients who are expected to benefit from statin therapy into "statin-benefit" groups. (See Table 9 in Chapter 8, "Cardiometabolic Disorders in Midlife Women.") Persons falling into each of the four statin-benefit groups are recommended for different intensity of statin therapy on the basis of the clinical characteristics of each statin-benefit group.

High-intensity statin therapy has been shown to reduce LDL-C levels by more than 50% on average and are recommended for persons with clinical ASCVD. Moderate-intensity statins lower LDL-C by 30% to 50%. Most data support intensive LDL-C lowering with statins in patients with stable ischemic heart disease; therefore, high-intensity statin therapy is indicated in the 2018 cholesterol guidelines for all adults with clinically established ASCVD. Moderate-intensity statin therapy may be used in patients with established ASCVD who cannot tolerate higher-dose statins or patients aged older than 75 years. For adults aged 20 to 75 years with severe hypercholesterolemia LDL-C of 190 mg/dL or more, high-intensity statin therapy is recommended. For adults aged 40 to 75 years with underlying DM, moderate-intensity statin therapy is recommended. For secondary prevention in adults aged 40 to 75 years with an LDL-C level of 70 mg/dL or more to less than 190 mg/dL, these guidelines provide recommendations for statin therapy based on the 10-year ASCVD risk calculation greater than 7.5% (Table 18).[184]

The USPSTF recommends use of low- to moderate-dose statin therapy for primary prevention when all these criteria are met: 1) age 40 to 75 years; 2) presence of one or more CVD risk factors (ie, dyslipidemia, DM, HTN, or smoking); and 3) calculated 10-year risk of a CV event of 10% or greater. The USPSTF recommends use of the same risk estimator proposed in the 2013 ACC/AHA cholesterol guidelines. The USPSTF found adequate evidence that the benefits of low- to moderate-dose statin therapy exceeded the harms in adults aged 40 to 75 years.[188]

Both of these recommendations are consistent with beneficial results reported from the Heart Outcomes Prevention Evaluation 3 trial that found that statin use in persons at intermediate risk of ASCVD without regard to baseline LDL-C levels reduced risk.[191] The USPSTF did not make a recommendation on the use of statins for the prevention of CVD events in adults aged 76 years or older because of inadequate evidence in this age group.[188]

On the basis of the evidence and guideline recommendations, there is a proposed algorithm for determination of statin use in postmenopausal women.[192] The algorithm serves as an initial work flow for determining a postmenopausal woman's underlying risk category with these potential categories: 1) clinical ASCVD risk; 2) LDL-C level alone; 3) age, LDL-C, and presence of DM; and 4) age, LDL-C without DM.[184]

Statin safety and adverse event profiles

Statin drugs are predominantly safe for use for most patients. However, AEs are major causes of statin dose reduction or complete discontinuation of therapy, leaving patients who would benefit from this treatment at persistent risk. Patients with multiple comorbidities may be subjected to AEs associated with long-term statin use. Thus, a discussion of statin AEs is important between patients and providers. The overall incidences of the most common statin-specific AEs are myalgias (3-5%), myopathy (0.1-0.2%), new-onset DM (9-27%), and hepatotoxicity (<1%).[193]

Muscle-related symptoms are the most common AEs related to statin dose reduction or discontinuation. The severity can range from mild to severe, such as cramps and tenderness, to loss of muscle strength. Four clinical presentations have been described by the National Lipid Association Statin Muscle Safety Task Force[194]:

Myalgias
Myalgias are marked by muscle pain and flu-like symptoms, with normal creatinine kinase (CK) levels.

Myopathy
Myopathy is muscle weakness with or without elevated CK levels. Risk factors associated with the development of myopathy include renal failure, female sex, hypothyroidism, renal or liver dysfunction, and concurrent use of medications that interact with statin metabolism causing higher-than-expected levels of statin in the blood stream.

Myositis
Myositis is muscle tenderness because of inflammation, marked by elevated CK levels and leukocytosis.

Myonecrosis
Myonecrosis is muscle injury with elevated CK levels. The most serious form of myonecrosis results in rhabdomyolysis,

Table 18. Summary of ACC/AHA Class I Recommendations for Statin Therapy for Secondary ASCVD Prevention

Statin-benefit group		Recommendation
Clinical ASCVD	Age ≤75 y	High intensity
	Associated AEs with high-intensity statin	Moderate intensity
Severe hypercholesterolemia (LDL-C ≥190 mg/dL)	Age 10-75 y	High intensity
DM	Age 40-75 y	Moderate intensity
ASCVD risk assessment	≥7.5% to <20%	Moderate intensity

ASCVD risk assessment requires risk discussion specific to the patient. ASCVD risk assessment >20% requires risk reduction goal of >50% LDL-C, which can be achieved with at least moderate- or high-intensity statin therapy.
Abbreviations: ACC, American College of Cardiology; AEs, adverse events; AHA, American Heart Association; ASCVD, atherosclerotic cardiovascular disease; DM, diabetes mellitus; LDL-C, low-density lipoprotein cholesterol.
Grundy SM, et al.[184]

a rare, severe form of myonecrosis that occurs in patients with an underlying genetic predisposition or extensive drug-drug interaction. To standardize the diagnosis of statin-associated muscle symptoms, the National Lipid Association Statin Muscle Safety Task Force created a statin-associated muscle symptoms clinical index to assess muscle symptoms as unlikely, possible, and probable.[194] The primary treatment for statin intolerance because of statin-associated muscle symptoms is discontinuation and rechallenge of statin therapy, either in a different dose of the same statin or a different statin.[195]

A large prospective cohort study from a primary care population in England and Wales evaluated the AEs collected from a database of patients who were newly prescribed statins between 2002 and 2008.[196] The most serious AEs noted included myopathy, acute renal failure, cataracts, esophageal cancer, and moderate to severe liver dysfunction. Moderate to serious liver dysfunction as an AE is very rare and not sex-specific. The highest risk in both sexes has been associated with fluvastatin. Women experience a dose-response effect, with higher doses associated with an incremental risk of liver dysfunction. The risk of liver dysfunction was observed to be highest in the first year of treatment, but this is often because of drug-drug interactions.[197] Overall there has been no confirmed link between liver dysfunction and statin use; thus, consensus from an International Lipid Expert Panel recommends only screening liver enzymes before statin therapy and only if symptoms occur after statin initiation.[198]

It is important for patients to discuss any new symptom as a perceived AE before discontinuing statin therapy. Adverse events can be managed by either decreasing the dose or switching to a different type of statin therapy,

but the provider-patient relationship is paramount. Self-discontinuation can lead to increased CVD risk, and healthcare providers need to be aware of any change in treatment. In an effort to address the challenges associated with managing patients who develop potential AEs, the ACC created the *ACC Statin Intolerance App* (acc.org/StatinIntoleranceApp) to help healthcare providers evaluate and treat patients who report muscle-related symptoms on statin therapy.

Last, the risk of new-onset DM associated with statin therapy is of major importance because of the inherent CVD risk associated with DM and dyslipidemia.[199] The risk of developing new-onset DM during statin therapy initiation is largely because of risk factors such as central obesity, increased waist circumference, elevated TG, hyperglycemia, and LDL-C associated with metabolic syndrome and insulin resistance. It appears that there is a direct relationship between the increase in metabolic syndrome risk factors and the risk of developing new-onset DM when initiating statin therapy. A large randomized, controlled primary prevention trial demonstrated that the benefit of CVD reduction and mortality benefit observed with statin therapy outweighed any harm of developing DM from statin therapy initiation.

REFERENCES

1. Trussell J, Aiken ARA, Micks E, Guthrie KA. Efficacy, safety, and personal considerations. In: Hatcher RA, Nelson AL, Trussell J, et al, eds. *Contraceptive Technology.* 21st ed. New York: Ayer; 2018:95-128.

2. Curtis KM, Peipert JF. Long-acting reversible contraception. *N Engl J Med.* 2017;376(5):461-468.

3. Curtis KM, Jatlaoui TC, Teppwr NK, et al. US Selected Practice Recommendations for Contraceptive Use, 2016. *MMWR Recomm Rep.* 2016;65(4):1-66.

4. Curtis KM, Tepper NK, Jatlaoui TC, et al. US Medical Eligibility Criteria for Contraceptive Use, 2016. *MMWR Recomm Rep*. 2016;65(3):1-103.

5. Winner B, Peipert JF, Zhao Q, et al. Effectiveness of long-acting reversible contraception. *N Engl J Med*. 2012;366(21):1998-2007.

6. Kavanaugh ML, Jerman J. Contraceptive method use in the United States: trends and characteristics between 2008, 2012, and 2014. *Contraception*. 2018;97(1):14-21.

7. Wu JP, Pickle S. Extended use of the intrauterine device: a literature review and recommendations for clinical practice. *Contraception*. 2014;89(6):495-503.

8. Eisenberg DL, Schreiber CA, Turok DK, Teal SB, Westhoff CL, Creinin MD; ACCESS IUS Investigators. Three-year efficacy and safety of a new 52-mg levonorgestrel-releasing intrauterine system. *Contraception*. 2015;92(1):10-16.

9. Schreiber CA, Teal SB, Blumenthal PD, Keder LM, Olariu AI, Creinin MD. Bleeding patterns for the Liletta levonorgestrel 52 mg intrauterine system. *Eur J Contracept Reprod Health Care*. 2018;23(2):116-120.

10. Hurskainen R, Teperi J, Rissanen P, et al. Clinical outcomes and costs with the levonorgestrel-releasing intrauterine system or hysterectomy for treatment of menorrhagia: randomized trial 5-year follow-up. *JAMA*. 2004;291(12):1456-1463.

11. Kaunitz AM, Meredith S, Inki P, Kubba A, Sanchez-Ramos L. Levonorgestrel-releasing intrauterine system and endometrial ablation in heavy menstrual bleeding: a systematic review and meta-analysis. *Obstet Gynecol*. 2009;113(5):1104-1116.

12. Petta CA, Ferriani RA, Abrao MS, et al. Randomized clinical trial of a levonorgestrel-releasing intrauterine system and a depot GnRH analogue for the treatment of chronic pelvic pain in women with endometriosis. *Hum Reprod*. 2005;20(7):1993-1998.

13. Depypere H, Inki P. The levonorgestrel-releasing intrauterine system for endometrial protection during estrogen replacement therapy: a clinical review. *Climacteric*. 2015;18(4):470-482.

14. Nelson A, Apter D, Hauck B, et al. Two low-dose levonorgestrel intrauterine contraceptive systems: a randomized controlled trial. *Obstet Gynecol*. 2013;122(6):1205-1213.

15. Gemzell-Danielsson K, Schellschmidt I, Apter D. A randomized, phase II study describing the efficacy, bleeding profile, and safety of two low-dose levonorgestrel-releasing intrauterine contraceptive systems and Mirena. *Fertil Steril*. 2012;97(3):616-622.e1-3.

16. Long-term reversible contraception. Twelve years of experience with the TCu380A and TCu220C. *Contraception*. 1997;56(6).341-352.

17. Hubacher D, Chen PL, Park S. Side effects from the copper IUD: do they decrease over time? *Contraception*. 2009;79(5):356-362.

18. Heinemann K, Reed S, Moehner S, Minh TD. Risk of uterine perforation with levonorgestrel-releasing and copper intrauterine devices in the European Active Surveillance Study on Intrauterine Devices. *Contraception*. 2015;91(4):274-279.

19. Madden T, McNicholas C, Zhao Q, Secura GM, Eisenberg DL, Peipert JF. Association of age and parity with intrauterine device expulsion. *Obstet Gynecol*. 2014;124(4):718-726.

20. McNicholas C, Swor E, Wan L, Peipert JF. Prolonged use of the etonogestrel implant and levonorgestrel intrauterine device: 2 years beyond Food and Drug Administration-approved duration. *Am J Obstet Gynecol*. 2017;216(6):586.e1-586.e6.

21. Zigler RE, McNicholas C. Unscheduled vaginal bleeding with progestin-only contraceptive use. *Am J Obstet Gynecol*.2017;216(5):443-450.

22. Kaunitz AM, Darney PD, Ross D, Wolter KD, Speroff L. Subcutaneous DMPA vs. intramuscular DMPA: a 2-year randomized study of contraceptive efficacy and bone mineral density. *Contraception*. 2009;80(1):7-17.

23. Schwallie PC, Assenzo JR. The effect of depo-medroxyprogesterone acetate on pituitary and ovarian function, and the return of fertility following its discontinuation: a review. *Contraception*. 1974;10(2):181-202.

24. Jain J, Jakimiuk AJ, Bode FR, Ross D, Kaunitz AM. Contraceptive efficacy and safety of DMPA-SC. *Contraception*. 2004;70(4):269-275.

25. Kaunitz AM, Peipert JF, Grimes DA. Injectable contraception: issues and opportunities. *Contraception*. 2014;89(5):331-334.

26. Lopez LM, Chen M, Mullins Long S, Curtis KM, Helmerhorst FM. Steroidal contraceptives and bone fractures in women: evidence from observational studies. *Cochrane Database Syst Rev*. 2015;(7):CD009849.

27. Lanza LL, McQuay LJ, Rothman KJ, et al. Use of depot medroxyprogesterone acetate contraception and incidence of bone fracture. *Obstet Gynecol*. 2013;121(3):593-600.

28. Trussell J, Guthrie KA, Schwarz EB. Much ado about little: obesity, combined hormonal contraceptive use and venous thrombosis. *Contraception*. 2008;77(3):143-146.

29. Horton LG, Simmons KB, Curtis KM. Combined hormonal contraceptive use among obese women and risk for cardiovascular events: a systematic review. *Contraception*. 2016;94(6):590-604.

30. Lidegaard Ø, Løkkegaard E, Jensen A, Skovlund CW, Keiding N. Thrombotic stroke and myocardial infarction with hormonal contraception. *N Engl J Med*. 2012;366(24):2257-2266.

31. Allen RH, Cwiak CA, Kaunitz AM. Contraception in women over 40 years of age. *CMAJ*. 2013;185(7):565-573.

32. Iversen L, Sivasubramaniam S, Lee AJ, Fielding S, Hannaford PC. Lifetime cancer risk and combined oral contraceptives: the Royal College of General Practitioners' Oral Contraception Study. *Am J Obstet Gynecol*. 2017;216(6):580.e1-580.e9.

33. Mørch LS, Skovlund CW, Hannaford PC, Iversen L, Fielding S, Lidegaard Ø. Contemporary hormonal contraception and the risk of breast cancer. *N Engl J Med*. 2017;377(23):2228-2239.

34. Nakajima ST, Archer DF, Ellman H. Efficacy and safety of a new 24-day oral contraceptive regimen of norethindrone acetate 1 mg/ethinyl estradiol 20 micro g (Loestrin 24 Fe). *Contraception*. 2007;75(1):16-22.

35. Archer DF, Nakajima ST, Sawyer T, et al. Norethindrone acetate 1.0 milligram and ethinyl estradiol 10 micrograms as an ultra low-dose oral contraceptive. *Obstet Gynecol*. 2013;122(3):601-607.

36. Vandever MA, Kuehl TJ, Sulak PJ, et al. Evaluation of pituitary-ovarian axis suppression with three oral contraceptive regimens. *Contraception*. 2008;77(3):162-170.

37. Fels H, Steward R, Melamed A, Granat A, Stanczyk FZ, Mishell DR Jr. Comparison of serum and cervical mucus hormone levels during hormone-free interval of 24/4 vs. 21/7 combined oral contraceptives. *Contraception*.2013;87(6):732-737.

38. Dinger J, Minh TD, Buttmann N, Bardenheuer K. Effectiveness of oral contraceptive pills in a large U.S. cohort comparing progestogen and regimen. *Obstet Gynecol*. 2011;117(1):33-40.

39. Pearlstein T B, Bachmann GA, Zacur HA, Yonkers KA. Treatment of premenstrual dysphoric disorder with a new drospirenone-containing oral contraceptive formulation. *Contraception*. 2005;72(6):414-421.

40. Yonkers KA, Brown C, Pearlstein TB, Foegh M, Sampson-Landers C, Rapkin A. Efficacy of a new low-dose oral contraceptive with drospirenone in premenstrual dysphoric disorder. *Obstet Gynecol*. 2005;106(3):492-501.

41. Bird ST, Pepe SR, Etminan M, Liu X, Brophy JM, Delaney JA. The association between drospirenone and hyperkalemia: a comparative-safety study. *BMC Clin Pharmacol*. 2011;11:23.

42. Dinger J, Shapiro S. Combined oral contraceptives, venous thromboembolism, and the problem of interpreting large but incomplete datasets. *J Fam Plann Reprod Health Care*. 2012;38(1):2-6.

43. US Food and Drug Administration. FDA Drug Safety Communication: updated information about the risk of blood clots in women taking birth control pills containing drospirenone [safety announcement]. Posted September 26, 2011. Updated February 13, 2018. www.fda.gov/Drugs/DrugSafety/ucm299305.htm?source=govdelivery. Accessed July 16, 2019.

44. Dinger J, Bardenheuer K, Heinemann K. Cardiovascular and general safety of a 24-day regimen of drospirenone-containing combined oral contraceptives: final results from the International Active Surveillance Study of Women Taking Oral Contraceptives. *Contraception*. 2014;89(4):253-263.

45. Jensen JT, Parke S, Mellinger U, Machlitt A, Fraser IS. Effective treatment of heavy menstrual bleeding with estradiol valerate and dienogest: a randomized controlled trial. *Obstet Gynecol.* 2011;117(4):777-787.

46. Jensen JT. Evaluation of a new estradiol oral contraceptive: estradiol valerate and dienogest. *Expert Opin Pharmacother.* 2010;11(7):1147-1157.

47. Scarabin PY, Oger E, Plu-Bureau G; EStrogen and THromboEmbolism Risk Study Group. Differential association of oral and transdermal oestrogen-replacement therapy with venous thromboembolism risk. *Lancet.* 2003;362(9382):428-432.

48. Edelman A, Micks E, Gallo MF, Jensen JY, Grimes DA. Continuous or extended cycle vs. cyclic use of combined hormonal contraceptives for contraception. *Cochrane Database Syst Rev.* 2014;(7):CD004695.

49. Kaunitz AM, Portman DJ, Hait H, Reape KZ. Adding low-dose estrogen to the hormone-free interval: impact on bleeding patterns in users of a 91-day extended regimen oral contraceptive. *Contraception.* 2009;79(5):350-355.

50. Portman DJ, Kaunitz AM, Howard B, Weiss H, Hsieh J, Ricciotti N. Efficacy and safety of an ascending-dose, extended-regimen levonorgestrel/ethinyl estradiol combined oral contraceptive. *Contraception.* 2014;89(4):299-306.

51. Sulak PJ, Kuehl TJ, Coffee A, Willis S. Prospective analysis of occurrence and management of breakthrough bleeding during an extended oral contraceptive regimen. *Am J Obstet Gynecol.* 2006;195(4):935-941.

52. Roumen FJ, Apter D, Mulders TM, Dieben TO. Efficacy, tolerability and acceptability of a novel contraceptive vaginal ring releasing etonogestrel and ethinyl oestradiol. *Hum Reprod.* 2001;16(3):469-475.

53. Abrams LS, Skee D, Natarajan J, Wong FA. Pharmacokinetic overview of Ortho Evra/Evra. *Fertil Steril.* 2002;77(2 suppl 2):S3-S12.

54. Ahrendt HJ, Nisand I, Bastianelli C, et al. Efficacy, acceptability and tolerability of the combined contraceptive ring, NuvaRing, compared with an oral contraceptive containing 30 microg of ethinyl estradiol and 3 mg of drospirenone. *Contraception.* 2006;74(6):451-457.

55. Creinin MD, Meyn LA, Borgatta L, et al. Multicenter comparison of the contraceptive ring and patch: a randomized controlled trial. *Obstet Gynecol.* 2008;111(2 pt 1):267-277.

56. van den Heuvel MW, van Bragt AJ, Alnabawy AK, Kaptein MC. Comparison of ethinylestradiol pharmacokinetics in three hormonal contraceptive formulations: the vaginal ring, the transdermal patch and an oral contraceptive. *Contraception.* 2005;72(3):168-174.

57. Cole JA, Norman H, Doherty M, Walker AM. Venous thromboembolism, myocardial infarction, and stroke among transdermal contraceptive system users. *Obstet Gynecol.* 2007;109(2 pt 1):339-346.

58. Dinger J, Mohner S, Heinemann K. Cardiovascular risk associated with the use of an etonogestrel-containing vaginal ring. *Obstet Gynecol.* 2013;122(4):800-808.

59. Kaunitz AM. Transdermal and vaginal estradiol for the treatment of menopausal symptoms: the nuts and bolts. *Menopause.* 2012;19(6):602-603.

60. Cleland K, Zhu H, Goldstuck N, Cheng L, Trussell J. The efficacy of intrauterine devices for emergency contraception: a systematic review of 35 years of experience. *Hum Reprod.* 2012;27(7):1994-2000.

61. Cleland K, Wood S. A tale of two label changes. *Contraception.* 2014;90(1):1-3.

62. Plan B One-Step [package insert]. Budapest, Hungary: Duramed Pharmaceuticals; 2009.

63. Piaggio G, von Hertzen H, Grimes DA, Van Look PF. Timing of emergency contraception with levnonorgestrel or the Yuzpe regimen. Task Force on Postovulatory Methods of Fertility Regulation. *Lancet.* 1999;353(9154):721.

64. Glasier AF, Cameron ST, Fine PM, et al. Ulipristal acetate versus levonorgestrel for emergency contraception: a randomised non-inferiority trial and meta-analysis. *Lancet.* 2010;375(9714):555-562. Erratum in: *Lancet.* 2014;384(9953):1504.

65. Glasier A, Cameron ST, Blithe D, et al. Can we identify women at risk of pregnancy despite using emergency contraception? Data from randomized trials of ulipristal acetate and levonorgestrel. *Contraception.* 2011;84(4):363-367.

66. Cibula D, Zikan M, Dusek L, Majek O. Oral contraceptives and risk of ovarian and breast cancers in *BRCA* mutation carriers: a meta-analysis. *Expert Rev Anticancer Ther.* 2011;11(8):1197-1207.

67. Friebel TM, Domchek SM, Rebbeck TR. Modifiers of cancer risk in *BRCA1* and *BRCA2* mutation carriers: systematic review and meta-analysis. *J Natl Cancer Inst.* 2014;106(6):dju091.

68. The NAMS 2017 Hormone Therapy Position Statement Advisory Panel. The 2017 hormone therapy position statement of The North American Menopause Society. *Menopause.* 2017;24(7):728-753.

69. Coelingh Bennink HJT, Verhoeven C, Zimmerman Y, Visser M, Foidart JM, Gemzell-Danielsson K. Pharmacodynamic effects of the fetal estrogen estetrol in postmenopausal women: results from a multiple-rising-dose study. *Menopause.* 2017;24(6):677-685.

70. Shifren JL, Davis SR. Androgens in postmenopausal women: a review. *Menopause.* 2017;24(8):970-979.

71. Lindsay R, Gallagher JC, Kleerekoper M, Pickar JH. Effect of lower doses of conjugated equine estrogens with and without medroxyprogesterone acetate on bone in early postmenopausal women. *JAMA.* 2002;287(20):2668-2676.

72. LaCroix AZ, Chlebowski RT, Manson JE, et al; WHI Investigators. Health outcomes after stopping conjugated equine estrogens among postmenopausal women with prior hysterectomy: a randomized controlled trial. *JAMA.* 2011;305(13):1305-1314.

73. Manson JE, Chlebowski RT, Stefanick ML, et al. Menopausal hormone therapy and health outcomes during the intervention and extended poststopping phases of the Women's Health Initiative randomized trials. *JAMA.* 2013;310(13):1353-1368.

74. Manson JE, Aragaki AK, Rossouw JE, et al; WHI Investigators. Menopausal hormone therapy and long-term all-cause and cause-specific mortality: the Women's Health Initiative randomized trials. *JAMA.* 2017;318(10):927-938.

75. Bhavnani BR, Nisker JA, Martin J, Aletebi F, Watson L, Milne JK. Comparison of pharmacokinetics of a conjugated equine estrogen preparation (premarin) and a synthetic mixture of estrogens (C.E.S.) in postmenopausal women. *J Soc Gyncecol Investig.* 2000;7(3):175-183.

76. Prestwood KM, Kenny AM, Kleppinger A, Kulldorff M. Ultralow-dose micronized 17beta-estradiol and bone density and bone metabolism in older women: a randomized controlled trial. *JAMA.* 2003;290(8):1042-1048.

77. Ettinger B, Ensrud KE, Wallace R, et al. Effects of ultralow-dose transdermal estradiol on bone mineral density: a randomized clinical trial. *Obstet Gynecol.* 2004;104(3):443-451.

78. Bachmann GA, Schaefers M, Uddin A, Utian WH. Lowest effective transdermal 17beta-estradiol dose for relief of hot flushes in postmenopausal women: a randomized controlled trial. *Obstet Gynecol.* 2007;110(4):771-779.

79. Shifren JL, Rifai N, Desindes S, McIlwain M, Doros G, Mazer NA. A comparison of the short-term effects of oral conjugated equine estrogens versus transdermal estradiol on C-reactive protein, other serum markers of inflammation, and other hepatic proteins in naturally menopausal women. *J Clin Endocrinol Metab.* 2008;93(5):1702-1710.

80. Goodman MP. Are all estrogens created equal? A review of oral vs. transdermal therapy. *J Womens Health (Larchmt).* 2012;21(2):161-169.

81. Canonico M, Carcaillon L, Plu-Bureau G, et al. Postmenopausal hormone therapy and risk of stroke: impact of the route of estrogen administration and type of progestogen. *Stroke.* 2016;47(7):1734-1741.

82. Laliberte F, Dea K, Duh MS, Kahler KH, Rolli M, Lefebvre P. Does the route of administration for estrogen hormone therapy impact the risk of venous thromboembolism? Estradiol transdermal system versus oral estrogen-only hormone therapy. *Menopause.* 2011;18(10):1052-1059.

83. Renoux C, Dell'aniello S, Garbe E, Suissa S. Transdermal and oral hormone replacement therapy and the risk of stroke: a nested case-control study. *BMJ*. 2010;340:c2519.

84. Santen RJ. Vaginal administration of estradiol: effects of dose, preparation and timing on plasma estradiol levels. *Climacteric*. 2015;18:121-134.

85. Suckling J, Lethaby A, Kennedy R. Local oestrogen for vaginal atrophy in postmenopausal women. *Cochrane Database Syst Rev*. 2006;CD001500.

86. Brisdelle [package insert]. Miami, FL: Noven; 2013.

87. Simon JA, Portman DJ, Kaunitz AM, et al. Low-dose paroxetine 7.5 mg for menopausal vasomotor symptoms: two randomized controlled trials. *Menopause*. 2013;20(10):1027-1035.

88. Effects of estrogen or estrogen/progestin regimens on heart disease risk factors in postmenopausal women. The Postmenopausal Estrogen/Progestin Interventions (PEPI) Trial. The Writing Group for the PEPI Trial. *JAMA*. 1995;273(3):199-208.

89. Schüssler P, Kluge M, Yassouridis A, et al. Progesterone reduces wakefulness in sleep EEG and has no effect on cognition in healthy postmenopausal women. *Psychoneuroendocrinology*. 2008;33(8):1124-1131.

90. Montplaisir J, Lorrain J, Denesle R, Petit D. Sleep in menopause: differential effects of two forms of hormone replacement therapy. *Menopause*. 2001;8(1):10-16.

91. Hitchcock CL, Prior JC. Oral micronized progesterone for vasomotor symptoms—a placebo-controlled randomized trial in healthy postmenopausal women. *Menopause*. 2012;19(8):886-893.

92. Warren MP, Biller BM, Shangold MM. A new clinical option for hormone replacement therapy in women with secondary amenorrhea: effects of cyclic administration of progesterone from the sustained-release vaginal gel Crinone (4% and 8%) on endometrial morphologic features and withdrawal bleeding. *Am J Obstet Gynecol*. 1999;180(1 pt 1):42-48.

93. Luo L, Luo B, Zheng Y, Zhang H, Li J, Sidell N. Oral and intrauterine progestogens for atypical endometrial hyperplasia. *Cochrane Database Syst Rev*. 2018;12:CD009458.

94. Ettinger B, Selby J, Citron JT, Vangessel A, Ettinger VM, Hendrickson MR. Cyclic hormone replacement therapy using quarterly progestin. *Obstet Gynecol*. 1994;83(5 pt 1):693-700.

95. Ettinger B, Pressman A, Van Gessel A. Low-dosage esterified estrogen opposed by progestin at 6-month intervals. *Obstet Gynecol*. 2001;98(2):205-211.

96. Odmark IS, Rixo M, Englund D, Risberg B, Jonsson B, Olsson SE. Endometrial safety and bleeding pattern during a five-year treatment with long-cycle hormone therapy. *Menopause*. 2005;12(6):699-707.

97. Steiner AZ, Xiang M, Mack WJ, et al. Unopposed estradiol therapy in postmenopausal women: results from two randomized trials. *Obstet Gynecol*. 2007;109(3):581-587.

98. Prempro [package insert]. Philadelphia, PA: Wyeth; 2009.

99. Furness S, Roberts H, Marjoribanks J, Lethaby A. Hormone therapy in postmenopausal women and risk of endometrial hyperplasia. *Cochrane Database Syst Rev*. 2012;(8):CD000402.

100. Casper RF, MacLusky NJ, Vanin C, Brown TJ. Rationale for estrogen with interrupted progestin as a new low-dose hormonal replacement therapy. *J Soc Gynecol Investig*. 1996;3(5):225-234.

101. Prefest [package insert]. North Wales, PA: Teva Women's Health; 2017.

102. Effects of hormone replacement therapy on endometrial histology in postmenopausal women. The Postmenopausal Estrogen/Progestin Interventions (PEPI) Trial. The Writing Group for the PEPI Trial. *JAMA*. 1996;275(5):370-375.

103. Jaakkola S, Lyytinen H, Pukkala E, Ylikorkala O. Endometrial cancer in postmenopausal women using estradiol-progestin therapy. *Obstet Gynecol*. 2009;14(6):1197-1204.

104. Brinton LA, Felix AS. Menopausal hormone therapy and risk of endometrial cancer. *J Steroid Biochem Mol Biol*. 2014;142:83-89.

105. Stute P, Neulen J, Wildt L. The impact of micronized progesterone on the endometrium: a systematic review. *Climacteric*. 2016;19(4):316-328.

106. Johnson JV, Davidson M, Archer D, Bachmann G. Postmenopausal uterine bleeding profiles with two forms of combined continuous hormone replacement therapy. *Menopause*. 2002;9(1):16-22.

107. Lyytinen H, Pukkala E, Ylikorkala O. Breast cancer risk in postmenopausal women using estradiol-progestogen therapy. *Obstet Gynecol*. 2009;113(1):65-73.

108. Chlebowski RT, Anderson GL, Gass M, et al; WHI Investigators. Estrogen plus progestin and breast cancer incidence and mortality in postmenopausal women. *JAMA*. 2010;304(15):1684-1692.

109. Fournier A, Berrino F, Clavel-Chapelon F. Unequal risks for breast cancer associated with different hormone replacement therapies: results from the E3N cohort study. *Breast Cancer Res Treat*. 2008;107(1):103-111. Erratum in: *Breast Cancer Res Treat*. 2008;107(2):307-308.

110. Crandall CJ, Aragaki AK, Chlebowski RT, et al. New-onset breast tenderness after initiation of estrogen plus progestin therapy and breast cancer risk. *Arch Intern Med*. 2009;169(18):1684-1691.

111. Cordina-Duverger E, Truong T, Anger A, et al. Risk of breast cancer by type of menopausal hormone therapy: a case-control study among post-menopausal women in France. *PLoS One*. 2013;8(11):e78016.

112. Archer DF, Lewis V, Carr BR, Olivier S, Pickar JH. Bazedoxifene/conjugated estrogens (BZA/CE): incidence of uterine bleeding in postmenopausal women. *Fertil Steril*. 2009;92(3):1039-1044.

113. Pinkerton JV, Harvey JA, Pan K, et al. Breast effects of bazedoxifene-conjugated estrogens: a randomized controlled trial. *Obstet Gynecol*. 2013;121(5):959-968.

114. Pinkerton JV, Harvey JA, Lindsay R, et al; SMART-5 Investigators. Effects of bazedoxifene/conjugated estrogens on the endometrium and bone: a randomized trial. *J Clin Endocrinol Metab*. 2014;99(2):E189-E198.

115. Pickar JH, Boucher M, Morgenstern D. Tissue selective estrogen complex (TSEC): a review. *Menopause*. 2018;25(9):1033-1045.

116. Schumaker SA, Legault C, Rapp SR, et al; WHIMS Investigators. Estrogen plus progestin and the incidence of dementia and mild cognitive impairment in postmenopausal women: the Women's Health Initiative Memory Study: a randomized controlled trial. *JAMA*. 2003;289(20):2651-2662.

117. Schumaker SA, Legault C, Kuller L, et al; Women's Health Initiative Memory Study. Conjugated equine estrogens and incidence of probable dementia and mild cognitive impairment in postmenopausal women: Women's Health Initiative Memory Study. *JAMA*. 2004;291(24):2947-2950.

118. Jacobson BC, Moy B, Colditz GA, Fuchs CS. Postmenopausal hormone use and symptoms of gastroesophageal reflux. *Arch Intern Med*. 2008;168(16):1798-1804.

119. Oskarsson V, Orsini N, Sadr-Azodi O, Wolk A. Postmenopausal hormone replacement therapy and risk of acute pancreatitis: a prospective cohort study. *CMAJ*. 2014;186(5):338-344.

120. Rossouw JE, Prentice RL, Manson JE, et al. Postmenopausal hormone therapy and risk of cardiovascular disease by age and years since menopause. *JAMA*. 2007;297(13):1465-1477. Erratum in: *JAMA*. 2008;299(12):1426.

121. Harman SM, Black DM, Naftolin F, et al. Arterial imaging outcomes and cardiovascular risk factors in recently menopausal women: a randomized trial. *Ann Intern Med* 2014;161:249-260.

122. Hodis HN, Mack WJ, Henderson VW, et al; ELITE Research Group. Vascular effects of early versus late postmenopausal treatment with estradiol. *N Engl J Med*. 2016;374(13):1221-1231.

123. Clarkson TB, Meléndez GC, Appt SE. Timing hypothesis for postmenopausal hormone therapy: its origin, current status, and future. *Menopause*. 2013;20(3):342-353.

124. Mikkola TS, Tuomikoski P, Lyytinen H, et al. Estradiol-based postmenopausal hormone therapy and risk of cardiovascular and all-cause mortality. *Menopause*. 2015;22(9):976-983.

125. Mikkola TS, Tuomikoski P, Lyytinen H, et al. Increased cardiovascular mortality risk in women discontinuing postmenopausal hormone therapy. *J Clin Endocrinol Metab*. 2015;100(12):4588-4594.

126. Boardman HM, Hartley L, Eisinga A, et al. Hormone therapy for preventing cardiovascular disease in post-menopausal women. *Cochrane Database Syst Rev.* 2015;(3):CD002229.

127. Salpeter SR, Walsh JM, Greyber E, Salpeter EE. Brief report: coronary heart disease events associated with hormone therapy in younger and older women. A meta-analysis. *J Gen Intern Med.* 2006;21(4):363-366.

128. Salpeter SR, Walsh JM, Greyber E, Ormiston TM, Salpeter EE. Mortality associated with hormone replacement therapy in younger and older women: a meta-analysis. *J Gen Intern Med.* 2004;19(7):791-804.

129. Salpeter SR, Cheng J, Thabane L, Buckley NS, Salpeter EE. Bayesian meta-analysis of hormone therapy and mortality in younger postmenopausal women. *Am J Med.* 2009;122(11):1016-1022.

130. Schierbeck LL, Rejnmark L, Tofteng CL, et al. Effect of hormone replacement therapy on cardiovascular events in recently postmenopausal women: randomized trial. *BMJ* 2012;345:e6409.

131. Oliver-Williams C, Glisic M, Shahzad S, et al. The route of administration, timing, duration and dose of postmenopausal hormone therapy and cardiovascular outcomes in women: a systematic review *Hum Reprod Update.* 2019;25(2):257-271.

132. Faubion SS, Kuhle CL, Shuster LT, Rocca WA. Long-term health consequences of premature or early menopause and considerations for management. *Climacteric.* 2015;18(4):483-491.

133. Stuenkel CA, Gass ML, Manson JE, et al. A decade after the Women's Health Initiative—the experts do agree. *Menopause.* 2012;19(8):846-847.

134. Stuenkel CA, Davis SR, Gompel A, et al. Treatment of symptoms of the menopause: an Endocrine Society clinical practice guideline. *J Clin Endocrinol Metab.* 2015;100(11):3975-4011.

135. Lindh-Astrand L, Bixo M, Hirschberg AL, Sundström-Poromaa I, Hammar M. A randomized controlled study of taper-down or abrupt discontinuation of hormone therapy in women treated for vasomotor symptoms. *Menopause.* 2010;17(1):72-79.

136. Ockene JK, Barad DH, Cochrane BB, et al. Symptom experience after discontinuing use of estrogen plus progestin. *JAMA.* 2005;294(2):183-193.

137. Crandall CJ, Hovey KM, Andrews CA, et al. Breast cancer, endometrial cancer, and cardiovascular events in participants who used vaginal estrogen in the Women's Health Initiative Observational Study. *Menopause.* 2018;25(1):11-20.

138. *Bio-Identicals: Sorting Myths From Facts* [FDA Consumer Update]. *Pharmwatch* web site. January 9, 2008. www.pharmwatch.org/strategy/bioidentical_myths.shtml. Accessed June 26, 2019.

139. Simon JA, Patsner B, Allen LV Jr, et al. *Understanding the Controversy: Hormone Testing and Bioidentical Hormones.* Proceedings from the Postgraduate Course presented prior to the 17th Annual Meeting of The North American Menopause Society. Nashville, TN: October 11, 2006.

140. Rosenthal MS. The Wiley Protocol: an analysis of ethical issues. *Menopause.* 2008;15(5):1014-1022.

141. Cirigliano M. Bioidentical hormone therapy: a review of the evidence. *J Womens Health (Larchmt).* 2007;16(5):600-631.

142. Bhavnani BR, Stanczyk FZ. Misconception and concerns about bioidentical hormones used for custom-compounded hormone therapy. *J Clin Endocrinol Metab.* 2012;97(3):756-759.

143. Sellers S, Utian WH. Pharmacy compounding primer for physicians: prescriber beware. *Drugs.* 2012;72(16):2043-2050.

144. US Food and Drug Administration. *FDA Announces New and Expanded Compounding Research Projects* [press release]. September 26, 2018. www.fda.gov/Drugs/DrugSafety/ucm621776.htm. Updated October 3, 2018. Accessed July 19, 2019.

145. US Food and Drug Administration. *FDA Takes Action Against Compounded Menopause Hormone Therapy Drugs.* January 10, 2008. www.fiercebiotech.com/biotech/fda-takes-action-against-compounded-menopause-hormone-therapy-drugs. Accessed July 16, 2019.

146. Gaudard AM, Silva de Souza S, Puga ME, Marjoribanks J, da Silva EM, Torloni MR. Bioidentical hormones for women with vasomotor symptoms. *Cochrane Database Syst Rev.* 2016;(8):CD010407.

147. Dresser JC. *FDA Provides Clarity on Use of Estriol by Section 503A Compounding Pharmacies* [blog post]. November 19, 2014. www.frierlevitt.com/articles/pharmacylaw/fda-provides-clarity-on-use-of-estriol-by-section-503a-compounding-pharmacies. Accessed July 16, 2019.

148. Gass ML, Stuenkel CA, Utian WH, LaCroix A, Liu JH, Shifren JL; North American Menopause Society (NAMS) Advisory Panel consisting of representatives of NAMS Board of Trustees and other experts in women's health. Use of compounded hormone therapy in the United States: report of The North American Menopause Society Survey. *Menopause.* 2015;22(12):1276-1284.

149. US Food and Drug Administration. *2018 Compounding Policy Priorities Plan.* January 2018. www.fda.gov/Drugs/GuidanceComplianceRegulatoryInformation/PharmacyCompounding/ucm592795.htm. Updated July 16, 2018. Accessed June 26, 2019.

150. US Department of Health and Human Services. Food and Drug Administration. Center for Drug Evaluation and Research (CDER). *Pharmacy Compounding of Human Drug Products Under Section 503A of the Federal Food, Drug, and Cosmetic Act.* Silver Spring, MD: US Department of Health and Human Services; 2016.

151. Lonard DM, O'Malley BW. The expanding cosmos of nuclear receptor coactivators. *Cell.* 2006;125(3):411-414.

152. Dutertre M, Smith CL. Molecular mechanisms of selective estrogen receptor modulator (SERM) action. *J Pharmacol Exp Ther.* 2000;295(2):431-437.

153. Gültekin E, Yidiz F. Introduction to phytoestrogens. In: Yidiz F, ed. *Phytoestrogens in Functional Foods.* Boca Raton, FL: CRC; 2006:3-16.

154. Karahalil B. Benefits and risks of phytoestrogens. In: Yidiz F, ed. *Phytoestrogens in Functional Foods.* Boca Raton, FL: CRC; 2006:209-242.

155. Jordan VC. Tamoxifen treatment for breast cancer: concept to gold standard. *Oncology (Williston Park).* 1997;11(2 suppl 1):7-13.

156. Fisher B, Costantino JP, Wickerham DL, et al. Tamoxifen for prevention of breast cancer: report of the National Surgical Adjuvant Breast and Bowel Project P-1 study. *J Natl Cancer Inst.* 1998;90(18):1371-1388.

157. Love RR, Mazess RB, Barden HS, et al. Effects of tamoxifen on bone mineral density in postmenopausal women with breast cancer. *N Engl J Med.* 1992;326(13):852-856.

158. Bouchard C. Selective estrogen receptor modulators and their effects on hot flashes: a dilemma. *Menopause.* 2011;18(5):477-479.

159. Fisher B, Costantino JP, Redmond CK, Fisher ER, Wickerham DL, Cronin WM. Endometrial cancer in tamoxifen-treated breast cancer patients: findings from the National Surgical Adjuvant Breast and Bowel Project (NSABP) B-14. *J Natl Cancer Inst.* 1994;86(7):527-537.

160. Ettinger B, Black DM, Mitlak BH, et al. Reduction of vertebral fracture risk in postmenopausal women with osteoporosis treated with raloxifene: results from a 3-year randomized clinical trial. Multiple Outcomes of Raloxifene Evaluation (MORE) investigators. *JAMA.* 1999;282(7):637-645.

161. Delmas PD, Ensrud KE, Adachi JD, et al; Multiple Outcomes of Raloxifene Evaluation Investigators. Efficacy of raloxifene on vertebral fracture risk reduction in postmenopausal women with osteoporosis: four-year results from a randomized clinical trial. *J Clin Endocrinol Metab.* 2002;87(8):3609-3617.

162. Cummings SR, Eckert S, Krueger KA, et al. The effect of raloxifene on risk of breast cancer in postmenopausal women: results from the MORE randomized trial. Multiple Outcomes of Raloxifene Evaluation. *JAMA.* 1999;281(23):2189-2197. Erratum in: *JAMA.* 1999;282(22):2124.

163. Martino S, Cauley JA, Barrett-Connor E, et al; CORE Investigators. Continuing outcomes relevant to Evista: breast cancer incidence in postmenopausal osteoporotic women in a randomized trial of raloxifene. *J Natl Cancer Inst.* 2004;96(23):1751-1761.

164. Vogel VG, Costantino JP, Wickerham DL, et al; National Surgical Adjuvant Breast and Bowel Project (NSABP). Effects of tamoxifen vs raloxifene on the risk of developing invasive breast cancer and other disease outcomes: the NSABP Study of Tamoxifen and Raloxifene (STAR) P-2 trial. *JAMA.* 2006;295(23):2727-2741. Erratum in: *JAMA.* 2006;296(24):2926; *JAMA.* 2007;298(9):973.

165. Parsons A, Merritt D, Rosen A, Heath H 3rd, Siddhanti S, Plouffe L Jr; Study Groups on the Effects of Raloxifene HCl With Low-Dose Premarin Vaginal Cream. Effect of raloxifene on the response to conjugated estrogen vaginal cream or nonhormonal moisturizers in postmenopausal vaginal atrophy. *Obstet Gynecol.* 2003;101(2):346-352.

166. Silverman SL, Christiansen C, Genant HK, et al. Efficacy of bazedoxifene in reducing new vertebral fracture risk in postmenopausal women with osteoporosis: results from a 3-year, randomized, placebo-, and active-controlled clinical trial. *J Bone Miner Res.* 2008;23(12):1923-1934.

167. Duggan ST, McKeage K. Bazedoxifene: a review of its use in treatment of postmenopausal osteoporosis. *Drugs.* 2011;71(16):2193-2212.

168. Christiansen C, Chestnut CH 3rd, Adachi JD, et al. Safety of bazedoxifene in a randomized, double-blind placebo- and active-controlled phase 3 study of postmenopausal women with osteoporosis. *BMC Musculoskelet Disord.* 2010;11:130.

169. Bachmann GA, Komi JO; Ospemifene Study Group. Ospemifene effectively treats vulvovaginal atrophy in postmenopausal women: results from a pivotal phase 3 study. *Menopause.* 2010;17(3):480-486.

170. Constantine GD, Goldstein SR, Archer DF. Endometrial safety of ospemifene: results of the phase 2/3 clinical development program. *Menopause.* 2015;22(1):36-43.

171. Wurz GT, Kao CJ, DeGregorio MW. Safety and efficacy of ospemifene for the treatment of dyspareunia associated with vulvar and vaginal atrophy due to menopause. *Clin Interv Aging.* 2014;9:1939-1950.

172. Kangas L, Unkila M. Tissue selectivity of ospemifene: pharmacologic profile and clinical implications. *Steroids.* 2013;78(12-13):1273-1280.

173. Harvey HA, Kimura M, Hajba A. Toremifene: an evaluation of its safety profile. *Breast.* 2006;15(2):142-157.

174. Fareston [package insert]. Memphis, TN: GTx, Inc; 2011.

175. Liu JH, Arredondo F. Menopause. In: Falcone T, Hurd WW, eds. *Clinical Reproductive Medicine and Surgery: A Practical Guide.* Philadelphia, PA: Mosby-Elsevier; 2017:164-193.

176. Pinkerton JV, Utian WH, Constantine GD, Olivier S, Pickar JH. Relief of vasomotor symptoms with the tissue-selective estrogen complex containing bazedoxifene/conjugated estrogens: a randomized, controlled trial. *Menopause.* 2009;16(6):1116-1124.

177. Goldberg T, Fidler B. Conjugated estrogens/bazedoxifene (DuaVee): a novel agent for the treatment of moderate-to-severe vasomotor symptoms associated with menopause and the prevention of postmenopausal osteoporosis. *P T.* 2015;40(3):178-182.

178. Kagan R, Williams RS, Pan K, Mirkin S, Pickar JH. A randomized, placebo- and active-controlled trial of bazedoxifene/conjugated estrogens for treatment of moderate to severe vulvar/vaginal atrophy in postmenopausal women. *Menopause.* 2010;17(2):281-289.

179. Gallagher JC, Palacios S, Ryan KA, et al. Effect of conjugated estrogens/bazedoxifene on postmenopausal bone loss: pooled analysis of two randomized trials. *Menopause.* 2016;23(10):1083-1091.

180. Cummings SR, Ensrud K, Delmas PD, et al; PEARL Study Investigators. Lasofoxifene in postmenopausal women with osteoporosis. *N Engl J Med.* 2010;362(8):686-696.

181. Goldstein SR, Neven P, Cummings S, et al. Postmenopausal Evaluation and Risk Reduction with Lasofoxifene (PEARL) trial: 5-year gynecological outcomes. *Menopause.* 2011;18(1):17-22.

182. Benjamin EJ, Virani SS, Callaway CW, et al; American Heart Association Council on Epidemiology and Prevention Statistics Committee and Stroke Statistics Subcommittee. Heart disease and stroke statistics—2018 update: a report from the American Heart Association. *Circulation.* 2018;137(12):e67-e492.

183. Yusuf S, Hawken S, Ounpuu S, et al; INTERHEART Study Investigators. Effect of potentially modifiable risk factors associated with myocardial infarction in 52 countries (the INTERHEART study): case-control study. *Lancet.* 2004;364(9438):937-952.

184. Grundy SM, Stone NJ, Bailey AL, et al. 2018 AHA/ACC/AACVPR/AAPA/ABC/ACPM/ ADA/AGS/APhA/ASPC/NLA/ PCNA guideline on the management of blood cholesterol. *Circulation.* 2019;139(25):e1082-e1143. Erratum in: *Circulation.* 2019;139(25):e1182-e1186.

185. Zipes DP, Libby P, Bonow RO, Mann DL, Tomaselli GF, Braunwald E, eds. *Braunwald's Heart Disease: A Textbook of Cardiovascular Medicine.* Eleventh edition. Philadelphia, PA: Elsevier/Saunders; 2019.

186. Chou R, Dana T, Blazina I, et al. Statin use for the prevention of cardiovascular disease in adults: a systematic review for the US Preventive Services Task Force [Internet]. Rockville, MD: Agency for Health Care Research and Quality (US); 2016 Nov. Report No: 1405206 EF-2.

187. Stone NJ, Robinson JG, Lichtenstein AH, et al; American College of Cardiology/American Heart Association Task Force on Practice Guidelines. 2013 ACC/AHA guideline on the treatment of blood cholesterol to reduce atherosclerotic cardiovascular risk in adults: a report of the American College of Cardiology/American Heart Association Task Force on Practice Guidelines. *Circulation.* 2014;129(25 suppl 2):S1-S45.

188. US Preventive Services Task Force, Bibbins-Domingo K, Grossman DC, et al. Statin use for the primary prevention of cardiovascular disease in adults: US Preventive Services Task Force recommendation statement. *JAMA.* 2016;316(19):1997-2007.

189. Randomised trial of cholesterol lowering in 4444 patients with coronary heart disease: the Scandinavian Simvastatin Survival Study (4S). *Lancet.* 1994;344(8934):1383-1389.

190. Lewis SJ, Sacks FM, Mitchell JS, et al. Effect of pravastatin on cardiovascular events in women after myocardial infarction: the Cholesterol and Recurrent Events (CARE) trial. *J Am Coll Cardiol.* 1998;32(1):140-146.

191. Yusuf S, Lonn E, Pais P, et al; HOPE-3 Investigators. Blood-pressure and cholesterol lowering in persons without cardiovascular disease. *N Engl J Med.* 2016;374(21):2032-2043.

192. Ziaeian B, Dinkler J, Guo Y, Watson K. The 2013 ACC/AHA cholesterol treatment guidelines: applicability to patients with diabetes. *Curr Diab Rep.* 2016;16(2):13.

193. Toth PP, Patti AM, Giglio RV, et al. Management of statin intolerance in 2018: still more questions than answers. *Am J Cardiovasc Drugs.* 2018;18(3):157-173.

194. Rosenson RS, Baker SK, Jacobson TA, Kopecy SL, Parker BA; the National Lipid Association's Muscle Safety Expert Panel. An assessment by the Statin Muscle Safety Task Force: 2014 update. *J Clin Lipidol.* 2014;8(3 suppl):S58-S71.

195. Guyton JR, Bays HE, Grundy SM, Jacobson TA; the National Lipid Association Statin Intolerance Panel. An assessment by the Statin Intolerance Panel: 2014 update. *J Clin Lipidol.* 2014;8(3 suppl):S72-S81.

196. Hippisley-Cox J, Coupland C. Unintended effects of statins in men and women in England and Wales: population based cohort study using the QResearch database. *BMJ.* 2010;340:c2197.

197. Bays H, Cohen DE, Chalasani N, Harrison SA; the National Lipid Association's Statin Safety Task Force. As assessment by the Statin Liver Safety Task Force: 2014 update. *J Clin Lipidol.* 2014; 8(3 suppl):S47-S57.

198. Banach M, Rizzo M, Toth PP, et al. Statin intolerance—an attempt at a unified definition. Position paper from an International Lipid Expert Panel. *Arch Med Sci.* 2015;11(1):1-23.

199. Ridker PM, Pradhan A, MacFadyen JG, Libby P, Glynn RJ. Cardiovascular benefits and diabetes risks of statin therapy in primary prevention: an analysis from the JUPITER trial. *Lancet.* 2012;380(9841):565-571.

Appendix

How to Evaluate Scientific Literature

As new studies are published, the evidence base increases for understanding the risks and benefits of treatment options. A basic understanding of the types of studies and the meaning of the analyses helps healthcare providers evaluate the evidence and implications for clinical practice. Readers in search of more sophisticated discussions are urged to consult current clinical epidemiology texts.

Types of studies

Two major types of studies are *experimental* and *observational*.[1,2] There are also meta-analyses, which pool the results of clinical trials or other types of studies into one analysis.

Experimental studies

In experimental studies, interventions and conditions are strictly defined and controlled by the investigators. In observational studies, investigators observe outcomes in relation to variables of interest. They do not assign participants to an exposure of interest. Types of experimental studies are randomized, controlled trials (RCTs), crossover trials, and quasi-experimental studies.

Randomized, controlled trials

Randomized, controlled trials are considered the strongest for therapeutic interventions. In RCTs, a group of participants with similar characteristics is identified (eg, low bone density). Each participant is then randomly assigned (similar to a flip of a coin; neither the participants nor the investigator chooses) to an *intervention group* (or groups) or to a *control group*. Participants typically have an equal and unbiased (random) chance of being assigned to each treatment under study. Randomized, controlled trials have the best chance of avoiding selection bias if the randomization is adequate and the study size is large. This is because known and unknown characteristics should be the same in each group. The baseline characteristics of the two groups should be presented and statistically compared in an RCT's final report. The Women's Health Initiative is an example of an RCT.

Randomized, controlled trials are best suited to situations in which exposure to treatment is modifiable, a legitimate uncertainty exists regarding benefit or harm of treatment, and outcomes are reasonably common. However, inclusion and exclusion criteria may limit the extrapolation of the results to other groups (limiting whether the results can be generalized).

The *power* of a trial is the likelihood that it will determine the effect of the intervention. The number of participants is determined when the trial is designed, based on the likelihood of the measured outcome events and the anticipated magnitude of the intervention's effect. If events do not occur as often as predicted, the trial may not have adequate power to determine the effect of the intervention.

The *Methods* section of the published trial results will describe how the investigator calculated the number of participants required and will quantify the range of effect the study can detect (eg, the study was powered to detect more than a 20% reduction in heart attacks). *Publication bias* favors small trials with positive outcomes. An international registry of clinical trials requires submission of the planned trial (including design, interventions, and prespecified outcomes) so that a full accounting of the status of trials that are not completed or are completed, regardless of their outcomes, can be assessed.

Depending on the intervention, participants and investigators may be purposefully *blinded* or *masked* (they do not know which treatment a participant is receiving). This helps reduce some forms of bias and the effects of the participant's or investigator's expectations of intervention benefit.

Classically, RCTs are used to assess for *efficacy* of the treatment in an ideal controlled setting. More often, an RCT will assess *effectiveness* (not efficacy) by studying the intervention under more usual circumstances. This is because a study for efficacy may not reflect its actual effectiveness in a real-world, clinical practice setting. Both these types of RCTs often use a relatively narrowly defined patient population. Even though an RCT is quite internally valid (ie, the study was done well), it may not be accurate to extrapolate (generalize) the results from one RCT to another patient population that was not studied in the trial.

Other important issues when evaluating the results of an RCT include checking to see whether all participants who started the trial were accounted for at trial conclusion and whether the groups were treated equally aside from the experimental intervention.

Crossover trials

Crossover trials allow participants to serve as their own controls. Participants are randomly assigned to one treatment arm and later switched to the other treatment arm. This crossover study methodology has often been used in trials to assess the efficacy of medications. The design is difficult to do well because of its potential for residual effects between interventions. Often there will be a *washout* period (time during which no intervention is given) between interventions.

Quasi-experimental studies

Quasi-experimental studies are of two general varieties. In one, two interventions are simultaneously compared in two groups of participants, but interventions are not randomized for any given participant (eg, two hospitals comparing two types of wound closure for the same type of surgery).

Another common quasi-experimental study is when participants serve as their own controls and the investigator controls the intervention. The intervention is neither randomized nor is there a control population to which the response can be compared. After baseline evaluation, the intervention is given and the participants are reevaluated to observe any changes in characteristics because of the intervention.

Observational studies

Types of observational studies include purely *analytic* (or *descriptive*) studies. Analytic studies (including cohort studies, case-control studies, and cross-sectional studies) have a nonrandomized control group (eg, women who did not use hormone therapy [HT] for any number of reasons would be compared with women who elected to use HT). What is sampled first—risk factor, outcome, or both risk factor and outcome—simultaneously determines which analytic study design is being used. Case reports and case series are not analytic because they do not have control comparisons. Observational studies can assess associations and correlations between exposures and outcomes, but they cannot confirm cause-and-effect relationships.

Cohort studies

Cohort studies (or longitudinal studies) begin with a defined group of participants (eg, persons of a certain age or those who work in a certain industry) called the *cohort*. These studies sample persons from the general population and determine whether they have exposures or risk factors of interest (eg, HT users vs nonusers). This cohort of persons is then followed over time to study a variety of outcomes. Data are collected in a similar manner on all participants from the beginning of the study (the *baseline*) and frequently at set intervals during follow-up. The Nurses' Health Study (NHS) is one of the best-known prospective (occurring over time) cohort studies.

These studies provide a clearer temporal sequence of exposures and outcomes than other analytic studies, are well suited for common exposures, and can study multiple exposures and outcomes. However, they can be time-consuming and expensive, they have the potential for many forms of bias, and participants may be lost during follow-up. When too many patients are lost, the validity of the study is compromised.

Cohort studies may follow relevant events as they occur over time (prospective), but they may also be performed in a historical or a concurrent (cross-sectional) manner. Evidence from prospective cohort studies is considered stronger than the other forms of analytic studies because data on exposures are collected before the outcomes occur.

The term *retrospective* is sometimes used when referring to a historical cohort study, and it can be confusing. If the data are easily accessible, the researcher can retrospectively evaluate a cohort that was followed in time, but the time was in the past moving forward (historical cohort), not progressing from current time onward (concurrent cohort). An example of a retrospective cohort is an occupational cohort with known exposure to a carcinogen or toxin in the remote past and whose participants have already accrued outcomes. In the NHS and the Framingham Study, information was gleaned in a concurrent and prospective fashion (in contrast to a historical cohort). All participants in each of these circumstances were followed longitudinally forward in some time frame.

Case-control studies

Case-control studies begin with an outcome or disease of interest (eg, myocardial infarction [MI], breast cancer) and then compare the characteristics or exposures of individual persons with the outcome *cases* to *controls* who do not have the outcome or disease of interest. Case-control studies are prone to many more forms of bias. A frequent one is *recall bias* (participants cannot remember exposures or risk factors accurately).

Matching participants for specific characteristics and defining strict eligibility criteria lessens, but cannot eliminate, the possibility that the results are *confounded*. For example, women who use HT are known to smoke less and lead generally healthier lifestyles. Hormone therapy users have less cardiovascular disease primarily because of better lifestyle habits rather than from any beneficial effect of HT use. Smoking or other lifestyle patterns can confound the results when observational studies analyze HT use and health outcomes. Matching cases and controls for smoking status (or adjusting for this variable) helps reduce this confounding.

Despite these limitations, case-control studies have many advantages. Because they begin with an outcome of interest, they can be performed efficiently and at less cost than cohort studies. They are important in situations in which it would be unethical to assign individual persons to an exposure (eg, chemotherapy) or when an outcome is rare (eg, X-chromosome abnormalities associated with primary ovarian insufficiency).

Cross-sectional studies

Cross-sectional studies are snapshots in time. Here, cases and controls are evaluated at the same time for both risk factors or characteristics and outcomes of interest. Cross-sectional studies are very useful for determining prevalence, for planning for healthcare needs, and for generating hypotheses.

Case reports and case series

Case reports and case series describe the experience of a single patient or series of patients. Such reports are useful in bringing new diseases or phenomena to the attention of the clinical and scientific community and for generating new hypotheses. However, lacking a control group, case reports or series without further study are only suggestive.

Many of these basic designs can be modified or combined, and many hybrid studies exist. An example is a case-control study within a cohort; this is a very useful study design and can provide many advantages, including cost efficiency.

Meta-analyses

This term describes an analytic technique used to pool the results of clinical trials or other types of studies (not only RCTs). Often, a meta-analysis is performed on a group of studies that are too small to have statistical significance by themselves but that may show significance when pooled. Specific criteria (eg, eligibility criteria of participants, follow-up rates, data quality) are established to determine which studies will be included in the analysis. Inasmuch as any biases present in the contributing studies will be present in the meta-analysis, the outcome of a meta-analysis is only as good as the studies included.

In general, meta-analyses are difficult to perform. They are best performed based on the original data obtained from each investigator from each individual study. International guidelines provide checklists to understand the quality of a meta-analysis of clinical trials (CONSORT guidelines).[3,4]

Analyzing study results

The bottom line in evaluating a study is: *What are the results?* The results of cohort studies and clinical trials are most frequently presented as a *relative risk* (RR)—the likely level of greater or lower risk (eg, for HT users vs nonusers). The RR can be determined because these study designs follow participants longitudinally, and risk (which is time-dependent) can be determined in each comparison group.

Rate/Risk

The term *rate* is the number of events per the number of participants per the time interval (eg, 44/10,000/y). Knowing the exact number of events over time is very useful, because this determines the risk.

The Council for International Organizations of Medical Sciences Task Force[5] has provided the nomenclature to guide the interpretation of risks:
- Rare = less than or equal to 10/10,000/y
- Very rare = less than or equal to 1/10,000/y

Rare outcomes would not be of such great concern to an individual woman making a decision about treatment. However, it is important to recognize that common exposures that produce rare outcomes can still have profound public health effects.

Relative risk

The RR is a ratio—the rate of disease or the outcome of interest in a group exposed to a potential risk factor or treatment or having a characteristic of interest, divided by the rate of disease of interest in an unexposed group (ie, those without the risk factor, treatment, or characteristic of interest). The RR should be used only for prospective studies.

Rate is used as above in both the numerator and the denominator. These are the numbers of events, per number of participant, per time interval (eg, 50/100,000/y). For example, if the annual rate of MI in women who smoke is 220 per 100,000, and the annual rate in women who do not smoke is 110 per 100,000, the RR associated with smoking is

$$RR = \frac{220}{100,000/y} \div \frac{110}{100,000/y} = 2.00$$

This means that compared with nonsmoking women, the risk of MI for a smoking woman is twice that of a nonsmoking woman in the study.

An RR less than 1.0 suggests that the factor decreases risk. For example, an RR of 0.50 means there is a 50% less chance (or risk) of the outcome studied in those with the risk factor versus those without the risk factor of interest. An RR of 0.3 means a 70% lower relative risk.

An RR greater than 1.0 suggests that the factor increases risk. For example, an RR of 1.2 means there is a 20% increase in risk in the group with the risk factor versus the group without the risk factor. An RR of 2.0 means double the risk.

Odds ratio

The odds ratio (OR) is an estimate used in many of the analytic studies. It best approximates the RR when the outcome is rare.

Confidence interval

The confidence interval (CI), usually cited with the RR or the OR, indicates with a certain degree of assurance the range within which lies the true magnitude of the measured effect. The CI has two components—the degree of certainty and the range (eg, 95% CI, 1.09-1.32). The point estimate (the RR or OR number) is the best mathematical estimate

from the data. Understanding the upper and lower limits of the range is often clinically useful. If the CI is *wide*, the reader's confidence in the validity of the RR would be less than if the CI is *narrow* (ie, closer to the value of the RR).

Often, a 95% CI is used. A 95% CI gives the range of values that have a 95% probability of containing the true RR or OR. When a 95% CI does not contain the number 1.0 (eg, 0.40-0.80 or 1.12-1.37), the measured RR or OR is statistically significant by at least $P<.05$. The CI is more clinically useful than the P value, because the CI helps the reader to understand the best estimate of the effect, and it also provides the mathematical estimated limits, which are useful in determining the best-case and worse-case scenarios.

P value

This term is the probability of obtaining the observed RR or OR (or a more extreme value) by chance (random sampling) alone. A P value of .01 means that there is a 1% mathematical probability that the observed difference between two groups occurred by chance. By convention, P is generally deemed statistically significant if below .05. This means that if 20 outcomes are evaluated in a single study, one of these outcomes is likely to show a positive result just because of chance alone ($P=.05$, or 1/20). By the time $P=.001$, the likelihood is only 1/1,000 that the results occurred by chance—in other words, the finding is more likely to be real.

It is important to remember that a study can be statistically significant and not clinically significant. However, if it is not statistically significant, it cannot reach clinical significance, and the result could be clinically nonsignificant or inconclusive. An example is when the study is underpowered.

Absolute risk/Attributable risk

The effect of RR on both a population and an individual basis depends on *incidence* (ie, the number of new cases in a given period). This can be quantified by the absolute risk or attributable risk (AR), which is the difference between the incidence rates in the exposed and unexposed groups—in other words, the *risk difference*. The AR quantifies the effect of exposure, providing a measure of its public health effect. For example, for the calculation presented earlier about the risk of MI in smoking women, the AR is

$$AR = \frac{220}{100,000/y} - \frac{110}{100,000/y} = \frac{110}{100,000/y}$$

This means that for every 100,000 women who smoke, there would be 110 additional cases of MI per year.

Often, AR is more clinically useful than RR in explaining risk to patients. FDA requires that the absolute risk reduction be included on the product information sheet.

Number needed to treat

To communicate this risk difference to patients, the number needed to treat (NNT) can be useful. The NNT is merely the reciprocal of the AR (ie, 1 divided by the AR). For example, in a 1-year study, if the rate of an outcome was 20 per 1,000 in an untreated group, and 10 per 1,000 in a treated group, the NNT is

$$NNT = \frac{1}{(20/1{,}000) - (10/1{,}000)} = \frac{1}{(10/1{,}000)} = \frac{1}{0.01} = 100$$

This means that for every 100 people treated, there would be 1 less negative outcome over the year.

REFERENCES

1. Koepsell TD, Weiss NS. *Epidemiologic Methods: Studying the Occurrence of Illness*. New York: Oxford University Press, 2003.

2. Porta M, ed. *A Dictionary of Epidemiology*. 5th ed. New York: Oxford University Press, 2008.

3. Moher D, Schulz KF, Altman D, for the CONSORT Group (Consolidated Standards of Reporting Trials). The CONSORT statement: revised recommendations for improving the quality of reports of parallel-group randomized trials. *JAMA*. 2001;285(15):1987-1991.

4. Stroup DF, Berlin JA, Morton SC, et al; Meta-analysis Of Observational Studies in Epidemiology (MOOSE) Group. Meta-analysis of observational studies in epidemiology: a proposal for reporting. *JAMA*. 2000;283(15):2008-2012.

5. World Health Organization. *Guidelines for Preparing Core Clinical-Safety Information on Drugs*. 2nd ed. Report of CIOMS Working Groups III and IV. Geneva: World Health Organization, 1999.

Index

Index

Index

330

Index

Index

Index

Continuing Medical Education Evaluation

To claim continuing medical education (CME) credit or pharmacotherapeutic hours, please read and study the entire *Clinician's Guide* and complete and submit the evaluation found at www.menopause.org/CG6_CME before September 25, 2022.

This information is included on the online evaluation for this enduring activity. Please be prepared to respond to these items because you must complete the entire evaluation when using the online form. You must use this link, www.menopause.org/CG6_CME, to submit for CME credit or pharmacotherapeutic hours. Do not mail your responses to these questions. **This can be completed online ONLY.**

Evaluation Questions

Please rate the level to which the learning objectives for *Menopause Practice: A Clinician's Guide*, 6th edition, were met.

Initiate discussion with patients on menopause and healthy aging, including its effect on quality of life and sexuality.
Not at all met   *Poorly met*   *Somewhat met*   *Mostly met*   *Completely met*

Perform appropriate clinical assessments to diagnose conditions of menopause and aging, assess health risks, and identify any contraindications to medications
Not at all met   *Poorly met*   *Somewhat met*   *Mostly met*   *Completely met*

Discuss a full range of management options with patients on the basis of their health risks, goals, and preferences
Not at all met   *Poorly met*   *Somewhat met*   *Mostly met*   *Completely met*

Collaborate with other healthcare professionals to offer effective, individualized therapy for menopause symptoms and conditions
Not at all met   *Poorly met*   *Somewhat met*   *Mostly met*   *Completely met*

Counsel and encourage patients to achieve a healthy lifestyle
Not at all met   *Poorly met*   *Somewhat met*   *Mostly met*   *Completely met*

Please rate your ability to apply the objectives BEFORE this activity and AFTER this activity.

BEFORE the activity
Very poor   *Poor*   *Fair*   *Good*   *Excellent*

AFTER the activity
Very poor   *Poor*   *Fair*   *Good*   *Excellent*

For each of the chapters in the *Clinician's Guide*, please describe any changes you plan to make in your practice as a result of information contained in the chapter. Responses to these questions are required in order to earn credit.

Chapter 1: Menopause. What changes will you make in your practice with the updated information in this chapter?

Chapter 2: Midlife Body Changes. What changes will you make in your practice to properly evaluate and manage your patients' midlife body changes?

Chapter 3: Vasomotor Symptoms. What changes will you make in your practice to properly evaluate and manage your patients' vasomotor symptoms?

Chapter 4: Common Genitourinary Symptoms in Midlife. What changes will you make in your practice to properly evaluate and manage your patients' genitourinary symptoms?

Chapter 5: Other Common Symptoms in Midlife. What changes will you make in your practice to properly evaluate and manage your patients' common midlife symptoms?

Chapter 6: Diseases Common in Midlife. What changes will you make in your practice to properly evaluate and manage your patients' common midlife diseases?

Chapter 7: Osteoporosis. What changes will you make in your practice to properly evaluate and manage your patients' osteoporosis?

Chapter 8: Cardiometabolic Disorders in Midlife. What changes will you make in your practice to properly evaluate and manage your patients' cardiometabolic disorders?

Chapter 9: Cancers Common in Midlife. What changes will you make in your practice to properly evaluate and manage your patients' common midlife cancers?

Chapter 10: Vitamins, Minerals, and Other Dietary Supplements. What changes will you make in your practice to properly evaluate and manage the use of vitamins, minerals, and other dietary supplements by your patients?

Chapter 11: Prescription Therapies. What changes will you make in your practice to properly evaluate and manage your patients' prescription therapies?

NAMS practice pea

Have you implemented any of these changes at this time?
Yes/No (if yes, please describe)

Have you noticed any change or improvement in the effectiveness, results, or outcomes of your patient care from what you implemented in your practice?

Have you seen any improvement or difference in the health of your patients as a result of what you learned or the changes you implemented?

Was this activity fair, balanced, and free of commercial bias?
Yes/No (if no, please indicate why not)

What is your profession?
Physician/Resident
Nurse
Nurse midwife
Nurse practitioner
Physician assistant
Pharmacist
Researcher
Psychologist/Other mental health
Dietician or Nutritionist
Product industry (eg, pharma)
Media/Publishing/Writing
Other